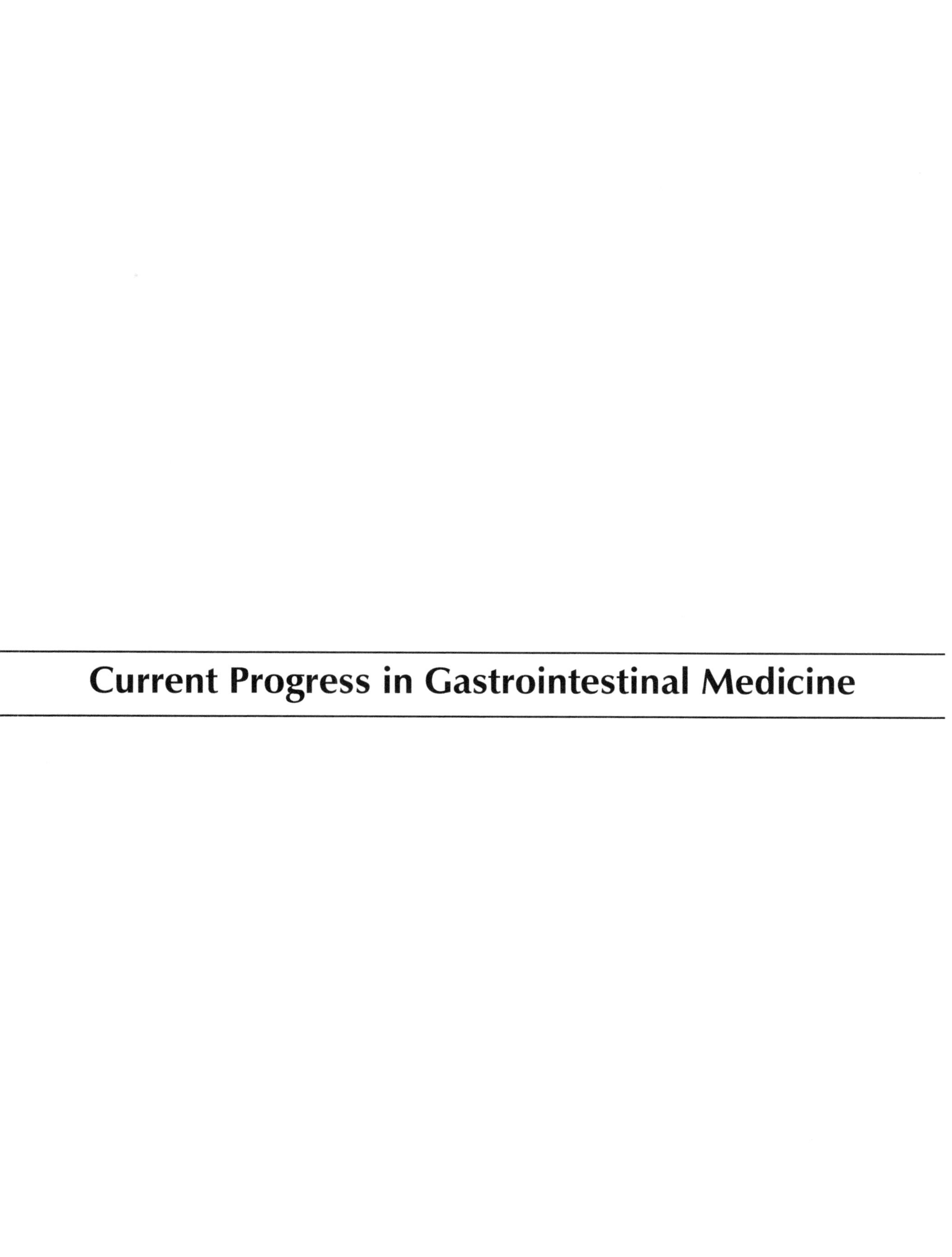

Current Progress in Gastrointestinal Medicine

Current Progress in Gastrointestinal Medicine

Editor: Ronald Graves

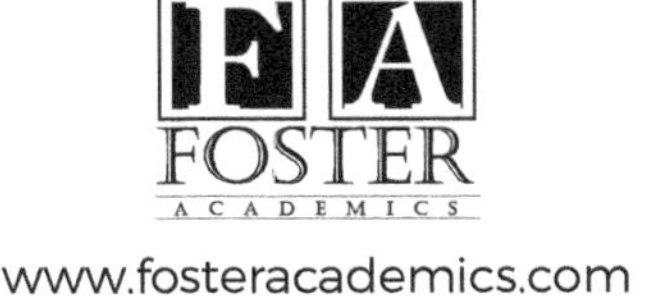

www.fosteracademics.com

www.fosteracademics.com

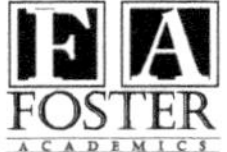

Cataloging-in-Publication Data

Current progress in gastrointestinal medicine / edited by Ronald Graves.
p. cm.
Includes bibliographical references and index.
ISBN 978-1-63242-657-4
1. Gastrointestinal system--Diseases. 2. Gastrointestinal system--Diseases--Diagnosis.
3. Gastrointestinal system--Diseases--Treatment. 4. Gastroenterology. I. Graves, Ronald.
RC801 .C87 2019
616.33--dc23

© Foster Academics, 2019

Foster Academics,
118-35 Queens Blvd., Suite 400,
Forest Hills, NY 11375, USA

ISBN 978-1-63242-657-4 (Hardback)

This book contains information obtained from authentic and highly regarded sources. Copyright for all individual chapters remain with the respective authors as indicated. All chapters are published with permission under the Creative Commons Attribution License or equivalent. A wide variety of references are listed. Permission and sources are indicated; for detailed attributions, please refer to the permissions page and list of contributors. Reasonable efforts have been made to publish reliable data and information, but the authors, editors and publisher cannot assume any responsibility for the validity of all materials or the consequences of their use.

Trademark Notice: Registered trademark of products or corporate names are used only for explanation and identification without intent to infringe.

Contents

Preface

Over the recent decade, advancements and applications have progressed exponentially. This has led to the increased interest in this field and projects are being conducted to enhance knowledge. The main objective of this book is to present some of the critical challenges and provide insights into possible solutions. This book will answer the varied questions that arise in the field and also provide an increased scope for furthering studies.

Gastroenterology is a branch of medicine that studies the functioning of the digestive system and the diseases related to it. Diseases affecting the internal organs from mouth to anus, along the alimentary canal are the areas of focus in this field. Physicians or specialists in this field are known as gastroenterologists. The techniques and medical procedures used by a gastroenterologist to diagnose and treat gastrointestinal diseases include endoscopy, colonoscopy, liver biopsy and endoscopic ultrasound. Endoscopy is one of the most common procedures used in the treatment of gastrointestinal diseases. In this procedure, an endoscope is used for the purpose of examining the interior of a hollow body organ. This book provides comprehensive insights into the field of gastrointestinal medicine. It consists of contributions made by international experts. It will help the readers in keeping pace with the rapid changes in this field.

I hope that this book, with its visionary approach, will be a valuable addition and will promote interest among readers. Each of the authors has provided their extraordinary competence in their specific fields by providing different perspectives as they come from diverse nations and regions. I thank them for their contributions.

Editor

1

Familial Abdominal and Intestinal Lipomatosis Presenting with Upper GI Bleeding

Yilmaz Bilgic,[1] Hasan Baki Altinsoy,[2] Nezahat Yildirim,[3] Ozkan Alatas,[2] Burhan Hakan Kanat,[4] and Abdurrahman Sahin[5]

[1]*Department of Gastroenterology, Faculty of Medicine, Inonu University, Malatya, Turkey*
[2]*Department of Radiology, Elazig Training and Research Hospital, Elazig, Turkey*
[3]*Department of Pathology, Elazig Training and Research Hospital, Elazig, Turkey*
[4]*Department of General Surgery, Elazig Training and Research Hospital, Elazig, Turkey*
[5]*Department of Gastroenterology, Elazig Training and Research Hospital, Elazig, Turkey*

Correspondence should be addressed to Abdurrahman Sahin; arahmansmd@yahoo.com

Academic Editor: Tetsuo Hirata

Although lipomas are encapsulated benign tumors, systemic lipomatosis defines infiltrative nonencapsulated tumors resembling normal adipose tissue. Abdominal lipomatosis and intestinal lipomatosis are different clinicopathological entities with similar clinical symptoms. We describe here a case presenting with upper gastrointestinal bleeding from eroded submucosal lipoma at duodenum secondary to intestinal lipomatosis and abdominal lipomatosis.

1. Introduction

Multiple systemic lipomatosis (MSL) is a rare disorder with unknown etiology, characterized by the accumulation of nonencapsulated adipose tissue at face, head, neck, upper and lower extremities, trunk, abdominal cavity, and pelvis [1]. Involvement of gastrointestinal (GI) tract and abdominal cavity is very rare. Abdominal and intestinal involvements present with abdominal pain, obstruction, intussusception, and GI bleeding. Abdominal lipomatosis might also cause distension, via intermittent obstruction and altering bowel transit time. Intestinal lipomatosis refers to having multiple submucosal lipomas at small intestine and colon. We describe here a case with bleeding duodenal lipoma related to intestinal lipomatosis and diffuse abdominal lipomatosis that is deforming stomach and proximal small bowel loops.

2. Case Presentation

A 35-year-old man was admitted to emergency department with one-day history of hematemesis and melena after taking nonsteroidal anti-inflammatory drug. He had no medical illness. He denied smoking, alcohol consumption. The height and weight of patient were 178 cm and 68 kg, respectively (body mass index: 21 kg/cm^2). On physical examination, blood pressure was 120/70 mmHg and pulse rate 86/min. There was a 2 cm mobile painless submucosal nodular lesion on the left neck. His abdomen was soft with no tenderness, rebound, mass lesion, or ascites. The patient was promptly given intravenous crystalloid and colloid fluid replacement; parenteral proton-pump inhibitor was administered. Initial laboratory values were as follows: leukocyte: 5800/mm^3, hemoglobin: 14.8 g/dL, platelet: 347.000/mm^3, prothrombin time: 12 sec, and INR: 1.05. Biochemical parameters were normal.

Upper gastrointestinal endoscopy revealed gastric and duodenal multiple submucosal mobile lesions with narrowing of antrum and constant deformation of duodenum. It was unable to proceed to the second part of duodenum with endoscope (Figure 1). Colonoscopic examination was normal. Abdominal magnetic resonance imaging (MRI) showed that diffuse lipomatosis of abdominal cavity extending to the mediastinum (Figure 2) and obliteration at the distal part of stomach, bulb, and proximal duodenum due to submucosal

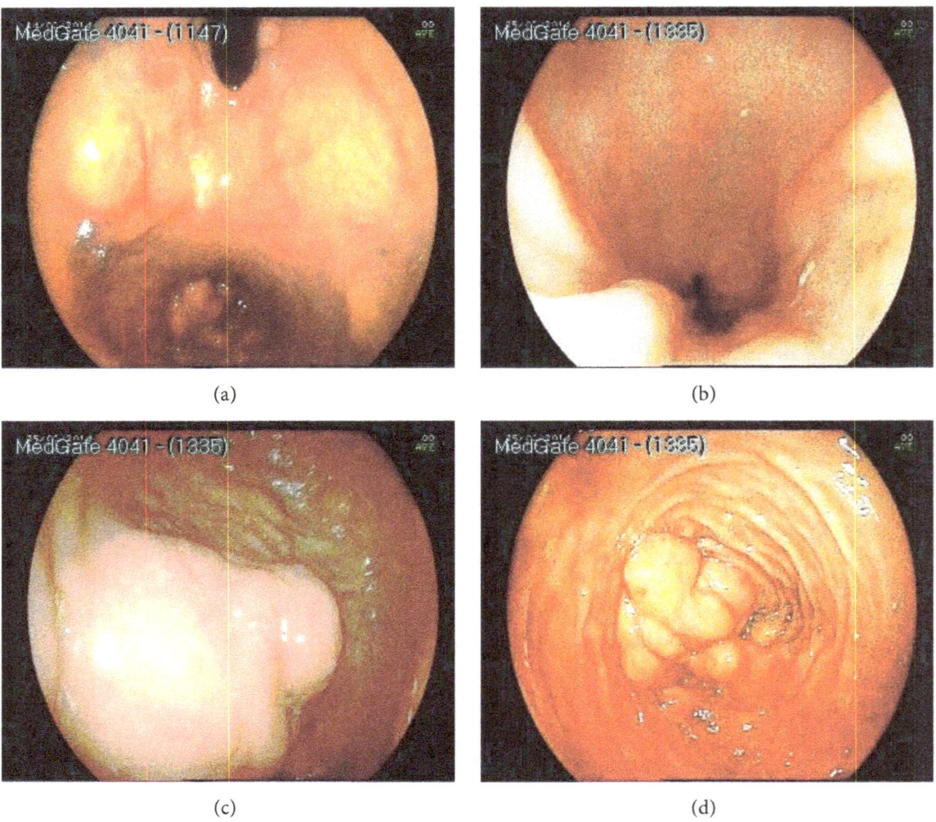

FIGURE 1: Endoscopic view of submucosal lesions: (a) fundus at retroflection position, (b) antrum and pylorus, (c) bulb and bleeding submucosal lesion, and (d) second part of duodenum.

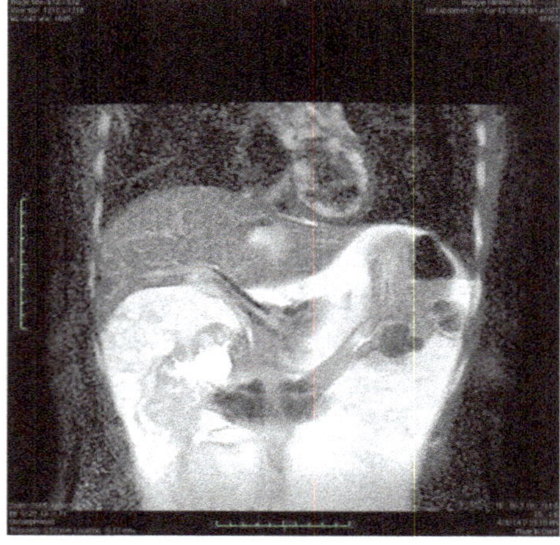

FIGURE 2: Coronal T2 weighted MR imaging of diffuse abdominal lipomatosis, luminal narrowing at distal part of stomach and bulb secondary to diffuse lipomatosis and antral submucosal lipoma with deplased intestinal loops.

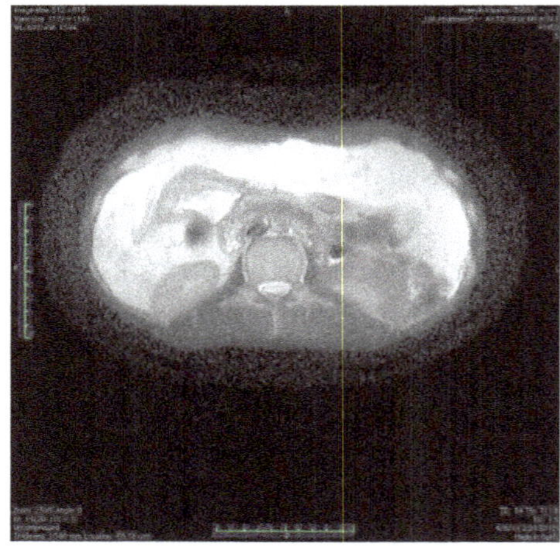

FIGURE 3: Axial T2 weighted MR imaging of abdominal cavity with diffuse abdominal lipomatosis, luminal obliteration of antrum and distal part of corpus due to lipoma and clustered intestinal loops at the right upper part of intestinal cavity.

lipomatous lesions with deplased small intestine loops to the right upper abdomen (Figure 3). Laboratory investigation showed fasting glucose 68 mg/dL, fasting insulin 1.18 mg/dL, triglyceride 53 mg/dL, low density lipoprotein 62 mg/dL, and high density lipoprotein 47 mg/dL. His father similarly has mobile nontender lesions at neck and right upper extremity. However, submucosal lesions were not detected on UGIE examination. Abdominal MRI of his father showed similarly

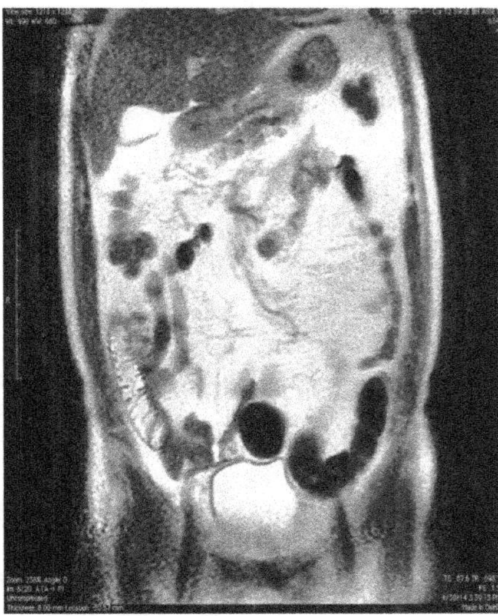

FIGURE 4: Coronal T2 weighted MR imaging with diffuse abdominal lipomatosis of the father of index case.

lipomatous tissue increase in abdominal cavity (Figure 4). Endoscopic biopsy of submucosal polypoid lesion was diagnosed as lipoma and trucut biopsy of diffuse mass lesion filling abdominal cavity was consistent with fibroadipose tissue.

3. Discussion

Multiple symmetrical lipomatosis affects mostly white men between 25 and 60 years of age. It may occur sporadically or familiarly [2]. Diffuse abdominal lipomatosis is a variant of MSL characterized by massive enlargement of abdomen by collection of large nonencapsulated lipomas [3]. This rare disease might be associated with dyslipidemia (high triglyceride, high HDL), insulin resistance, hyperuricemia, macrocytic anemia, and peripheral neuropathy [2]. Several etiological factors are assumed in the development of lipomatosis such as embryonic displacement of adipose tissue, congenital predisposition, degenerative disease with disturbance of fat metabolism, postchemotherapeutic fat deposition, chronic inflammation such as chronic inflammatory bowel disease, low-grade infection, and hamartomatous syndromes and alcohol [4]. Alcohol consumption is common coexisting factor that causes folate deficiency, macrocytic anemia and promote lipomas through effects on adiposities [1].

In MSL, adipocytes have increased lipoprotein lipase activity and a defect in adrenergic lipolysis. Adipogenesis in MSL is not a consequence of energy excess but it is an active hyperplastic proliferation of subcutaneous adipose tissue. This kind of behavior of some adipocytes in several subcutaneous areas in MSL suggests that the energy unrelated adipogenesis could contribute to the expansion of adipose tissue [5]. Chen et al. demonstrated abdominal and subcutaneous adipose tissue accumulation did not induce glucose and lipid metabolism dysfunction in MSL [6]. Our patient supports this finding, as not to have dyslipidemia, glucose intolerance, or alcohol consumption. Furthermore, father of the patient had lipoma on the neck and increased fat tissue in the abdominal cavity at MRI, similarly. Familial tendency to the accumulation of fat in the abdominal cavity might be the cause of MSL in this case.

Diffuse abdominal lipomatosis and intestinal lipomatosis are two distinct clinical entities. Abdominal lipomatosis refers to massive infiltrative nonencapsulated fat accumulation. However, intestinal lipomatosis defines the presence of multiple lipomas. Gastrointestinal lipomas occur predominantly in the large intestine (especially right sided) and then decreasing prevalence in the small bowel, stomach, and esophagus [7]. We found multiple gastric and duodenal lipomas at upper GI endoscopic examination. We did not detect lipomas via colonoscopic examination or radiologically at distal part of small intestine and colon. On the contrary of the literature, our patient has lipomas at stomach and small intestine. Abdominal lipomatosis and intestinal lipomatosis present together in our patient. Abdominal lipomatosis might be asymptomatic as in the father of index case.

Intestinal lipomatosis related GI bleeding revealed coexistence of these two very rare diseases. In patients presenting with obstructive symptoms, paroxysmal abdominal pain, or GI hemorrhage, endoscopic treatment including endoscopic submucosal dissection, endoscopic snare resection, or surgical intervention might be definitive treatment [8, 9]. With conservative management, bleeding stopped spontaneously and did not recur. Although imaging studies demonstrated compression of upper small bowel and stomach, the patient did not suffer from distension, intermittent abdominal pain, or other obstructive symptoms. This patient should be followed closely for obstructive symptoms. In case of obstructive findings, surgical resection is the treatment of choice.

Consent

Written informed consents were obtained from the patients who participated in this study.

References

[1] A. H. Zargar, B. A. Laway, S. R. Masoodi et al., "Diffuse abdominal lipomatosis," *Journal of Association of Physicians of India*, vol. 51, pp. 621–622, 2003.

[2] N. Lomartire, F. Ciocca, C. Di Stanislao, G. Bologna, and M. Giuliani, "Multiple symmetrical lipomatosis (MSL): a clinical case and a review of the literature," *Annali Italiani di Chirurgia*, vol. 70, no. 2, pp. 259–263, 1999.

[3] W. D. Craig, J. C. Fanburg-Smith, L. R. Henry, R. Guerrero, and J. H. Barton, "Fat-containing lesions of the retroperitoneum: radiologic-pathologic correlation," *Radiographics*, vol. 29, no. 1, pp. 261–290, 2009.

[4] I. H. Jeong and Y. H. Maeng, "Gastric lipomatosis," *Journal of Gastric Cancer*, vol. 10, no. 4, pp. 254–258, 2010.

[5] V. Pandzic Jaksic and M. Sucic, "Multiple symmetric lipomatosis—a reflection of new concepts about obesity," *Medical Hypotheses*, vol. 71, no. 1, pp. 99–101, 2008.

[6] K. Chen, Y. Xie, P. Hu, S. Zhao, and Z. Mo, "Multiple symmetric lipomatosis: substantial subcutaneous adipose tissue accumulation did not induce glucose and lipid metabolism dysfunction," *Annals of Nutrition and Metabolism*, vol. 57, no. 1, pp. 68–73, 2010.

[7] A. J. Taylor, E. T. Stewart, and W. J. Dodds, "Gastrointestinal lipomas: a radiologic and pathologic review," *American Journal of Roentgenology*, vol. 155, no. 6, pp. 1205–1210, 1990.

[8] R. M. S. Moreno, D. A. H. Ramirez, M. M. Navarro, C. R. S. Lozano, and R. M. Gen, "Multiple intestinal lipomatosis. Case report," *Cirugía y Cirujanos*, vol. 78, no. 2, pp. 163–165, 2010.

[9] Y.-D. T. Tzeng, S.-I. Liu, M.-C. Yang, and K.-T. Mok, "Bowel obstruction with intestinal lipomatosis," *Digestive and Liver Disease*, vol. 44, no. 2, p. e4, 2012.

2

Unawareness of a Prolonged Retained Capsule Endoscopy: The Importance of Careful Follow-Up and Cooperation between Medical Institutions

Susumu Saigusa,[1,2] Masaki Ohi,[1,2] Hiroki Imaoka,[1,2] Tadanobu Shimura,[1,2] Ryo Uratani,[1,2] Yasuhiro Inoue,[1,2] and Masato Kusunoki[2]

[1] *Department of Surgery, Wakaba Hospital, 28-13 Minami-Chuo, Tsu, Mie 514-0832, Japan*
[2] *Department of Gastrointestinal and Pediatric Surgery, 2-174 Edobashi, Tsu, Mie 514-8507, Japan*

Correspondence should be addressed to Susumu Saigusa; saigusa@wakabahsp.jp

Academic Editor: Haruhiko Sugimura

A 50-year-old man with anemia was referred to our hospital to undergo capsule endoscopy (CE), which revealed small intestinal ulcers. After 5 months of CE, he returned because of recurrent anemia without abdominal symptoms. Abdominal X-ray and computed tomography showed capsule retention in the small intestine at the pelvic cavity. The capsule remained at the same place for 7 days. We performed capsule retrieval by laparoscopy-assisted surgery with resection of the involved small intestine, including an ileal stricture. Resected specimen showed double ulcers with different morphologies, an ulcer scar with stricture, and a wide ulcer at the proximal side of the others. Each ulcer had different histopathological findings such as the degree of fibrosis and monocyte infiltration. These differences led us to consider that the proximal ulcer may have been secondarily induced by capsule retention. Our experience indicated that careful follow-up and the cooperation between medical institutions after CE examination should be undertaken for patients with incomplete examination, unknown excretion of the capsule, and/or ulcerative lesions despite the lack of abdominal symptoms. Additionally, a retained CE remaining over long periods and at the same place in the small intestine may lead to secondary ulceration.

1. Introduction

Capsule endoscopy (CE) is an innovative and noninvasive tool for investigating small bowel pathology. In recent years, the number of CE examination is increasing. The capsule is usually excreted with feces within 24–48 hours [1]. However, capsule retention, which is defined as having a capsule remain in the digestive tract for a minimum of 2 weeks, is known as one of the complications of CE. The rate of capsule retention has been reported to be less than 1.5% [2–4]. Capsule retention has the risk of bowel obstruction and perforation [4–9]. We report a case of CE retention for 5 months due to ileal ulcer with severe stricture without awareness.

2. Case Report

A 50-year-old man with gradually worsening anemia and suspected small bowel bleeding was referred to our hospital to undergo CE because esophagogastroduodenoscopy and total colonoscopy did not reveal the source of the gastrointestinal bleeding. His oral medications included several psychoactive drugs and iron preparations but not nonsteroidal anti-inflammatory drugs. He had no history of abdominal surgery. We did not perform patency examination before CE because we assessed low possibility of severe stenosis and inflammatory bowel disease based upon his clinical history and abdominal X-ray examination. CE (PillCam SB2 system, Given Imaging, Yokneam, Israel) demonstrated several ulcers at the small intestine, but the capsule did not reach the cecum during the recording time (stomach transit time: 220 minutes). These results were sent to his primary care doctor. Five months after the CE examination, he was referred again for the recurrence of anemia. Abdominal X-ray examination revealed that the capsule was retained at the pelvic cavity (Figure 1(a)). Follow-up abdominal X-ray examination after 7 days demonstrated that the capsule remained in exactly

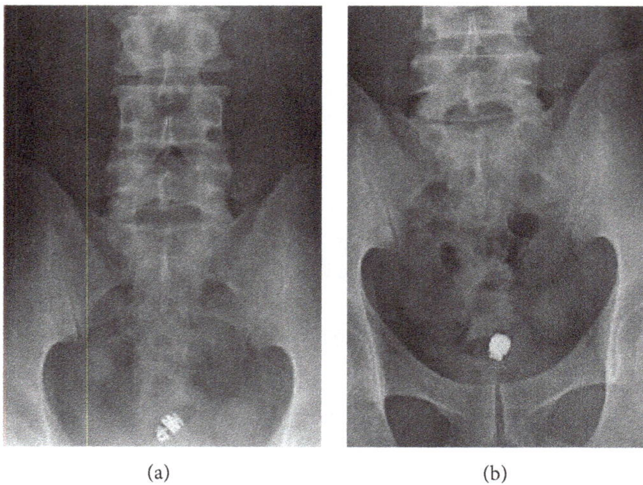

(a) (b)

Figure 1: Abdominal X-ray image visualizing a CE capsule in the pelvic cavity. The capsule retention might have been overlooked if the range of the X-ray image had shifted slightly (a). Follow-up X-ray after 7 days revealed that the capsule remained at the same place (b).

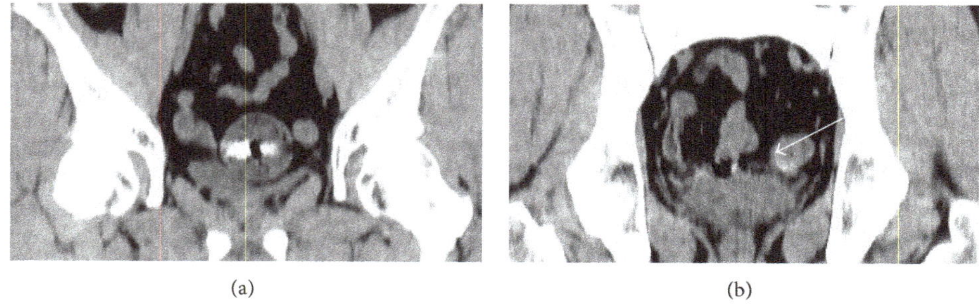

(a) (b)

Figure 2: Coronal view by CT showed CE capsule retention in the small intestinal lumen with dilatation and fluid collection (a), and the finding was suspicious for stenosis ((b), arrow).

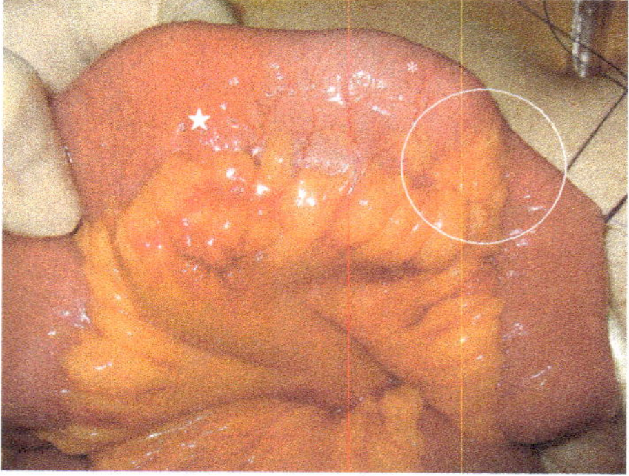

Figure 3: Operative findings. Retained CE capsule (∗). Reddened serosa (star). Stenosis with the wrapping-sign and caliber change (inside the circle).

the same part but was rotatable (Figure 1(b)). Computed tomography (CT) showed that the capsule seemed to be floating in the small intestinal lumen with dilatation and fluid collection proximal to the capsule (Figure 2(a)). Additionally, the CT coronal view indicated findings suspicious for stenosis distal to the capsule (Figure 2(b)). The patient had had regular bowel movements and no abdominal complaints for the past 5 months. He could not confirm that the capsule was egested because he failed to monitor his stools. After proper informed consent was obtained, we retrieved the capsule by laparoscopy-assisted surgery. The patient declined endoscopic approach and treatments. Laparoscopic instruments were placed through 3 trocars. The CE was laparoscopically detected approximately 50 cm from the end of the ileum. After fluoroscopic confirmation, the part of the ileum with the capsule was moved outside the abdominal cavity, and we made the following observations around the area of retention: the fat-wrapping sign and a caliber change were observed distal to the capsule, with reddened serosa proximal to the capsule. The capsule could not pass through this stricture (Figure 3). The small intestine was extensively evaluated, and no other abnormalities were found. We resected approximately 30 cm of ileum and performed a functional end-to-end anastomosis. An ulcer scar with stricture was macroscopically observed, and a wide ulcer was observed at the proximal side of the lesion (Figure 4). On histopathological examination, the lesions were determined to be a nonspecific ulcer (Ul III) with fibrosis, formation of lymphoid follicles, and infiltration of monocytes and neutrophils to the subserosa, without evidence of malignancy,

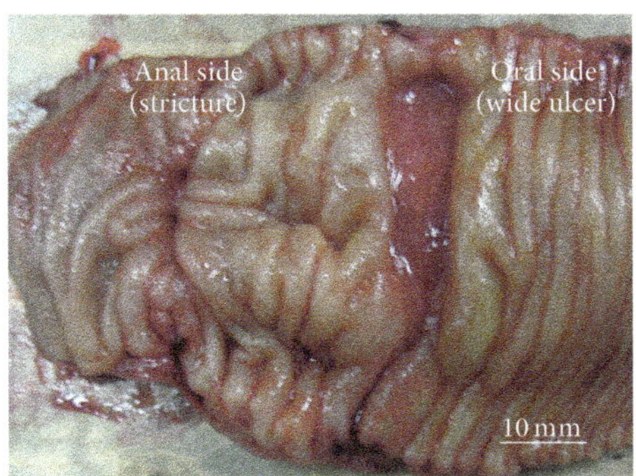

FIGURE 4: Resected lesion showed double ulcers. There was a wide ulcer at the proximal side of the ulcer scar.

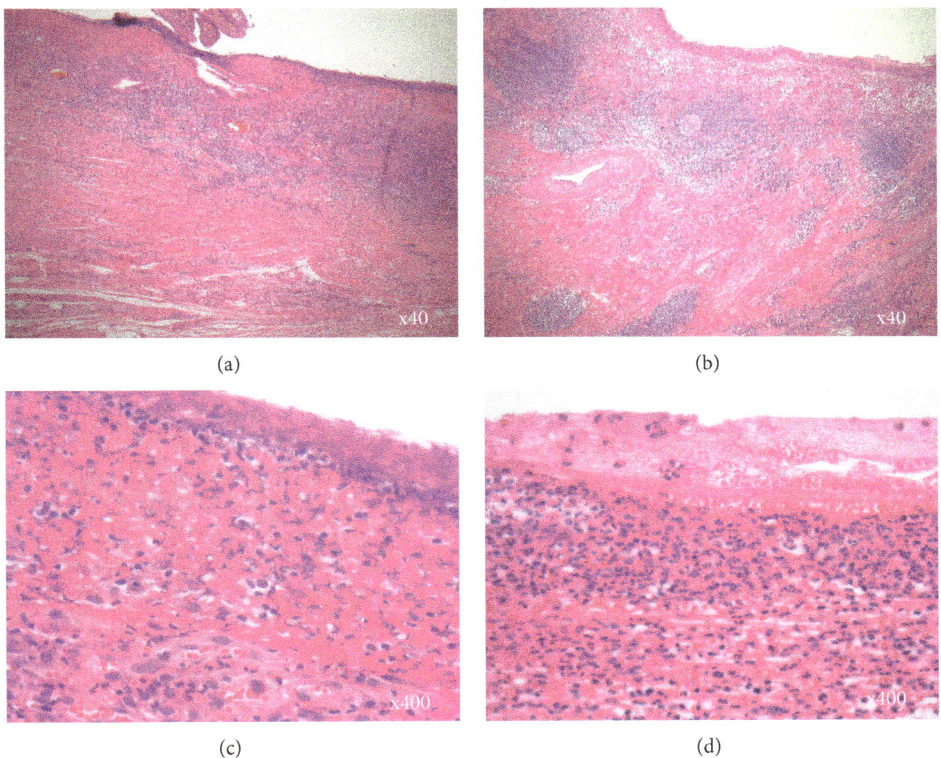

FIGURE 5: Histopathological examination revealed that an ulcer scar at the distal side had mainly fibrosis ((a) and (c)), while lymphoid follicles, infiltration of monocytes, and neutrophils were more noticeable in the wide ulcer on the proximal side ((b) and (d)). Hematoxylin-eosin staining. Original magnification 40x: (a) and (b); 400x: (c) and (d).

inflammatory bowel disease, or tuberculosis (Figure 5). The patient's postoperative course was uneventful, and he was discharged on the postoperative day 8. There was no evidence of progression of anemia at a follow-up visit conducted 7 months after surgery.

3. Discussion

An incomplete examination means that there is failure of the capsule to reach the cecum during the recording time. It has been reported that the rate of incomplete examination ranges from 16.5 to 20% [3, 4]. In our case, the patient had an incomplete examination and subsequently failed to determine if the capsule was egested. Moreover, his primary care doctor did not perform an X-ray examination because the patient remained asymptomatic for 5 months after CE examination despite a severe ileal stricture caused by a simple ulcer. It has been reported that most patients with CE retention remain asymptomatic [2–4, 10, 11]. Our case indicated that follow-up X-ray examination after CE should routinely be performed for patients with incomplete examination and unknown capsule excretion despite a lack of abdominal symptoms, and the cooperation between medical institutions is essential.

Although there were many reports of capsule retention of long duration [4, 12, 13], we think that the retained CE should be retrieved if spontaneous or pharmaceutical manipulation, the rates of spontaneous or pharmaceutical-manipulated passage of retained capsules have been reported to vary from 15 to 65.6% [3, 14], is ineffective to egest it because there are several reports of retained capsule causing intestinal obstruction and perforation [5, 6, 8, 9]. Surgical retrieval is often required secondary to an underlying pathologic process causing a stricture or obstruction although double-balloon endoscopy has been reported as one of the effective approaches for the retrieval of retained CE [15, 16]. We removed the retained CE by laparoscopy-assisted surgery. Laparoscopic detection of the retained CE and the intestinal abnormality were easy and useful. Moreover, definitive surgery to resect the culprit stricture was performed. Except in cases of known or suspected Crohn's disease, laparoscopy-assisted surgery may be the first choice for the retrieval of retained CE in the small intestine because this procedure can simultaneously allow for diagnosis and treatment.

In the current case, histopathological examination revealed double ulcers of nonspecific cause without evidence of malignancies, Crohn's disease, or tuberculosis. A comparison of the 2 ulcers histopathologically found that an ulcer scar at the distal side had mainly fibrosis (Figures 5(a) and 5(c)), while lymphoid follicles and monocyte infiltration were more noticeable in the wide ulcer on the proximal side (Figures 5(b) and 5(d)). These differences in the degree of inflammation led us to suspect that the wide ulcer at the proximal side of the stricture may have been secondarily induced by the capsule retention and resulted in the recurrence of anemia. However, our verifications are insufficient to clarify whether the proximal ulcer is truly caused by capsule retention because we could not detect the multinucleate giant cells, which is known as the foreign body response [17, 18], in the wide ulcer on the proximal side.

In conclusion, our experience indicated that careful follow-up after CE examination should be undertaken for patients with incomplete examination, unknown excretion of the capsule, and/or ulcerative lesions despite the lack of abdominal symptoms, and the cooperation between medical institutions is essential with increasing CE examination. Additionally, a prolonged CE retention in the same part of the small intestine should be retrieved because it may further endanger the patient with more "ammunition" for secondary ulceration and perforation.

Consent

Written informed consent was obtained from the patient for publication of this case report and accompanying images.

References

[1] M. Muñoz-Navas, "Capsule endoscopy," *World Journal of Gastroenterology*, vol. 15, pp. 1584–1586, 2009.

[2] F. Li, S. R. Gurudu, G. De Petris et al., "Retention of the capsule endoscope: a single-center experience of 1000 capsule endoscopy procedures," *Gastrointestinal Endoscopy*, vol. 68, no. 1, pp. 174–180, 2008.

[3] Z. Liao, R. Gao, C. Xu, and Z.-S. Li, "Indications and detection, completion, and retention rates of small-bowel capsule endoscopy: a systematic review," *Gastrointestinal Endoscopy*, vol. 71, no. 2, pp. 280–286, 2010.

[4] C. M. Höög, L.-Å. Bark, J. Arkani, J. Gorsetman, O. Broström, and U. Sjöqvist, "Capsule retentions and incomplete capsule endoscopy examinations: an analysis of 2300 examinations," *Gastroenterology Research and Practice*, vol. 2012, Article ID 518718, 7 pages, 2012.

[5] G. D. de Palma, S. Masone, M. Persico et al., "Capsule impaction presenting as acute small bowel perforation: a case series," *Journal of Medical Case Reports*, vol. 6, article 121, 2012.

[6] P. González Carro, J. Picazo Yuste, S. Fernández Díez, F. Pérez Roldán, and O. Roncero Garciá-Escribano, "Intestinal perforation due to retained wireless capsule endoscope," *Endoscopy*, vol. 37, no. 7, article 684, 2005.

[7] R. Srai, L. Tullie, A. Wadoodi, and M. Saunders, "Capsule endoscopy: a dangerous but diagnostic tool," *BMJ Case Reports*, vol. 2013, 2013.

[8] A. P. Skovsen, J. Burcharth, and S. K. Burgdorf, "Capsule endoscopy: a cause of late small bowel obstruction and perforation," *Case Reports in Surgery*, vol. 2013, Article ID 458108, 2 pages, 2013.

[9] S. Um, H. Poblete, and J. Zavotsky, "Small bowel perforation caused by an impacted endocapsule," *Endoscopy*, vol. 40, no. 2, pp. E122–E123, 2008.

[10] A. S. Cheifetz and B. S. Lewis, "Capsule endoscopy retention: is it a complication?" *Journal of Clinical Gastroenterology*, vol. 40, no. 8, pp. 688–691, 2006.

[11] X.-Y. Yang, C.-X. Chen, B.-L. Zhang et al., "Diagnostic effect of capsule endoscopy in 31 cases of subacute small bowel obstruction," *World Journal of Gastroenterology*, vol. 15, no. 19, pp. 2401–2405, 2009.

[12] D. Cave, P. Legnani, R. de Franchis, and B. S. Lewis, "ICCE consensus for capsule retention," *Endoscopy*, vol. 37, no. 10, pp. 1065–1067, 2005.

[13] M. Bhattarai, P. Bansal, and Y. Khan, "Longest duration of retention of video capsule: a case report and literature review," *World Journal of Gastrointestinal Endoscopy*, vol. 5, pp. 352–355, 2013.

[14] J. H. Cheon, Y.-S. Kim, I.-S. Lee et al., "Can we predict spontaneous capsule passage after retention? A nationwide study to evaluate the incidence and clinical outcomes of capsule retention," *Endoscopy*, vol. 39, no. 12, pp. 1046–1052, 2007.

[15] S. J. B. van Weyenberg, S. T. V. Turenhout, G. Bouma et al., "Double-balloon endoscopy as the primary method for small-bowel video capsule endoscope retrieval," *Gastrointestinal Endoscopy*, vol. 71, no. 3, pp. 535–541, 2010.

[16] K. Makipour, A. N. Modiri, A. Ehrlich et al., "Double balloon enteroscopy: effective and minimally invasive method for removal of retained video capsules," *Digestive Endoscopy*, 2014.

[17] J. M. Anderson, A. Rodriguez, and D. T. Chang, "Foreign body reaction to biomaterials," *Seminars in Immunology*, vol. 20, no. 2, pp. 86–100, 2008.

[18] A. K. McNally and J. M. Anderson, "Macrophage fusion and multinucleated giant cells of inflammation," *Advances in Experimental Medicine and Biology*, vol. 713, pp. 97–111, 2011.

3

Characteristics of Small Bowel Polyps Detected in Cowden Syndrome by Capsule Endoscopy

Keita Saito, Eiki Nomura, Yu Sasaki, Yasuhiko Abe, Nana Kanno, Naoko Mizumoto, Rika Shibuya, Kazuhiro Sakuta, Makoto Yagi, Kazuya Yoshizawa, Daisuke Iwano, Takeshi Sato, Shoichi Nishise, and Yoshiyuki Ueno

Department of Gastroenterology, Faculty of Medicine, Yamagata University, 2-2-2 Iida-Nishi, Yamagata 990-9585, Japan

Correspondence should be addressed to Eiki Nomura; nom_e@yahoo.co.jp

Academic Editor: Matteo Neri

Cowden syndrome is an uncommon, autosomal dominant disease characterized by multiple hamartomas and hyperplastic lesions in the skin, mucous membrane, brain, breast, thyroid, and gastrointestinal tract. About 30% of Cowden syndrome cases are reportedly complicated by malignant diseases. Hamartomatous polyps occur throughout the gastrointestinal tract, the most common sites being the stomach, colon, esophagus, and duodenum. Small bowel polyps can occur in Cowden syndrome; however, they are difficult to detect by conventional examination, including double-contrast X-ray study. Here, we report three cases of Cowden syndrome with small bowel polyps, which were detected by capsule endoscopy. The small bowel polyps of Cowden syndrome frequently occur at the oral end of the small bowel, especially in the duodenum and jejunum, and their color is similar to that of the surrounding mucosa; additionally, the polyps are relatively small (2–5 mm). Capsule endoscopy is useful for detecting small bowel polyps in Cowden syndrome.

1. Introduction

Cowden syndrome is an uncommon, autosomal dominant disease characterized by multiple hamartomas and hyperplastic lesions of the skin, mucous membrane, brain, breast, thyroid, and gastrointestinal tract [1, 2]. Its incidence is estimated to be one in 200,000–250,000 [3]. About 30% of Cowden syndrome cases are reportedly complicated by malignant tumors [4].

The incidence of gastrointestinal polyps is 65.6% in the esophagus, 75% in the stomach, 36.5% in the duodenum, and 65.6% in the colon [5]. The small bowel polyps can occur in Cowden syndrome; however, the characteristics of these polyps are unclear, and they are difficult to detect by conventional examination, including double-contrast X-ray study [6].

We report three cases of Cowden syndrome with small bowel polyps, which were detected by capsule endoscopy (CE), and describe the characteristic findings of the small bowel polyps in this syndrome.

2. Case Reports

2.1. Case 1. A 46-year-old man was referred to our hospital for hematochezia. He had no significant medical history and family history. He had multiple facial papules and small, whitish gingival papilloma. A colonoscopy revealed multiple rectosigmoid colon polyps, predominantly located in the lower rectum (Figure 1(a)). Esophagogastroduodenoscopy (EGD) showed whitish polypoid lesions in the esophagus (Figure 1(b)) and multiple gastric polyps (Figure 1(c)). Biopsy specimens from the gastric and rectal polyps revealed hamartomatous changes and hyperplasia. The esophageal polyps were diagnosed histopathologically as glycogenic acanthosis. The facial papules were diagnosed as trichilemmomas by histopathological examination. He was diagnosed with

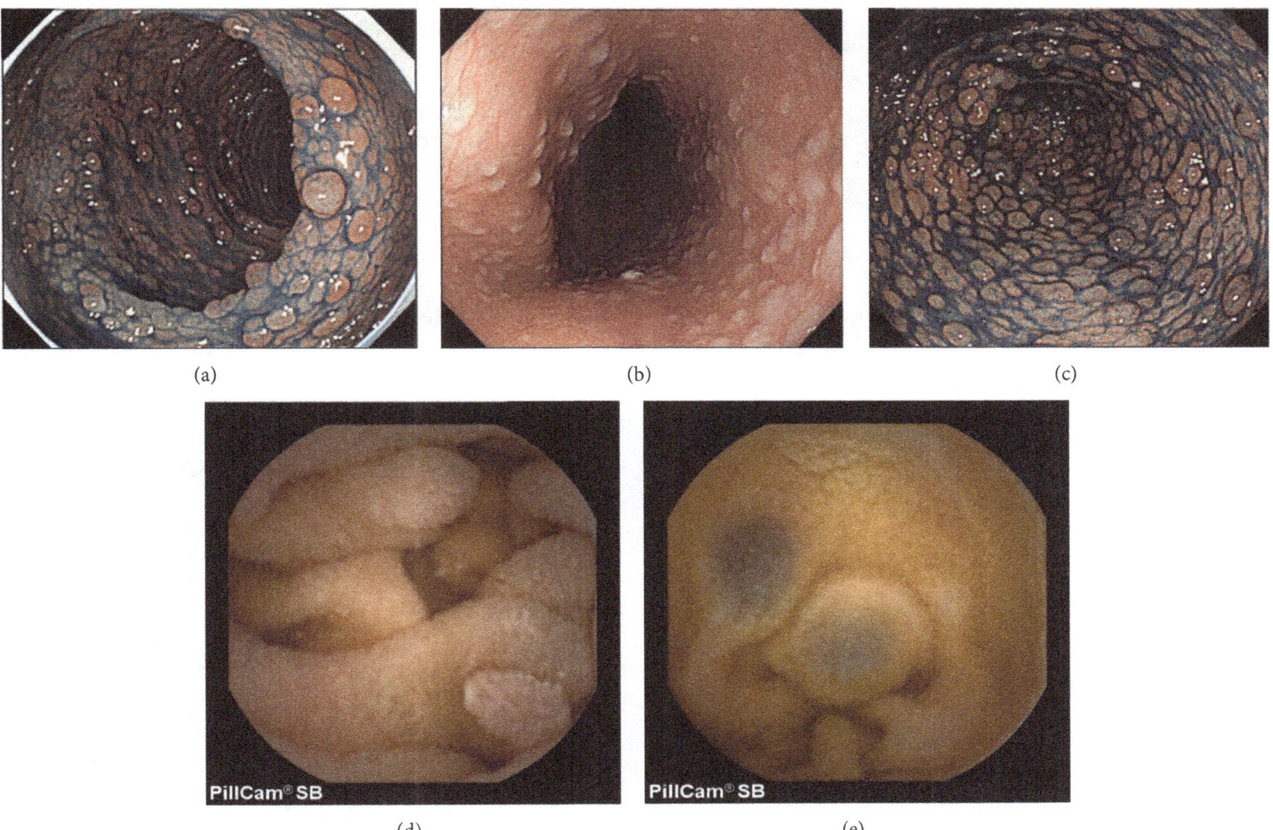

(a) (b) (c) (d) (e)

FIGURE 1: Endoscopic views of Case 1. (a) Colonoscopy revealed multiple rectal polyps. (b) Esophagogastroduodenoscopy (EGD) showed whitish polypoid lesions in the esophagus. (c) EGD showed multiple gastric polyps. (d) Capsule endoscopy revealed multiple polypoid lesions similar in color to the surrounding mucosa in the jejunum, with their diameters of 2–5 mm. (e) Capsule endoscopy revealed hemangiomas in the jejunum.

Cowden syndrome in accordance with the criteria of the International Cowden Consortium [7]. CE was performed to examine the small bowel and revealed multiple polypoid lesions that were similar in color to the surrounding mucosa; their diameters ranged from 2 to 5 mm at the distal end of the duodenum and jejunum (Figure 1(d)). The polyps were sparse, although their numbers were higher in the jejunum. Several hemangiomas were also observed in the jejunum (Figure 1(e)). They were more frequently observed at the oral end of the small bowel. The duodenal polyps were histopathologically diagnosed as being hamartomatous. No further malignant complications were observed; the patient was followed up in our hospital.

2.2. Case 2. A 60-year-old woman was referred to our hospital for further examination of multiple gastric polyps. She had a past history of breast fibroadenoma and thyroid goiter. She had oral papilloma, esophageal glycogenic acanthosis, and polyposis in the stomach, duodenum, and colon as observed by endoscopic examination. Histological assessment of the biopsy specimens revealed that the gastric and colonic polyps were hamartomatous, and she was diagnosed with Cowden syndrome. CE revealed many polyps of normal color that ranged from 2 to 5 mm in size in the small bowel (Figure 2). These polyps were sparse but were more frequently observed in the jejunum.

2.3. Case 3 (Daughter of Case 2). A 27-year-old woman received gastrointestinal examination after her mother's diagnosis with Cowden syndrome. EGD revealed esophageal multiple glycogenic acanthosis and duodenal polyps, but no significant lesions were found in the stomach, unlike her mother. A colonoscopy revealed small hamartomatous polyps in the rectum. She had bilateral tonsil papilloma, multiple thyroid cysts, and breast lipoma. She was diagnosed with Cowden syndrome. CE revealed minimal polyps of normal color, which ranged from 2 to 3 mm in size, from the duodenum to the oral end of the jejunum (Figure 3). We did not find any significant lesions in the ileum or malignant tumors in her body.

3. Discussion

Cowden syndrome, also known as multiple hamartoma syndrome, was first described in 1963 by Lloyd and Dennis [1]. This uncommon syndrome is characterized by multiple

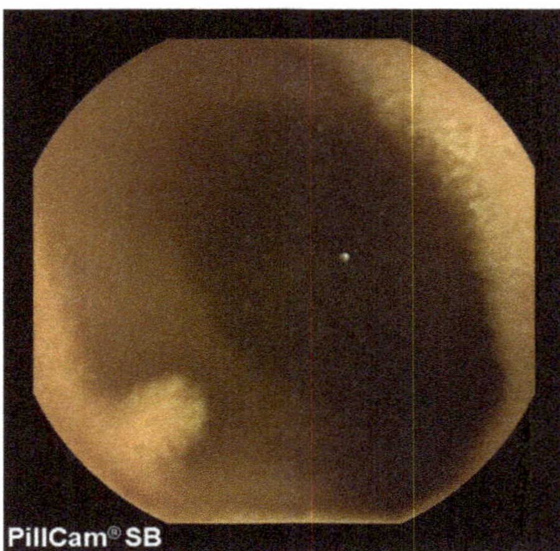

Figure 2: Capsule endoscopy revealed polyps of normal color in the jejunum.

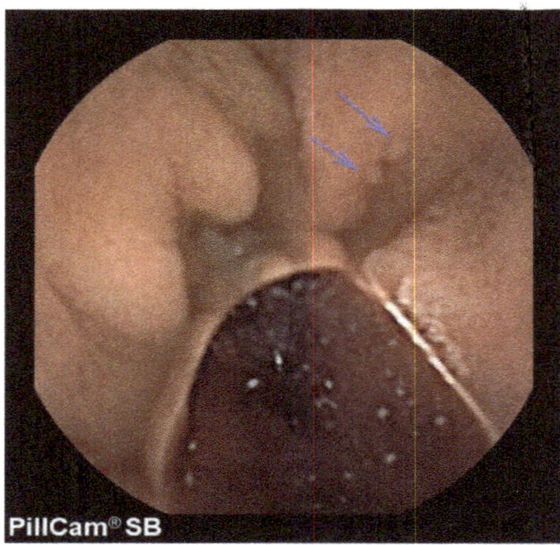

Figure 3: Capsule endoscopy revealed minimal polyps of normal color in the duodenum.

hamartomas and hyperplastic lesions of the whole body [2]. About 30% of Cowden syndrome cases are reportedly complicated by malignant diseases, including breast cancer, thyroid cancer, endometrium cancer, renal cell cancer, colorectal cancer, and melanoma [2–4].

Cowden syndrome is an autosomal dominant disorder that has been linked to germline mutations in the *PTEN* (phosphatase and tensin homolog) gene located on chromosome 10q23.3 [3]. Approximately 80% of patients with classically defined Cowden syndrome carry the *PTEN* gene [8], which acts as a negative regulator of the PI3-kinase signaling pathway by catalyzing the dephosphorylation of PIP3 [9]. *PTEN* hamartoma tumor syndrome incorporates several rare diseases that develop secondary to germline mutations within the *PTEN* gene. Component syndromes include Cowden syndrome and Bannayan-Riley-Ruvalcaba syndrome, which many now consider to be a single entity with age-related phenotypic presentations [10]. In our patients, genetic analysis was not performed.

The diagnosis of Cowden syndrome was originally made based on skin examination and family history [11]. However, the original diagnostic criteria of the International Cowden Consortium are now commonly used [7]. The presence of gastrointestinal polyposis is considered as a minor criterion owing to the lack of systematic studies to determine its true frequency and histology [12]. Nonetheless, in reality, it is a very common finding, with an estimated prevalence of up to 80% in patients with Cowden syndrome. In particular, esophageal polyps composed of glycogenic acanthosis are reportedly characteristic of Cowden syndrome [13, 14]. All three cases reported here fulfilled the criteria of the International Cowden Consortium. Gastric polyposis was found in Cases 1 and 2 and rectal polyposis and esophageal polyposis were found in all three. Esophageal polyposis was histopathologically shown to be composed of glycogenic acanthosis.

Small bowel polyps can arise in Cowden syndrome. However, the characteristics of these polyps are unclear, and they are difficult to detect with conventional examination, including double-contrast X-ray study, due to the small size of the polyps and the fact that they do not protrude much [6]. These polyps have been histopathologically found to be hamartomatous or hyperplastic polyps [2]. CE allows for endoscopic imaging of the entire small bowel without discomfort [15]. Three previous case reports have demonstrated small bowel polyps in Cowden syndrome using CE [6, 16, 17]. Nakaji et al. performed CE on a 24-year-old man with Cowden syndrome and observed multiple polypoid lesions that ranged from 3 to 5 mm in size in the small bowel, with the number of these polyps increasing from the jejunum to the terminal ileum [6]. Further, Riegler et al. reported a 53-year-old female with four minimal polyps in different tracts of the jejunum and vascular ectasia in the ileum as detected by CE [16]. Additionally, Hatogai et al. reported that small bowel polyps in Cowden syndrome are more clearly visualized using contrast image CE [17]. To our knowledge, there have been no previous case series of small bowel polyps in Cowden syndrome as demonstrated by CE. In our series, small bowel polyps were detected in all three cases. In Case 1, multiple polypoid lesions were found of a similar color to the surrounding mucosa, with their diameters ranging from 2 to 5 mm in the duodenum and jejunum. The polyps were sparse, although their numbers were higher in the jejunum. Several hemangiomas were also observed in the jejunum. Hemangiomas were frequently observed at the oral end of the small intestine. Many polyps of normal color, ranging from 2 to 5 mm in size, were observed in the small bowel in Case 2, mostly in the jejunum. Minimal polyps were seen in the duodenum to the jejunum in Case 3. Histopathological examination revealed hamartomatous polyps in all three cases, which needed to be biopsied.

In all the three cases, preparation for CE consisted solely of fasting (no solid food, only clear liquids) for 12 h prior to the procedure, and polyethylene glycol solution was not used; nonetheless, we obtained relatively clear images from the jejunum to the terminal ileum. It was reported that ileal involvement is not rare [12] and that polyp density increased aborally [6]; however, Riegler et al. [16] showed jejunal polyps, not ileal polyps, in Cowden syndrome. The quality of bowel preparation and imaging could affect polyp detection by CE; nevertheless, we think that there were more jejunal polyps than ileal polyps in our patients. Further examinations are needed to clarify the most common sites for small bowel polyps in Cowden syndrome.

We did not detect any malignant diseases in the three cases. However, Cowden syndrome is associated with increased susceptibility to malignant diseases, and periodic follow-up examination and early diagnosis are necessary.

In summary, we described the characteristics of small bowel polyps in Cowden syndrome using CE. Small bowel polyps in Cowden syndrome are frequently observed at the oral end of the small bowel, especially in the duodenum and jejunum, and their color is similar to that of the surrounding mucosa; additionally, the polyps are relatively small (2–5 mm). CE is useful for detecting polyps in the small bowel in Cowden syndrome.

References

[1] K. M. Lloyd II and M. Dennis, "Cowden's disease. A possible new symptom complex with multiple system involvement," *Annals of Internal Medicine*, vol. 58, pp. 136–142, 1963.

[2] R. Pilarski, "Cowden syndrome: a critical review of the clinical literature," *Journal of Genetic Counseling*, vol. 18, no. 1, pp. 13–27, 2009.

[3] M. R. Nelen, H. Kremer, I. B. M. Konings et al., "Novel PTEN mutations in patients with Cowden disease: absence of clear genotype-phenotype correlations," *European Journal of Human Genetics*, vol. 7, no. 3, pp. 267–273, 1999.

[4] K. Ushio, T. Ishikawa, and T. Hukutomi, "Cowden's disease (multiple hamartoma syndrome)—recent knowledge and problems," *Clinical Oncology*, vol. 44, pp. 1024–1032, 1998.

[5] M. Kato, A. Mizuki, T. Hayashi et al., "Cowden's disease diagnosed through mucocutaneous lesions and gastrointestinal polyposis with recurrent hematochezia, unrevealed by initial diagnosis," *Internal Medicine*, vol. 39, no. 7, pp. 559–563, 2000.

[6] K. Nakaji, Y. Nakae, and S. Suzumura, "Enteric manifestations of Cowden syndrome," *Internal Medicine*, vol. 49, no. 8, pp. 795–796, 2010.

[7] C. Eng, "Will the real Cowden syndrome please stand up: revised diagnostic criteria," *Journal of Medical Genetics*, vol. 37, no. 11, pp. 828–830, 2000.

[8] D. J. Marsh, V. Coulon, K. L. Lunetta et al., "Mutation spectrum and genotype-phenotype analyses in Cowden disease and Bannayan-Zonana syndrome, two hamartoma syndromes with germline *PTEN* mutation," *Human Molecular Genetics*, vol. 7, no. 3, pp. 507–515, 1998.

[9] T. Maehama and J. E. Dixon, "The tumor suppressor, PTEN/MMAC1, dephosphorylates the lipid second messenger, phosphatidylinositol 3,4,5-triphosphate," *The Journal of Biological Chemistry*, vol. 273, no. 22, pp. 13375–13378, 1998.

[10] D. J. Marsh, J. B. Kum, K. L. Lunetta et al., "PTEN mutation spectrum and genotype-phenotype correlations in Bannayan-Riley-Ruvalcaba syndrome suggest a single entity with Cowden syndrome," *Human Molecular Genetics*, vol. 8, no. 8, pp. 1461–1472, 1999.

[11] O. S. Salem and W. D. Steck, "Cowden's disease (multiple hamartoma and neoplasia syndrome). A case report and review of the English literature," *Journal of the American Academy of Dermatology*, vol. 8, no. 5, pp. 686–696, 1983.

[12] B. Heald, J. Mester, L. Rybicki, M. S. Orloff, C. A. Burke, and C. Eng, "Frequent gastrointestinal polyps and colorectal adenocarcinomas in a prospective series of PTEN mutation carriers," *Gastroenterology*, vol. 139, no. 6, pp. 1927–1933, 2010.

[13] P. S. Kay, R. M. Soetikno, R. Mindelzun, and H. S. Young, "Diffuse esophageal glycogenic acanthosis: an endoscopic marker of Cowden's disease," *The American Journal of Gastroenterology*, vol. 92, no. 6, pp. 1038–1040, 1997.

[14] K. Umemura, S. Takagi, Y. Ishigaki et al., "Gastrointestinal polyposis with esophageal polyposis is useful for early diagnosis of Cowden's disease," *World Journal of Gastroenterology*, vol. 14, no. 37, pp. 5755–5759, 2008.

[15] G. Iddan, G. Meron, A. Glukhovsky, and P. Swain, "Wireless capsule endoscopy," *Nature*, vol. 405, no. 6785, pp. 417–418, 2000.

[16] G. Riegler, I. Esposito, P. Esposito et al., "Wireless capsule enteroscopy (Given) in a case of Cowden syndrome," *Digestive and Liver Disease*, vol. 38, no. 2, pp. 151–152, 2006.

[17] K. Hatogai, N. Hosoe, H. Imaeda et al., "Role of enhanced visibility in evaluating polyposis syndromes using a newly developed contrast image capsule endoscope," *Gut and Liver*, vol. 6, no. 2, pp. 218–222, 2012.

4

A Rare Cause of Acute Abdomen: Perforation of Double Meckel's Diverticulum

İlhan Tas,[1] Serdar Culcu,[1] Yigit Duzkoylu,[2] Sadik Eryilmaz,[1] Mehmet Mehdi Deniz,[3] and Deniz Yilmaz[4]

[1] *General Surgery Clinic, Cizre Dr. Selahattin Cizrelioglu State Hospital, Şırnak, Turkey*
[2] *General Surgery Clinic, Islahiye State Hospital, Gaziantep, Turkey*
[3] *General Surgery Clinic, Bayrampasa State Hospital, Istanbul, Turkey*
[4] *Pathology Department, Cizre Dr. Selahattin Cizrelioglu State Hospital, Şırnak, Turkey*

Correspondence should be addressed to Yigit Duzkoylu; dryigit@gmail.com

Academic Editor: Yoshihiro Moriwaki

Meckel's diverticulum is the most common congenital anomaly of the gastrointestinal tract. In this report, we aimed to represent a case of intestinal perforation, caused by double Meckel's diverticulum, which is a very rare entity in surgical practice. The patient was a 20-year-old Caucasian man, admitted to hospital with complaints of abdominal pain, nausea, and vomitting during the last 3 days. Physical examination indicated tenderness, rebound, and guarding in the right lower quadrant of abdomen. Abdominal X-ray revealed a few air-liquid levels in the left upper quadrant. In the operation, 2 Meckel's diverticula were observed, one at the antimesenteric side, at 70 cm distance to the ileocecal valve, approximately in 3 cm size, and the other between the mesenteric and antimesenteric sides, approximately in 5 cm size. The first one had been perforated at the tip and wrapped with omentum. A 30 cm ileal resection, including both diverticula with end-to-end anastomosis, was performed. The diagnosis of symptomatic Meckel's diverticulum is considerably hard, especially when it is complicated. Diverticulectomy or segmentary resections are therapeutic options. In patients with acute abdomen clinic, Meckel's diverticulum and its complications should be kept in mind, and the intestines should be observed for an extra diverticulum for caution although it is a very rare condition.

1. Introduction

Meckel's diverticulum is the most common congenital anomaly of the gastrointestinal tract, with the incidence of 1–3% [1–4]. Incomplete obliteration of the omphalomesenteric duct in intrauterine period is thought to be the main etiologic factor [1, 5]. Preoperative diagnosis is compelling especially in uncomplicated cases. Meckel's diverticulum is symptomatic in 4–6% of the patients [5, 6]. The ratio of men to women in symptomatic cases is reported to be 3/1 [2, 7]. Most common complications include ulceration, intestinal obstruction, hemorrhage, perforation, intussusception, vesicodiverticular fistula, and malignancy [3, 8, 9]. In our study, we aimed to report a rare case of double Meckel's diverticulum, resulting in intestinal perforation, mentioning the diagnosis, treatment, and postoperative results.

2. Case

The patient was a 20-year-old Caucasian male, admitted to the Emergency Clinic 3 days ago, diagnosed as non-specific abdominal pain, and discharged with symptomatic treatment. Later he was admitted to General Surgery Clinic with clinical signs of acute abdomen. He had neither any comorbidities, nor any specificities in his history.

In his physical examination, blood pressure was found to be 120/70 mmHg, pulse was 86/minutes, respiration rate was 16/minutes, and the temperature was 36.8°C. There were tenderness, guarding, and rebound in the right lower quadrant of abdomen. Digital rectal examination was normal. In his laboratory findings, WBC was found to be 11.200, hemoglobin was 12.8 g/dL, and platelet count was 133.000. Abdominal X-ray revealed a few air-liquid levels in the left

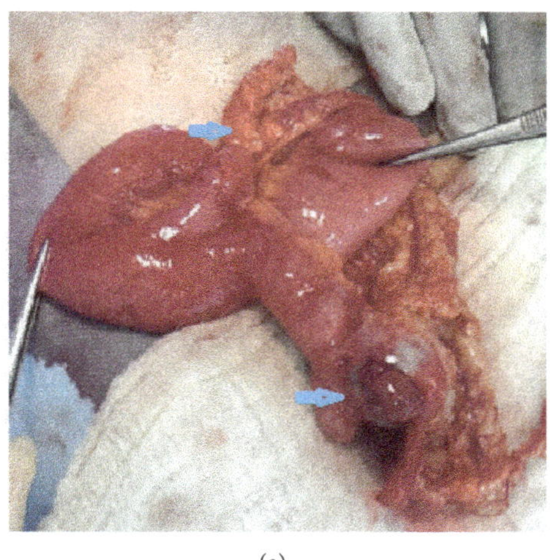
(a)

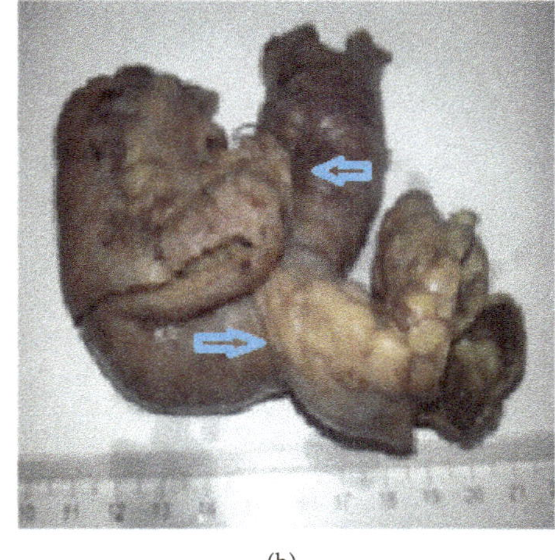
(b)

FIGURE 1: (a) Double Meckel's diverticulum, one wrapped with omentum. (b) Two diverticula, located in the resected material; the right one is inflamed.

upper quadrant. In abdominal ultrasonography, intestinal ansae were found to be dilated at the lower quadrants, and a noncompressible appendix in 6 mm thickness was observed at the right lower quadrant.

Following adequate hydration and double antibiotic prophylaxis with 1 gr of ceftriaxone and 500 mg of metronidazole, the patient was taken to operation at emergency conditions. Following a Mc Burney incision, appendix was found to be inflamed, with extensive reactional free fluid in the cavity. After performing appendectomy, a mass was palpated in the abdomen, and intestinal ansae were taken out of the abdomen for exploration. Two diverticula were observed, one on the antimesenteric side, at 70 cm distance to the ileocecal valve, in 3 cm size, and the second one between the mesenteric and antimesenteric sides, in 5 cm size. The first diverticulum was found to be perforated at the tip and wrapped with omentum (Figure 1). An ileal resection of 30 cm, including the diverticula and end-to-end anastomosis, was performed, because the abdominal cavity was not contaminated. A drainage tube was inserted into the rectovesical pouch.

Gaita discharge started on the postoperative second day, and oral intake was allowed on the fourth day. The patient was discharged on postoperative sixth day without any complications. Histopathologic examination revealed perforation signs in the larger diverticulum with heterotopic gastric mucosa and active inflammation hemorrhage and edema in the smaller one (Figure 2).

3. Discussion

Meckel's diverticulum is the most frequent congenital anomaly of the gastrointestinal tract, resulting from the incomplete atrophy of the omphalomesenteric duct [1–3, 5, 10]. Heterotopic tissues such as gastric, duodenal, colonic ones and rarely pancreatic mucosa can be found in the diverticula, as well as the anatomically normal intestinal mucosa [9, 10]. They are found in 15–50% of the cases and more often in symptomatic patients [10]. Preoperative diagnosis is rare in uncomplicated cases, and the diverticulum is usually observed incidentally, during other procedures for various reasons [11]. "Rule of twos" is characteristic for Meckel's diverticulum, which includes the prevalence in 2% of the population; it is usually diagnosed under the age of 2; it is in 2-inches size and 2 cm diameter, 2 feets proximal to the valve, twice frequent in men, and symptomatic in 2% of the patients [11, 12].

Double Meckel's diverticulum is a rare condition, and the first study was reported by Emre et al., representing 5 cases with double diverticula [1]. In our case, the rare entity is the observation of double Meckel's diverticulum and perforation in one of them. Although preoperative diagnosis may be compelling, and the most frequently used modalities are computerized tomography (CT), Technetium-99 m pertechnetate scintigraphy, and double-balloon enteroscopy, which is superior to the others [13], scintigraphy has the capability of observing ectopic gastric mucosa but may have false positive and negative results at high rates [10].

In our case, we performed an emergent operation with the initial diagnosis of acute appendicitis, relying on the physical examination findings and Meckel's diverticulum was observed incidentally. The most useful imaging method is CT in the diagnosis of intestinal obstruction, which is a possible complication of the disease [12]. Laparoscopy may also be useful, in both diagnosis and treatment [10]. Surgery is the gold standard treatment option in symptomatic patients. Diverticulectomy or segmentary resection with anastomosis is the surgical options. Mortality rates are reported to be 1.6–7.7% [6]. Laparoscopic procedures have taken conventional operations' place in the recent years, providing two different surgical options, intracorporeal laparoscopy and TULA (transumbilical laparoscopic-assisted Meckel's diverticulectomy), which are useful in both diagnosis and treatment. The most important disadvantage of the former technique is to leave heterotopic tissue at the distal parts, especially when it is performed with staplers [10].

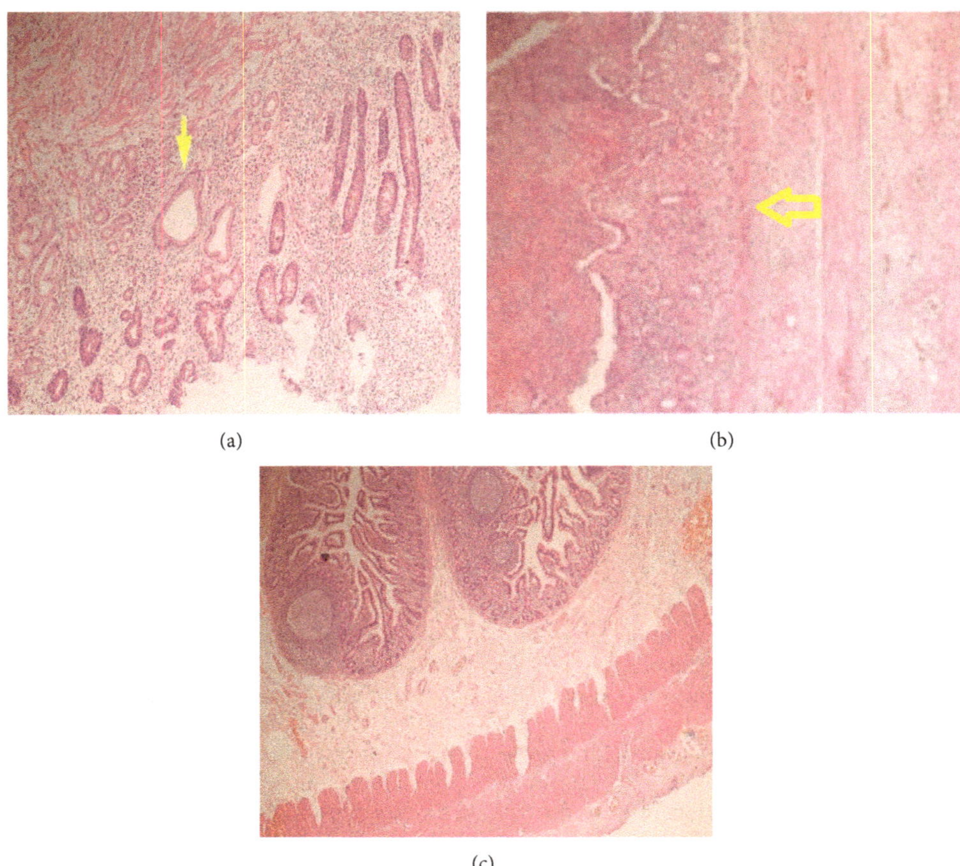

FIGURE 2: (a) Gastric mucosa (arrow), at the side of ulcerated intestinal mucosa (HE ×100). (b) Ulcerated intestinal wall (HE ×200). (c) Histopathology of the second diverticulum (HE ×200).

4. Conclusion

In patients with clinical signs of acute abdomen, Meckel's diverticulum and its potential complications should be kept in mind, especially when any reasons that can explain the clinical findings of the patient are not observed intraoperatively.

References

[1] A. Emre, S. Akbulut, M. Yilmaz, M. Kanlioz, and B. E. Aydin, "Double Meckel's diverticulum presenting as acute appendicitis: a case report and literature review," *The Journal of Emergency Medicine*, vol. 44, no. 4, pp. e321–e324, 2013.

[2] I. Wani, V. Šnábel, G. Naikoo et al., "Encountering Meckel's diverticulum in emergency surgery for ascaridial intestinal obstruction," *World Journal of Emergency Surgery*, vol. 5, article 15, 2010.

[3] M. Bouassida, M. Mongi Mighri, K. Trigui et al., "Meckel's diverticulum: an exceptional cause of vesicoenteric fistula: case report and literature review," *Pan African Medical Journal*, vol. 15, no. 9, 2013.

[4] S. Madhyastha, V. L. Prabhu, V. Saralaya, and Prakash, "Meckel's diverticulum. A case report," *International Journal of Morphology*, vol. 25, no. 3, pp. 519–522, 2007.

[5] K. Uppal, R. S. Tubbs, P. Matusz, K. Shaffer, and M. Loukas, "Meckel's diverticulum: a review," *Clinical Anatomy*, vol. 24, no. 4, pp. 416–422, 2011.

[6] M. J. Soltero and A. H. Bill, "The natural history of Meckel's diverticulum and its relation to incidental removal: a study of 202 cases of diseased Meckel's diverticulum, found in King County, Washington, over a fifteen year period," *The American Journal of Surgery*, vol. 132, no. 2, pp. 168–173, 1976.

[7] A. Cotirlet, R. Anghel, E. Tincu, S. Rau, I. Motoc, and E. Popa, "Perforation of Meckel's diverticulum by foreign body, a rare complication," *Chirurgia*, vol. 108, pp. 411–413, 2013.

[8] J. Sagar, V. Kumar, and D. K. Shah, "Meckel's diverticulum: a systematic review," *Journal of the Royal Society of Medicine*, vol. 99, no. 10, pp. 501–505, 2006.

[9] M. I. Beyrouti, M. Ben Amar, R. Beyrout, and M. Abid, "Complication du diverticule de Meckel, a propose de 42 cas," *La Tunisie Médicale*, vol. 87, no. 4, pp. 253–256, 2009.

[10] M. Fukushima, C. Kawanami, S. Inoue, A. Okada, Y. Imai, and T. Inokuma, "A case series of Meckel's diverticulum: usefulness of double-balloon enteroscopy for diagnosis," *BMC Gastroenterology*, vol. 14, no. 1, article 155, 2014.

[11] A. Altaf and H. Aref, "A case report: cecal volvulus caused by Meckel's diverticulum," *International Journal of Surgery Case Reports*, vol. 5, no. 12, pp. 1200–1202, 2014.

[12] M. Murruste, "Torsion of Meckel's diverticulum as a cause of small bowel obstruction: a case report," *World Journal of Gastrointestinal Surgery*, vol. 6, no. 10, pp. 204–207, 2014.

[13] A. Papparella, F. Nino, C. Noviello et al., "Laparoscopic approach to Meckel's diverticulum," *World Journal of Gastroenterology*, vol. 20, no. 25, pp. 8173–8178, 2014.

5

Gastric Emphysema a Spectrum of Pneumatosis Intestinalis: A Case Report and Literature Review

Guillermo López-Medina,[1] Roxana Castillo Díaz de León,[2] Alberto Carlos Heredia-Salazar,[1] and Daniel Ramón Hernández-Salcedo[1]

[1] *Hospital Angeles Clinica Londres, Durango No. 50, Roma Norte, Cuauhtémoc, 06700 Ciudad de México, DF, Mexico*
[2] *Hospital Angeles Mocel, Gregorio V. Gelati 29, San Miguel Chapultepec, Miguel Hidalgo, 11850 Ciudad de México, DF, Mexico*

Correspondence should be addressed to Guillermo López-Medina; dr.guillermolopezmedina@gmail.com

Academic Editor: Haruhiko Sugimura

The finding of gas within the gastric wall is not a disease by itself, rather than a sign of an underlying condition which could be systemic or gastric. We present the case of a woman identified with gastric emphysema secondary to the administration of high doses of steroids, with the purpose of differentiating emphysematous gastritis versus gastric emphysema due to the divergent prognostic implications. Gastric emphysema entails a more benign course, opposed to emphysematous gastritis which often presents as an acute abdomen and carries a worse prognosis. Owing to the lack of established diagnostic criteria, computed tomography is the assessment method of choice. Currently no guidelines are available for the management of this entity, since the evidence is limited to a few case series and a considerable number of single case reports.

1. Introduction

Radiologic detection of gas within the wall of the gastric chamber is not an entity per se but a sign of an underlying disease [1]. Described for the first time in 1889 by Fraenkel, a variety of names have been given to this condition: interstitial emphysema, intramural emphysema, gastric emphysema, emphysematous gastritis, gastric pneumatosis, and pneumatosis cystoides intestinalis; however, based on underlying cause and anatomical situation they are considered distinct pathologies carrying for a different treatment and prognosis [1, 2].

2. Case Report

We present a 44-year-old woman with history of mixed connective tissue disease, who was hospitalized due to exacerbation of her underlying condition for which she was treated with high dose pulses of methylprednisolone. Two days after discharge she arrives back to the emergency room, complaining mainly of abdominal pain located on upper quadrants, not related to food ingestion, associated with vomiting of gastric content in four occasions and one liquid stool free from mucus or blood. At admission with stable vital signs, without acute abdomen or other relevant findings revealed on physical examination, stool specimens, blood analyses, and cultures analyses were requested in search for infectious origin, resulting negative. The plain abdominal X-ray showed a radiolucent image in the left upper quadrant (Figure 1), which was also observed on the plain chest X-ray (Figure 2), subsequently a computed tomography (CT) scan with double contrast of the abdomen, documented the presence of air in the gastric wall (Figures 3, 4, and 5).

Fasting was indicated as well as management with proton bomb inhibitor and broad spectrum antibiotic ampicillin/sulbactam. After twelve hours of close monitoring, the patient persisted nauseous and vomiting, therefore, underwent a liberating mucotomy via superior endoscopy, without complications and minimum bleeding. However, 24 hours later the patient continued presenting abdominal

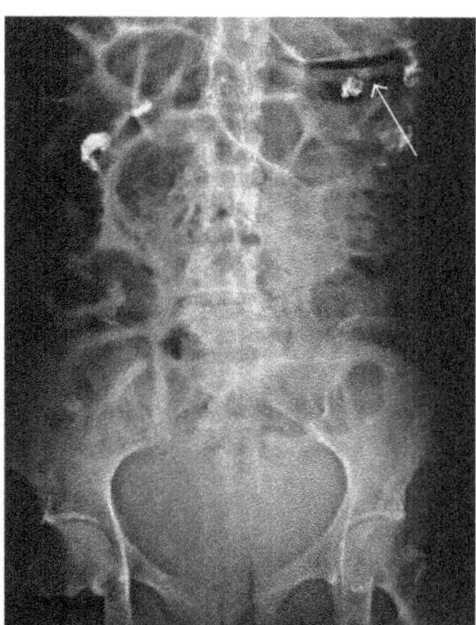

FIGURE 1: Plain abdominal X-ray. Radiolucent image in the upper left abdominal quadrant, showing the presence of air within the wall of the stomach (arrow).

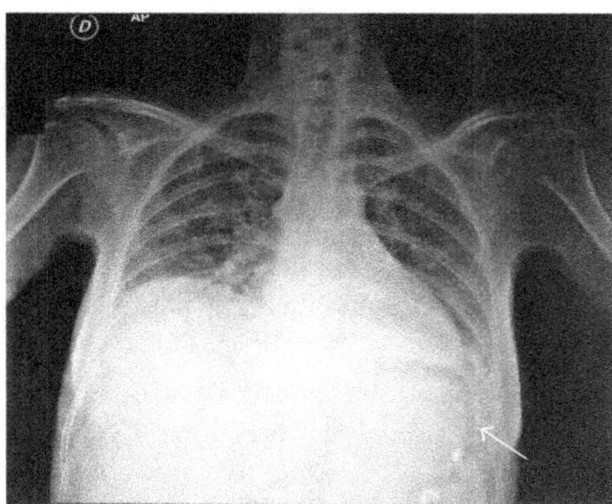

FIGURE 2: Plain chest X ray. Radiolucent image below the left diaphragm showing the presence of air within the wall of the stomach (arrow).

pain and under the suspicion of gastric perforation, due to the presence of right subdiaphragmatic air on a chest X-ray, she was taken to the operating room for an exploratory laparotomy revealing free hematic fluid in the abdominal cavity; methylene blue dye was instilled into the gastric lumen without evidence of dye extravasation, concluding the absence of perforation, considering the procedure complete. Afterwards the evolution was torpid showing signs of rheumatologic activity associated to acute pulmonary deterioration that led to the patient's death due to a possible hemorrhagic alveolitis.

3. Discussion

The pathogenesis of this disease has been debated for decades; however, it may be approached through the questions, where did the gas come from? And how did it get there? Based on these are how three mechanisms of origin are proposed: (1) intraluminal, (2) bacterial production, and (3) gas of pulmonary origin [3].

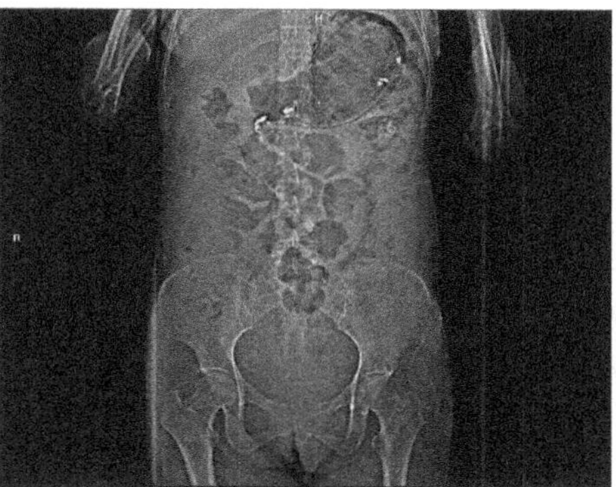

FIGURE 3: Abdominal scout image from a computed tomography.

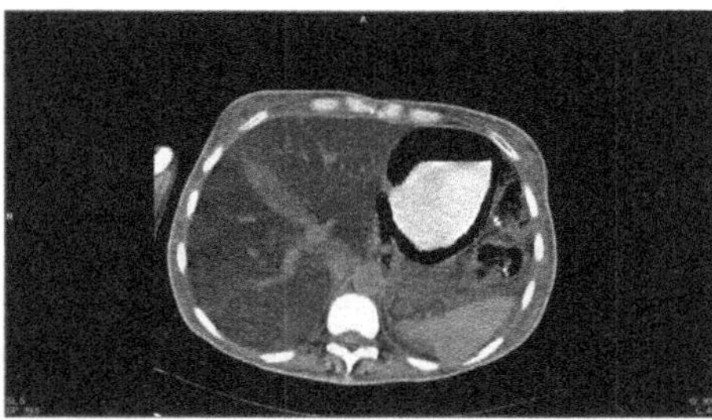

FIGURE 4: Computed axial tomography of the abdomen with oral contrast agent enhancing the stomach.

Intestinal pneumatosis is referred to the presence of gas within the wall of the gastrointestinal tract and it can appear in any site from stomach to the rectum [4]. The stomach is the least common site of presentation; one retrospective study identified only 18 cases during a period of 15 years [5]. Another study in 2004 by Hawn MT, Canon CL, and Lockhart ME et al. reported a casuistry of 86 patients with intestinal pneumatosis, being the colonic localization the most frequent counting for 50%, while the gastric location counted hardly 9%, with a mortality rate of 38% reported for this last one [6]. Emphasizing on the gastric chamber, it can be classified into two categories: emphysematous gastritis and gastric emphysema or gastric pneumatosis [7]. Nevertheless there are no clear and universal definitions available to distinguish each.

It has been postulated that emphysematous gastritis is produced by gas forming bacteria and gastric emphysema by air dissecting the wall [8], through several mechanisms either traumatic, mechanic, or inflammatory [9]; it is important to mention that emphysematous gastritis and gastric emphysema entail contrasting prognosis, the latter being more benign [8].

When the origin of the gas is intraluminal, pneumatosis can occur even alongside an intact mucosa, with intraluminal high pressure accounted as the responsible mechanism. In the context of an injured mucosa, because of trauma or inflammation, a normal intraluminal pressure may be present or a combination of both [3].

In the case gas derives from bacteria, the theory of counterperfusion-supersaturation has been postulated,

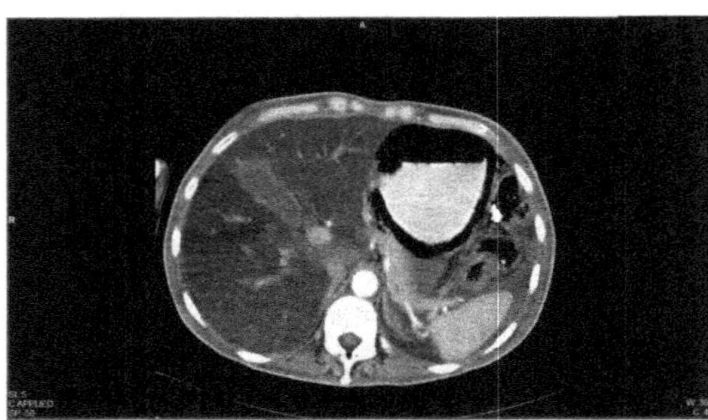

FIGURE 5: Computed axial tomography of the abdomen with oral and intravenous contrast agent enhancing the stomach during the arterial phase.

and it sustains that the production of nitrogen by intraluminal bacteria overflows the plasma concentration producing a plasma-intraluminal gradient and causing a diffusion of nitrogen into submucosal vessels which would explain the gas pattern found through the blood vessels in the border of the mesentery [3].

A pulmonary source has also been debated. The proposed theory is that air travels from an alveolar rupture into the blood vessels up to the gastrointestinal tract. Nevertheless the absence of interstitial emphysema in the mesentery has called this theory into question, giving place to a hypothesis of an increase in intraabdominal pressure hence intraluminal pressure, frequently seen in chronic cough patients causing transmural migration of air [3].

Resuming the etiopathogenesis of this entity, some causes can be mentioned in referral to gastric processes associated to injury of the mucous wall of the stomach. It is well known that acute gastric distension can result in gastric emphysema, emphysematous gastritis, or necrosis. Massive distension causes ischemia with extension of intraluminal gas in to the wall [10]. The ingestion of caustic substances, primarily acids more than alkalis promote corrosive lesions altering the gastric wall in various degrees of depth [11]. Also there have been reported cases of caustic gastritis coursing without gastric emphysema and yet gas within portal venous system [12]. Perforating ulcers, upper endoscopy procedures, such as argon plasma coagulation, installation of intragastric catheters, or biliary stents, are diverse precedents of lesion that can complicate with mobilization of intraluminal gas to submucous spaces [11]. Evidence exists of gastric bezoars associated with this disease as well as distension due to the administration of positive pressure through a bag-mask device during cardiopulmonary resuscitation [13–15], in addition to a case secondary to a diabetic gastropathy in a patient with type 1 diabetes [16].

Pneumatosis can also result from a variety of extragastric processes, which favor air migration thru the wall of the colon despite maintaining intact. That being said we can include chronic pulmonary obstructive disease, polymyositis, perforated appendicitis, small bowel volvulus, intestinal infarction, gangrenous cholecystitis, superior mesenteric artery syndrome, cholangiocarcinoma, parastomal hernia, and multiple episodes of vomiting. In relation to drug related background, it has been linked to chemotherapy agents such as cyclophosphamide, adriamycin, and vincristine, in addition to high doses of dexamethasone in one case report [5, 17–23].

Clinical manifestations are usually nonspecific, presenting with nausea, vomit occasionally resistant to antiemetics, mild to severe abdominal pain, abdominal distension, haematemesis, or melena; presentation as an acute abdomen is rare [2]. Most frequently reported cases follow an acute-subacute course [5, 16, 17, 23] and findings at physical examination rarely support the diagnosis [3].

Among the image battery available, computed tomography (CT) of the abdomen is the method of choice since it can detect a minimum amount of air inside the wall of the gastrointestinal tract and evaluate the abdominal cavity. Gastric emphysema is presented as a hypodense lineal or curve fringe on the gastric wall along with distension, without evidence of thickening of the wall. Occasionally pneumoperitoneum may be detected, in contrast to emphysematous gastritis where a streaky and linear pattern distribution of air and gastric wall thickening are characteristic, or air in some other bowel or biliary tract can be found [5, 17, 24]. In a simple X-ray of the abdomen, stomach is distended and outlined with linear gas shadows in the gastric wall. These stripes or streaks can be single or double, with round areas of radiolucency a few millimeters wide and parallel to the border of the stomach [17]. Within endoscopic findings we can come across a pebble-like gastric mucous that only traduces the presence of air bubbles [25].

There is no available standard treatment for this condition; most of the reported cases have been treated in a conservative manner. A retrospective study by Morris et al. [26] included 97 patients with intestinal pneumatosis, 46% involving colon, 27% small bowel, 14% affecting the whole gastrointestinal tract including the portal venous system, 7% small bowel and colon, and 5% located on the stomach; they reported a mortality of 16% in the group who received surgical treatment contrasting with a 6% mortality rate reported for the group who received conservative treatment. In stable patients a clinical improvement or resolution of the emphysema within 72 hours has been reported with the use of nasogastric catheter for decompression [10]. Algorithms for the management of intestinal pneumatosis have been proposed, however, without emphasis on gastric emphysema so their application is limited [27, 28].

The prognosis of gastric emphysema is usually benign with spontaneous resolution even without a specific treatment [3]. More so, a reported case of recurrent gastric emphysema by two distinct mechanisms, where managed in a conservative way obtaining a favorable outcome [29]. Nevertheless mortality associated to emphysematous gastritis is documented from 61% as far as 100% [2, 9].

4. Conclusion

Gastric emphysema and emphysematous gastritis are spectrum of intestinal pneumatosis; both belong to the least common forms of presentation, with different etiopathogenic possibilities (traumatic, inflammatory, or mechanic), systemic impact, intraabdominal findings, and prognosis and with a distinctive feature of gastric emphysema that in most cases yields more indolent behavior. It is maintained as a misunderstood pathology, in great part since most of the evidence derives from single case reports and series in a significant number of clinical scenarios.

The main suspicion in the presented case was an inflammatory cause which was sustained by the presence of hematic ascites, not rare in patients with connective tissue diseases. The implemented measures of endoscopic mucotomy plus coverage by board spectrum antibiotics turned out in a positive impact regarding the gastrointestinal aspect, unlike the rest of the progression of her base rheumatologic disease.

Authors' Contribution

All authors have contributed in terms of material, images, and review of the final document.

References

[1] F. P. Agha, "Gastric emphysema: an etiologic classification," *Australasian Radiology*, vol. 28, no. 4, pp. 346–352, 1984.

[2] T. H. Loi, J. See, R. K. Diddapur, and J. R. Issac, "Emphysematous gastritis: a case report and a review of literature," *Annals of the Academy of Medicine Singapore*, vol. 36, no. 1, pp. 72–73, 2007.

[3] S. D. St Peter, M. A. Abbas, and K. A. Kelly, "The spectrum of pneumatosis intestinalis," *Archives of Surgery*, vol. 138, no. 1, pp. 68–75, 2003.

[4] S. Donovan, J. Cernigliaro, and N. Dawson, "Pneumatosis intestinalis: a case report and approach to management," *Case Reports in Medicine*, vol. 2011, Article ID 571387, 5 pages, 2011.

[5] S. Majumder, G. Trikudanathan, K. Moezardalan, and J. Cappa, "Vomiting-induced gastric emphysema: a rare self-limiting condition," *The American Journal of the Medical Sciences*, vol. 343, no. 1, pp. 92–93, 2012.

[6] M. T. Hawn, C. L. Canon, M. E. Lockhart et al., "Serum lactic acid determines the outcomes of CT diagnosis of pneumatosis of the gastrointestinal tract," *The American Surgeon*, vol. 70, no. 1, pp. 19–24, 2004.

[7] R. D'Cruz and S. Emil, "Gastroduodenal emphysema," *Journal of Pediatric Surgery*, vol. 43, no. 11, pp. 2121–2123, 2008.

[8] E. M. Pauli, J. M. Tomasko, V. Jain, C. E. Dye, and R. S. Haluck, "Multiply recurrent episodes of gastric emphysema," *Case Reports in Surgery*, vol. 2011, Article ID 587198, 3 pages, 2011.

[9] M. Krier, R. B. Jeffrey Jr., and S. Banerjee, "Troubles with stomach bubbles? or not?" *Digestive Diseases and Sciences*, vol. 54, no. 5, pp. 919–921, 2009.

[10] S. A. Khan, E. Boko, H. A. Khookhar, S. Woods, and A. H. Nasr, "Acute gastric dilatation resulting in gastric emphysema following postpartum hemorrhage," *Case Reports in Surgery*, vol. 2012, Article ID 230629, 4 pages, 2012.

[11] P. T. Johnson, K. M. Horton, B. H. Edil, E. K. Fishman, and W. W. Scott, "Gastric pneumatosis: the role of CT in diagnosis and patient management," *Emergency Radiology*, vol. 18, no. 1, pp. 65–73, 2011.

[12] M. Lewin, M. Pocard, S. Caplin, A. Blain, J.-M. Tubiana, and R. Parc, "Benign hepatic portal venous gas following caustic ingestion," *European Radiology*, vol. 12, supplement 3, pp. S59–S61, 2002.

[13] K. N. Chintapalli, "Gastric bezoar causing intramural pneumatosis," *Journal of Clinical Gastroenterology*, vol. 18, no. 3, pp. 264–265, 1994.

[14] H. Reuter, C. Bangard, F. Gerhardt, S. Rosenkranz, and E. Erdmann, "Extensive hepatic portal venous gas and gastric emphysema after successful resuscitation," *Resuscitation*, vol. 82, no. 2, pp. 238–239, 2011.

[15] C. Lai, W. Chang, P. Liang, W. Lien, H. Wang, and W. Chen, "Pneumatosis intestinalis and hepatic portal venous gas after CPR," *The American Journal of Emergency Medicine*, vol. 23, no. 2, pp. 177–181, 2005.

[16] S. V. Cherian, S. Das, L. Khara, and A. S. Garcha, "Gastric emphysema associated with diabetic gastroparesis," *Internal Medicine*, vol. 50, no. 16, p. 1777, 2011.

[17] N. A. Zenooz, M. R. Robbin, and V. Perez, "Gastric pneumatosis following nasogastric tube placement: a case report with literature review," *Emergency Radiology*, vol. 13, no. 4, pp. 205–207, 2007.

[18] Y. Sakamoto, K. Mashiko, H. Matsumoto, Y. Hara, N. Kutsukata, and Y. Yamamoto, "Gastric pneumatosis and portal venous gas in superior mesenteric artery syndrome," *Indian Journal of Gastroenterology*, vol. 25, no. 5, pp. 265–266, 2006.

[19] J. S. Tuck and L. H. Boobis, "Interstitial emphysema of the stomach due to perforated appendicitis," *Clinical Radiology*, vol. 38, no. 3, pp. 315–317, 1987.

[20] J. E. Lim, G. L. Duke, and S. R. Eachempati, "Superior mesenteric artery syndrome presenting with acute massive gastric dilatation, gastric wall pneumatosis, and portal venous gas," *Surgery*, vol. 134, no. 5, pp. 840–843, 2003.

[21] T. Zander, V. Briner, F. Buck, and R. Winterhalder, "Gastric pneumatosis following polychemotherapy," *European Journal of Internal Medicine*, vol. 18, no. 3, pp. 251–252, 2007.

[22] C. Ilyas, A. L. Young, M. Lewis, A. Suppia, R. Gerotfeke, and E. P. Perry, "Parastomal hernia causing gastric emphysema," *Annals of the Royal College of Surgeons of England*, vol. 94, no. 2, pp. e72–e73, 2012.

[23] J. Chou, Y. Tseng, and C. Tseng, "A rare complication of chemotherapy in a 56-year-old patient," *Gastroenterology*, vol. 139, no. 4, pp. e1–e2, 2010.

[24] Y.-L. Chang, Y.-Y. Lu, C.-C. Huang, and H.-H. Chiu, "Gastrointestinal: gastric emphysema and pneumoperitoneum with spontaneous resolution," *Journal of Gastroenterology and Hepatology*, vol. 26, no. 4, p. 786, 2011.

[25] D. E. Grayson, R. M. Abbott, A. D. Levy, and P. M. Sherman, "Emphysematous infections of the abdomen and pelvis: a pictorial review," *Radiographics*, vol. 22, no. 3, pp. 543–561, 2002.

[26] M. S. Morris, A. C. Gee, S. D. Cho et al., "Management and outcome of pneumatosis intestinalis," *The American Journal of Surgery*, vol. 195, no. 5, pp. 679–682, 2008.

[27] A. J. Greenstein, S. Q. Nguyen, A. Berlin et al., "Pneumatosis intestinalis in adults: Management, surgical indications, and risk factors for mortality," *Journal of Gastrointestinal Surgery*, vol. 11, no. 10, pp. 1268–1274, 2007.

[28] E. Wayne, M. Ough, A. Wu et al., "Management algorithm for pneumatosis intestinalis and portal venous gas: treatment and outcome of 88 consecutive cases," *Journal of Gastrointestinal Surgery*, vol. 14, no. 3, pp. 437–448, 2010.

[29] M. Kalina and M. Rubino, "Recurrent gastric emphysema," *American Surgeon*, vol. 75, no. 11, pp. 1149–1151, 2009.

Treatment of Hepatic Epithelioid Hemangioendothelioma: Finding Uses for Thalidomide in a New Era of Medicine

Matthew P. Soape, Rashmi Verma, J. Drew Payne, Mitchell Wachtel, Fred Hardwicke, and Everardo Cobos

Texas Tech University Health Sciences Center, 3601 4th Street, Lubbock, TX 79430, USA

Correspondence should be addressed to Matthew P. Soape; m.soape@me.com

Academic Editor: Gregory Kouraklis

Hepatic epithelioid hemangioendothelioma (HEH) is extremely rare, occurring in 1 to 2 per 100,000, with chemotherapy options not well defined. Our case involved a 49-year-old female who had hepatic masses and metastasis to the lungs with a liver biopsy revealing HEH. After developing a rash from sorafenib, thalidomide was started with the progression of disease stabilized. Resection is only an option in 10% of the cases; therefore, chemotherapy is the only line of treatment. Newer chemotherapy alternatives are targeting angiogenesis via the vascular endothelial growth factor. Thalidomide was first used as an antiemetic, but, sadly, soon linked to phocomelia birth defects. Given the mechanism of action against angiogenesis, thalidomide has a valid role in vascular tumors. In conclusion, the use of thalidomide as chemotherapy is novel and promising, especially in the setting of a rare vascular liver tumor such as HEH.

1. Introduction

Vascular in origin, hepatic epithelioid hemangioendothelioma (HEH) is an extremely rare diagnosis; therefore, treatment for this malignancy has not been well defined. Much of the data on HEH are in case studies and small case series with treatment usually confined to only a few options. Given the vascular nature of this cancer, thalidomide has been used with some degree of success. In the mid-twentieth century, thalidomide was used for morning sickness in pregnant women, and their babies developed well-documented phocomelia birth defects.

From those horrific malformations, continued investigation into the explanation of thalidomide involvement has led to a better understanding of its harmful effects on angiogenesis. With this discovery, the careful use of the medication has been employed as chemotherapy in cancers such as HEH. In this case report, we present a female diagnosed with metastatic HEH who has been successfully treated with thalidomide chemotherapy.

2. Case Report

We present a 49-year-old Hispanic female originally seen in the ER for atypical chest pain needing cardiac evaluation. Patient presented months back with chest pain that started early the morning of admission, intermittent in nature, worsened with deep inspiration, and radiated to her back. No abdominal pain was noted, but she did complain of associated nausea, diaphoresis, fatigue, and dizziness. She also reported 30-pound weight loss in the last month with no change in appetite discussed. Past medical history was only significant for type 2 diabetes mellitus. Family history was significant for coronary artery disease in her father and stomach cancer in her mother. No pertinent surgical history was given. She denied any tobacco, alcohol, and illicit drug use.

Full cardiac evaluation, including EKG, cardiac marker testing, and chest X-ray, was negative. Upon further review of her chart, 3 years prior to this presentation, a computed tomography (CT) of the abdomen and pelvis was ordered by an urgent care physician secondary to abdominal pain. It showed multiple hypodense masses in the right and left

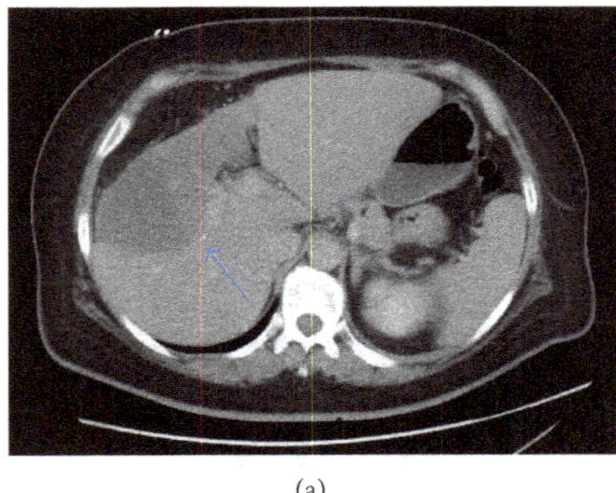

(a)

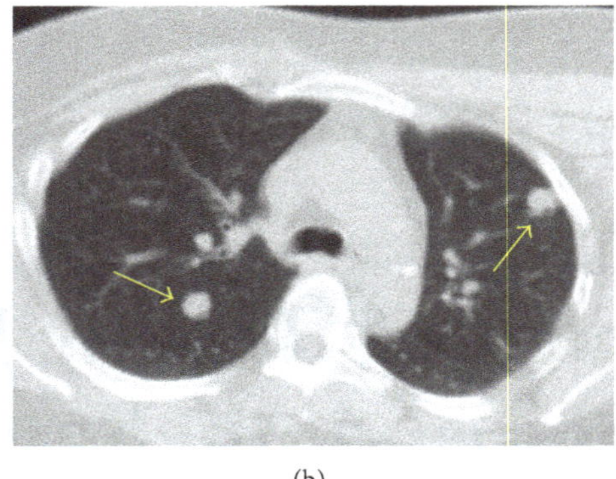

(b)

FIGURE 1: (a) Computed tomography (CT) of the abdomen showing a large hepatic mass, measuring 12 cm × 5.5 cm and designated by the blue arrow. (b) CT of the chest showing metastatic nodules, designated by yellow arrows.

lobe of the liver. The largest one showed a lobulated margin measuring 6.7 cm × 5.5 cm. The masses did not show typical characteristics of hemangioma or simple hepatic cyst. Also noted were fatty liver changes. There was no older study for comparison at that time. A short term repeat CT scan was recommended but she was lost to follow-up. During this admission, CT abdomen with intravenous contrast showed hepatic masses, largest being 12 cm × 5.5 cm, and development of small pulmonary nodules worrisome for metastasis (Figure 1). Small lucencies within the thoracolumbar spine were also found and thought to be focal areas of osteopenia, but metastasis could not be excluded.

Initial gastrointestinal evaluation revealed normal bilirubin, PT, PTT, and INR. Hepatitis B and hepatitis C were both negative. She did exhibit elevated alkaline phosphatase of 311 IU/L and elevated cancer markers, including CEA of 6.0 ng/mL, CA 19-9 of 74.8 units/mL, and CA 125 of 36.3 units/mL. Ultrasound guided liver biopsy was elected at this time and pathology was consistent with HEH (Figure 2). Oncology was then consulted and surgical resection was deferred in the setting of metastatic disease to the lungs. She was started on the oral multikinase inhibitor sorafenib (Nexavar) but soon developed a worsening rash. Thalidomide 200 mg nightly was started in its place with the patient tolerating therapy for the past 10 months. One year after her diagnosis, a repeat CT scan of the abdomen showed increased size of the right and left lobe pulmonary mass lesions, ranging from 4 mm to 7 mm. The largest mass in the liver had also increased to a size of 13.2 cm × 7.1 cm. However, her laboratory values including bilirubin and alkaline phosphatase have been stable; therefore, thalidomide has been continued.

3. Discussion

The term epithelioid hemangioma was coined by Weiss and Enzinger in 1982 to describe a distinct entity, a soft tissue vascular tumor of endothelial origin with a clinical course intermediate between benign hemangioma and malignant angiosarcoma [1]. This malignant hemangioma is extremely rare, occurring in only <1 to 2 per 100,000 patients with a female to male sex ratio of 1.5 to 1 [2]. Presentation is commonly asymptomatic, as in our patient, where she was evaluated for chest pain with no reported abdominal pain. 87% of patients presented with bilobar and multifocal disease, and 37% of patients presented with extrahepatic involvement [3]. Both multifocal and extrahepatic involvements were observed in our patient. HEH is usually a low grade malignant tumor with a slow progression phenotype. HEH, in contrast to many other types of primary liver tumor, does not arise in a background of chronic liver disease. Speculated risk factors include oral contraceptives, vinyl chloride, and hepatitis B infection [4], none of which was admitted by the patient, and hepatitis panel was negative. Histology is characterized as vascular endothelium in origin. Histology shows nests and cords of spindle to epithelioid cells embedded in a hyaline and myxoid stroma with closer examination of cells having prominent cytoplasmic vacuoles with a characteristic signet ring formation [5]. Immunohistochemical stains are positive for endothelial markers such as CD31, CD34, and Factor XIII related antigen [5]. Our case showed positive stains for both CD34 and Factor XIII related antigen.

In regard to treatment, resection is preferable with a 75% 5-year survival rate. However, resection is usually only an option in 10% of the cases [3]. Therefore, chemotherapy is the only available option in most cases. Other procedure treatments for HEH are limited to liver-liver transplant and transcatheter arterial chemoembolization (TACE). As in our case, metastatic disease had already been confirmed with pulmonary involvement, making resection not a viable option. In the past, chemotherapy agents employed have been doxorubicin, vincristine, interferon-alpha, 5-FU, and thalidomide. A newer chemotherapy alternative includes vascular endothelial growth factor (VEGF) targeted therapy. Angiogenesis in malignancy relies on VEGF and fibroblast growth factors (FGFs). Angiogenesis and malignancy association has numerous proposed mechanisms but the most accepted is an overexpression of VEGF [6].

In 1957, thalidomide was first released in West Germany. It was intended as a hypnotic and sedative medication but soon found favor working against nausea in morning sickness during pregnancy. Common side effects include somnolence, edema, hypotension, myelosuppression, peripheral neuritis,

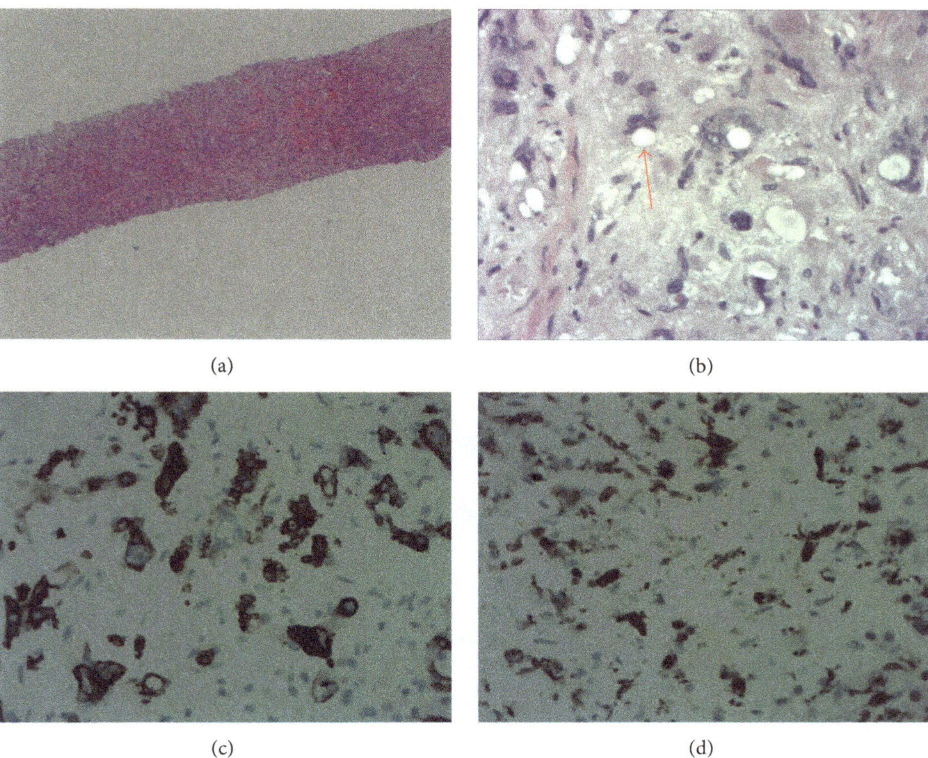

FIGURE 2: (a) Replacing hepatocytes is tumor with sometimes large, often spindled, aberrant nuclei amid abundant light pink, feathery matrixes (H&E, 100x). (b) Uniformly dark, cancerous nuclei, sometimes huge, lie in variably colored cytoplasm, often not evident. Cancer cells lie in isolation and in epithelioid groups. At the arrowhead, a group lies about a vacuole, which is a vascular lumen (H&E, 400x). (c) Cancer cell cytoplasm often expresses CD34, which emphasizes the epithelioid pattern (DAB, 400x). (d) Many cancer cell nuclei, often juxtaposed to vacuoles, express Factor XIIIa (DAB, 400x). Gold bars are 200 μ long.

interstitial lung disease, and pneumonia. Sadly, thalidomide was also discovered to have a high association with birth defects such as phocomelia, a malformation of limbs. The phocomelia was severe with formation of the limbs appearing to be stunted and underdeveloped. 10,000 children were thought to be affected before it was taken off the market. One proposed teratogenic mechanism includes halting of angiogenesis by inhibition of fibroblastic growth factor (bFGF) and/or VEGF, which has been verified with in vivo studies [7]. Cereblon inactivation has also been suggested as a possible mechanism. This protein has a positive regulatory effect via ubiquitination on FGF8 and FGF10. FGF8 has a direct effect on limb formation. As indicated in a 2009 study, limb formation is thought to be highly susceptible due to the limb's "relatively immature, highly angiogenic vessel network" [8]. Thalidomide has been shown to be a well-tolerated medication. Two recent case reports of patients diagnosed with HEH demonstrate thalidomide tolerance factor, controlling the disease progression over an extended amount of time (as long as 109 months) [9, 10].

Other than its effects on vascular growth, thalidomide also inhibits tumor necrosis factor (TNF)-α, various interleukins (IL-6, IL-10, and IL-12) production, and NF-κB and COX-2 activity. It modulates the production of IFN-γ and enhances the production of IL-2, IL-4, and IL-5 by immune cells. It also increases lymphocyte count, costimulates T cells, and modulates natural killer cell cytotoxicity [11]. Due to these regulatory factors, thalidomide has been recently used to treat multiple myeloma and erythema nodosum leprosum. It is also being investigated in therapeutic strategy for vascular malformations and hereditary hemorrhagic telangiectasia [12].

In conclusion, both the diagnosis of HEH and the use of thalidomide in a vascular mediated tumor are extremely rare. Given the mechanism of action against angiogenesis, thalidomide does show some benefit in treatment for such cancers. Furthermore, given the direction of cell receptor and/or growth factor guided chemotherapy, thalidomide may hold promising future derivatives that can better target malignant hepatic hemangiomas and other malignancies.

Consent

Informed consent was obtained from the patient.

Authors' Contribution

Rashmi Verma provided editorial and writing assistance to the paper. Drew Payne provided editorial and writing assistance to the paper. Mitchell Wachtel provided writing assistance to the paper, especially regarding figures. Fred Hardwicke was the attending physician in the case and provided editorial assistance to the paper. Everardo Cobos provided editorial assistance to the paper.

References

[1] S. W. Weiss and F. M. Enzinger, "Epitheloid hemangioendothelioma: a vascular tumor often mistaken for a carcinoma," *Cancer*, vol. 50, no. 5, pp. 970–981, 1982.

[2] B. G. Taal and O. Visser, "Epidemiology of neuroendocrine tumours," *Neuroendocrinology*, vol. 80, no. 1, pp. 3–7, 2004.

[3] A. Mehrabi, A. Kashfi, H. Fonouni et al., "Primary malignant hepatic epithelioid hemangioendothelioma: a comprehensive review of the literature with emphasis on the surgical therapy," *Cancer*, vol. 107, no. 9, pp. 2108–2121, 2006.

[4] E. J. Grossman and J. M. Millis, "Liver transplantation for non-hepatocellular carcinoma malignancy: indications, limitations, and analysis of the current literature," *Liver Transplantation*, vol. 16, no. 8, pp. 930–942, 2010.

[5] H. R. Makhlouf, K. G. Ishak, and Z. D. Goodman, "Epithelioid hemangioendothelioma of the liver: a clinicopathologic study of 137 cases," *Cancer*, vol. 85, no. 3, pp. 562–582, 1999.

[6] F. A. Scappaticci, "Mechanisms and future directions for angiogenesis-based cancer therapies," *Journal of Clinical Oncology*, vol. 20, no. 18, pp. 3906–3927, 2002.

[7] R. J. D'Amato, M. S. Loughnan, E. Flynn, and J. Folkman, "Thalidomide is an inhibitor of angiogenesis," *Proceedings of the National Academy of Sciences of the United States of America*, vol. 91, no. 9, pp. 4082–4085, 1994.

[8] C. Therapontos, L. Erskine, E. R. Gardner, W. D. Figg, and N. Vargesson, "Thalidomide induces limb defects by preventing angiogenic outgrowth during early limb formation," *Proceedings of the National Academy of Sciences of the United States of America*, vol. 106, no. 21, pp. 8573–8578, 2009.

[9] C. Raphael, E. Hudson, L. Williams, J. F. Lester, and P. M. Savage, "Successful treatment of metastatic hepatic epithelioid hemangioendothelioma with thalidomide: a case report," *Journal of Medical Case Reports*, vol. 4, article 413, 2010.

[10] F. Salech, S. Valderrama, B. Nervi et al., "Thalidomide for the treatment of metastatic hepatic epithelioid hemangioendothelioma: a case report with a long term follow-up," *Annals of Hepatology*, vol. 10, no. 1, pp. 99–102, 2011.

[11] S. Singhal and J. Mehta, "Thalidomide in cancer," *Biomedicine & Pharmacotherapy*, vol. 56, no. 1, pp. 4–12, 2002.

[12] F. Lebrin, S. Srun, K. Raymond et al., "Thalidomide stimulates vessel maturation and reduces epistaxis in individuals with hereditary hemorrhagic telangiectasia," *Nature Medicine*, vol. 16, no. 4, pp. 420–428, 2010.

7

Acute Onset Collagenous Colitis with Unique Endoscopic Findings

Rintaro Moroi, Katsuya Endo, Masatake Kuhroha, Hisashi Shiga, Yoichi Kakuta, Yoshitaka Kinouchi, and Tooru Shimosegawa

Division of Gastroenterology, Department of Internal Medicine, Tohoku University Graduate School of Medicine, 1-1 Seiryo, Aoba-ku, Sendai 980-8574, Japan

Correspondence should be addressed to Rintaro Moroi; rinta@med.tohoku.ac.jp

Academic Editor: Özlem Yönem

We experienced a rare case of 72-year-old woman with acute onset collagenous colitis (CC) induced by lansoprazole. The patient developed acute abdominal pain, watery diarrhea, and melena that are quite rare in usual CC. We could find the characteristic colonoscopic findings such as active long liner ulcers in the patient. We also observed the healing courses of these unique findings. Our case indicates two important points of view. (1) CC sometimes develops with acute onset symptoms which resemble those of ischemic colitis. (2) Colonoscopy would be useful and necessary to distinguish acute onset CC and ischemic colitis.

1. Introduction

Microscopic colitis (MC) is a disease characterized by chronic, nonbloody watery diarrhea and few or no endoscopic abnormalities [1]. MC comprises two histological subtypes, collagenous colitis (CC) and lymphocytic colitis (LC). Both diseases are characterized by the presence of an inflammatory infiltrate in the lamina propria but differentiated by having either a thickened collagen band in CC or an increased amount of intraepithelial lymphocytes in LC [2]. It is reported that there are much more LC patients in western countries than in Japan. In Japan, there are few LC patients, and CC is much more common [3]. Particularly, the cases of CC induced by lansoprazole are reported to be increasing in Japan [3–8] in recent years.

In the original description, MC has few or no endoscopic abnormalities [9, 10]. However, in recent years, some unique endoscopic findings have been reported in CC patients mainly by Japanese endoscopists. Several case reports described that mucosal abnormalities such as longitudinal ulcer [3, 4, 8, 11, 12], mucosal tears [13, 14], nodular appearance [15], abnormal vascular patterns [10, 16–18], or edema [18] were recognized in CC patients. These findings could be specific for CC suggesting that the original definition of CC in which there are few or no endoscopic abnormalities has to be changed.

CC is originally described as presenting with chronic diarrhea. Actually, most of the CC patients gradually develop chronic continuing watery diarrhea. In CC patients, acute onset symptoms such as acute abdominal pain and melena are thought to be rare. In recent years, a few acute onset cases have been reported [4, 8, 12]. However, the clinical courses and endoscopic findings of acute onset CC are not well understood because of the small number of the patients.

We experienced a rare case of lansoprazole-induced CC with acutely developed abdominal pain and melena. We could also find the characteristic endoscopic findings in this patient and observe the healing courses of these unique findings. In this report, we described the details of clinical courses and endoscopic findings of the patient and made a literature review.

2. Case Report

A 72-year-old woman started to take lansoprazole for treatment of the firstly diagnosed reflux esophagitis. At about three months after the first administration of lansoprazole,

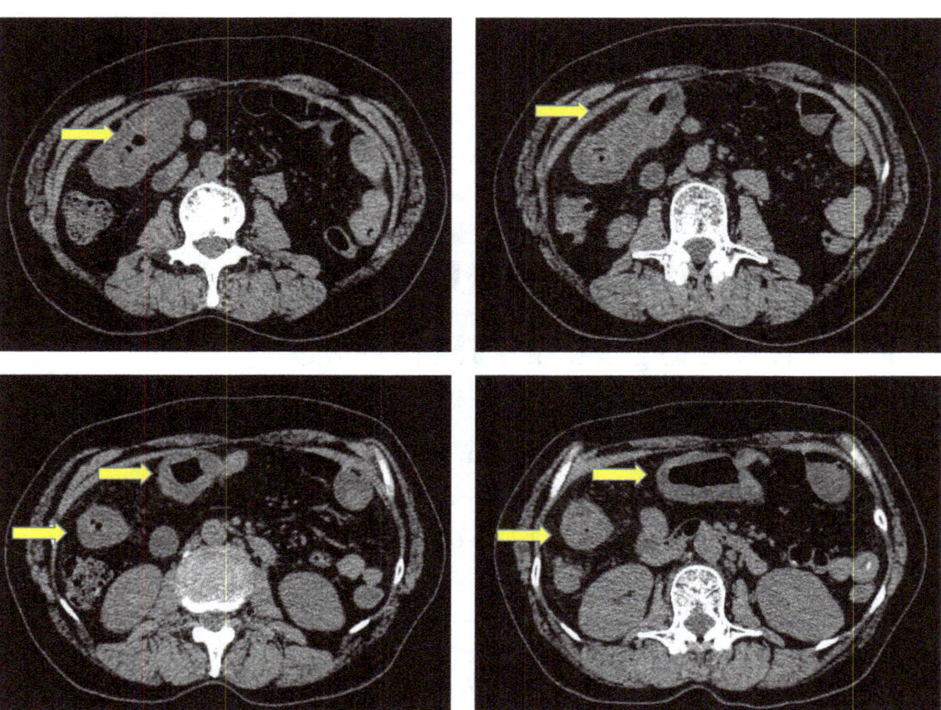

FIGURE 1: Abdominal computed tomography test revealed the slight edema of the ascending to transverse colon.

TABLE 1: Laboratory data on admission.

WBC	7300/μL	AST	22 IU/L	PT	105.1%
Seg	81%	ALT	30 IU/L	APTT	26.6 sec
Eosino	1%	ALP	198 IU/L		
Baso	0%	TP	5.4 g/dL	IgG	378 mg/dL
Lymph	9%	Alb	3.4 g/dL	IgA	153 mg/dL
Mono	9%	BUN	11 mg/dL	IgM	109 mg/dL
RBC	491 × 104/μL	Cr	0.9 mg/dL	IgG4	6.5 mg/dL
Hb	15.8 g/dL	Na	142 mEq/L	IgE	85.2 IU/mL
Ht	45.4%	K	3.7 mEq/L	sIL-2R	177 U/mL
Plt	26.4 × 104/μL	Cl	105 mEq/L	ANA	Negative
		CRP	0.1 mg/dL		

WBC: white blood cell, Seg: segmented neutrophils, Eosino: eosinophils, Baso: basophil, Lymph: lymphocytes, Mono: monocytes, RBC: red blood cells, Hb: hemoglobin, Ht: hematocrit, Plt: platelets, AST: aspartate aminotransferase, ALT: alanine aminotransferase, ALP: alkaline phosphatase, TP: total protein, Alb: albumin, BUN: blood urea nitrogen, Cr: creatinine, Na: sodium, K: potassium, Cl: chloride, CRP: C-reactive protein, PT: prothrombin time, APTT: activated partial thromboplastin time, IgG: immunoglobulin G, IgA: immunoglobulin A, IgM: immunoglobulin M, IgE: immunoglobulin E, IgG4: immunoglobulin G4, sIL-2R: soluble interleukin-2 receptor, and ANA: antinuclear antigen.

she suddenly complained of abdominal pain, watery diarrhea, and hematochezia. Therefore, she was admitted to our hospital urgently. Laboratory data revealed white blood cells were 9900/μL; C-reactive protein was 0.9 mg/mL. Other laboratory data are almost within normal range (Table 1). Abdominal computed tomography test (CT) revealed slight edema of the ascending to transverse colon (Figure 1). Because the bloody stool was observed, we performed urgent colonoscopy in order to detect the origin of bleeding. Colonoscopic findings revealed two liner long ulcers in the transverse colon. Neither edema nor reddening was observed around these ulcers (Figures 2(a) and 2(b)). Because of the pain, we could not insert the endoscope into the cecum and the ascending colon. From the descending colon to the rectum, the appearances of the mucosa were normal, and the pool of watery-bloody stool was observed (Figures 2(c) and 2(d)). Although the endoscopic findings were atypical, ischemic colitis was suspected from the clinical symptoms such as acute onset abdominal pain and hematochezia. The patient was conservatively treated with intravenous fluids and was given nothing by mouth. Abdominal pain and bloody diarrhea disappeared in several days. However, watery diarrhea (7~8 times/day) emerged and continued. We followed up the patient as an outpatient. A second colonoscopy was performed two months after the first colonoscopy. Although the liner ulcers dramatically tended to be healed (Figure 3(a)), mucosal tear occurred when biopsy specimen was taken from the ascending colon (Figure 3(b)). Histological findings of the biopsy specimen revealed the thickened collagen band in the subepithelial layer (Figure 4). Therefore, we diagnosed this patient with CC. We stopped administrating lansoprazole because the drug was considered to cause her CC possibly. After stopping the drug, watery diarrhea gradually disappeared in subsequent three months. A third colonoscopy was performed six months after the second colonoscopy. Liner ulcers were completely healed and

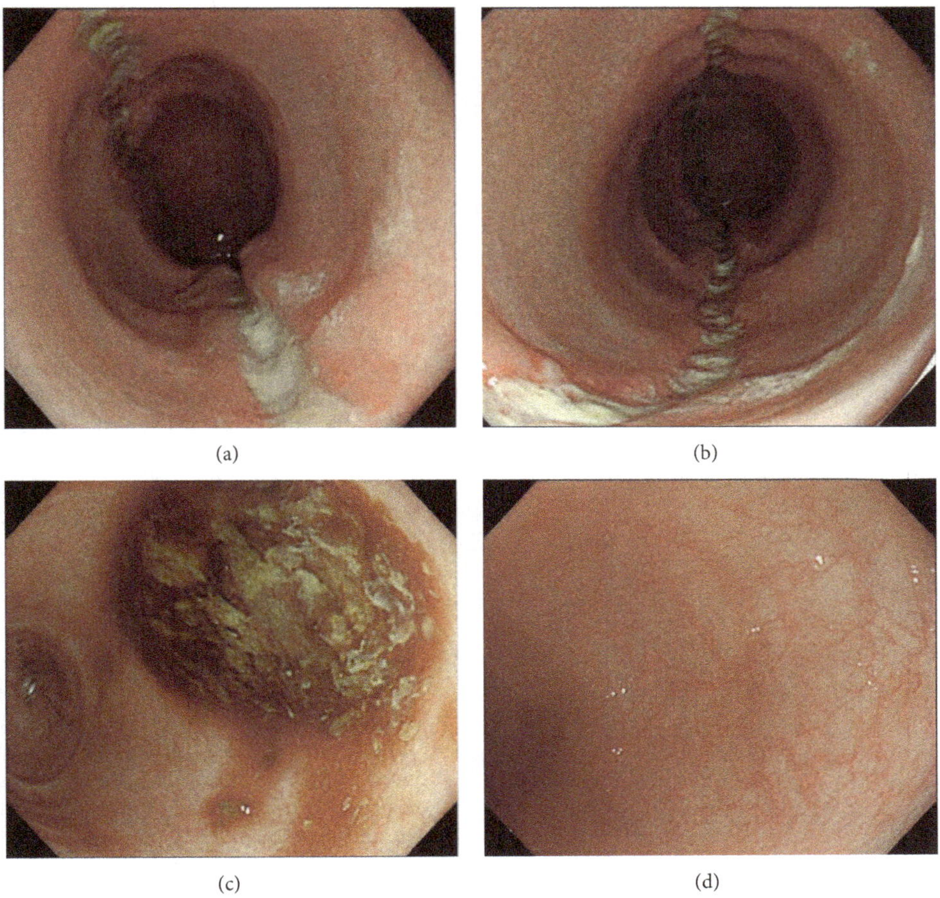

(a) (b) (c) (d)

FIGURE 2: (a, b) Two long linear ulcers were observed in the transverse colon. Neither edema nor reddening was observed around these ulcers. (c, d) From the descending colon to the rectum, the appearances of the mucosa were normal, and the pool of watery-bloody stool was observed.

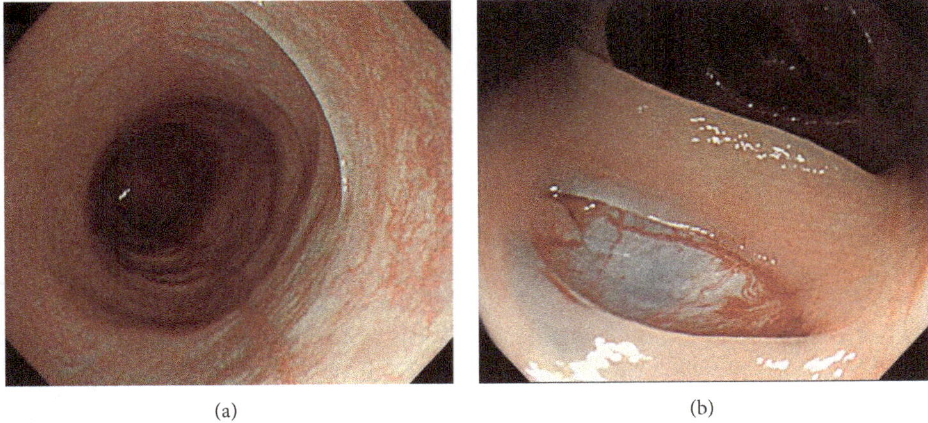

(a) (b)

FIGURE 3: (a) A second colonoscopy was performed two months after the first colonoscopy. The liner ulcers dramatically tended to be healed. (b) Mucosal tear occurred when biopsy specimen was taken from the ascending colon.

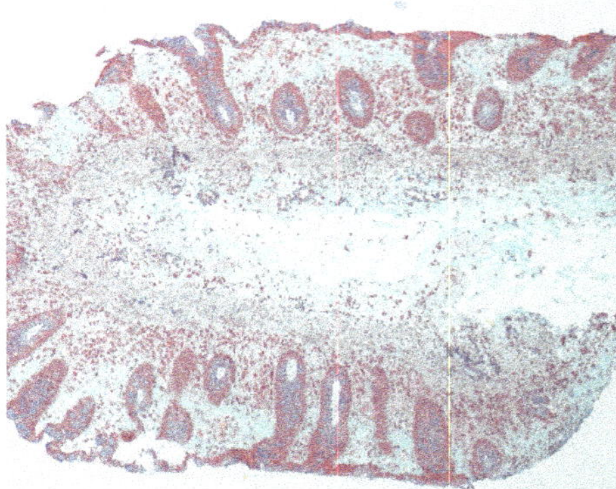

Figure 4: Histological findings of the biopsy specimen revealed the thickened collagen band in the subepithelial layer (Masson trichrome ×100).

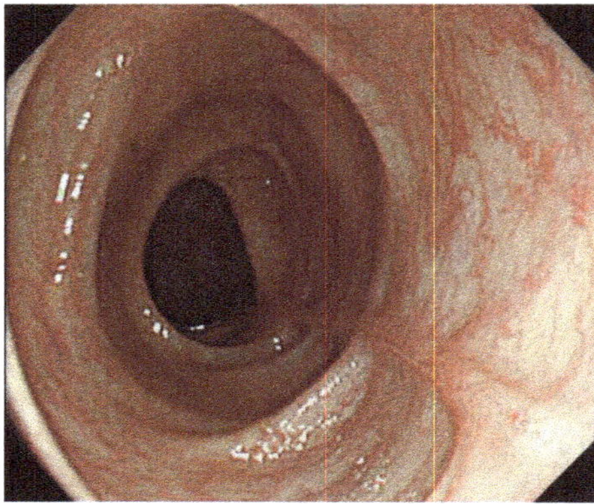

Figure 5: The colonoscopy performed 6 months after stopping lansoprazole showed that liner ulcers were completely healed and became scarred.

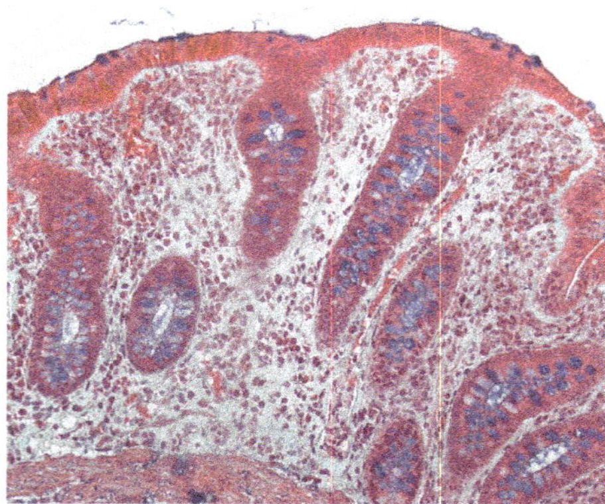

Figure 6: Disappearance of collagen band was confirmed from the histological findings of the ascending colon biopsy specimen (Masson trichrome ×400).

became scarred (Figure 5). Disappearance of collagen band was also confirmed from the histological findings of the biopsy specimen (Figure 6). Therefore, we concluded her CC was completely healed only by stopping the administration of lansoprazole.

3. Discussion

CC is a distinct clinicopathologic entity characterized by chronic watery diarrhea and the subepithelial deposition of collagen band [19]. The disease usually develops gradually with chronic watery diarrhea. Mechanisms of chronic diarrhea in CC have been considered as follows: (1) reduced net absorption of sodium and chloride, (2) some component of active secretion of chloride, and (3) barrier of water reabsorption due to collagen band [20]. In CC patients, acute onset symptoms such as abdominal pain or melena are quite rare. According to the database searches, only 3 cases with acute symptoms have been reported [4, 8, 12] (Table 2). In these 3 cases, acutely developed abdominal pain was observed in all cases, and bloody stool was observed in 2 of 3 cases. All 3 cases had longitudinal ulcer on endoscopic findings. Our case was also a very rare case of CC complaining of acute onset abdominal pain, watery diarrhea, and hematochezia. The present case had unique endoscopic findings which are similar to those in the previous reports. Thus the acute onset CC seems to have common clinical characteristics and endoscopic findings. Here, we have to recognize that clinical symptoms of acute onset CC resemble those of ischemic colitis. When a patient complains of acute abdominal pain with bloody stool, CC should be considered in the differential diagnosis of ischemic colitis. It is important to perform colonoscopy because it could be difficult to distinguish CC from ischemic colitis only by the clinical symptoms.

Endoscopic findings of collagenous colitis are generally thought as no or minimal abnormalities. However, some recent reports have revealed that mucosal abnormalities, such as longitudinal ulcer [3, 4, 8, 11, 12], mucosal tears [13, 14], nodularity, abnormal vascular pattern [10, 16–18], or edema [18], were characteristic endoscopic findings of CC. As for the endoscopic findings of acute onset cases, hemorrhagic, sharply demarcated-longitudinal ulcers were observed [4, 8, 12]. The endoscopic findings of our case also showed active long liner ulcers similar to those of previous reports. In our case, the mucosal tear was also observed when taking the biopsy specimen. Several previous reports assumed that subepithelial collagen deposits cause the mucosal stiffness and friability [13, 21]. The liner ulcers and mucosal tears in our case could possibly be induced by the mucosal fragility caused by the depositions of collagen band. We hypothesized that mucosal stiffness and friability split the membrane sharply in acute phase which led to the acute abdominal pain and hematochezia. According to the previous reports and the experience of our case, active liner longitudinal ulcer would be a specific feature in acute onset CC. Here, we have to focus on the differences between CC and ischemic colitis in endoscopic findings. As previously described, the longitudinal ulcer of acute onset CC resembles that of ischemic colitis. The shortcoming with this case report is that we did not take a biopsy specimen at the first time endoscopy. However, the differences can be observed between two diseases. In common, ischemic colitis presents the longitudinal ulcers accompanied by circumferential mucosal edema [22]. On the other hand, acute onset CC presents sharply demarcated long liner ulcers without any edema or redness. Therefore, it can

TABLE 2: The list of case reports developing with acute abdomen.

Case number	Year	Symptoms	Colonoscopic findings	Cause (duration)	Treatment	Treatment responses
1	Yusuke et al., 2009 [4]	Abdominal pain, hematochezia, diarrhea	Liner ulcers (S/C)	LPZ induced (2 months)	Stopping LPZ	Good
2	Kitagawa et al., 2013 [8]	Abdominal pain, hematochezia	Liner ulcers (D/C, S/C)	LPZ induced (unknown)	Stopping LPZ	Good
3	Takanashi et al., 2010 [12]	Abdominal pain, diarrhea, vomit	Liner ulcers (T/C-S/C)	LPZ induced (1 month)	Stopping LPZ	Good
4	Our case	Abdominal pain, hematochezia, diarrhea	Liner ulcers (T/C)	LPZ induced (3 months)	Stopping LPZ	Good

be possible to distinguish two diseases from these endoscopic findings. We think endoscopic examination might be not only useful, but also necessary to differentiate acute onset CC from ischemic colitis.

In conclusion, we experienced a rare case of lansoprazole-induced collagenous colitis with acutely developed abdominal pain and melena. We could also find the characteristic endoscopic findings in the patient and observe the healing courses of these unique findings. Our case indicates two important points of view. (1) CC sometimes develops with acute onset symptoms such as acute abdominal pain and melena which resemble those of ischemic colitis. (2) Acute onset CC could have characteristic active liner ulcers in the colon. Therefore, colonoscopy would be useful and necessary to distinguish acute onset CC and ischemic colitis.

Although our case and previous reports figured out the characteristics of acute onset CC, additional cases should be needed to understand the disease in detail.

References

[1] A. Münch, D. Aust, J. Bohr et al., "Microscopic colitis: Current status, present and future challenges: statements of the European Microscopic Colitis Group," *Journal of Crohn's and Colitis*, vol. 6, no. 9, pp. 932–945, 2012.

[2] M. A. Rasmussen and L. K. Munck, "Systematic review: are lymphocytic colitis and collagenous colitis two subtypes of the same disease—microscopic colitis?" *Alimentary Pharmacology and Therapeutics*, vol. 36, no. 2, pp. 79–90, 2012.

[3] J. Umeno, T. Matsumoto, S. Nakamura et al., "Linear mucosal defect may be characteristic of lansoprazole-associated collagenous colitis," *Gastrointestinal Endoscopy*, vol. 67, no. 7, pp. 1185–1191, 2008.

[4] H. Yusuke, T. Jun, M. Naotaka, T. Yuichi, E. Yutaka, and I. Kazuaki, "Lansoprazole-associated collagenous colitis: unique presentation, similar to ischemic colitis," *Endoscopy*, vol. 41, supplement 2, pp. E281–E282, 2009.

[5] Y. Sasatomi, M. Takahata, Y. Abe et al., "Case of suspicious lansoprazole-associated collagenous colitis in ANCA-associated nephritis," *The Japanese Journal of Nephrology*, vol. 52, no. 2, pp. 141–146, 2010.

[6] T. Ozeki, N. Ogasawara, S. Izawa et al., "Protein-losing enteropathy associated with collagenous colitis cured by withdrawal of a proton pump inhibitor," *Internal Medicine*, vol. 52, no. 11, pp. 1183–1187, 2013.

[7] S. Saito, T. Tsumura, H. Nishikawa et al., "Clinical characteristics of collagenous colitis with linear ulcerations," *Digestive Endoscopy*, vol. 26, no. 1, pp. 69–76, 2014.

[8] T. Kitagawa, K. Sato, Y. Yokouchi, K. Tominaga, S. Ito, and I. Maetani, "A case of Lansoprazole-associated collagenous colitis with longitudinal ulcer," *Journal of Gastrointestinal and Liver Diseases*, vol. 22, no. 1, article 9, 2013.

[9] J. Bohr, C. Tysk, S. Eriksson, H. Abrahamsson, and G. Järnerot, "Collagenous colitis: a retrospective study of clinical presentation and treatment in 163 patients," *Gut*, vol. 39, no. 6, pp. 846–851, 1996.

[10] P. Katsinelos, I. Katsos, K. Patsiaoura, P. Xiarchos, I. Goulis, and N. Eugenidis, "A new endoscopic appearance of collagenous colitis," *Endoscopy*, vol. 29, no. 2, p. 135, 1997.

[11] E. Nomura, H. Kagaya, K. Uchimi et al., "Linear mucosal defects: a characteristic endoscopic finding of lansoprazole-associated collagenous colitis," *Endoscopy*, vol. 42, supplement 2, pp. E9–E10, 2010.

[12] K. Takanashi, S. Minami, N. Miyajima et al., "A case of collagenous colitis appearing acute abdomen due to colonic longitudinal ulcers," *Gastroenterological Endoscopy*, vol. 52, no. 11, pp. 3133–3139, 2010 (Japanese).

[13] M. Cruz-Correa, F. Milligan, F. M. Giardiello et al., "Collagenous colitis with mucosal tears on endoscopic insufflation: a unique presentation," *Gut*, vol. 51, no. 4, p. 600, 2002.

[14] R. R. Smith and A. Ragput, "Mucosal tears on endoscopic insufflation resulting in perforation: an interesting presentation of collagenous colitis," *Journal of the American College of Surgeons*, vol. 205, no. 5, p. 725, 2007.

[15] A. Saleem, P. A. Brahmbhatt, S. Khan, M. Young, and G. D. LeSage, "Microscopic colitis with macroscopic endoscopic findings," *Case Reports in Medicine*, vol. 2013, Article ID 461485, 2 pages, 2013.

[16] S. Kakar, D. S. Pardi, and L. J. Burgart, "Colonic ulcers accompanying collagenous colitis: implication of nonsteroidal anti-inflammatory drugs," *The American Journal of Gastroenterology*, vol. 98, no. 8, pp. 1834–1837, 2003.

[17] J.-P. Richieri, H.-P. Bonneau, N. Cano, J. Di Costanzo, and J. Martin, "Collagenous colitis: an unusual endoscopic appearance," *Gastrointestinal Endoscopy*, vol. 39, no. 2, pp. 192–194, 1993.

[18] A. Katanuma, T. Kodama, T. Tamaki et al., "Collagenous colitis," *Internal Medicine*, vol. 34, no. 3, pp. 195–198, 1995.

[19] C. G. Lindstrom, "'Collagenous colitis' with watery diarrhoea—a new entity?" *Pathologia Europaea*, vol. 11, no. 1, pp. 87–89, 1976.

[20] N. Bürgel, C. Bojarski, J. Mankertz, M. Zeitz, M. Fromm, and J. Schulzke, "Mechanisms of diarrhea in collagenous colitis," *Gastroenterology*, vol. 123, no. 2, pp. 433–443, 2002.

[21] A. Sherman, J. J. Ackert, R. Rajapaksa, A. B. West, and T. Oweity, ""Fractured Colon": an endoscopically distinctive lesion associated with colonic perforation following colonoscopy in patients with collagenous colitis," *Journal of Clinical Gastroenterology*, vol. 38, no. 4, pp. 341–345, 2004.

[22] C. W. Scowcroft, R. A. Sanowski, and R. A. Kozarek, "Colonoscopy in ischemic colitis," *Gastrointestinal Endoscopy*, vol. 27, no. 3, pp. 156–161, 1981.

8

Concurrent Esophageal Dysplasia and Leiomyoma

Asim Shuja[1] and Khalid A. Alkimawi[2]

[1] *Department of Medicine, St. Elizabeth's Medical Center, Brighton, MA 02135, USA*
[2] *Department Gastroenterology, Tufts Medical Center, 800 Washington Street Boston, MA 02111, USA*

Correspondence should be addressed to Khalid A. Alkimawi; kalkimawi@tuftsmedicalcenter.org

Academic Editor: Yoshiro Kawahara

Esophageal leiomyomas (ELMs) are rare but described in the literature. They are usually benign and do not require resection unless they are large and symptomatic. Most of such masses arise from the muscularis mucosa. It is very uncommon to find epithelial dysplasia overlying a subepithelial leiomyoma. A review of the literature reveals only one prior case of ELM with an overlying epithelia dysplasia and here we report a second case.

1. Introduction

Leiomyoma (LM) is the most common benign esophageal tumor [1]. It is usually small, asymptomatic, and slow growing. Studies like esophagogastroduodenoscopy (EGD), barium swallow, computed tomography (CT) of the chest, and endoscopic ultrasound (EUS) may aid in diagnosis. Biopsies should not be obtained if LMs are covered by endoscopically normal mucosa, as this may interfere with surgical removal as well as the fact that they have negligible malignant transformation. Surgery is indicated if lesions are large and symptomatic in the form of dysphagia. These tumors are positive for desmin and smooth muscle actin (SMA) stains [2]. It is important to differentiate LM from esophageal gastrointestinal stromal tumor (GIST) because of higher malignancy potential of the latter. LM with overlying squamous cell carcinoma has been reported, but a subepithelial lesion (i.e., LM) with epithelial dysplasia is extremely rare. From our literature review, we report a second case of such kind [3].

2. Case Report

A 72-year-old male with history of GERD and Barrett's esophagus presented with an incidental finding of a subepithelial nodule in the gastroesophageal (GE) junction, found on surveillance EGD (Figures 1(a) and 1(b)). GE junction biopsy revealed intramucosal adenocarcinoma and high grade dysplasia, without lymphangioplastic invasion. An endoscopic mucosal resection (EMR) was done and successful ablation of the Barrett's mucosa was performed using multipolar electrocoagulation. The subsequent endoscopy showed normal mucosa and biopsies were negative for any pathology (Figures 2(a) and 2(b)). Three months later, a repeated EGD showed reappearance of a small nodule at the GE junction at the site of previous EMR (Figure 3(a)). This time, the mucosal biopsy was positive for intestinal metaplasia and severe high grade dysplasia. EUS was performed in order to determine the depth and nature of the nodule. It showed an 11.0 mm × 5.0 mm oval, homogenous, hypoechoic mass arising from the mucosa (Figure 3(b)). Fine-needle aspiration biopsy was negative for malignancy. Repeated EMR was performed only for the nodule to recur after few months again, with histological examination of GE junction again revealing high grade dysplasia and adenocarcinoma *in situ* (Figures 4(a) and 4(b)). Histopathology of the esophageal nodule showed superficial fragments of dysplastic mucosa, with spindle cells and no mitotic activity (Figures 5(a), 5(b), and 5(c)). Immunohistochemical analysis revealed cells negative for CD117 (C-Kit) and positive for desmin and SMA (Figures 6(a), 6(b), and 6(c)). A diagnosis of severe dysplasia overlying a small LM from the muscularis mucosa was made. An endoscopic *en bloc* resection was done for removal of the lesion (Figures 7(a) and 7(b)). No procedural complications were observed.

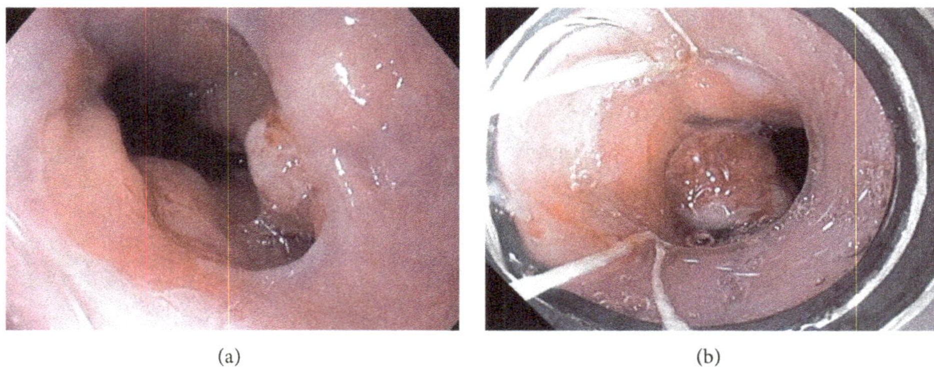

(a) (b)

Figure 1: (a) Esophagus: a tongue of Barrett's was found in the distal third of the esophagus. (b): A nodule was found in the GE junction. A mucosal resection (using a Duette EMR kit) was performed, with success.

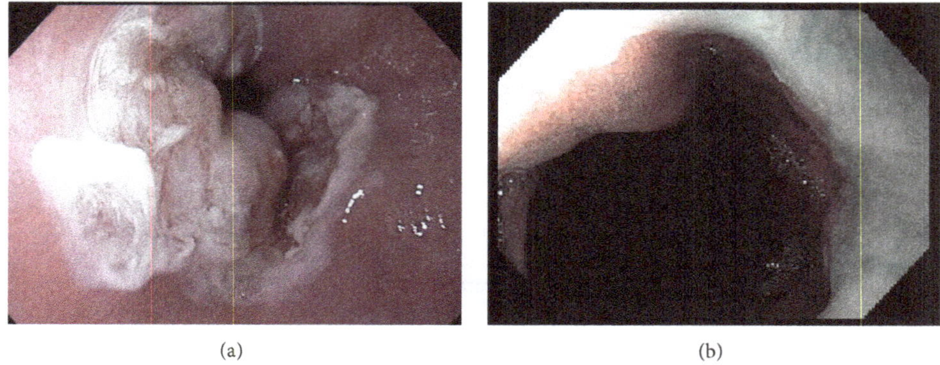

(a) (b)

Figure 2: (a) Scar was found in the area of previous mucosal resection. Ablation of Barrett's mucosa was performed with multipolar electrocoagulation with success. (b) A tongue of columnar appearing mucosa was found in the esophagus spanning 1 cm: no residual columnar appearing mucosa.

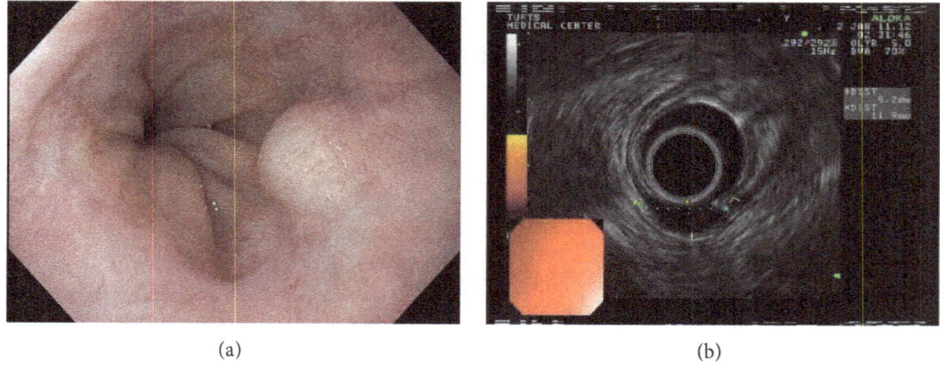

(a) (b)

Figure 3: (a) Reappearance of submucosal nodule at the GE junction. (b) EUS: 11 mm × 5 mm nodule arising from the mucosa.

3. Discussion

ELM was first well described by von Rahden et al. in 2004 [1]. Although it is the most common benign intramural tumor of the esophagus, it is still very rare, with an incidence of 0.006 to 0.1% on autopsy series data [2]. It is 50 times less common than esophageal carcinoma [4]. ELMs account for approximately 12% of all GI leiomyomas [5]. It is typically found in the 20–60-year-age group with male preponderance (M 2 : 1 F) [6]. Lower third of the esophagus (50%) is the most common site of involvement, followed by the middle third (40%) and upper third (10%), which is consistent with the normal anatomical distribution of smooth muscle within the esophageal wall [7]. The size of the LMs can range from less than 0.5 cm (microleiomyomas) to as large as 30 cm. These tumors rarely cause symptoms when they are smaller than 5 cm in diameter. Large tumors can cause dysphagia, vague retrosternal discomfort, and so forth [2]. In extreme

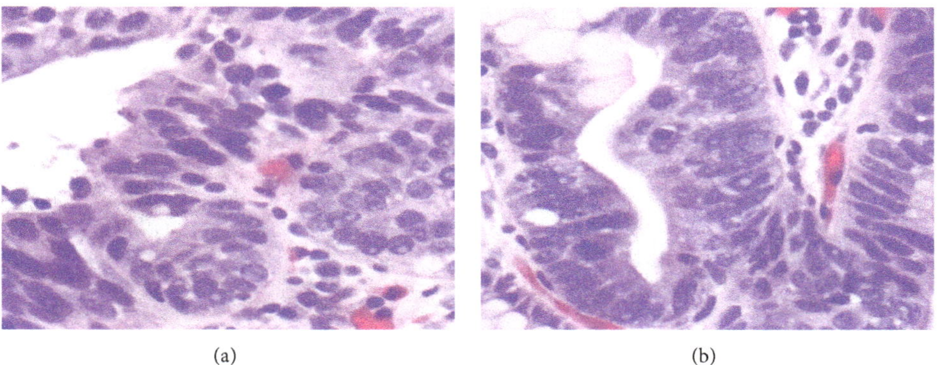

(a) (b)

Figure 4: (a) GE junction mucosa with focal intestinal metaplasia and extensive high grade dysplasia/adenocarcinoma *in situ*. (b) High grade dysplasia extends to one margin and detached fragments of high grade dysplasia are also present.

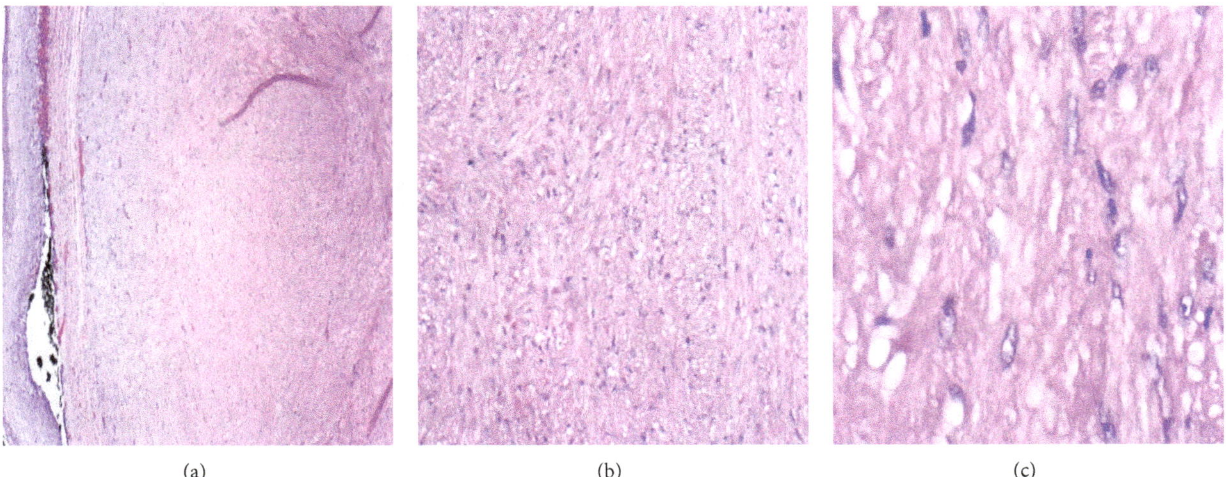

(a) (b) (c)

Figure 5: (a) Esophageal LM arising from muscularis mucosa. (b, c) ELM is composed of intersecting bland spindle cells with no mitosis or nuclear atypia.

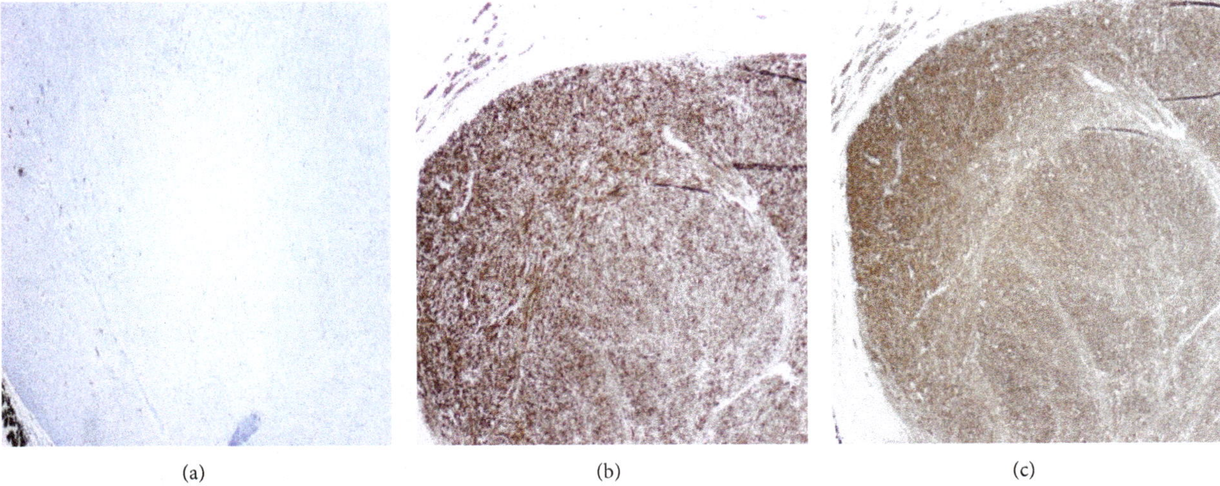

(a) (b) (c)

Figure 6: (a) ELM negative for CD117 (C-Kit). (b, c) LM diffusely and strongly positive for desmin and SMA stain, respectively.

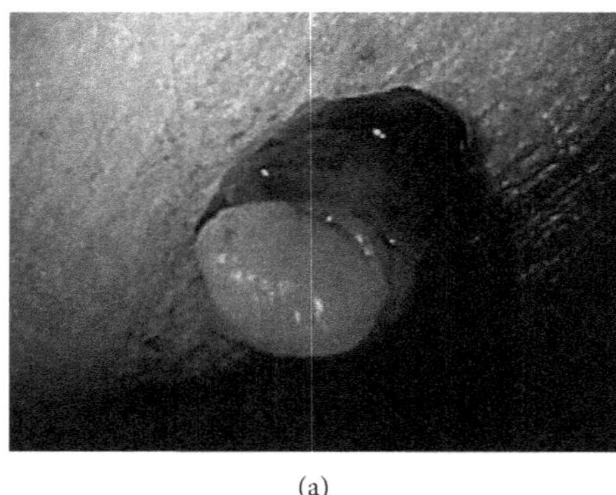

(a)

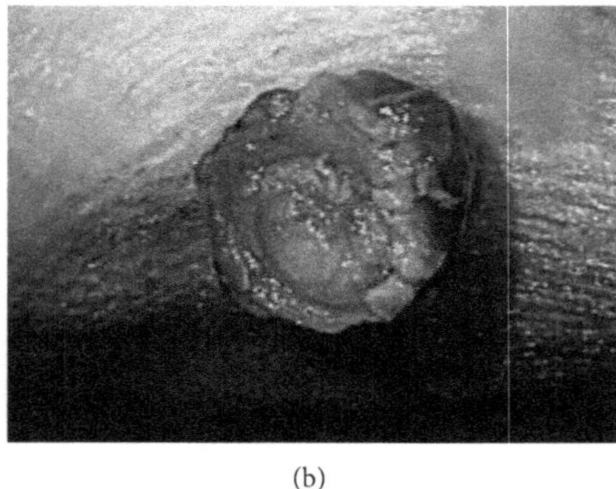

(b)

FIGURE 7: (a, b) 8 mm firm nodule in the distal third/GE junction. It was removed via endoscopic mucosal resection.

cases where severe esophageal obstruction is caused by a LM, weight loss and muscle wasting may be observed [8].

EGD, EUS, CT of chest, and so forth may aid in diagnosis. On endoscopy, LM is identified as a submucosal, freely movable mass with intact mucosa [9]. EUS finding of leiomyoma, homogenous, and hypoechoic mass is the key for differentiating leiomyoma from invasive cancer [10]. LMs may occur in the muscularis propria layer but is most common in the muscularis mucosa of the esophagus [11]. If a LM is suspected and the overlying mucosa is normal, biopsy should be avoided, for it is likely to be nondiagnostic and may increase intraoperative complications [12]. Microscopically, they have low cellularity and are composed of interlacing fascicles of bland spindle-shaped smooth muscle cells. There is minimal nuclear atypia and no rare mitotic activity seen. The characteristic morphology makes the histological diagnosis of esophageal LM relatively easy, and usually no immunohistologic studies (IHS) are required. However, in cases where there is moderate cellularity with some nuclear atypia, other tumors such as GIST and schwannoma are included in the differential diagnosis. IHS for SMA and desmin show positive staining in LM and they are negative for CD117 (C-Kit), CD34, or S100. Although GIST of the esophagus is even rarer, it is important to differentiate it from LM, because esophageal GIST is a more aggressive tumor [11]. In contrast to LM, GISTs are positive for CD117 and CD34 [12–14]. Malignant transformation is extremely rare. In review of 800 cases in the world literature, only two (0.2%) cases were documented to show malignant transformation [2].

Treatment for ELMs depends on multiple factors, including tumor size, location, appearance, and the patient's symptoms and overall conditions [15, 16]. Asymptomatic patients can be monitored by endoscopy and radiology [17]. The indications for surgical treatment include unremitting symptoms, progressive increase in tumor size, mucosal ulceration, the need to obtain histological diagnosis, and facilitation of other esophageal procedures [11]. Recurrence of the ELM is extremely rare [18].

The coexistence of an epithelial lesion and a subepithelial lesion is rare. To our knowledge, twelve patients in ten case reports with carcinoma located in the mucosa overlying a benign tumor have been reported [19–21]. All of these cases were squamous cell carcinoma. However, from our experience, this is the second case of epithelial dysplasia overlying a LM in the esophagus. It is difficult to understand whether these dysplastic changes were related to his underlying LM or they were a precursor to his Barrett's. Nodule was removed via EMR, and surveillance EGD performed 6 months later did not show recurrence of the mesenchymal tumor nor showed any dysplastic changes in the mucosa. We speculate that the coincidence of LM and epithelial dysplasia is a very rare finding which needs proper surveillance.

4. Conclusions

In conclusion, leiomyomas of the esophagus can rarely be found underneath a severely dysplastic mucosa. Endoscopic removal is a suitable option for lesions arising from muscularis mucosa, if detected early.

Authors' Contribution

Asim Shuja reviewed, designed, edited, and organized the report; Khalid A. Alkimawi edited the report and served as the fellow/clinical instructor for the patient.

References

[1] B. H. A. von Rahden, H. J. Stein, H. Feussner, and J. R. Siewert, "Enucleation of submucosal tumors of the esophagus: minimally invasive versus open approach," *Surgical Endoscopy and Other Interventional Techniques*, vol. 18, no. 6, pp. 924–930, 2004.

[2] C. J. Mutrie, D. M. Donahue, J. C. Wain et al., "Esophageal leiomyoma: a 40-year experience," *Annals of Thoracic Surgery*, vol. 79, no. 4, pp. 1122–1125, 2005.

[3] S. Y. Ahn and S. W. Jeon, "Endoscopic resection of co-existing severe dysplasia and a small esophageal leiomyoma," *World Journal of Gastroenterology*, vol. 19, no. 1, pp. 137–140, 2013.

[4] T. Arnorsson, C. Aberg, and T. Aberg, "Benign tumours of the oesophagus and oesophageal cysts," *Scandinavian Journal of Thoracic and Cardiovascular Surgery*, vol. 18, no. 2, pp. 145–150, 1984.

[5] C. K. Choong and B. F. Meyers, "Benign esophageal tumors: introduction, incidence, classification, and clinical features," *Seminars in Thoracic and Cardiovascular Surgery*, vol. 15, no. 1, pp. 3–8, 2003.

[6] T. Kabuto, K. Taniguchi, T. Iwanaga, T. Terasawa, R. Tateishi, and H. Taniguchi, "Diffuse leiomyomatosis of the esophagus," *Digestive Diseases and Sciences*, vol. 25, no. 5, pp. 388–391, 1980.

[7] A. Punpale, A. Rangole, N. Bhambhani et al., "Leiomyoma of esophagus," *Annals of Thoracic and Cardiovascular Surgery*, vol. 13, no. 2, pp. 78–81, 2007.

[8] E. A. Rendina, F. Venuta, E. O. Pescarmona et al., "Leiomyoma of the esophagus," *Scandinavian Journal of Thoracic and Cardiovascular Surgery*, vol. 24, no. 1, pp. 79–82, 1990.

[9] Y. Wang, R. Zhang, Z. Ouyang, D. Zhang, L. Wang, and D. Zhang, "Diagnosis and surgical treatment of esophageal leiomyoma," *Chinese Journal of Oncology*, vol. 24, no. 4, pp. 394–396, 2002.

[10] T. W. Rice, "Benign esophageal tumors: esophagoscopy and endoscopic esophageal ultrasound," *Seminars in Thoracic and Cardiovascular Surgery*, vol. 15, no. 1, pp. 20–26, 2003.

[11] W. Jiang, T. W. Rice, and J. R. Goldblum, "Esophageal leiomyoma: experience from a single institution," *Diseases of the Esophagus*, vol. 26, no. 2, pp. 167–174, 2013.

[12] L. S. Lee, S. Singhal, C. J. Brinster et al., "Current management of esophageal leiomyoma," *Journal of the American College of Surgeons*, vol. 198, no. 1, pp. 136–146, 2004.

[13] S. Suster, "Gastrointestinal stromal tumors," *Seminars in Diagnostic Pathology*, vol. 13, no. 4, pp. 297–313, 1996.

[14] I. Pidhorecky, R. T. Cheney, W. G. Kraybill, and J. F. Gibbs, "Gastrointestinal stromal tumors: current diagnosis, biologic behavior, and management," *Annals of Surgical Oncology*, vol. 7, no. 9, pp. 705–712, 2000.

[15] G. F. Hatch III, L. Wertheimer-Hatch, K. F. Hatch et al., "Tumors of the esophagus," *World Journal of Surgery*, vol. 24, no. 4, pp. 401–411, 2000.

[16] E. Rijcken, C. M. Kersting, N. Senninger, and M. Bruewer, "Esophageal resection for giant leiomyoma: report of two cases and a review of the literature," *Langenbeck's Archives of Surgery*, vol. 394, no. 4, pp. 623–629, 2009.

[17] I. Glanz and M. Grunebaum, "The radiological approach to leiomyoma of the oesophagus with a long term follow up," *Clinical Radiology*, vol. 28, no. 2, pp. 197–200, 1977.

[18] R. J. Standerfer and M. Paneth, "Recurrent leiomyoma of the oesophagus," *Thorax*, vol. 37, no. 6, pp. 478–479, 1982.

[19] H. Kuwano, N. Sadanaga, M. Watanabe, M. Yasuda, T. Nozoe, and K. Sugimachi, "Esophageal squamous cell carcinoma occurring in the surface epithelium over a benign tumor," *Journal of Surgical Oncology*, vol. 59, no. 4, pp. 268–272, 1995.

[20] T. Iizuka, H. Kato, H. Watanabe, M. Itabashi, and T. Hirota, "Superficial carcinoma of the esophagus coexisting with esophageal leiomyoma: a case report and review of the Japanese literature," *Japanese Journal of Clinical Oncology*, vol. 14, no. 1, pp. 115–122, 1984.

[21] R. Ishihara, S. Yamamoto, S. Yamamoto et al., "Endoscopic resection of the esophageal squamous cell carcinoma overlying leiomyoma," *Gastrointestinal Endoscopy*, vol. 67, no. 4, pp. 745–747, 2008.

Tumor Necrosis Factor Alpha Inhibition for Inflammatory Bowel Disease after Liver Transplant for Primary Sclerosing Cholangitis

Ravish Parekh,[1] **Ahmed Abdulhamid**,[1] **Sheri Trudeau**,[2] **and Nirmal Kaur**[1]

[1]*Department of Gastroenterology and Hepatology, Henry Ford Health System, Detroit, MI, USA*
[2]*Department of Public Health Sciences, Henry Ford Health System, Detroit, MI, USA*

Correspondence should be addressed to Nirmal Kaur; nkaur1@hfhs.org

Academic Editor: Warwick S. Selby

Background. Outcome data regarding the use of tumor necrosis factor alpha inhibitors (anti-TNFα) in patients with inflammatory bowel disease (IBD) after liver transplant (LT) for primary sclerosing cholangitis (PSC) are scant. *Methods.* We performed a retrospective chart review to investigate outcomes among a series of post-liver-transplant PSC/IBD patients receiving anti-TNFα therapy at Henry Ford Health System ((HFHS), Detroit, MI). *Results.* A total of five patients were treated with anti-TNFα agents for IBD after LT for PSC from 1993 through 2015. Two patients were treated with adalimumab, and three were treated with infliximab. Three patients were hospitalized with severe posttransplant infections. Two patients developed posttransplant lymphoproliferative disease (PTLD); one of these patients died due to complications of PTLD. *Conclusion.* Anti-TNFα treatment following LT worsened the disease course in our patients with concurrent PSC/IBD and led to serious complications and surgical intervention. Larger studies are needed to evaluate the side effects and outcomes of the use of such agents in this patient population. Until then, clinicians should have a high threshold to use anti-TNFα therapy in this setting.

1. Introduction

The co-occurrence of inflammatory bowel disease (IBD) and primary sclerosing cholangitis (PSC) is a well-documented phenomenon. Although there are no epidemiological studies regarding the prevalence of concurrent PSC/IBD, as many as 90% of patients with PSC may have underlying IBD [1, 2]. No medical therapy has yet been proven to affect the natural progression of PSC and therefore, liver transplant (LT) remains the mainstay of therapy for patients with advanced cirrhosis secondary to the disease; without transplant, the mean survival of patients with PSC is 10–12 years [3–5]. Compared to patients with IBD alone, patients with cooccurring PSC/IBD generally present with a different clinical course, mainly characterized by a high prevalence of pancolitis with rectal sparing and backwash ileitis [6].

In recent years, multiple agents have been approved for the treatment of IBD. However, tumor necrosis factor alpha inhibitors (anti-TNFα) remain widely used, given their widespread demonstrated efficacy in moderate, severe, and refractory IBD [7, 8]. However, the risks and benefits of these agents in PSC/IBD patients after liver transplant are yet to be determined. We examined the clinical course of PSC/IBD patients receiving liver transplants and treated with anti-TNFα agents.

2. Methods

This study was approved by the HFHS Institutional Review Board; requirements for written informed consent were waived due to the deidentified nature of the study. A retrospective chart review of our patient database was performed, using International Classification of Diseases, version 9 (ICD-9) codes related to Crohn's disease (555.0, 555.1, 555.9), ulcerative colitis (556.9), PSC (576.1), and LT (V42.7). Using this method, we identified five patients with concurrent PSC/IBD who underwent liver transplantation and also received anti-TNFα therapy at HFHS between 1993 and 2015. Three trained gastroenterologists (RP, AAH, and NK) performed retrospective chart review for data including demographic data (sex, age, and race); hospital admissions (indications); medical treatment, including prednisone escalation for IBD; endoscopy results; surgery; and infectious complications. The aim of the study was to assess the clinical effectiveness (defined as the absence of symptoms and endoscopic remission) and safety of biologic therapy in this clinical scenario.

3. Results

A total of five post-LT PSC/IBD patients were treated with anti-TNFα agents from 1993 through 2015 at HFHS. Two patients were treated with adalimumab, and three were treated with infliximab. See summary results in Table 1.

3.1. Subject 1. A 9-year-old white male was diagnosed with pancolonic Crohn's disease and responded well to treatment with prednisone, azathioprine, and then methotrexate. Two years following his IBD diagnosis, the patient was found to have primary sclerosing cholangitis with bridging fibrosis and cirrhosis. At age 17, the patient received a deceased donor liver transplant, after which he received mycophenolate mofetil and cyclosporine for immunosuppression. Following the transplant, the patient underwent multiple hospitalizations for cholangitis, perihepatic abscess secondary to methicillin-resistant Staphylococcus aureus (MRSA), cytomegalovirus (CMV) viremia, cellulitis, and esophageal candidiasis. The patient's posttransplant course was also complicated by worsening Crohn's colitis, treated with adalimumab. Despite this therapy, however, his colitis continued to worsen. He subsequently developed toxic megacolon and underwent a subtotal abdominal colectomy with end-ileostomy for refractory colitis. For approximately 5 months following his colectomy, the patient had marked improvement in pain, appetite, and functional status. He subsequently began to develop strictures at the ileostomy site secondary to active colitis with small bowel involvement, requiring multiple office visits for dilation of the ileostomy site. The patient was eventually hospitalized with worsening abdominal pain. Endoscopic ultrasound with biopsy showed malignant lymphoma, consistent with posttransplant lymphoproliferative disease (PTLD). Despite treatment with rituximab and corticosteroids, the patient continued to decompensate and eventually expired due to complications of PTLD.

3.2. Subject 2. A white female patient was diagnosed with ulcerative colitis at age 18, and PSC at age 20. The patient's colitis symptoms were initially well-controlled with azathioprine and mesalamine. At age 25, the patient received a living-donor liver transplant subsequent to PSC; posttransplant immunosuppressant treatment included tacrolimus and azathioprine in addition to mesalamine. Following transplant, the patient experienced symptoms of worsening colitis, with frequent flare-ups requiring multiple courses of high-dose prednisone for disease control. Despite the steroid treatments, the patient's symptoms continued to worsen. Subsequent treatment with infliximab resulted in marked improvement in her symptoms. However, the patient's course was complicated by pancytopenia. She continued to have active IBD symptoms following her transplant.

3.3. Subject 3. A white male patient was diagnosed with ulcerative colitis at age 29 and responded well to ASA and azathioprine therapy. He was diagnosed with PSC at age 32 and received a deceased donor liver transplant at age 41. He had a history of recurrent clostridium difficile infections requiring fecal transplantation prior to the transplant. Following liver transplant, the patient was hospitalized for MRSA bacteremia, pneumonia with severe sepsis, recurrent MRSA pneumonia, and recurrent clostridium difficile infections. However, despite treatment with azathioprine, his colitis symptoms began to worsen posttransplant and required escalation of prednisone dose. Azathioprine was subsequently discontinued and infliximab started in response to worsening colitis. Prednisone therapy was tapered off due to side effects. At of the end of follow-up, the patient was maintained on infliximab and budesonide; his UC was in clinical remission.

3.4. Subject 4. A white female patient was diagnosed with ulcerative colitis at age 26 and PSC at age 33. Prior to transplant, the patient was maintained on mesalamine and her UC was under good control, with no evidence of active colitis on colonoscopy. The patient's PSC was initially asymptomatic but quickly deteriorated, with multiple hospital admissions for episodes of cholangitis. At age 48, she received a liver transplant from a deceased donor for end-stage liver disease secondary to PSC. Posttransplant, the patient was started on mycophenolate mofetil, tacrolimus, and prednisone for immunosuppression. Her course was complicated by acute cellular rejection, which was treated with an increased dose of corticosteroids. The patient also experienced worsening of colitis. Mesalamine therapy was reinitiated with poor response; treatment was changed to infliximab, but symptoms continued to worsen. Her course was further complicated by clostridium difficile colitis, which did not respond to antibiotics and subsequently required a fecal transplant. Due to uncontrolled colitis with worsening symptoms, the patient underwent a colectomy with ileostomy, with marked improvement in her symptoms and overall health following surgery.

3.5. Subject 5. A white male patient was diagnosed with Crohn's disease at age 29 and PSC at age 33. Prior to liver transplant, the patient's Crohn's disease was in remission, maintained on adalimumab. Following transplant of a deceased donor liver at age 45, the patient was continued on adalimumab, with tacrolimus added for immunosuppression. His posttransplant course was complicating by posttransplant lymphoproliferative disease (PTLD); 9 months after transplant, adalimumab was discontinued. The patient was started on cyclophosphamide for his PTLD with interval improvement in disease activity on his most recent PET scan.

Table 1: Five patients with inflammatory bowel disease, primary sclerosing cholangitis, and liver transplant treated with antitumor necrosis factor alpha agents.

	IBD type	Age at IBD onset	Age at PSC onset	Age at LT	Pre-LT TNFα agent	Liver donor status	Post-LT TNFα agent	Concomitant immunosuppression	Complications	IBD disease activity
Patient 1: white male	Crohn's	9	11	17	None	Deceased	Adalimumab	Cyclosporine; mycophenolate mofetil	C. diff colitis, esophageal candidiasis, CMV viremia, PTLD, Death	Hospital admission; prednisone escalation; colectomy
Patient 2: white female	UC	18	20	25	None	Living unrelated	Infliximab	Tacrolimus; azathioprine	Pancytopenia	Hospital admission; prednisone escalation; active colitis
Patient 3: white male	UC	29	32	41	None	Deceased	Infliximab	Tacrolimus	MRSA bacteremia; pneumonia with sepsis; C. diff. colitis.	Hospital admission; prednisone escalation; active colitis
Patient 4: white female	UC	26	33	48	None	Deceased	Infliximab	Tacrolimus; mycophenolate mofetil	Acute rejection; C. diff colitis	Hospital admission; colectomy
Patient 5: white male	Crohn's	29	33	45	Adalimumab	Deceased	Adalimumab	Tacrolimus	PTLD	Active colitis

IBD: inflammatory bowel disease; PSC: primary sclerosing cholangitis; LT: liver transplant; TNFα: tumor necrosis factor alpha; C. diff: Clostridium difficile; CMV: cytomegalovirus; PTLD: posttransplant lymphoproliferative disease; UC: ulcerative colitis.

The patient's Crohn's disease symptoms remained under good control, with multiple colonoscopies showing no evidence of flare-ups of his disease. However, the patient's course was further complicated by acute cellular rejection and recurrence of PTLD. At last follow-up, the patient was maintained on mycophenolate, tacrolimus, and prednisone therapy, in addition to cyclophosphamide for PTLD. The addition of mesalamine has provided only partial relief from symptoms.

4. Discussion

Our patient experience suggests that anti-TNFα agents appear to be both relatively unsafe for patients with IBD after liver transplant and less effective at mitigating the disease than in patients without liver disease or transplant. Two patients went on to require a colectomy for severe colitis with immediate improvement in symptoms following the surgery. While our patients did well after colectomy, undergoing such a major operation in the post-LT setting is a high-risk scenario that should ideally be avoided. These outcomes demonstrate that these anti-TNFα agents can be poorly effective in the post-LT setting, in stark contrast to the known effectiveness of these therapies in patients without transplant.

Our study also demonstrates the severity of anti-TNFα-related complications in the post-LT setting. After transplant, three of five patients treated with anti-TNFα agents developed serious infections, including clostridium difficile colitis, esophageal candidiasis, CMV viremia, MRSA bacteremia, and community acquired pneumonia requiring multiple hospitalizations. In addition, two patients developed PTLD while being treated with an anti-TNFα agent, and one patient died due to this condition. This relatively high rate of such severe and potentially fatal complications is disproportionate to what is generally observed with anti-TNFα agents and suggests an underlying pathophysiology that is specific to the post-LT setting.

A previous study (n = 8) [9] of anti-TNFα agents in PSC/IBD patients reported similar outcomes. Four patients developed opportunistic infections (esophageal candidiasis, Clostridium difficile colitis, community acquired bacterial pneumonia, and cryptosporidiosis); one patient developed PTLD. This is consistent with our own observations; it is possible that anti-TNFα agents increase risk of PTLD among these patients. In contrast, however, that study also observed improvement in IBD-related clinical outcomes as well as mucosal healing. Another similar study (n = 6) [10] described significant improvement in IBD-related symptoms in four patients following the use of infliximab therapy.

Our case series is limited by the small number of patients observed; although this is a reflection of the relative rarity of IBD/PSC-LT in the population, we are hesitant to generalize the results to a whole population. Furthermore, given the variation in both the IBD subtype (Crohn's disease versus ulcerative colitis), the timing and type of anti-TNFα agents that each patient received, and the posttransplant immunosuppressive regimens used, it is difficult to isolate the effects of the anti-TNFα treatment [11] on disease activity. In particular, it is important to note that tacrolimus and immunosuppressive medications may also contribute to the risk of adverse clinical outcomes, especially infections, observed among these patients [12].

In summary, this case report illustrates that—despite widespread use of anti-TNFα agents in patients with refractory IBD—clinicians should exercise caution when employing these medications in the treatment of patients after liver transplant. Given the potential for significant complications, choice of immunosuppressive therapy and IBD treatment should be carefully considered; patients should be counseled regarding the possibility of an IBD exacerbation prior to transplant and monitored closely afterward. Further, large-scale studies are needed to evaluate the safety and efficacy of anti-TNFα therapies in IBD/PSC patients.

References

[1] K. Bambha, W. R. Kim, J. Talwalkar et al., "Incidence, Clinical Spectrum, and Outcomes of Primary Sclerosing Cholangitis in a United States Community," *Gastroenterology*, vol. 125, no. 5, pp. 1364–1369, 2003.

[2] O. Fausa, E. Schrumpf, and K. Elgjo, "Relationship of inflammatory bowel disease and primary sclerosing cholangitis," *Seminars in Liver Disease*, vol. 11, no. 1, pp. 31–39, 1991.

[3] J. J. W. Tischendorf, H. Hecker, M. Krüger, M. P. Manns, and P. N. Meier, "Characterization, outcome, and prognosis in 273 patients with primary sclerosing cholangitis: a single center study," *American Journal of Gastroenterology*, vol. 102, no. 1, pp. 107–114, 2007.

[4] U. Broomé, R. Olsson, L. Lööf et al., "Natural history and prognostic factors in 305 Swedish patients with primary sclerosing cholangitis," *Gut*, vol. 38, no. 4, pp. 610–615, 1996.

[5] R. H. Wiesner, P. M. Grambsch, E. R. Dickson et al., "Primary sclerosing cholangitis: Natural history, prognostic factors and survival analysis," *Hepatology*, vol. 10, no. 4, pp. 430–436, 1989.

[6] E. V. Loftus Jr., G. C. Harewood, C. G. Loftus et al., "PSC-IBD: a unique form of inflammatory bowel disease associated with primary sclerosing cholangitis," *Gut*, vol. 54, no. 1, pp. 91–96, 2005.

[7] J. F. Colombel, W. J. Sandborn, and W. Reinisch, "Infliximab, azathioprine, or combination therapy for Crohn's disease," *The New England Journal of Medicine*, vol. 362, no. 15, pp. 1383–1395, 2010.

[8] J. Costa, F. Magro, D. Caldeira, J. Alarcão, R. Sousa, and A. Vaz-Carneiro, "Infliximab reduces hospitalizations and surgery interventions in patients with inflammatory bowel disease: A systematic review and meta-analysis," *Inflammatory Bowel Diseases*, vol. 19, no. 10, pp. 2098–2110, 2013.

[9] A. B. Mohabbat et al., "Anti-tumour necrosis factor treatment of inflammatory bowel disease in liver transplant recipients," *Alimentary pharmacology & therapeutics*, vol. 36, no. 6, pp. 569–574, 2012.

[10] A. Sandhu, T. Alameel, C. H. Dale, M. Levstik, and N. Chande, "The safety and efficacy of antitumour necrosis factor-alpha therapy for inflammatory bowel disease in patients post liver transplantation: A case series," *Alimentary Pharmacology & Therapeutics*, vol. 36, no. 2, pp. 159–165, 2012.

[11] S. Singh, E. V. Loftus, and J. A. Talwalkar, "Inflammatory bowel disease after liver transplantation for primary sclerosing cholangitis," *American Journal of Gastroenterology*, vol. 108, no. 9, pp. 1417–1425, 2013.

[12] European FK506 Multicentre Liver Study Group, "Randomised trial comparing tacrolimus (FK506) and cyclosporin in prevention of liver allograft rejection," *The Lancet*, vol. 344, no. 8920, pp. 423–428, 1994.

10

IgG4-Seronegative Autoimmune Pancreatitis and Sclerosing Cholangitis

Allon Kahn,[1] Anitha D. Yadav,[2] and M. Edwyn Harrison[2]

[1] *Department of Medicine, Mayo Clinic, Scottsdale, AZ, USA*
[2] *Division of Gastroenterology and Hepatology, Mayo Clinic, Scottsdale, AZ, USA*

Correspondence should be addressed to M. Edwyn Harrison; harrison.m@mayo.edu

Academic Editor: Haruhiko Sugimura

IgG4-related disease is a relatively novel clinical entity whose gastrointestinal manifestations include type 1 autoimmune pancreatitis (AIP) and IgG4-associated sclerosing cholangitis. The presence of elevated serum IgG4 is suggestive but not essential for the diagnosis of type 1 AIP and is a pervasive feature of the proposed diagnostic criteria. The differential diagnosis of type 1 AIP includes malignant conditions, emphasizing the importance of a deliberate, comprehensive evaluation. Management of patients with a suggestive clinical presentation, but without serum IgG4 elevation, is difficult. Here we present three cases of IgG4-seronegative AIP and sclerosing cholangitis that responded to empiric steroid therapy and discuss approach considerations. These cases demonstrate the value of meticulous application of existing diagnostic algorithms to achieve a clinical diagnosis and avoid surgical intervention.

1. Introduction

Type 1 autoimmune pancreatitis (AIP) and immunoglobulin G4- (IgG4-) associated sclerosing cholangitis (IgG4-SC) are pancreatic and biliary manifestations of IgG4-related disease, respectively. Recently, IgG4-related disease has emerged as a novel clinical entity characterized by multiorgan infiltration of IgG4-positive cells, storiform fibrosis, and elevated serum IgG4 levels. Several diagnostic criteria have been proposed in the last decade based on radiology, histopathology, serology, and response to steroids [1–3]. However, the diagnosis still remains challenging. Often the differential diagnosis for AIP/IgG4-SC includes malignant conditions such as pancreatic cancer and cholangiocarcinoma, placing patients at risk for unnecessary surgery for a more benign condition.

Current clinical diagnostic criteria for type 1 AIP/IgG4-SC involve elevated serum IgG4 concentrations (>135 mg/dL). The reported sensitivity of increased serum IgG4 levels in AIP ranges from 68% to 81% [1, 4]. Hence, in patients with normal serum IgG4 levels, a thorough workup including pancreatic and biliary imaging, histology, and identification of extrapancreatic manifestations aids in accurate diagnosis. Here we describe three cases of serum IgG4 negative type 1 AIP/IgG4 SC that responded to a trial of steroid therapy, allowing for the avoidance of surgery.

2. Case 1

An 80-year-old Caucasian man with a history of resected prostate adenocarcinoma and hyperlipidemia presented with complaints of pruritus, anorexia, fatigue, 20 pound weight loss, and painless jaundice. He denied abdominal pain, melena, or hematochezia. His vital signs were within normal limits and physical examination revealed only jaundice. There was no history of significant alcohol use.

Laboratory workup revealed an elevated total bilirubin 8.5 mg/dL, direct bilirubin 5.2 mg/dL, alkaline phosphatase 372 IU/L, alanine aminotransferase (ALT) 299 IU/L, aspartate aminotransferase (AST) 143 IU/L, amylase 70 μ/L, and lipase 54 μ/L. His platelet count was 258 and International Normalized Ratio (INR) 0.9. Carbohydrate antigen (CA) 19-9 was 175 U/mL and carcinoembryonic antigen (CEA) level 1.1 ng/mL. Total IgG was 1,550 mg/dL and IgG4 levels were 51.8 (reference range 2.4–121). Other serologic tests included anti-neutrophil antibody (ANA), anti-smooth muscle antibody (ASMA), and anti-mitochondrial antibody (AMA), all

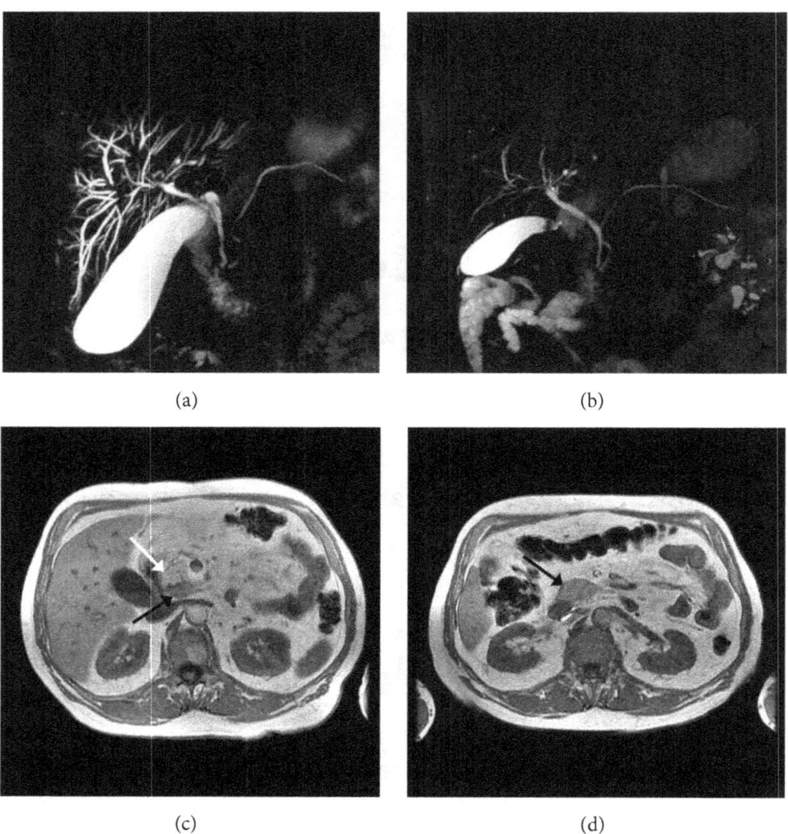

Figure 1: MRCP findings: Case 1. (a) Narrowing and stricture of the common bile duct with dilated intrahepatic ducts. (b) Resolution of intrahepatic duct dilation and CBD narrowing after steroid therapy. (c) 2.7 cm hypointense lesion in the pancreatic head (black arrow) near a region of normal pancreatic parenchyma (white arrow). (d) Resolution after steroid therapy. The pancreatic parenchyma is homogeneous and isointense with the adjacent liver.

of which were negative. A computed tomography (CT) of the abdomen demonstrated diffuse intrahepatic biliary ductal dilatation. Magnetic resonance imaging (MRI) revealed an area of enhancement concerning for neoplasm at the biliary confluence, narrowing of the central right and left intrahepatic bile ducts and intrahepatic biliary duct dilation (Figure 1(a)). Diffuse pancreatic enhancement was noted. An ERCP was performed and demonstrated a complex narrow biliary stricture involving both right and left hepatic ducts and extending to the common hepatic duct, consistent with type 4 pattern cholangiography [5]. Biliary brushings and FISH were negative for malignancy. IgG4 immunostaining of biliary brushing specimen was not pursued. Subsequently our patient underwent three ERCPs with biliary dilation/stent exchange and biliary brushings for cytology and FISH, all of which revealed no evidence of malignancy.

Six months after initial presentation, a repeat MRI was obtained which demonstrated a new 2.7 cm mass at the posterior aspect of the head of the pancreas extending into the uncinate process (Figure 1(c)). An endoscopic ultrasound with fine needle aspiration was performed and revealed benign pancreatic ductal cells and acini in addition to fragments of chronically inflamed stromal material. IgG4 immunostaining showed rare IgG4-positive inflammatory cells and was felt to be inconclusive. Periampullary mucosal biopsies showed small bowel mucosa without diagnostic abnormality. Incidentally, a CT of the chest revealed bilateral hilar, paratracheal and mediastinal enlarged lymph nodes, small pulmonary nodules, and ground glass opacities.

After a thorough negative workup for malignancy, based on the available clinical, radiological, and extrapancreatic presentation, a diagnosis of type 1 AIP and IgG4-SC was suspected. The patient was started on 40 mg of prednisone and continued for 4 weeks and gradually tapered. His symptoms abated and a follow-up MRI performed demonstrated complete resolution of the pancreatic mass and biliary strictures (Figures 1(b) and 1(d)). With this clinical and radiologic response, the patient was diagnosed with IgG4-related SC and the symptoms have not recurred after 3 years of follow-up.

3. Case 2

A 45-year-old gentleman with prior history of small duct primary sclerosing cholangitis and Crohn's disease presented with symptoms of abdominal pain, pruritus, dark urine, and jaundice. Laboratory analysis showed an AST of 152, ALT of 158, alkaline phosphatase of 531, total bilirubin of 5.6, direct bilirubin of 3.8, total protein of 7.4, albumin of 4.0, lipase of

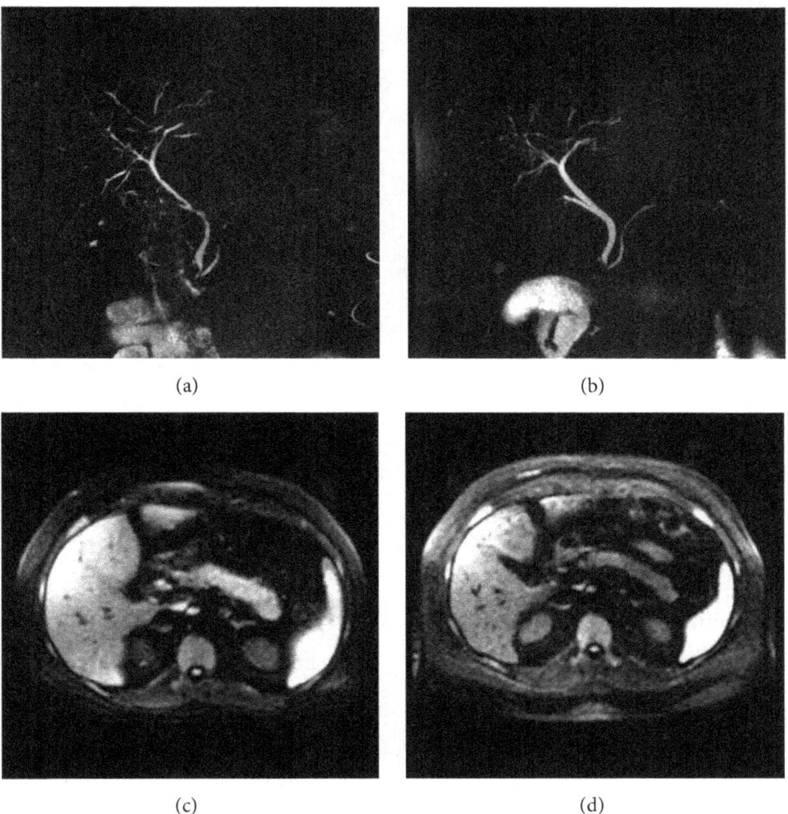

Figure 2: MRCP findings: Case 2. (a) Extrahepatic bile duct narrowing. (b) Resolution after steroid therapy. (c) Diffusion restriction shows hyperintensity and edema in the pancreatic tail. (d) Resolution after steroid therapy.

157, amylase of 82, CA of 19-9 194, CEA of 2.9, total IgG of 1620, and IgG4 of 53.3. MRI of the abdomen demonstrated diffuse enlargement of the body and the tail of the pancreas. No focal enhancing pancreatic mass was identified. MRCP revealed new irregular narrowing of the common hepatic duct, upper common bile duct beaded dilatation, and narrowing of the intrahepatic bile ducts (Figures 2(a) and 2(c)). Several prominent porta hepatis lymph nodes were noted.

An ERCP was performed and revealed mild intrahepatic biliary strictures and moderately severe common bile duct stricture, most consistent with a type 2 cholangiogram [5]. Sphincterotomy and dilation were performed and brushings were obtained. Biliary brushings revealed reactive epithelial cells and FISH was negative for malignancy; IgG4 immunostaining was not performed. Based on the clinical findings and parenchymal and ductal imaging, a diagnosis of autoimmune pancreatitis and IgG4-SC was made and patient was initiated on prednisone 60 mg daily. Within 2 weeks of initiating steroid therapy, his laboratory tests show significant improvement with resolution of cholestasis and MRCP showed significant improvement in intrahepatic and extrahepatic bile duct changes with resolution of pancreatic enlargement (Figures 2(b) and 2(d)). A decision was made to continue immunosuppressive therapy and he was started on mycophenolate 500 mg twice daily (prior history of Imuran-induced pancreatitis). His steroids were tapered gradually and stopped with no subsequent relapse.

4. Case 3

A 52-year-old gentleman presented to the gastroenterology clinic with a history of acute pancreatitis and complaints of abdominal pain. He denied abnormal weight loss or alcohol use. Laboratory analysis showed an amylase of 495, lipase of 1305, bilirubin of 2.8, AST of 658, ALT of 533, and alkaline phosphatase of 65. He was diagnosed with acute pancreatitis and treated conservatively. Abdominal MR imaging revealed segmental biliary dilatation from the bifurcation proximally to the right and left system with CBD stricture. The common hepatic duct was 10 mm and the CBD distally was 2.5 mm. The pancreatic duct was unremarkable. Additionally, there was significant retroperitoneal adenopathy and diffuse pulmonary nodules on the imaging.

An ERCP was performed and revealed a 2.5 cm high-grade stricture in the distal common bile duct, consistent with type 1 cholangiogram [5]. Brushing and biopsies were taken and a biliary stent was placed. A CA 19-9 at the time was 37. The biliary biopsies and FISH were negative for malignancy. IgG4 immunostaining of biliary brushings demonstrated occasional, scattered positive cells of indeterminate clinical significance. An EUS performed revealed a hypoechoic mass in the head of the pancreas (measuring 26 × 18 mm) and the body (measuring 22 × 22 mm). Pancreatic biopsies showed mild atypical epithelial cells. Serum total IgG was elevated at 2,430, but IgG4 level was normal at 41.2. On follow-up, he was noted to have enlarged submandibular salivary glands. Given a negative diagnostic workup, a CT guided biopsy of submandibular glands was pursued which confirmed chronic inflammatory infiltrate with numerous IgG4 positive plasma cells. A diagnosis of type 1 AIP and IgG4-SC was made and the patient was treated with prednisone 40 mg daily. He was also started on Imuran 150 mg daily and his prednisone was slowly tapered and stopped. The patient improved clinically, his laboratory parameters normalized, and repeat imaging showed dramatic improvement in biliary strictures with a normal-appearing pancreas.

5. Discussion

IgG4-related disease is a multiorgan fibroinflammatory disorder characterized by organ infiltration with lymphoplasmacytic cells rich in IgG4, storiform fibrosis, obliterative phlebitis, elevated serum IgG4 levels, and response to steroids. Two types of AIP have been described in the literature. Type 1 AIP is related to IgG4-related disease, while type 2 (idiopathic duct centric pancreatitis) is associated with a distinct characteristic histological pattern and is usually not accompanied by extrapancreatic manifestations [6]. Type 1 AIP is prevalent worldwide and typically affects middle-aged and elderly men. The most common presentation of type 1 AIP is obstructive jaundice. Other symptoms can include abdominal pain, weight loss, and anorexia [7]. Additionally, AIP can present as acute and chronic pancreatitis and could closely mimic pancreatic cancer. The commonest extrapancreatic manifestation of type 1 AIP is IgG4-SC, which can mimic cholangiocarcinoma. Other extrapancreatic manifestations include salivary gland enlargement, lymphadenopathy, pulmonary disease with nodules, hydronephrosis, and retroorbital disease [8].

In our current series, we describe three patients with type 1 AIP and IgG4-SC with normal serum IgG4 levels in whom steroid treatment was successful and surgery was entirely avoided. Each of these cases provides lessons in the diagnosis of IgG4-SC in patients with normal IgG4 levels. In Case 1, cholangiocarcinoma was suspected on the basis of clinical findings and compatible radiologic findings on CT, MR, and ERCP. However, a thorough and measured approach to diagnosis led to four ERCPs with biliary brushings and FISH, which were negative for malignancy. This allowed the patient to defer needless surgery. Follow-up MRI after six months revealed a new pancreatic mass which would not be expected with cholangiocarcinoma, and pulmonary nodules and mediastinal lymphadenopathy were seen on CT imaging, suggesting extrapancreatic involvement. When an EUS with FNA of the pancreatic mass did not reveal malignancy, but rather a chronic stromal infiltrate, the combination of pathologic findings and extrapancreatic involvement led to a trial of prednisone. With dramatic clinical and radiologic response to steroids, the diagnosis of type 1 AIP was made and surgery was avoided.

In Case 2, the patient presented with abdominal pain and jaundice. Imaging showed diffuse enlargement of the pancreas, as well as biliary strictures and pulmonary nodules. Serological tests were negative for IgG4, and histology and FISH were negative from ERCP brushings. Based on clinical and radiological presentation, a diagnosis of AIP was considered and empiric treatment was initiated with steroids. The patient responded well, with resolution of pancreatic enlargement and biliary strictures on imaging.

In our 3rd case, the patient presented with a diagnosis of acute pancreatitis of unknown etiology. His abdominal imaging, however, revealed biliary strictures which raised the question of an uncommon cause of pancreatitis. By carefully pursuing this clinical clue, misdiagnosis was avoided. Two ERCPS with biliary brushings and FISH were negative for malignancy, and EUS demonstrated pancreatic masses in the head and the body of the pancreas, biopsies of which were also negative for malignancy. The subsequent detection of an enlarged submandibular gland allowed a diagnostic biopsy that demonstrated chronic inflammatory infiltrate with numerous IgG4 positive plasma cells. This patient also was treated successfully with steroids, and continues on Imuran with no relapse.

The diagnosis of AIP is challenging and a number of diagnostic criteria (Japan, Italy, the United States, and Korea) have been proposed in the recent years. The HISORt criteria proposed by the Mayo Clinic to diagnose AIP include histology, imaging findings, elevated serum IgG4 levels, other organs involvement, and response to steroids [1]. In order to unify the disparate diagnostic criteria, a multinational group convened in 2011 and developed International Consensus Diagnostic Criteria (ICDC) for AIP [3]. The ICDC criteria are based on the following parameters: pancreatic parenchymal imaging, pancreatic ductal imaging (ERCP), serum IgG4 level, other organs involvement, histology of the pancreas, and response to steroid treatment. These parameters may provide level 1 (highly suggestive) or level 2 (supportive) evidence that will aid in definitive diagnosis and are associated with well-defined diagnostic algorithms.

The ICDC criteria can still be successfully applied in cases of seronegative IgG4-associated AIP and IgG4-SC. In Case 1, MRI pancreatography findings were indeterminate for AIP. A thorough evaluation for possible malignancy was negative. Pancreatic ductal imaging was normal. ERCP revealed level 1 findings, but serology was negative and no additional organ involvement (OOI) was noted. Two level 1 criteria were not met, so EUS-guided pancreatic biopsy was performed and was inconclusive. Because of the presence of a single level 1 OOI, steroid trial was pursued and resulted in radiographic and symptomatic resolution, supporting a diagnosis of type 1 AIP. In Case 2, initial MR pancreatography was typical for type 1 AIP. There was a single level 1 OOI criterion (multiple proximal and distal CBD strictures); thus, a steroid trial was pursued and resulted in substantial improvement, confirming the diagnosis. In Case 3, neither pancreatic parenchymal imaging nor ductal imaging was typical for AIP. However, level 1 OOI findings were seen on ERCP. A pancreatic biopsy was thus performed and yielded inconclusive findings. At this point, a steroid trial would have been reasonable; however, the interval development of submandibular gland enlargement allowed for establishment of definitive histological diagnosis.

The typical histological findings in type 1 AIP are comprised of abundant infiltration of lymphocytes, IgG4 positive plasma cells (greater than 10 IgG4 positive cells per high power field), fibrosis in periductal and interlobular areas, and obliterative phlebitis [9]. Tissue samples obtained with EUS-guided pancreatic trucut biopsies provide accurate histological diagnosis as compared to FNA alone [10]. However, if tissue samples are not available, the diagnosis can be made with the aid of imaging studies, extrapancreatic involvement, and response to steroids [2, 11]. In our series, two patients did not have definitive histopathological findings of lymphoplasmacytic infiltrate with IgG4 cells. Yet, based on the collateral evidence, all patients were treated with steroids and immunosuppressive medications and thus surgery was avoided.

Increased serum IgG4 levels (>135 mg/dL) have been frequently described in patients with type 1 AIP and have been included as a part of diagnostic criteria. Hamano and colleagues first described an association between elevated IgG4 and AIP in 2001 and reported the sensitivity and specificity of elevated IgG4 for AIP as 95 and 97%, respectively [12]. However, subsequent studies of larger AIP patient cohorts demonstrated IgG4 seropositivity in as few as 76% [13]. Thus, further estimates of sensitivity and specificity for AIP diagnosis have been shown to vary widely and are reported as low as 62 and 59%, respectively [14]. This heterogeneity is largely attributable to the application of disparate diagnostic criteria in study design, a fact which prompted the ICDC's creation. Ultimately, the sole elevation of serum IgG4 is inadequate to establish a definitive diagnosis of AIP. Some have suggested that it may play a clearer role in the differentiation of AIP from malignancy, particularly at higher cutoff levels where specificity is enhanced [14].

It has also been suggested that IgG4-seronegative AIP may behave as a different clinicopathologic entity. When compared to IgG4-seropositive patients, those with negative serology are more likely to be female, present with abdominal pain or acute pancreatitis, and demonstrate segmental pancreatic body and/or tail enlargement [15, 16]. They are less likely to present with obstructive jaundice and less frequently require maintenance immunosuppression, owing to a lower relapse rate [17]. In this way, IgG4 level may serve as a prognostic biomarker. Patients with IgG4 seropositivity are also noted to have a higher prevalence of extrapancreatic manifestations of IgG4-related disease, particularly lacrymal and salivary gland involvement and hilar lymphadenopathy [17]. In contrast to this data, all of our IgG4-seronegative patients were male and presented with extrapancreatic disease (i.e., IgG4-SC and submandibular involvement), with 2 of 3 presenting with obstructive jaundice and requiring maintenance immunosuppression. This divergence from previously documented patterns is likely a manifestation of the observational quality of existing data and the heterogeneous clinical course of this relatively novel disease.

In Cases 1 and 3, pancreatic imaging was not suggestive of typical features for AIP, while cholangiography suggested the presence of IgG4-SC. While AIP and IgG4-SC often coexist, it is important to recognize that they are likely distinct, if closely related, manifestations of the single overarching clinical entity of IgG4-related disease. Several studies have reported histologically proven IAC (i.e., lymphoplasmacytic infiltrate, storiform fibrosis, and obliterative phlebitis on resection specimen) in the absence of any clinical or radiographic evidence of AIP [18–20]. As was seen in our cases and is corroborated by the ICDC algorithms, biliary findings suspicious for IgG4-SC without characteristic evidence of AIP should not lead one away from a meticulous evaluation for IgG4-related disease.

The diagnosis of isolated IgG4-SC is challenging and IgG4 serology alone is inadequate to establish the diagnosis, as has been previously discussed. The sensitivity of IgG4 for IgG4-SC diagnosis has been estimated as 74%, a level comparable to estimates in AIP [18]. Several of the reported cases of isolated IgG4-SC demonstrate borderline elevations in IgG4 [20] and elevation of IgG4 in other stricturing biliary disorders, such as PSC, has been observed [21]. The addition of IgG4 immunostaining is often critical to accurate identification. Ampullary, hepatic, or biliary duct biopsies have been demonstrated as useful modalities, with relatively variable sensitivities (24–80%), but high specificities (91–100%) for the diagnosis of IAC [22].

Although our goal is early identification and treatment of benign IgG4-related disease and avoidance of surgery, it should be emphasized that the misdiagnosis of AIP/IgG4-SC in the setting of pancreatic cancer or cholangiocarcinoma must be strictly avoided [23]. In a recent UK study evaluating long-term outcomes in patients with AIP/IgG4-SC, 13 of 115 patients (11%) were diagnosed with a malignancy before or after the diagnosis of AIP [8]. Hence, caution should be exercised to rule out malignancy prior to embarking on investigations aimed at diagnosing AIP/IgG4-SC. On the other hand, the reported incidence of benign disease after pancreatoduodenectomy for a presumed malignancy is 5–13% and the incidence of AIP in the benign resected specimens is 30–43% [24]. Hence, diagnosis of AIP should be made cautiously taking into account all other collateral information such as characteristic imaging findings, serologic parameters, extrapancreatic involvement, and perhaps treatment with a short course of steroids prior to considering surgery. In our case series, we engaged in a thorough evaluation to exclude malignancy and include other findings within the spectrum of IgG4-related disease before diagnosis and initiation of steroid therapy.

Type 1 AIP/IgG4-SC typically responds dramatically to steroids. In our series we treated all patients with prednisone 40 mg daily for 4 weeks and tapered by 5 mg/week with close clinical follow-up, liver function tests, and imaging studies. In addition, all patients required biliary drainage procedures. Even though disease relapse is common with type 1 AIP, (30%–50%) none of our patients had clinical or biochemical relapse [25, 26]. However, in our series two out of 3 patients are maintained on immunosuppressive therapy (Imuran or mycophenolate).

In summary, our case series highlights the benefit of early recognition and medical treatment of IgG4-negative type 1 AIP and IgG4-SC. Despite normal IgG4 levels, a diagnosis of IgG4-related AIP and IgG4-SC should be considered when there is a typical clinical presentation, the presence of characteristic pancreatobiliary imaging findings, and extrapancreatic involvement. When IgG4-related AIP is recognized without elevation of IgG4, the patient can be spared morbidity associated with unnecessary surgical treatment by initiating a steroid trial and monitoring patients carefully.

References

[1] S. T. Chari, T. C. Smyrk, M. J. Levy et al., "Diagnosis of autoimmune pancreatitis: the Mayo clinic experience," *Clinical Gastroenterology and Hepatology*, vol. 4, no. 8, pp. 1010–1016, 2006.

[2] M. Otsuki, J. B. Chung, K. Okazaki et al., "Asian diagnostic criteria for autoimmune pancreatitis: consensus of the Japan-Korea symposium on autoimmune pancreatitis," *Journal of Gastroenterology*, vol. 43, no. 6, pp. 403–408, 2008.

[3] T. Shimosegawa, S. T. Chari, L. Frulloni et al., "International consensus diagnostic criteria for autoimmune pancreatitis: guidelines of the international association of pancreatology," *Pancreas*, vol. 40, no. 3, pp. 352–358, 2011.

[4] J. K. Ryu, J. B. Chung, S. W. Park et al., "Review of 67 patients with autoimmune pancreatitis in Korea: a multicenter nationwide study," *Pancreas*, vol. 37, no. 4, pp. 377–385, 2008.

[5] T. Nakazawa, I. Naitoh, K. Hayashi et al., "Diagnostic criteria for IgG4-related sclerosing cholangitis based on cholangiographic classification," *Journal of Gastroenterology*, vol. 47, no. 1, pp. 79–87, 2012.

[6] G. Klöppel, S. Detlefsen, S. T. Chari, D. S. Longnecker, and G. Zamboni, "Autoimmune pancreatitis: the clinicopathological characteristics of the subtype with granulocytic epithelial lesions," *Journal of Gastroenterology*, vol. 45, no. 8, pp. 787–793, 2010.

[7] A. Raina, D. Yadav, A. M. Krasinskas et al., "Evaluation and management of autoimmune pancreatitis: experience at a large US center," *The American Journal of Gastroenterology*, vol. 104, no. 9, pp. 2295–2306, 2009.

[8] M. T. Huggett, E. L. Culver, M. Kumar et al., "Type 1 autoimmune pancreatitis and IgG4-related sclerosing cholangitis is associated with extrapancreatic organ failure, malignancy, and mortality in a prospective UK cohort," *American Journal of Gastroenterology*, vol. 109, pp. 1675–1683, 2014.

[9] V. Deshpande, Y. Zen, J. K. Chan et al., "Consensus statement on the pathology of IgG4-related disease," *Modern Pathology*, vol. 25, no. 9, pp. 1181–1192, 2012.

[10] N. Mizuno, V. Bhatia, W. Hosoda et al., "Histological diagnosis of autoimmune pancreatitis using EUS-guided trucut biopsy: a comparison study with EUS-FNA," *Journal of Gastroenterology*, vol. 44, no. 7, pp. 742–750, 2009.

[11] S. T. Chari, N. Takahashi, M. J. Levy et al., "A diagnostic strategy to distinguish autoimmune pancreatitis from pancreatic cancer," *Clinical Gastroenterology and Hepatology*, vol. 7, no. 10, pp. 1097–1103, 2009.

[12] H. Hamano, S. Kawa, A. Horiuchi et al., "High serum IgG4 concentrations in patients with sclerosing pancreatitis," *The New England Journal of Medicine*, vol. 344, no. 10, pp. 732–738, 2001.

[13] R. P. Sah, S. T. Chari, R. Pannala et al., "Differences in clinical profile and relapse rate of type 1 versus type 2 autoimmune pancreatitis," *Gastroenterology*, vol. 139, no. 1, pp. 140–148, 2010.

[14] R. Sadler, R. W. Chapman, D. Simpson et al., "The diagnostic significance of serum IgG4 levels in patients with autoimmune pancreatitis: a UK study," *European Journal of Gastroenterology and Hepatology*, vol. 23, no. 2, pp. 139–145, 2011.

[15] T. Kamisawa, K. Takuma, T. Tabata et al., "Serum IgG4-negative autoimmune pancreatitis," *Journal of Gastroenterology*, vol. 46, no. 1, pp. 108–116, 2011.

[16] A. Ghazale, S. T. Chari, T. C. Smyrk et al., "Value of serum IgG4 in the diagnosis of autoimmune pancreatitis and in distinguishing it from pancreatic cancer," *The American Journal of Gastroenterology*, vol. 102, no. 8, pp. 1646–1653, 2007.

[17] S. Kawa, T. Ito, T. Watanabe et al., "The utility of serum IgG4 concentrations as a biomarker," *International Journal of Rheumatology*, vol. 2012, Article ID 198314, 4 pages, 2012.

[18] A. Ghazale, S. T. Chari, L. Zhang et al., "Immunoglobulin G4-associated cholangitis: clinical profile and response to therapy," *Gastroenterology*, vol. 134, no. 3, pp. 706–715, 2008.

[19] Y. Zen, K. Harada, M. Sasaki et al., "IgG4-related sclerosing cholangitis with and without hepatic inflammatory pseudotumor, and sclerosing pancreatitis-associated sclerosing cholangitis: do they belong to a spectrum of sclerosing pancreatitis?" *The American Journal of Surgical Pathology*, vol. 28, no. 9, pp. 1193–1203, 2004.

[20] H. Hamano, S. Kawa, T. Uehara et al., "Immunoglobulin G4-related lymphoplasmacytic sclerosing cholangitis that mimics infiltrating hilar cholangiocarcinoma: part of a spectrum of autoimmune pancreatitis?" *Gastrointestinal Endoscopy*, vol. 62, no. 1, pp. 152–157, 2005.

[21] F. D. Mendes, R. Jorgensen, J. Keach et al., "Elevated serum IgG4 concentration in patients with primary sclerosing cholangitis," *American Journal of Gastroenterology*, vol. 101, no. 9, pp. 2070–2075, 2006.

[22] Y. Zen and Y. Nakanuma, "IgG4 cholangiopathy," *International Journal of Hepatology*, vol. 2012, Article ID 472376, 6 pages, 2012.

[23] T. B. Gardner, M. J. Levy, N. Takahashi, T. C. Smyrk, and S. T. Chari, "Misdiagnosis of autoimmune pancreatitis: a caution to clinicians," *American Journal of Gastroenterology*, vol. 104, no. 7, pp. 1620–1623, 2009.

[24] H. J. Asbun, K. Conlon, L. Fernandez-Cruz et al., "When to perform a pancreatoduodenectomy in the absence of positive histology? A consensus statement by the International Study Group of Pancreatic Surgery," *Surgery*, vol. 155, no. 5, pp. 887–892, 2014.

[25] T. Kamisawa, T. Shimosegawa, K. Okazaki et al., "Standard steroid treatment for autoimmune pancreatitis," *Gut*, vol. 58, no. 11, pp. 1504–1507, 2009.

[26] S. T. Chari and J. A. Murray, "Autoimmune pancreatitis, part II: the relapse," *Gastroenterology*, vol. 134, no. 2, pp. 625–628, 2008.

11

Focal Intramucosal Adenocarcinoma Occurring in Gastric Hyperplastic Polyps: Two Case Reports

Keisuke Taniuchi,[1,2] **Mitsuo Okada,**[1] **and Hiroshi Sakaeda**[1]

[1]*Department of Gastroenterology, Chikamori Hospital, Kochi 780-8522, Japan*
[2]*Department of Endoscopic Diagnostics and Therapeutics, Kochi Medical School, Kochi University, Nankoku 783-8505, Japan*

Correspondence should be addressed to Keisuke Taniuchi; ktaniuchi@kochi-u.ac.jp

Academic Editor: Christoph Vogt

Gastric hyperplastic polyps are generally considered benign lesions, although rare cases of adenocarcinoma have been reported. Two cases of intramucosal adenocarcinoma originating from gastric hyperplastic polyps that were successfully removed by endoscopic mucosal resection or endoscopic submucosal dissection are reported. On pathological examination, adenocarcinoma limited to the hyperplastic foveolar epithelial mucosa of the gastric hyperplastic polyps was observed.

1. Introduction

Hyperplastic polyps (HPs) are the most common type of polypoid lesion of the stomach. Until recently, gastric HPs were considered to be insignificant in terms of potential malignant transformation, and the incidence of malignant change has been reported to be relatively low, with an average of only 2.1% in large series [1]. There have been increasing numbers of reports of dysplasia and carcinoma arising within HPs, with rates of occurrence varying from 1.5% to 4.5% [2]. Gastric HPs larger than 1 cm are said to have an increased risk of malignant transformation [3]. Therefore, HPs are sufficiently common to warrant careful attention because of their association with dysplasia and gastric cancer.

HPs are inflammatory proliferations of gastric foveolar cells. The classic association of gastric HPs has been with mucosal atrophy, whether caused by *Helicobacter pylori* (*H. pylori*) infection or autoimmune gastritis [4]. In recent years, the proportion of gastric HPs occurring in the setting of normal or reactive gastric mucosa with no evidence of current or prior *H. pylori* infection has been increasing [5]. Carcinomas arising in relation to gastric HPs are usually well differentiated, although some cases of poorly differentiated and signet-ring carcinomas have been reported [6].

Two cases of gastric HP with intramucosal adenocarcinoma are presented. In these cases, the neoplastic transformation occurred in the hyperplastic foveolar epithelium of the gastric HPs.

2. Case Report

Case 1. A 73-year-old woman was found to have a gastric HP on the posterior wall of the gastric antrum during a screening esophagogastroduodenoscopy (EGD) performed in April 2010. She had no symptoms, and her family history was unremarkable. The HP was 15 mm in size and classified as type II (Yamada classification). Thereafter, she underwent annual EGDs. The EGD performed 3 years later revealed that the gastric HP remained the same size (Figures 1(a) and 1(b)); a biopsy revealed mild dysplasia in the hyperplastic foveolar epithelium of the gastric HP. The following EGD, performed 4 years later, revealed a significant increase in size, to 20 mm, and the lesion was classified as type III (Yamada classification) (Figures 1(c) and 1(d)). At this time, a biopsy revealed focal adenocarcinoma in the HP. Routine laboratory examination results were within normal limits, and the serum carcinoembryonic antigen (CEA) level was not elevated. The polyp was resected *en bloc* by endoscopic submucosal

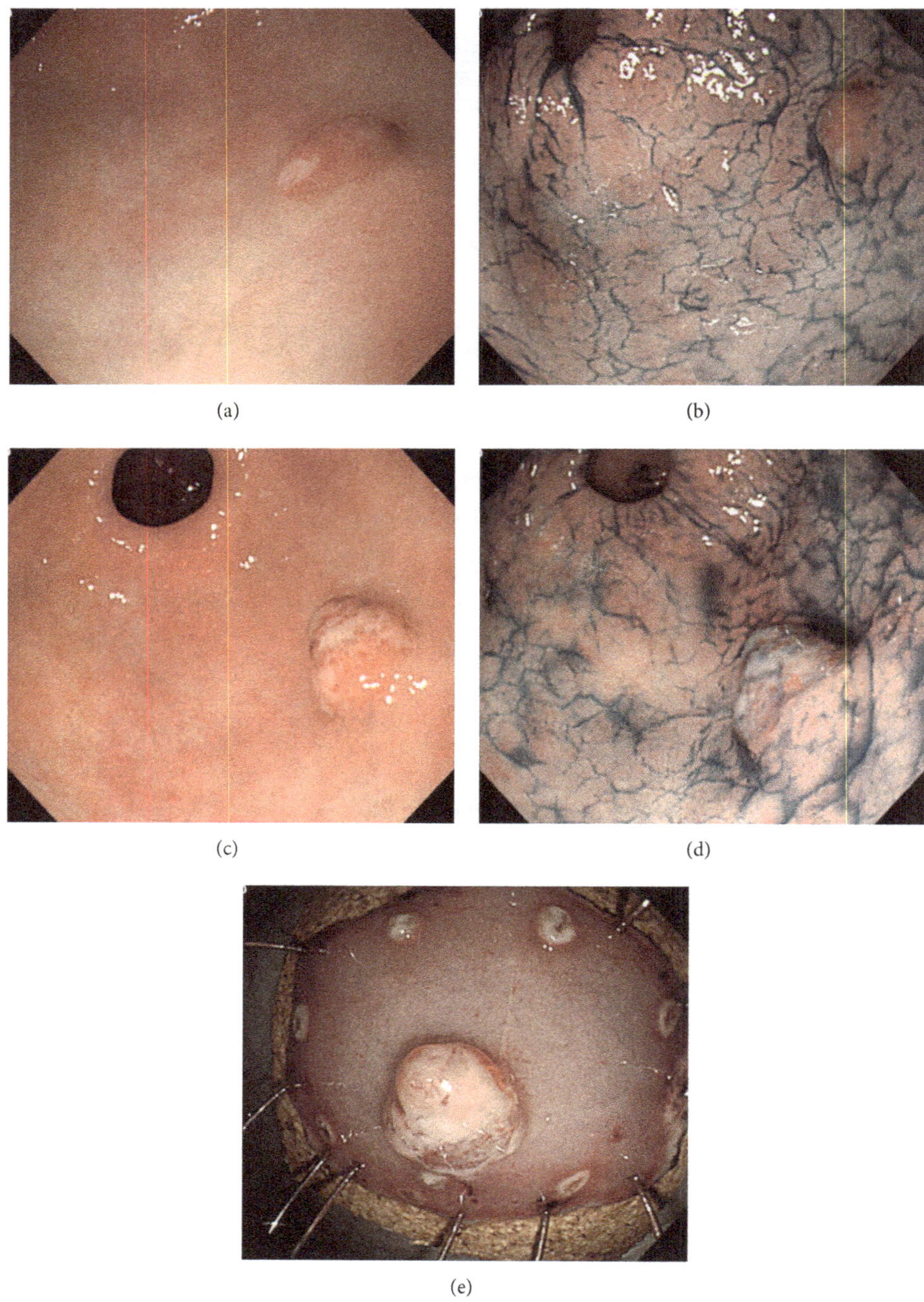

Figure 1: Case 1, endoscopic examination. EGD examination in April 2013 ((a) white-light endoscopy; (b) white-light endoscopy with indigo-carmine dye staining). EGD examination in April 2014, when an initial diagnosis of focal cancer within gastric HP was made ((c) white-light endoscopy; (d) white-light endoscopy with indigo-carmine dye staining). Endoscopic findings after *en bloc* resection by ESD (e). EGD: esophagogastroduodenoscopy; HP: hyperplastic polyp; ESD: endoscopic submucosal dissection.

dissection (ESD) performed with a hook knife (Figure 1(e)). The resected specimen revealed well-differentiated adenocarcinoma limited to the mucosa around the elongated, grossly distorted, branching, and dilated hyperplastic foveolae lying in an edematous stroma rich in vasculature and small, haphazardly distributed, smooth muscle bundles with dysplastic foci (Figures 2(a)–2(d)). The lesion was 20 mm in maximum diameter, and it was completely removed with an excision margin greater than 2 mm that was free of tumor cells. The polyp with focal adenocarcinoma was classified as early stomach cancer, pT1a(M), Tub1, ly0, v0, pN0, pM0, and pStage IA, in accordance with the Japanese Classification of Gastric Carcinoma (JCGC). Histopathological assessment of biopsy specimens collected from the mucous membrane of

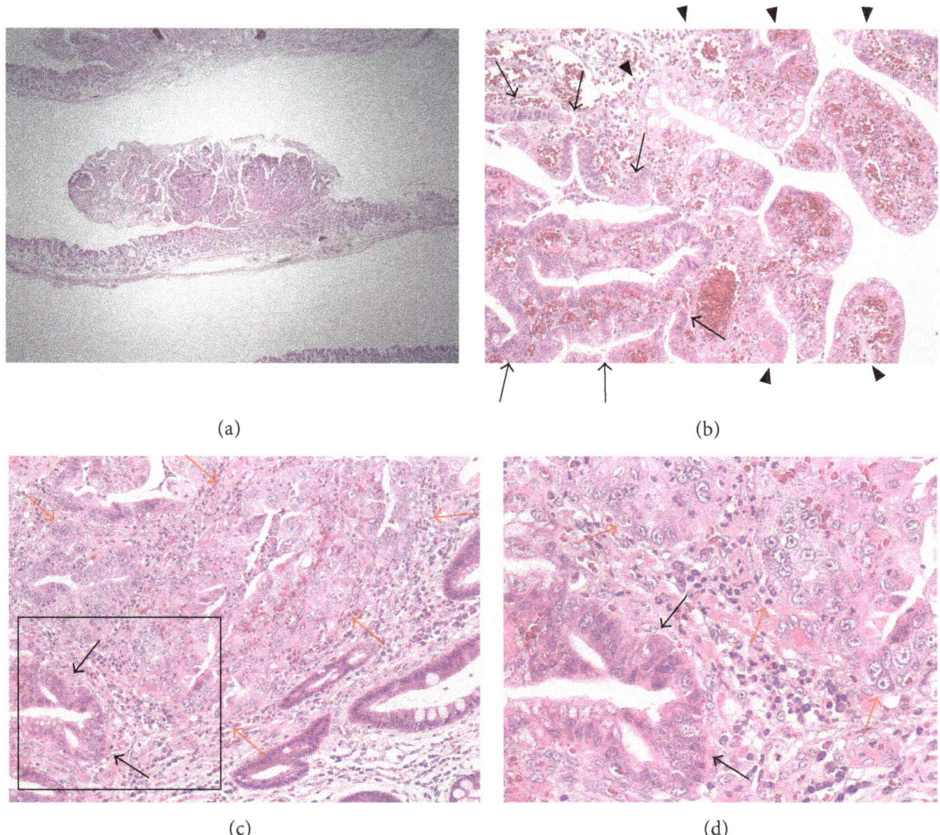

FIGURE 2: Case 1, histopathological findings. (a) Resected specimen obtained by endoscopic ESD (H&E, ×4). (b) Foci of tubular adenoma with mild dysplasia (between the arrows) in the setting of HP (between arrowheads) are noted (H&E, ×20). (c) Foci of carcinomatous transformation (between red arrows) adjacent to the adenomatous lesion (black arrows) in sequence are observed (H&E, ×20). (d) The black box in (c) depicts the position of the enlarged section. Red arrows: foci of carcinomatous transformation; black arrows: adenomatous lesion. ESD: endoscopic submucosal dissection; HP: hyperplastic polyp.

the antrum and body of the stomach showed chronic gastritis with no *H. pylori* infection. Serum anti-*H. pylori* antibody was less than 3 U/mL.

Case 2. A 66-year-old woman was found to have a gastric HP on the posterior wall of the proximal gastric body during a screening EGD performed in October 2011. She had no symptoms. Her family history was unremarkable, and she was a housekeeper. The HP was classified as type IV (Yamada classification). Thereafter, she underwent annual EGDs. The EGD performed 3 years later (Figures 3(a) and 3(b)) revealed the gastric HP to be unchanged in size, 20 mm, compared to the EGD performed 2 years later, when a biopsy had revealed no dysplasia or cancer cells. However, a biopsy taken at this time revealed focal adenocarcinoma in the HP. Routine laboratory examination results were within normal limits, and the serum CEA level was not elevated. The polyp was resected by endoscopic mucosal resection (EMR) using a submucosal saline injection technique for reduction of iatrogenic thermal injury, and, to increase the probability of a truly curative complete resection, the polyp was lifted up and removed *en bloc* with a diathermic loop (Figures 3(c) and 3(d)). The lesion was 20 mm in maximum diameter, and the resection margin was free of tumor cells. The resected specimen revealed focal well-differentiated adenocarcinoma limited to the mucosa around the hyperplastic foveolae lying in a vascular edematous stroma (Figures 4(a) and 4(b)). No dysplasia, intestinal metaplasia, or *H. pylori* infection was identified in the benign gastric epithelium of the polyp. The lesion was classified as early stomach cancer, pT1a(M), Tub1, ly0, v0, pN0, pM0, and pStage IA, according to the JCGC. Histopathological assessment of biopsy specimens collected from the mucous membrane of the antrum and the body of the stomach showed chronic gastritis with no *H. pylori* infection. Serum anti-*H. pylori* antibody was less than 3 U/mL.

In the present cases, the HPs were removed completely by ESD or EMR and the patients did not require any additional surgery because the tumors were limited to the mucosal layer.

3. Discussion

Two cases of rare focal adenocarcinoma arising in gastric HPs were presented. There have recently been increasing numbers

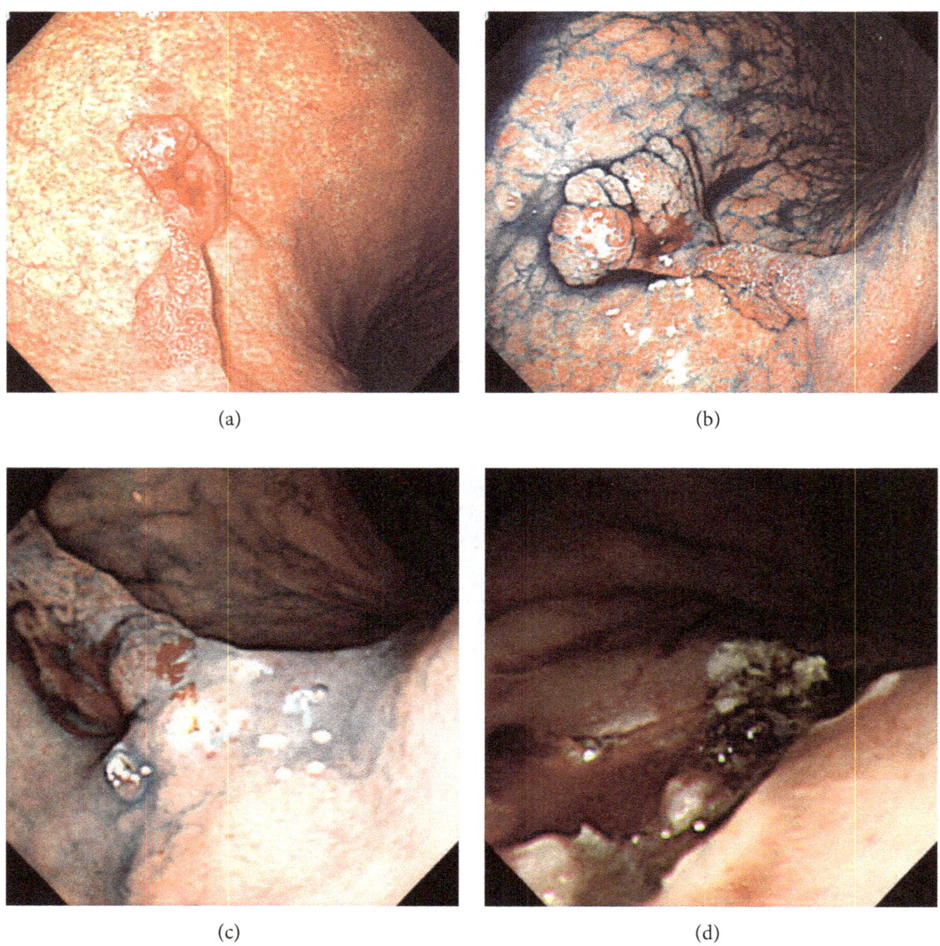

(a) (b) (c) (d)

Figure 3: Case 2, endoscopic examination. EGD examination in October 2014, when an initial diagnosis of focal cancer within gastric HP was made ((a) white-light endoscopy; (b) white-light endoscopy with indigo-carmine dye staining). Endoscopic findings after *en bloc* resection by EMR (c, d). EGD: esophagogastroduodenoscopy; HP: hyperplastic polyp; EMR: endoscopic mucosal resection.

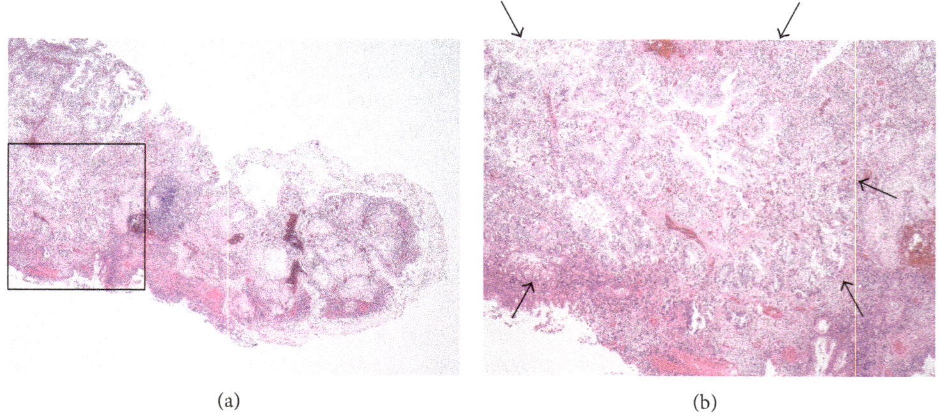

(a) (b)

Figure 4: Case 2, histopathological findings. (a) Resected specimen obtained by endoscopic EMR (H&E, ×4). (b) The black box in (a) indicates the region shown in the enlarged image. Foci of carcinomatous transformation (between arrows) in the setting of HP are observed (H&E, ×20). EMR: endoscopic mucosal resection; HP: hyperplastic polyp.

of reports of dysplasia and carcinoma arising within gastric HPs. During the malignant transformation of gastric HPs, cancer may spontaneously occur in the lesion through multistep carcinogenesis, such as via the hyperplasia-adenoma (dysplasia)-adenocarcinoma sequence [7]. Chromosomal aberrations, microsatellite instability, and p53 mutations were found to be mutually exclusive in adenomatous areas arising in gastric HPs; hence, there has been speculation regarding whether these could be alternate pathways of gastric carcinogenesis [1, 8, 9]. However, whether gastric HP carcinoma usually arises from a precancerous lesion or *de novo* remains unknown [2]. Current Case 1 had focal dysplasia situated close to the focal adenocarcinoma, which appears to confirm the theory of malignant conversion of HPs, that is, hyperplasia-dysplasia-adenocarcinoma. In contrast, current Case 2 had only adenocarcinoma cells without accompanying adenoma or other types of cancer cells. This case supports the existing hypothesis of a sequential progression from a benign HP to cancer. HPs have been reported in association with various types of chronic gastritis, particularly with autoimmune gastritis [10] and in *H. pylori* gastritis [11]; however, both gastric HPs in this report arose from chronic gastritis without intestinal metaplasia or *H. pylori* infection. Therefore, the settings of both cases were similar. The mechanism of carcinogenesis within gastric HPs is uncertain, but the present cases suggest that carcinoma can arise from dysplasia and from hyperplastic foveolar epithelium within gastric HPs.

HPs are usually asymptomatic and are typically found incidentally during routine endoscopic examination [12], as with the current asymptomatic gastric HP cases. Focal adenocarcinomas in these HPs were diagnosed by endoscopic biopsy during careful follow-up observation with EGD. Since attempts to identify molecular changes in gastric HPs have been hampered by the small number of reported cases, a marker for the malignant transformation of these lesions has not yet been found. Therefore, the most important prognostic factor is size: those larger than 1 cm are said to have an increased risk of malignant transformation [9, 13]. Accordingly, the potential association of HP with gastric cancer should generally be taken into consideration, and endoscopists should aggressively obtain biopsy specimens from gastric HPs larger than 1 cm in size. Since the results of biopsy specimen analysis may be falsely negative, all gastric HPs exceeding 2 cm (or, according to some opinions, even 5 mm) in size should always be resected [14]. Other authors recommend the resection of gastric HPs that are larger than 1 cm in size to obtain an accurate diagnosis [15, 16].

The current cases illustrate that gastric HP may be associated with gastric cancer and that the biopsy-first approach is reasonable, because it allows definitive diagnosis and planning of treatment according to pathology results after consultation with the patient. The decision of whether endoscopic or surgical resection is needed must be made, and the endoscopist should consider careful follow-up and/or complete removal of all HPs that measure 1 cm or more.

References

[1] W.-L. Zea-Iriarte, I. Sekine, M. Itsuno et al., "Carcinoma in gastric hyperplastic polyps. A phenotypic study," *Digestive Diseases and Sciences*, vol. 41, no. 2, pp. 377–386, 1996.

[2] R. Jain and R. Chetty, "Gastric hyperplastic polyps: a review," *Digestive Diseases and Sciences*, vol. 54, no. 9, pp. 1839–1846, 2009.

[3] D. J. Morais, A. Yamanaka, J. M. R. Zeitune, and N. A. Andreollo, "Gastric polyps: a retrospective analysis of 26,000 digestive endoscopies," *Arquivos de Gastroenterologia*, vol. 44, no. 1, pp. 14–17, 2007.

[4] K. Dirschmid, C. Platz-Baudin, and M. Stolte, "Why is the hyperplastic polyp a marker for the precancerous condition of the gastric mucosa?" *Virchows Archiv*, vol. 448, no. 1, pp. 80–84, 2006.

[5] Y. H. Shaib, M. Rugge, D. Y. Graham, and R. M. Genta, "Management of gastric polyps: an endoscopy-based approach," *Clinical Gastroenterology and Hepatology*, vol. 11, no. 11, pp. 1374–1384, 2013.

[6] C.-H. Wu, M.-J. Chen, W.-H. Chang, Y.-J. Chan, H.-Y. Wang, and S.-C. Shih, "Signet-ring type adenocarcinoma arising from a tiny gastric polyp," *Gastrointestinal Endoscopy*, vol. 67, no. 4, pp. 724–725, 2008.

[7] J. Imura, S. Hayashi, K. Ichikawa et al., "Malignant transformation of hyperplastic gastric polyps: an immunohistochemical and pathological study of the changes of neoplastic phenotype," *Oncology Letters*, vol. 7, no. 5, pp. 1459–1463, 2014.

[8] A. M. M. F. Nogueira, F. Cameiro, R. Seruca et al., "Microsatellite instability in hyperplastic and adenomatous polyps of the stomach," *Cancer*, vol. 86, no. 9, pp. 1649–1656, 1999.

[9] K. Murakami, H. Mitomi, K. Yamashita, S. Tanabe, K. Saigenji, and I. Okayasu, "p53, but not c-Ki-ras, mutation and down-regulation of p21WAF1/CIP1 and cyclin D1 are associated with malignant transformation in gastric hyperplastic polyps," *American Journal of Clinical Pathology*, vol. 115, no. 2, pp. 224–234, 2001.

[10] S. Hirasaki, S. Suzuki, H. Kanzaki, K. Fujita, S. Matsumura, and E. Matsumoto, "Minute signet ring cell carcinoma occurring in gastric hyperplastic polyp," *World Journal of Gastroenterology*, vol. 13, no. 43, pp. 5779–5780, 2007.

[11] N. Ljubičić, M. Banić, M. Kujundžić et al., "The effect of eradicating *Helicobacter pylori* infection on the course of adenomatous and hyperplastic gastric polyps," *European Journal of Gastroenterology and Hepatology*, vol. 11, no. 7, pp. 727–730, 1999.

[12] A. F. Goddard, R. Badreldin, D. M. Pritchard, M. M. Walker, and B. Warren, "The management of gastric polyps," *Gut*, vol. 59, no. 9, pp. 1270–1276, 2010.

[13] T. Yao, M. Kajiwara, S. Kuroiwa et al., "Malignant transformation of gastric hyperplastic polyps: alteration of phenotypes, proliferative activity, and p53 expression," *Human Pathology*, vol. 33, no. 10, pp. 1016–1022, 2002.

[14] R. N. Sharaf, A. K. Shergill, R. D. Odze et al., "Endoscopic mucosal tissue sampling," *Gastrointestinal Endoscopy*, vol. 78, no. 2, pp. 216–224, 2013.

[15] A.-R. Han, C. O. Sung, K. M. Kim et al., "The clinicopathological features of gastric hyperplastic polyps with neoplastic transformations: a suggestion of indication for endoscopic polypectomy," *Gut and Liver*, vol. 3, no. 4, pp. 271–275, 2009.

[16] S. W. Carmack, R. M. Genta, D. Y. Graham, and G. Y. Lauwers, "Management of gastric polyps: a pathology-based guide for gastroenterologists," *Nature Reviews Gastroenterology and Hepatology*, vol. 6, no. 6, pp. 331–341, 2009.

12

Nodular Esophageal Xanthoma: A Case Report and Review of the Literature

Ahmed Dirweesh,[1] Muhammad Khan,[1] Sumera Bukhari,[1] Cheryl Rimmer,[2] and Robert Shmuts[3]

[1] *Department of Internal Medicine, Seton Hall University, Hackensack Meridian School of Medicine, Saint Francis Medical Center, Trenton, NJ, USA*
[2] *Department of Pathology, Our Lady of Lourdes Hospital, Willingboro, NJ, USA*
[3] *Department of Gastroenterology, Our Lady of Lourdes Hospital, Willingboro, NJ, USA*

Correspondence should be addressed to Ahmed Dirweesh; adirweesh@stfrancismedical.org

Academic Editor: Chia-Tung Shun

Xanthomas are localized nonneoplastic lesions within tissues that may manifest as papules, plaques, or nodules. These lesions can be found anywhere along the gastrointestinal tract, commonly in the stomach and colon, and rarely in the small intestine and esophagus. Esophagogastroduodenoscopy (EGD) with biopsy is the gold standard tool for diagnosis. Here, we report a rare case of a lower solitary nodular esophageal xanthoma in an elderly black female. Correspondingly, all cases of esophageal xanthomas reported in the English medical literature were reviewed and presented with the reported case.

1. Introduction

Xanthoma (Greek word xanthos meaning "yellow") is an uncommon nonneoplastic lesion resulting from the accumulation of foamy lipid-laden histiocytic cells that can appear anywhere in the body. Most commonly, xanthomas are seen in the skin and tendons, while visceral xanthomas are uncommon. However, their histopathological features are identical regardless of location [1]. The gastrointestinal xanthomas were first described in 1887 as "lipid-laden macrophages in gastric mucosa." The importance and etiology of gastrointestinal xanthomas remain largely unclear [2]. Understanding the endoscopic and pathologic features of these lesions is crucial for their detection and as a differential diagnosis of other pathologies as that may help physicians to appropriately manage these lesions.

2. Case Presentation

A 60-year-old African American female presented with complaints of early satiety. She denied difficulty or pain with swallowing, reflux, vomiting, or regurgitation. She had a past medical history of diabetes mellitus, hypertension, hyperlipidemia, and tubular colonic adenoma. She also had an upper GI series showing questionable delayed esophageal drainage and thickening of esophageal folds concerning possible underlying delayed emptying and possible gastroparesis. She denied tobacco and drug use and consumes alcohol on rare occasions. On examination, vital signs were within normal ranges, and BMI was 36. The rest of the physical examination was normal. Based on her presenting complaints, she underwent an esophagogastroduodenoscopy (EGD) and a gastric emptying scan. EGD was positive for a polyp/nodule at the z-line together with a 1 cm hiatus hernia and gastritis (Figure 1).

Biopsy of the esophageal nodule showed numerous foamy histiocytes in the lamina propria consistent with xanthoma (Figures 2(a), 2(b), and 2(c)).

3. Discussion

Gastrointestinal xanthomas are rare, smooth, yellowish tumor-like benign lesions. They can be incidentally discovered in the upper gastrointestinal tract during endoscopy [3].

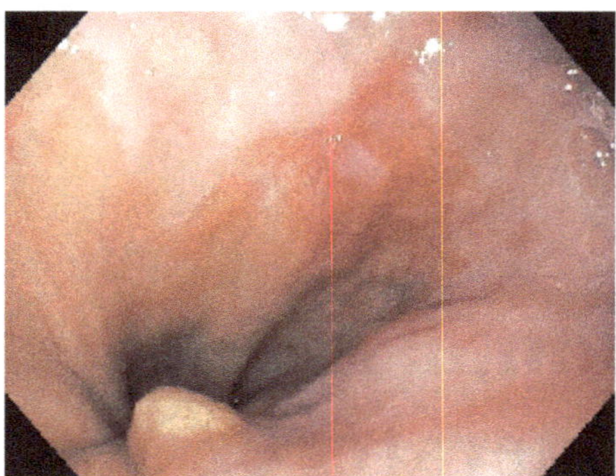

FIGURE 1: EGD showing a polyp (nodule) at the z-line.

The incidence of upper gastrointestinal xanthomas was reported as 0.23% [2]. Though the incidence in the upper gastrointestinal tract may vary among endoscopy series, the most frequent location is the stomach [3], followed by the duodenum and esophagus. One study showed the most common location of ectopic xanthoma in the gastrointestinal tract was the stomach (76%), followed by the esophagus (12%) and duodenum (12%) [2]. Xanthomas are considered as the sign of aging by few authors as the incidence of xanthomas increases with age. The incidence of 53.3% is in the age group of 40–60 years, although it can be seen in people of all ages [2].

Xanthomas are usually asymptomatic and can go undetected if the patient has no associated GI lesions. Their presence may be a manifestation of a metabolic disturbance, such as hyperlipidemia, or can be associated with other conditions such as previous radiotherapy, chemotherapy, and infection [cytomegalovirus (CMV) colitis and disseminated mycobacterium avium intracellulare (MAI)] in immunosuppressed patients (AIDS) [17]. However, it usually represents an isolated phenomenon. The correlation between lipid metabolism disorders and gastrointestinal tract xanthoma is not obvious [18, 19]. Many clinicians believe that yellowish plaque in the gastric mucosa is a benign lesion, and it has no clinical significance. But it can be mistakenly missed for a malignant underlying condition until unless proven by negative biopsy. It is important to distinguish xanthoma on endoscopy from other yellowish lesions such as carcinoid tumor, granular cell tumors, and ectopic sebaceous glands (ESGs).

It has been proposed that a proportion of gastric xanthomas may be provoked by *H. pylori* infection. Arima et al. reported that the prevalence of *H. pylori* infection was significantly higher in patients with gastric xanthomas compared to those without the disease [8, 9].

During endoscopy, xanthomas are shown to be small (1-2 mm) single or multiple yellow, orange, or white well-demarcated sessile macules with irregular outlines that rarely exceed 5 mm [1] though the larger lesions can be seen which may be nodular and elevated [6]. Microscopically, they are composed of compactly aggregated nests of large periodic acid-Schiff- (PAS-) negative round cells with small nuclei and foamy cytoplasm [1]. Most cells are histiocytes, although few other cells like plasma cells, smooth muscle cells, and Schwann cells may add to the entire picture [2].

The importance and etiology of gastrointestinal xanthomas remain largely unclear [2]. Few theories have been proposed by authors, explaining the possible trigger or etiology behind the pathogenesis of xanthomas. Mucosal injury has been presumed to contribute significantly to their pathogenesis as it yields lipid-containing debris, ultimately phagocytized by histiocytes forming foam cells [1]. This hypothesis would clarify why gastric xanthomas seem, by all accounts, to be more successive than esophageal xanthomas, as traumatism and irritation might be better endured by esophageal squamous epithelium than by gastric columnar epithelium [10]. Biliary reflux could be a fundamental etiological part [6].

The clinical significance of xanthomas arises due to the resemblance of features on endoscopy with other benign or malignant lesions. Understanding the endoscopic and pathologic features of xanthomas and other lesions is crucial for their detection and differential diagnosis as that may help physicians to appropriately manage these lesions. Differential diagnosis includes poorly differentiated carcinoma, storage diseases, infections (Whipple disease, mycobacterium, and AIDS), macroglobulinemia, and muciphages. The clinical picture together with the past medical history, symptoms of storage diseases, AIDS, and/or macroglobulinemia, is essential. In addition, special stains such as Gram, Ziehl-Neelsen, Gomori methenamine silver, PAS, and PAS-Diastase and immunohistochemistry for cytokeratin AE1–AE3 can be helpful [17].

Benign esophageal lesions have a broad range of clinical and pathologic features. The prevalence of benign esophageal tumors is under 0.5%, but they signify 20% of esophageal neoplasms on autopsy. With the widespread use of endoscopy, radiologic imaging, and increased awareness of the disease, these lesions could be detected more often [15]. Tsai et al. studied 2,997 patients and observed the frequency of benign epithelial and subepithelial lesions occurring in esophagus. In epithelial lesions, the frequency of occurrence was in the following order: glycogenic acanthosis, heterotopic gastric mucosa, squamous papilloma, hyperplastic polyp, ectopic sebaceous gland, and xanthoma. In subepithelial lesions, the order was as follows: hemangioma, leiomyoma, dysphagia aortica, and granular cell tumor [15].

Esophageal xanthomas, like all upper gastrointestinal tract xanthomas, are asymptomatic, the patients being usually investigated for other conditions. The first reported case occurred in the upper esophagus and was defined as "lipid islands" in 1984 by Remmele and Engelsing [4]. To the best of our knowledge, from 1984 to present, only 21 cases (including the presented one) have been reported (Table 1).

Data from Table 1 reflect the fact that most of these lesions were solitary, were less than 1 cm in size, and could be identified in all the three parts of the esophagus. The largest one of all was reported by Salamanca et al. as a verruciform growth in the upper esophagus in an elderly patient with a history of radiation exposure [12].

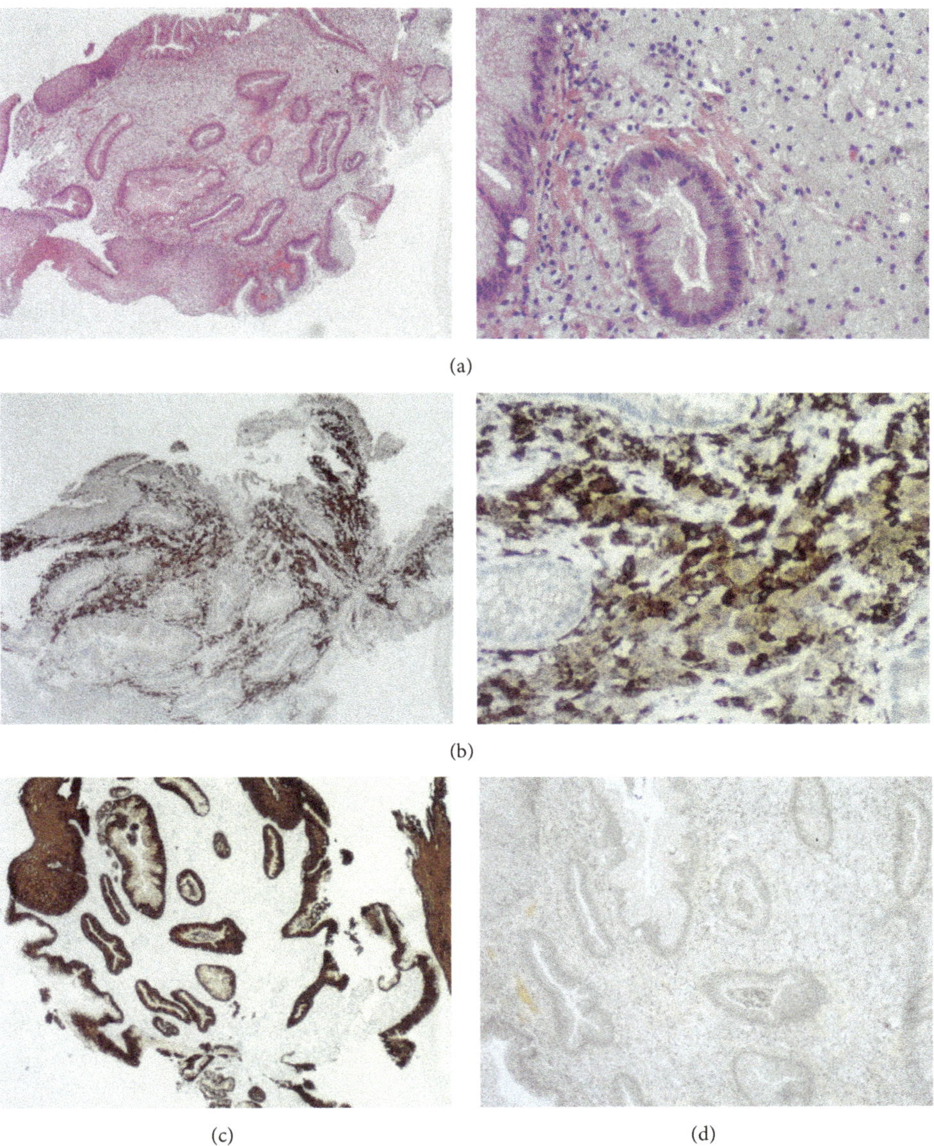

FIGURE 2: (a) Squamous and gastric mucosa with foamy histiocytes in the lamina propria (low and high power). (b) CD68 stain (low and high power) staining histiocytes brown in lamina propria. (c) A negative AE1/AE3 stain ruling out an epithelial lesion (carcinoma) as shown by staining the epithelium but the histiocytes in the lamina propria were negative. (d) A negative mucicarmine special stain ruling out signet ring cell carcinoma.

Esophageal xanthomas have to be grossly distinguished from ectopic sebaceous glands and small subepithelial tumors such as carcinoid and granular cell tumor because most of the reported esophageal xanthomas are yellowish or white mucosal elevated lesions. In terms of microscopic findings, signet ring cell carcinoma, which contains round cells with abundant cytoplasm, should be distinguished. While signet ring cell carcinoma has an eccentrically located nucleus because of the intracellularly abundant mucin, xanthoma has a centrally located and small nucleus. Accumulation of foamy histiocytes of xanthoma could be a clue for the differential diagnosis. In questionable cases, immunohistochemical stains for CD68 can be performed, which indicates a histiocytic origin, another characteristic finding of xanthoma [1]. Besides, esophageal malignancy and ectopic sebaceous glands do not commonly stain with Lugol's solution; consequently, endoscopists should be aware of these lesions for the differential diagnosis [20, 21]. The differential diagnosis becomes clearly inconclusive when biopsies are taken too superficially, permitting just assessment of the epithelium. It is in this way imperative that in any event some lamina propria is available in the biopsy example.

4. Conclusion

In spite of the fact that the etiology and clinical significance of gastrointestinal xanthomas are still obscure, determination of these lesions is imperative since they might coexist

Table 1: Characteristics of reported esophageal xanthomas.

Number	Author(s)	Sex/age (years)	Location	Number of lesions	Size (mm)	Macroscopic findings	Associated medical history
(1)	Remmele and Engelsing [4]	Male/54	Upper	1	10	Yellow spot	Gastrectomy
(2)	Stolte and Seifert [5]	Male/45	Middle	3	<1	Yellow flat elevations	Hyperlipidemia, diabetes mellitus
(3)	Vimala et al. [6]	Female/37	Lower	Multiple	2–5	Yellowish nodular	Gastric xanthoma
(4)	Hirokawa et al. [1]	Female/52	Lower	1	2	Yellowish granular	Duodenal ulcer
(5)	Hirokawa et al. [1]	Male/67	Lower	1	2	Yellow spots	Hepatocellular carcinoma, hypertension
(6)	Herrera-Goepfert et al. [7]	Male/61	Middle	1	5	Verruciform	Non-Hodgkin lymphoma of the testis
(7)	Gencosmanoglu et al. [2]	Not specified	Not specified	Multiple	<5	Yellow-white colored plaques	Not specified
(8)	Gencosmanoglu et al. [2]	Not specified	Not specified	1	<5	Yellow-white colored plaques	Not specified
(9)	Gencosmanoglu et al. [2]	Male/49	Lower	1	3	Yellowish elevated granular lesion	Atrophic gastritis
(10)	Arima [8]	Male/74	Middle	1	4	Yellowish white patch	Not specified
(11)	Arima [8]	Male/74	Upper	1	2	Whitish protruding lesion	Not specified
(12)	Licci et al. [9]	Male/49	Upper	1	3	Verruciform	Not specified
(13)	Becheanu et al. [10]	Male/72	Lower	1	3	Yellowish elevated granular lesion	Atrophic gastritis
(14)	Arima [8]	Female/56	Lower	1	4	Yellowish elevated lesion	Biermer anemia, antral hyperplastic polyp with focal adenocarcinoma, atrophic gastritis
(15)	Min et al. [11]	Female/74	Middle	1	3	Verruciform	Atrophic gastritis, hyperlipidemia, dementia
(16)	Salamanca et al. [12]	Male/70	Upper	1	20	Verruciform	Hypertension, HCV, hemochromatosis, glottis cancer, hepatocellular carcinoma, tracheal cancer
(17)	Park et al. [13]	Male/67	Lower	1	2	White-yellowish elevated lesion	Ileocecal lymphoma
(18)	Bang et al. [14]	Male/70	Upper	1	3	Yellowish granular elevated lesion	Gastric and duodenal ulcer
(19)	Tsai et al. [15]	Male/62	Middle and lower	Multiple	2–10	Well-defined, fern-like, and yellowish lesions	Not specified
(20)	Díaz Del Arco et al. [16]	Female/56	Lower	1	13	Sessile polyp with white vascular surface	Segmental pneumonectomy for bronchiectasis, partial fundoplication for GERD
(21)	Our case	Female/60	Lower	1	1	Polyp/nodule	Diabetes, hypertension, hyperlipidemia, tubular colonic adenoma

with malignant lesions. Having endoscopic resection of all granular cell tumors and squamous papillomas in light of the fact that, while uncommon, these lesions have malignant potential is suggestive.

References

[1] M. Hirokawa, R. Takenaka, A. Takahashi et al., "Esophageal xanthoma: report of two cases and a review of the literature," *Journal of Gastroenterology and Hepatology*, vol. 18, no. 9, pp. 1105–1108, 2003.

[2] R. Gencosmanoglu, E. Sen-Oran, O. Kurtkaya-Yapicier, and N. Tozun, "Xanthelasmas of the upper gastrointestinal tract," *Journal of Gastroenterology*, vol. 39, no. 3, pp. 215–219, 2004.

[3] E. Kaiserling, H. Heinle, H. Itabe, T. Takano, and W. Remmele, "Lipid islands in human gastric mucosa: morphological and immunohistochemical findings," *Gastroenterology*, vol. 110, no. 2, pp. 369–374, 1996.

[4] W. Remmele and B. Engelsing, "Lipid island of the esophagus. Case report," *Endoscopy*, vol. 16, no. 6, pp. 240–241, 1984.

[5] M. Stolte and E. Seifert, "Lipid islets in the esophagus," *Leber Magen Darm*, vol. 15, no. 4, pp. 137–139, 1985.

[6] R. Vimala, V. Ananthalakshmi, M. Murthy, T. R. Shankar, and V. Jayanthi, "Xanthelasma of esophagus and stomach," *Indian Journal of Gastroenterology*, vol. 19, no. 3, p. 135, 2000.

[7] R. Herrera-Goepfert, M. Lizano-Soberón, and M. Garcia-Perales, "Verruciform xanthoma of the esophagus," *Human Pathology*, vol. 34, no. 8, pp. 814–815, 2003.

[8] M. Arima, "Esophageal xanthoma: report of two cases," *Stomach Intest*, vol. 43, pp. 317–320, 2008.

[9] S. Licci, S. M. A. Campo, and P. Ventura, "Verruciform xanthoma of the esophagus: an uncommon entity in an unusual site," *Endoscopy*, vol. 42, supplement 2, article E330, 2010.

[10] G. Becheanu, M. Dumbrava, T. Arbanas, M. Diculescu, N. Hoyeau-Idrissi, and J.-F. Fléjou, "Esophageal xanthoma—report of two new cases and review of the literature," *Journal of Gastrointestinal and Liver Diseases*, vol. 20, no. 4, pp. 431–433, 2011.

[11] K.-W. Min, J.-S. Koh, K. G. Lee, H. C. Kim, K.-S. Jang, and S. S. Paik, "Verruciform xanthoma arising in the mid esophagus," *Digestive Endoscopy*, vol. 24, no. 5, article 387, 2012.

[12] J. Salamanca, I. Alemany, G. Sosa, F. Pinedo, S. Hernando, and P. Martín-Acosta, "Esophageal verruciform xanthoma following radiotherapy," *Gastroenterologia y Hepatologia*, vol. 35, no. 5, pp. 317–320, 2012.

[13] H. S. Park, K. Y. Jang, and W. S. Moon, "Incidental esophageal xanthoma in a patient with ileocecal lymphoma," *Digestive Endoscopy*, vol. 25, no. 1, pp. 92–93, 2013.

[14] C. S. Bang, Y. S. Kim, G. H. Baik, and S. H. Han, "Xanthoma of the esophagus," *Clinical Endoscopy*, vol. 47, no. 4, pp. 358–361, 2014.

[15] S.-J. Tsai, C.-C. Lin, C.-W. Chang et al., "Benign esophageal lesions: endoscopic and pathologic features," *World Journal of Gastroenterology*, vol. 21, no. 4, pp. 1091–1098, 2015.

[16] C. Díaz Del Arco, Á. Álvarez Sánchez, and M. J. Fernández Aceñero, "Non-gastric gastrointestinal xanthomas: case series and literature review," *Journal of Gastrointestinal and Liver Diseases*, vol. 25, no. 3, pp. 389–394, 2016.

[17] L. E. Barrera-Herrera, F. Arias, P. A. Rodríguez-Urrego, and M. A. Palau-Lázaro, "Small bowel obstruction due to intestinal Xanthomatosis," *Case Reports in Pathology*, vol. 2015, Article ID 231830, 4 pages, 2015.

[18] S. Y. Yi, "Dyslipidemia and H pylori in gastric xanthomatosis," *World Journal of Gastroenterology*, vol. 13, no. 34, pp. 4598–4601, 2007.

[19] T. Niemann, H. P. Marti, S. H. Duhnsen, and G. Bongartz, "Pulmonary schistosomiasis-imaging features," *Journal of Radiology Case Reports*, vol. 4, no. 9, pp. 37–43, 2010.

[20] Y. S. Kim, S. Y. Jin, and C. S. Shim, "Esophageal ectopic sebaceous glands," *Clinical Gastroenterology and Hepatology*, vol. 5, no. 1, article A23, 2007.

[21] D. S. Cho, H. K. Park, S. K. Park et al., "An esophageal xanthoma diagnosed by upper gastrointestinal endoscopy," *The Korean Journal of Medicine*, vol. 75, supplement 3, pp. S784–S786, 2008.

Acute Cholangitis following Biliary Obstruction after Duodenal OTSC Placement in a Case of Large Chronic Duodenocutaneous Fistula

Yaseen Alastal,[1] Tariq A. Hammad,[1] Mohamad Nawras,[1] Basmah W. Khalil,[1] Osama Alaradi,[2] and Ali Nawras[2]

[1]*Department of Internal Medicine, University of Toledo Medical Center, Toledo, OH 43614, USA*
[2]*Department of Gastroenterology and Hepatology, University of Toledo Medical Center, Toledo, OH 43614, USA*

Correspondence should be addressed to Ali Nawras; ali.nawras@utoledo.edu

Academic Editor: Christoph Vogt

Over-the-Scope Clip system, also called "Bear Claw," is a novel endoscopic modality used for closure of gastrointestinal defect with high efficacy and safety. We present a patient with history of eosinophilic gastroenteritis and multiple abdominal surgeries including Billroth II gastrectomy complicated by a large chronic duodenocutaneous fistula from a Billroth II afferent limb to the abdominal wall. Bear Claw clip was used for closure of this fistula. The patient developed acute cholangitis one day after placement of the Bear Claw clip. Acute cholangitis due to papillary obstruction is a potential complication of Bear Claw placement at the dome of the duodenal stump (afferent limb) in patient with Billroth II surgery due to its close proximity to the major papilla.

1. Introduction

Over-the-Scope Clip (OTSC) system, also called "Bear Claw," is a novel endoscopic modality used for closure of gastrointestinal defect. Current retrospective studies suggest high efficacy and safety of the device. Herein we present a patient who developed acute cholangitis one day after placement of Bear Claw clip for closure of duodenocutaneous fistula from the afferent enteric limb of Billroth II. This complication is unreported in the literature after placement of Bear Claw clip.

2. Case Presentation

28-year-old female patient with history of eosinophilic gastroenteritis and multiple abdominal surgeries including Billroth II gastrectomy referred to our hospital for treatment of duodenocutaneous fistula. She had large chronic duodenocutaneous fistula measuring about 0.8 cm in diameter extending from Billroth II afferent limb to the abdominal wall. Multiple previous attempts to close the fistula have failed. The patient was scheduled for elective cutaneous and enteric closure of the fistula with fibrin glue and Bear Claw endoclip placement, respectively. During the procedure, a pediatric colonoscope was introduced into the blind enteric limb; the major papilla was identified 3-4 cm proximal to the dome of the blind limb. India ink was injected through the cutaneous orifice of the fistula to localize the internal orifice in the dome of the blind limb (Figure 1). A 0.035 inch × 450 cm guide wire was introduced through the cutaneous orifice and advanced into the blind enteric limb under endoscopic and fluoroscopic guidance; the guide wire was grasped with rat tooth biopsy forceps. The pediatric colonoscope was then withdrawn with the guide wire. Subsequently, the scope was changed to an adult gastroscope. An 11/6 t Bear Claw endoclip was secured on the tip of the gastroscope; then the gastroscope with the Bear Claw endoclip was reintroduced over the guide wire into the afferent duodenal limb. The enteric orifice of the fistula was suctioned inside the cap of the Bear Claw with the wire still inside the fistula and scope channel (Figure 2). Once the fistula site at the dome of the afferent limb was seen filling the cap, the guide wire was removed and the clip was deployed successfully closing the enteric orifice of the fistula (Figure 3) (the attached video demonstrates the key portions of Bear Claw placement procedure in our patient). The position

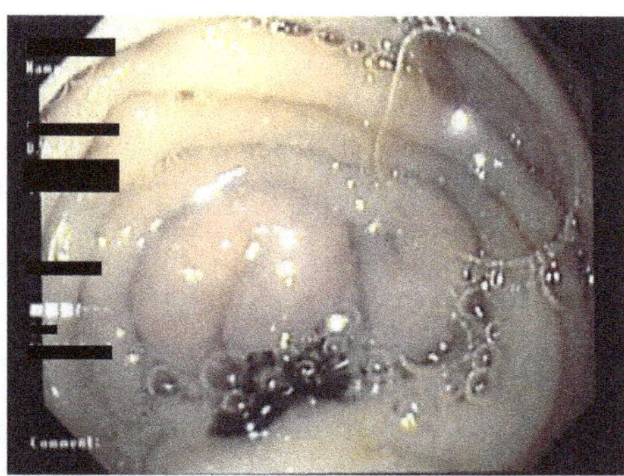

FIGURE 1: Spot draining from the internal fistula orifice at the dome of the blind limb of Billroth II after injecting it percutaneously.

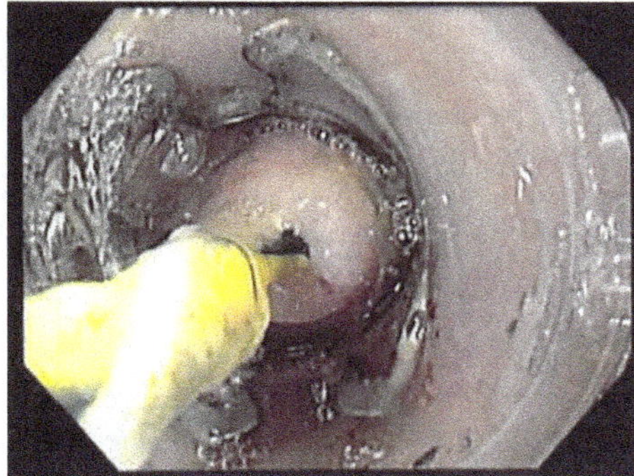

FIGURE 2: Enteric orifice of the fistula suctioned inside the cap of the Bear Claw with the guide wire still inside the fistula locating in the center.

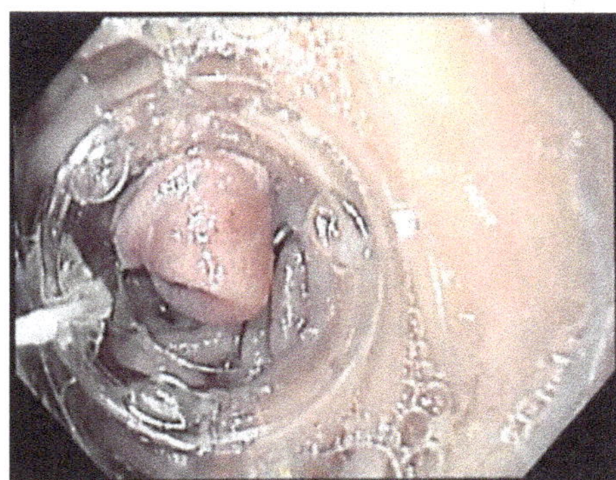

FIGURE 3: Bear Claw clip deployed at the enteric orifice of the fistula within the afferent limb.

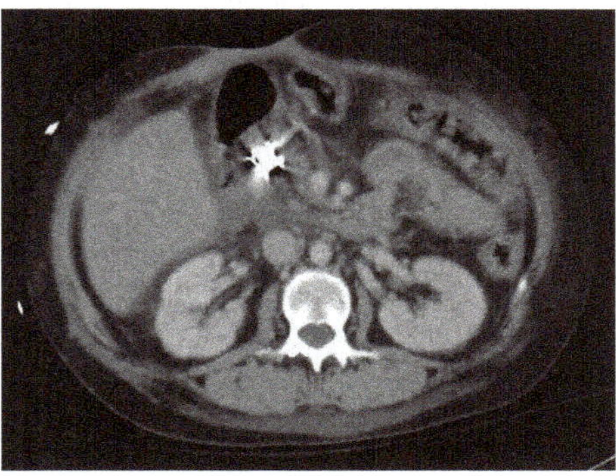

FIGURE 4: Bear Claw clip placed in the afferent loop of the Billroth II with mild edema surrounding this region.

of the Bear Claw endoclip was confirmed endoscopically and fluoroscopically. Subsequently, the cutaneous orifice was identified and injected with fibrin glue. The patient tolerated the procedure well without immediate complications and was discharged home for outpatient follow-up. On the next day, the patient developed fever, jaundice, changes in mental status, and abdominal pain. Her vital signs were as follows: blood pressure: 124/68, pulse rate: 151 beats per minutes, temperature: 40.1°C, and respiratory rate: 28 per minute. Abdominal examination revealed diffuse tenderness. Laboratory work showed white blood cell counts of 5×10^9/L (normal range: 4–10 $\times 10^9$/L), direct bilirubin of 3.3 mg/dL (normal range: 0–0.3 mg/dL), and Alkaline phosphatase, aspartate, and alanine aminotransferase levels of 255 U/L (normal range: 45–115 U/L), 272 U/L (normal range: 8–48 U/L), and 134 U/L (normal range: 7–55 U/L), respectively. Amylase and lipase were normal. Abdominal ultrasound revealed dilation of the common bile duct (1.2 cm) with intrahepatic biliary dilation. Abdominal CT scan showed mild edema surrounding the endoclip in the afferent loop of the Billroth II with no definite abscess or fluid collection (Figure 4). The pancreas was normal. HIDA scan suggested biliary obstruction. The patient was diagnosed with acute cholangitis secondary to biliary obstruction due to Bear Claw placement close to the major papilla grasping adjacent tissue. She was managed with empirical antibiotics and supportive care. Upon patient's family preference, percutaneous transhepatic cholangiography (PTC) was done rather than ERCP. PTC showed diffuse dilation of the biliary tree down to the papilla. Percutaneous transhepatic drainage was performed and the guide wire was advanced into the duodenum through the major papilla adjacent to the Bear Claw clip which was causing partial obstruction (Figure 5). An 8 French pigtail catheter was placed down to the duodenum. As a result, the patient had clinical and laboratory improvement. Five months later, the fistula did not close completely and the patient underwent laparotomy repair which involved dissection of the fistula from the surrounding adhesions and duodenotomy around it, followed by excision of the tract and the attached duodenal wall. The Bear Claw was not palpable on the duodenal wall during surgery which suggested spontaneous migration before surgery. The duodenal stump was sutured and covered with omental patch. The patient had an uneventful postoperative recovery with no recurrence of fistula after surgery.

3. Discussion

Therapeutic endoscopic procedures are rapidly evolving in the field of gastroenterology and have been showing promising results as minimal invasive interventions for treating gastrointestinal (GI) pathologies. Over-the-Scope Clip (OTSC)

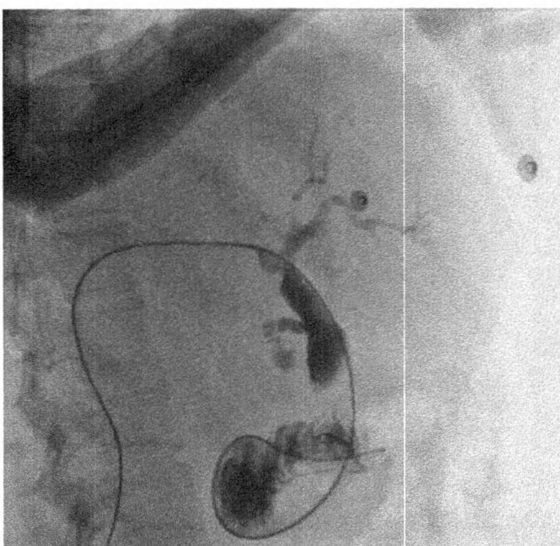

FIGURE 5: Percutaneous transhepatic cholangiography showed diffuse dilation of the biliary tree and the guide wire passing through the major papilla just adjacent to the Bear Claw clip.

system is one of this novel endoscopic modalities which was approved in Europe in 2009 and then by the US Food and Drug Administration (FDA) in 2010 [1]. OTSC system has been used mainly in closure of luminal gastrointestinal defects like fistulas and perforation but other uses have been described like treatment of bleeding lesions, resection of submucosal neoplasms, and stents fixation [2]. When compared to standard endoclips, it showed more efficacy and better safety for closure of gastrostomies up to 18 mm in diameter [3]. This is because of its ability to grasp more tissues up to the entire thickness of the visceral wall and applying a greater compression force [1]. Overall success rates of OTSC in the literature range from 75% to 100% for closure of iatrogenic gastrointestinal perforations, 38% to 100% for closure of gastrointestinal fistulas, 50% to 100% for anastomotic leaks, and 71% to 100% for bleeding lesions [4]. According to an international multicenter retrospective study of 188 patients who underwent attempted OTSC placement for GI defects, the rate of successful closure of perforations (90%) and leaks (73.3%) was significantly higher than that of fistulae (42.9%) [5]. At this time, the safety of the device cannot be assessed accurately as most of published studies are case reports and retrospective studies, with no long term follow-up studies. However, most of the current case series did not report any complication after using the Bear Claw [3, 6–8]. A prospective multicenter study by Voermans et al. reported one patient who developed esophageal perforation while introducing the endoscope with the OTSC. They related that to the OTSC cap which has 2 mm protruding plastic rim that might make it slightly more traumatic than standard plastic caps widely used for rubber band ligation [9]. The same study also reported a patient with persistent perforation secondary to clip detachment after he underwent OTSC for colonic perforation after polypectomy; subsequently he died secondary to peritonitis [9]. Surace et al. reported one complication in their case series related to the delivery system of the clip as the anchor was blocked within the clip resulting in inability to be immediately withdrawn; then it was removed endoscopically after 7 days [10]. Acute cholangitis is a serious condition which has not been reported in the literature as a complication of this procedure. We describe the first case report of acute cholangitis developed directly after Bear Claw endoclip placement for closure of duodenocutaneous fistula in patient with Billroth II surgery. In our patient the enteric site of the fistula was at the dome of the blind enteric loop of Billroth II which is also the site of biliary tract drainage. The close proximity between the enteric site of the fistula and the major papilla within the afferent limb can explain the reason for developing this complication. Deploying a Bear Claw clip at the end of the afferent limb carries a risk of either complete obstruction of the major papilla by direct occlusion from the clip itself or partial obstruction by inducing edema at the surrounding tissue (as in our case). Deployment of Bear Claw clip in the duodenum has been described in the literature, as Haito-Chavez et al. included 11 cases in their retrospective analysis who underwent Bear Claw placement in the duodenum but there was no procedure related complication [5]. However none of the Bear Claw clips was reported to be deployed in the afferent limb (duodenal stump) of patient with Billroth II surgery.

Duodenocutaneous fistulae closure is considered a therapeutic challenge. With the internal orifice being at the afferent limb of Billroth II, this adds more difficulty into closing this fistula endoscopically. Only one case report in the literature described endoscopic closure of an iatrogenic duodenocutaneous fistula in a Billroth II afferent limb [11]. In this case report, endoscopist successfully used three standard endoclips to approximate the fistula opening which resulted from pinpoint duodenotomy defect occurring during dissection. Our reported case is the first case in the literature to use Bear Claw clip for closure of duodenocutaneous fistula from a Billroth II afferent limb. The reason for using Bear Claw endoclip instead of standard endoclip in our patient was related to the characteristics of the fistula. It was chronic, persistent despite multiple previous attempts of closure and relatively too large to be fully contained with the standard endoclip. In our case, the Bear Claw placement was unsuccessful in closing the fistula. To the best of our knowledge, clinical success rates of chronic fistula closure were poor compared to acute phase, and delayed closure remains challenging [12]. Additionally, the fistula leakage was large which decreased the chance of successful closure. Endoscopic vacuum therapy (EVT) is a new technique which was introduced in the last few years as an alternative treatment for esophageal perforation and some other postoperative leakages [13]. It involves placement of an endoscopic vacuum polyurethane sponge under direct endoscopic visualization followed by transnasal application of external vacuum. A very few successful treatments have been reported, adapting EVT by intraluminal approach to close duodenal leakage and guide biliary secretion [14, 15]. One report described an endoscopic pull-through technique where the polyurethane foam drainage was introduced through a visible percutaneous abdominal drainage site [16]. In our case, this technique could have been utilized to introduce the vacuum sponge onto the defect zone given the large defect size and high drainage output, which might help in healing the duodenocutaneous fistula.

We faced some technical challenges in performing this procedure. One of these challenges was advancing the gastroscope with the Bear Claw secured to the tip of the scope into the afferent limb. This was facilitated with wire guidance advanced percutaneously through the fistula and grasped with forceps and pulled into the scope channel. Another challenge was the mobility of the afferent limb which could have altered the suctioned position of the duodenal wall within the cap of the clip prior to deploying it despite the wire guidance. Moreover, despite using a guide wire to stabilize the suctioned portion of the duodenal stump to avoid the papilla, the endoclip was still deployed close to the papilla. Perhaps using the anchor might have stabilized the suctioned portion better than the guide wire. Also, Gentle care needs to be taken applying additional suction, especially when fistula is underlying nearby biliary tract. Endoscopist should be careful with placement of OTSC in the afferent limb of Billroth II surgery as it can directly or indirectly result in papillary obstruction and acute cholangitis.

4. Conclusion

Over-the-Scope Clip system is a new endoscopic modality with high efficacy and safety in closure of duodenocutaneous fistulas. Acute cholangitis due to papillary obstruction is a potential complication of OTSC placement at the dome of the duodenal stump (afferent limb) in patient with Billroth II surgery due to its close proximity to the major papilla.

Consent

Consent was obtained from the patient per our institution policy.

Authors' Contribution

Yaseen Alastal and Tariq A. Hammad contributed equally to this paper.

References

[1] S. Banerjee, B. A. Barth, Y. M. Bhat et al., "Endoscopic closure devices," *Gastrointestinal Endoscopy*, vol. 76, no. 2, pp. 244–251, 2012.

[2] K. Mönkemüller, S. Peter, J. Toshniwal et al., "Multipurpose use of the 'bear claw' (over-the-scope-clip system) to treat endoluminal gastrointestinal disorders," *Digestive Endoscopy*, vol. 26, no. 3, pp. 350–357, 2014.

[3] D. V. Renteln, M. C. Vassiliou, and R. I. Rothstein, "Randomized controlled trial comparing endoscopic clips and over-the-scope clips for closure of natural orifice transluminal endoscopic surgery gastrotomies," *Endoscopy*, vol. 41, no. 12, pp. 1056–1061, 2009.

[4] S. Singhal, K. Changela, H. Papafragkakis, S. Anand, M. Krishnaiah, and S. Duddempudi, "Over the scope clip: technique and expanding clinical applications," *Journal of Clinical Gastroenterology*, vol. 47, no. 9, pp. 749–756, 2013.

[5] Y. Haito-Chavez, J. K. Law, T. Kratt et al., "International multicenter experience with an over-the-scope clipping device for endoscopic management of GI defects (with video)," *Gastrointestinal Endoscopy*, vol. 80, no. 4, pp. 610–622, 2014.

[6] T. H. Kothari, G. Haber, N. Sonpal, and N. Karanth, "The over-the-scope clip system—a novel technique for gastrocutaneous fistula closure: the first North American experience," *Canadian Journal of Gastroenterology*, vol. 26, no. 4, pp. 193–195, 2012.

[7] N. Nishiyama, H. Mori, H. Kobara et al., "Efficacy and safety of over-the-scope clip: including complications after endoscopic submucosal dissection," *World Journal of Gastroenterology*, vol. 19, no. 18, pp. 2752–2760, 2013.

[8] M. C. Sulz, R. Bertolini, R. Frei, G. M. Semadeni, J. Borovicka, and C. Meyenberger, "Multipurpose use of the over-the-scope-clip system ('Bear claw') in the gastrointestinal tract: Swiss experience in a tertiary center," *World Journal of Gastroenterology*, vol. 20, no. 43, pp. 16287–16292, 2014.

[9] R. P. Voermans, O. Le Moine, D. von Renteln et al., "Efficacy of endoscopic closure of acute perforations of the gastrointestinal tract," *Clinical Gastroenterology and Hepatology*, vol. 10, no. 6, pp. 603–608, 2012.

[10] M. Surace, P. Mercky, J.-F. Demarquay et al., "Endoscopic management of GI fistulae with the over-the-scope clip system (with video)," *Gastrointestinal Endoscopy*, vol. 74, no. 6, pp. 1416–1419, 2011.

[11] M. T. Voellinger, R. Knodell, and N. Choueiri, "Enterocutaneous fistula from a billroth II afferent limb: successful closure with endoclips," *ACG Case Reports Journal*, vol. 1, no. 2, pp. 76–78, 2014.

[12] R. Mennigen, N. Senninger, and M. G. Laukoetter, "Novel treatment options for perforations of the upper gastrointestinal tract: endoscopic vacuum therapy and over-the-scope clips," *World Journal of Gastroenterology*, vol. 20, no. 24, pp. 7767–7776, 2014.

[13] M. Bludau, A. H. Hölscher, T. Herbold et al., "Management of upper intestinal leaks using an endoscopic vacuum-assisted closure system (E-VAC)," *Surgical Endoscopy*, vol. 28, no. 3, pp. 896–901, 2014.

[14] T. Schorsch, C. Müller, and G. Loske, "Pancreatico-gastric anastomotic insufficiency successfully treated with endoscopic vacuum therapy," *Endoscopy*, vol. 45, supplement 2, pp. E141–E142, 2013.

[15] G. Loske, T. Schorsch, and C. T. Mueller, "Endoscopic intraluminal vacuum therapy of duodenal perforation," *Endoscopy*, vol. 42, no. 2, p. E109, 2010.

[16] A. Fischer, H. J. Richter-Schrag, J. Hoeppner, A. Braun, and S. Utzolino, "Endoscopic intracavitary pull-through vacuum treatment of an insufficient pancreaticogastrostomy," *Endoscopy*, vol. 46, no. 1, pp. E218–E219, 2014.

14

Intestinal Amyloidosis in Common Variable Immunodeficiency and Rheumatoid Arthritis

T. Meira,[1] R. Sousa,[1] A. Cordeiro,[2] R. Ilgenfritz,[3] and P. Borralho[3]

[1]*Gastroenterology Department, Hospital Garcia de Orta E.P.E., Avenida Torrado da Silva, 2801-951 Almada, Portugal*
[2]*Rheumatology Department, Hospital Garcia de Orta E.P.E., Avenida Torrado da Silva, 2801-951 Almada, Portugal*
[3]*Anatomical Pathology Department, Hospital Garcia de Orta E.P.E., Avenida Torrado da Silva, 2801-951 Almada, Portugal*

Correspondence should be addressed to T. Meira; tania_meira@hotmail.com

Academic Editor: Özlem Yönem

We present a case of reactive amyloidosis that developed secondary to common variable immunodeficiency and rheumatoid arthritis. A 66-year-old woman, with prior history of common variable immunodeficiency and rheumatoid arthritis, was referred to our clinic for chronic diarrhea investigation. The patient was submitted to colonoscopy with ileoscopy, which did not show relevant endoscopic alterations. However, undertaken biopsies revealed amyloid deposition. Since amyloidosis with GI involvement is a rare cause of chronic diarrhea, this pathology should be considered in etiologic investigation, especially when associated with chronic inflammatory diseases.

1. Introduction

Amyloidosis is a rare disease resulting from extracellular deposition of insoluble fibrillar proteins, subclassified as primary when fibrils result from monoclonal light chain fragments deposition and as secondary when the accumulated material is serum amyloid A [1]. In the past, the main cause for AA amyloidosis was chronic infectious diseases, such as tuberculosis. Nowadays, 50% of cases are due to chronic inflammatory diseases, with rheumatoid arthritis (RA) being the most frequent one, followed by ankylosing spondylitis and psoriatic arthritis [2].

In secondary subclassification, amyloidosis histological gastrointestinal (GI) involvement is very common, although clinically overt disease is rare [2]. On the contrary, in primary amyloidosis GI involvement occurs less frequently, once only 8% have amyloid tissue infiltration and 1% of patients have GI symptoms [3].

We report an unusual case of intestinal AA amyloidosis in a patient with common variable immunodeficiency and rheumatoid arthritis.

2. Case Report

A 66-year-old female with history of pleuropulmonary tuberculosis in 1979 and a thymoma in 2006 was submitted to resection and adjuvant radiotherapy. Since 2006, the patient has been investigated for recurrent respiratory tract infection. According to the complementary investigation conducted, our patient was submitted to a chest computed tomography, which showed bilateral interstitial thickening and bronchiectasis in the right hemithorax (Figure 1), leading to the conclusion of being radiation pneumonitis.

Also in 2006, she was referred to Rheumatology clinics for arthritis and rheumatoid factor and antinuclear antibody positives. Laboratory studies revealed the following: high serum value of C-reactive protein (CRP) 22 mg/dL (normal range: <0.1) and decreased immunoglobulins, IgG 593 mg/dL (normal range: 700–1000), IgA 40 mg/dL (normal range: 70–400), and IgM 8 mg/dL (normal range: 40–230). After exclusion of other rheumatic conditions, the diagnosis of rheumatoid arthritis was assumed. Due to high articular activity, immunomodulation was introduced starting with

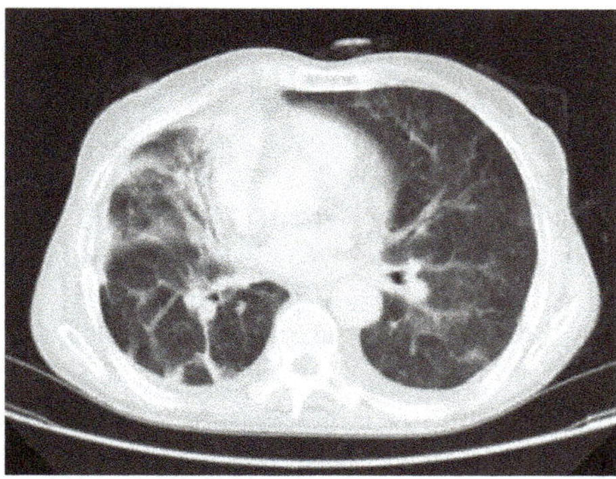

Figure 1: Chest computed tomography: bilateral interstitial thickening and bronchiectasis in the right hemithorax.

increasing doses of sulphasalazine, up to 3 g per day (patient refused methotrexate), hydroxychloroquine, naproxen up to 1000 mg per day, deflazacort 6 mg/day, alendronic acid 70 mg/week, and calcium, resulting in partial improvement of arthritis. She was referred to Hematology that confirmed the diagnosis as Common Variable Immunodeficiency, initiating a monthly treatment with intravenous human immunoglobulin.

Two years after the diagnosis, the patient had worsened articular activity and developed watery diarrhea, with average stools frequency of up to 4 to 5 times a day with no blood, mucus, or pus, along with intermittent abdominal pain. She denied fever, hematic losses, anorexia, weight loss, and profuse sweating. Abdominal physical examination was unremarkable and laboratory findings revealed the following: no anemia, thrombocytosis of 487000 platelets/L (normal values: 120–44000), erythrocyte sedimentation rate (ESR) 28 mm/h (normal value: 0–15), and 3.6 mg/dL of CRP. Microbiologic and parasitological analyses of the stools were negative. HIV and anti-CMV IgM serologies were negative. The colonoscopy with ileoscopy showed an accentuated vascular pattern along the colon, with no other significant changes. Biopsies were obtained from different colon segments. Microscopically, deposition of amorphous hyaline material that infiltrated the submucosa wall in colon with hematoxylin-eosin was observed. Congo red staining allowed detection of green birefringence on fibrils (Figure 2). Immunohistochemistry showed marking of AA proteins, confirming a reactive amyloidosis (Figures 3 and 4). Additional investigation was performed having excluded renal involvement by amyloidosis, with no changes in proteinuria and creatinine clearance.

The patient became asymptomatic after controlling RA activity with the addition of Tocilizumab, a biologic agent (TB reactivation excluded: chest CT, bronchofiberscopy, and cultures), and has been kept under surveillance without GI symptoms.

3. Discussion

Common variable immunodeficiency (CVID) is the most symptomatic primary antibody deficiency, characterized by hypogammaglobulinemia, leading primarily to recurrent pulmonary or GI infections [4]. Such as in our case, where the patient had recurrent pulmonary infection after treatment for thymoma, these complications may be present at the onset or may appear later.

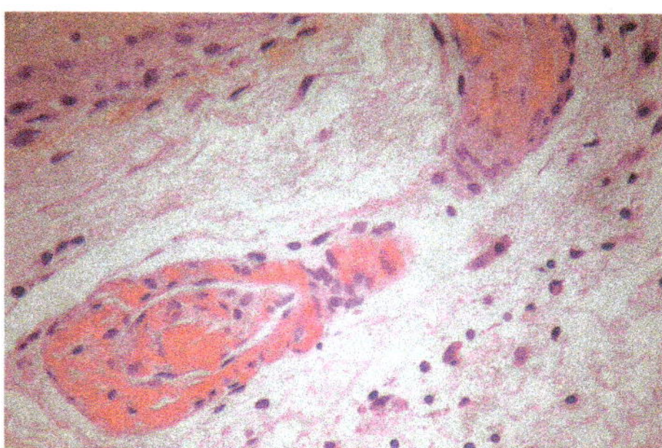

Figure 2: Perivascular amyloid deposit in colon submucosa (Congo red staining without polarization).

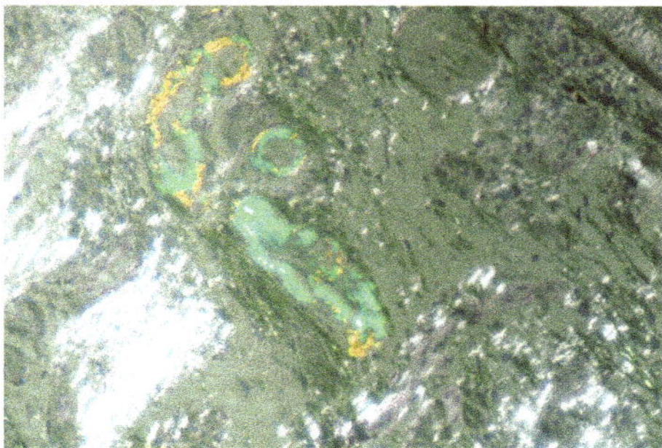

Figure 3: Perivascular amyloid deposit in colon submucosa (Congo red staining, with polarization).

In about 20% of the cases, common variable immunodeficiency is also associated with autoimmune diseases, such as rheumatoid arthritis [5]. In our case, the RA diagnostic was established simultaneously with CVID. While the pathogenesis of autoreactivity is unknown for CVID subjects in general, and to a greater extent for those with autoimmunity, there is a loss of switched memory B cells [5].

The incidence of gastrointestinal diseases in CVID group has a considerable relevance, referred to be between 20 and 60%, with the chronic diarrhea being the most common presentation of this disease [6]. Between 6 and 10% of CVID patients develop inflammatory bowel disease-like disorder and a poor group develop celiac enteropathy like lymphoma, gastric adenocarcinoma, and intestinal amyloidosis. The alterations on immune mediators such as impaired antibody production, disruption on T-cell function, and defects in innate immunity could be responsible for GI disease observed in CVID patients [6]. The secondary amyloidosis is a rather rare complication of the CVID; a time frame of 8 to 14 years between the AA amyloidosis diagnostic and the CVID inflammatory condition is seldom observed [7]. All amyloidosis CVID cases have recurrent infections, which was also observed in our patient, consisting in a relevant condition supposed to be related to amyloidosis progression [7]. The intravenous immunoglobulin administration decreased our

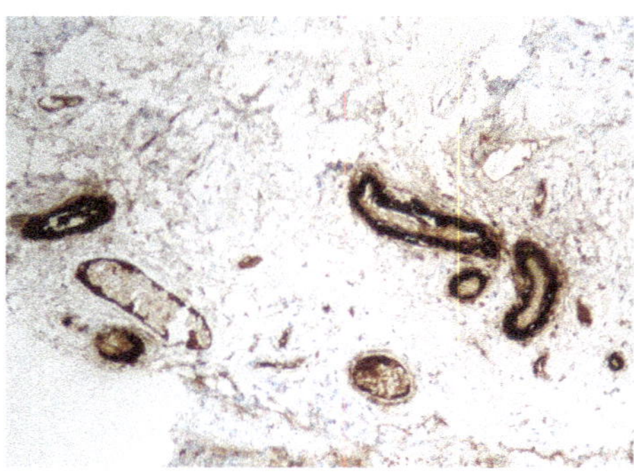

FIGURE 4: Immunolabeling pattern with monoclonal anti-amyloid A antibody (mcl clone).

patient's episodes of pulmonary infections but not the GI symptoms.

Recently, LRP12 mutations were found in patients with intestinal amyloidosis and CVID, which denotes the complex association between immunodeficiency and autoinflammatory disease [8].

Rheumatoid arthritis can either be associated with CVID or be an independent condition for amyloidosis development, which was not possible to determine in our case. Nowadays, RA is known to be one of the most common causes of AA amyloidosis, with a prevalence between 10 and 29% of patients with such disorder, varying according to different previous studies [9], usually associated with long duration (7 to 10 years) and uncontrolled rheumatoid arthritis. Our patient had a short duration and nonerosive arthritis at amyloidosis diagnosis, which however could have been a subclinical disease. Rheumatoid arthritis therapeutics aims to achieve disease remission by suppressing inflammation and immunological dysregulation [10]. Sulphasalazine was initially chosen instead of methotrexate, either due to the patient's refusal of that drug or due to the potentially limiting pulmonary drug toxicity. However, articular inflammatory activity was recurrently observed, requiring a more potent therapeutic approach.

Due to the history of pulmonary tuberculosis and immunomodulator therapy, mycobacterium intestinal infection should be excluded. The patient did not present clinical evidence of pulmonary tuberculosis and had normal chest X-ray. However, 76% of intestinal tuberculosis cases may occur in asymptomatic patients. The absence of granuloma or alcohol-acid-resistant bacilli at colonic biopsy leads to disregarding such hypothesis [11].

Independently of the trigger for secondary AA, there are unspecific gastrointestinal symptoms, varying from gastrointestinal haemorrhage to chronic intestinal dysmotility, or malabsorption caused by colon mucosa infiltration and bacterial overgrowth, or even exudative gastroenteropathy. Its endoscopic appearance derives from colon mucosa infiltration, more frequent at the descendent duodenum followed by stomach, colon, and esophagus. Intestinal mucosa may present itself slightly granular and friable erosions, ulcerations, and submucosa hematomas; nevertheless, polypoid or nodular lesions can rarely occur [1, 12]. Intestinal biopsies are diagnostic of AA amyloidosis in 75–95% of cases and it should be performed even in the presence of normal appearing mucosa [13].

Several studies have focused on genetic factors, with prognostic significance, which might increase susceptibility to AA, aiming to identify patients that would benefit from more aggressive treatments. To date, SAA genotype is the only established variable that significantly affects the risk of AA development. SSA genotype was not evaluated in our patient [14].

The aim of symptomatic treatment is to control the underlying disease. In cases of severe diarrhea and exudative gastroenteropathy, the use of steroids, octreotide, or immunosuppressors should be considered [14].

Our patient had two pathologic entities that can be associated with amyloidosis, common variable immunodeficiency and rheumatoid arthritis, both contributing to the development of intestinal amyloidosis. The perception of which pathology had a more significant contribution to amyloid substances intestinal deposition was unachievable. However, the previous history of pulmonary tuberculosis, along with recurrent pulmonary infections during the course of CVID and the CVID itself which led to RA development, may be in the origin of the amyloid deposition.

In conclusion, when investigating unknown etiology of chronic diarrhea, associated with chronic inflammatory disease, the biopsies are essentials, permitting the diagnosis of rare intestinal amyloidosis, allowing a clinical and therapeutic estimate, and significantly contributing to patient's quality of life.

References

[1] A. Hokama, "Endoscopic and histopathological features of gastrointestinal amyloidosis," *World Journal of Gastrointestinal Endoscopy*, vol. 3, no. 8, article 157, 2011.

[2] P. T. Sattianayagam, P. N. Hawkins, and J. D. Gillmore, "Systemic amyloidosis and the gastrointestinal tract," *Nature Reviews Gastroenterology and Hepatology*, vol. 6, no. 10, pp. 608–617, 2009.

[3] D. M. Menke, R. A. Kyle, C. R. Fleming, J. T. Wolfe III, P. J. Kurtin, and W. A. Oldenburg, "Symptomatic gastric amyloidosis in patients with primary systemic amyloidosis," *Mayo Clinic Proceedings*, vol. 68, no. 8, pp. 763–767, 1993.

[4] A. Aghamohammadi, A. Farhoudi, M. Moin et al., "Clinical and immunological features of 65 Iranian patients with common variable immunodeficiency," *Clinical and Diagnostic Laboratory Immunology*, vol. 12, no. 7, pp. 825–832, 2005.

[5] C. Cunningham-Rundles, "Autoimmune manifestations in common variable immunodeficiency," *Journal of Clinical Immunology*, vol. 28, no. S1, pp. 42–45, 2008.

[6] A. Shradha, S. Paul, H. Noam, C.-R. Charlotte, and M. Lloyd, "Characterization of immunologic defects inpatientes with common variable immunodeficiency with inttesinal disease," *Inflammatory Bowel Diseases*, vol. 17, no. 1, pp. 251–259, 2011.

[7] A. K. Kadiroğlu, Y. Yıldırım, Z. Yılmaz et al., "A rare cause of secondary amyloidosis: common variable immunodeficiency disease," *Case Reports in Nephrology*, vol. 2012, Article ID 860208, 4 pages, 2012.

[8] S. Borte, M. H. Celiksoy, V. Menzel et al., "Novel *NLRP*12 mutations associated with intestinal amyloidosis in a patient diagnosed with common variable immunodeficiency," *Clinical Immunology*, vol. 154, no. 2, pp. 105–111, 2014.

[9] P. Wiland, R. Wojtala, J. Goodacre, and J. Szechinski, "The prevalence of subclinical amyloidosis in Polish patients with rheumatoid arthritis," *Clinical Rheumatology*, vol. 23, no. 3, pp. 193–198, 2004.

[10] I. M. Fernández, A. M. F. Rodríguez, and S. G. Pérez, "Use of etanercept in amyloidosis secondary to rheumatoid arthritis: a report of two cases," *Reumatologia Clinica*, vol. 7, no. 6, pp. 397–400, 2011.

[11] A. F. Çelik, M. R. Altiparmak, G. E. Pamuk, Ö. N. Pamuk, and F. Tabak, "Association of secondary amyloidosis with common variable immune deficiency and tuberculosis," *Yonsei Medical Journal*, vol. 46, no. 6, pp. 847–850, 2005.

[12] L. B. Lovat, M. B. Pepys, and P. N. Hawkins, "Amyloid and the gut," *Digestive Diseases*, vol. 15, no. 3, pp. 155–171, 1997.

[13] S. Tada, M. Iida, A. Iwashita et al., "Endoscopic and biopsy findings of the upper digestive tract in patients with amyloidosis," *Gastrointestinal Endoscopy*, vol. 36, no. 1, pp. 10–14, 1990.

[14] L. Obici and G. Merlini, "AA amyloidosis: basic knowledge, unmet needs and future treatments," *Swiss Medical Weekly*, vol. 142, Article ID w13580, 2012.

15

Coccidioidomycosis Masquerading as Eosinophilic Ascites

Kourosh Alavi, Pradeep R. Atla, Tahmina Haq, and Muhammad Y. Sheikh

Division of Gastroenterology and Hepatology, University of California San Francisco, 1st Floor, Endoscopy Suite, 2823 Fresno Street, Fresno, CA 93721, USA

Correspondence should be addressed to Muhammad Y. Sheikh; msheikh@fresno.ucsf.edu

Academic Editor: Yoshihiro Moriwaki

Endemic to the southwestern parts of the United States, coccidioidomycosis, also known as "Valley Fever," is a common fungal infection that primarily affects the lungs in both acute and chronic forms. Disseminated coccidioidomycosis is the most severe but very uncommon and usually occurs in immunocompromised individuals. It can affect the central nervous system, bones, joints, skin, and, very rarely, the abdomen. This is the first case report of a patient with coccidioidal dissemination to the peritoneum presenting as eosinophilic ascites (EA). A 27-year-old male presented with acute abdominal pain and distention from ascites. He had eosinophilia of 11.1% with negative testing for stool studies, HIV, and tuberculosis infection. Ascitic fluid exam was remarkable for low serum-ascites albumin gradient (SAAG), PMN count >250/mm^3, and eosinophils of 62%. Abdominal imaging showed thickened small bowel and endoscopic testing negative for gastric and small bowel biopsies. He was treated empirically for spontaneous bacterial peritonitis, but no definitive diagnosis could be made until coccidioidal serology returned positive. We noted complete resolution of symptoms with oral fluconazole during outpatient follow-up. Disseminated coccidioidomycosis can present in an atypical fashion and may manifest as peritonitis with low SAAG EA. The finding of EA in an endemic area should raise the suspicion of coccidioidal dissemination.

1. Introduction

Eosinophilic ascites (EA) is generally a rare finding in clinical practice. When present, it is most commonly associated with migrant parasitic infections, neoplasms, peritoneal dialysis, and eosinophilic gastroenteritis (EGE) [1, 2]. Previous cases described in the literature indicate that intra-abdominal coccidioidomycosis (IAC) can clinically present in a variety of ways ranging from an incidentally found asymptomatic indolent form to a full-blown acute abdominal process and may even mimic an occult malignancy [3–5]. We propose in this report that an even more rare cause of EA is IAC with peritoneal involvement. To the best of our knowledge, this is the first report of its kind.

2. Case Report

A 27-year-old male immigrant from Mexico (BMI of 25.3 kg/m^2) with past medical history of constipation presented to the emergency room (ER) with abdominal pain, distention, and difficulty in breathing. His symptoms started 9 days prior to the visit. He had two prior ER visits for abdominal pain that was attributed to constipation but the symptoms persisted even after he had bowel movements. Associated symptoms included fatigue, dry cough for one month, and weight loss. He usually weighs around 130 pounds and reports weight loss of about 20 pounds. He denied fever, chills, night sweats, nausea, bloody stool, diarrhea, headache, or chest pain. He admitted to heavy alcohol use but quit about 4 months ago. There was no history of recent travel, sick contacts, transfusions, allergy, smoking, and illicit drug use. His physical exam was significant for distended abdomen with tense ascites and diffuse tenderness. There were no stigmata of chronic liver disease and no evidence of pedal edema. He weighed 125 pounds on initial presentation; however, his weight loss was apparent after paracentesis with 115 pounds after the removal of 4 liters of ascitic fluid. Abnormal laboratory values and the results for the paracentesis are listed in Tables 1 and 2.

Abdominal imaging with ultrasound and computed tomography (CT) scan showed ascites and thickened small bowel wall without evidence of bowel obstruction, cirrhosis,

TABLE 1: Laboratory characteristics.

Parameter	Value	Normal range
Complete blood count		
HGB	13.9 g/dL	13.5–17.5 g/dL
Platelet	457 K/μL	150–450 K/μL
Lymphocytes	13.7%	25–45%
Eosinophils	11.1%	0–6%
Electrolytes		
Bicarbonate	29 mEq/L	22–28 mEq/L
Calcium (ionized)	3.43 mg/dL	4.4–5.4 mg/dL
Liver function		
Albumin	3.2 g/dL	3.5–5.5 g/dL
Globulin	4.0 g/dL	2–3.5 g/dL
Iron		
Ferritin	387 ng/mL	20–250 ng/mL
Serum iron	23 μg/dL	65–177 μg/dL
TIBC	193 μg/dL	250–370 μg/dL
Iron saturation	12%	20–50%
Coagulation profile		
PT	14.7 sec	12–14.7 sec
INR	1.1	0.8–1.1
Miscellaneous		
Lipase	18 U/L	12–53 U/L
CRP	88 mg/L	<1 mg/L
ESR	46 mm	<15 mm/hr
LDH		
Serum IgE	530 IU/mL	0–380 IU/mL
HIV screen (ELISA)	Nonreactive	Nonreactive
Anti-cocci antibody	Positive	Negative
Quantiferon-TB Gold	Negative	Negative
Urinalysis		
Protein	50 mg/dL	Negative
Ketones	4+	Negative
Stool analysis		
Ova and parasite	Negative	Negative
Cultures	Negative	Negative

Only abnormal lab values are listed. HGB: hemoglobin; TIBC: total iron binding capacity; CRP: C-reactive protein; ESR: erythrocyte sedimentation rate; PT: prothrombin time; INR: international normalized ratio; LDH: lactate dehydrogenase; HIV: human immunodeficiency virus; ELISA: enzyme-linked immunosorbent assay.

TABLE 2: Characteristics of ascitic fluid.

Parameter	Value
Appearance	Hazy
Color	Yellow
Volume	1000 mL
White blood cells	4095 mm^3
Red blood cells	1884 mm^3
Neutrophils	7%
Lymphocyte	25%
Monocyte	1%
Macrocyte	3%
Eosinophils	62%
Mesothelial cells	2%
Culture	No growth
Gram stain	No organism
Protein	5.2 gm/dL
Albumin	2.2 g/dL
Amylase	11 U/L
Lactate dehydrogenase	118 IU/L
Glucose	47 mg/dL
Cytology	No malignancy

splenomegaly, and portal or hepatic venous thrombosis. Additionally, atelectasis of the lung bases (especially on the left) was seen on imaging. Transthoracic echocardiogram of the heart was normal.

Differential diagnoses considered were SBP and tuberculous peritonitis. Curiously due to the elevated ascitic fluid eosinophils of 62% we also considered parasitic infections, hypereosinophilic syndrome (HES), and eosinophilic gastroenteritis (EGE) as other possible etiologies. Additionally, because our patient was from an endemic area for coccidioidomycosis, disseminated infection with peritoneal involvement was considered as well and the necessary serological tests were requested on presentation while other etiologies were being evaluated.

We started empiric treatment with antibiotics (Ceftriaxone) for SBP with modest clinical improvement. Disseminated tuberculosis was ruled out following a negative Quantiferon-Gold TB test, absence of typical symptoms, and negative ascitic fluid results. Parasitic infections were also ruled out following a negative stool test for ova and parasite. Moreover, HES was unlikely as there was no evidence of organ failure.

We pursued upper gastrointestinal endoscopy and repeated with push enteroscopy to evaluate for EGE. However, gastric and duodenal biopsies were negative for malignancy, increased eosinophils, and Helicobacter pylori infection. Jejunal biopsies were negative for malignancy, ulcer, abnormal inflammation, or Giardia-like organisms.

Subsequent to these and a host of other negative diagnostic test results (Table 3), the existence of marked EA in our young patient, who had no history of any liver disease, allergy, or drug use, especially in the setting of significant weight loss, became worrisome for an occult malignancy. Therefore, a bone marrow biopsy was added to the plan; however, it was never done since the patient's clinical condition continued to improve on SBP treatment. In retrospect, our concern for malignancy was grounded since there is evidence that extrapulmonary coccidioidomycosis can occasionally mimic symptoms of an occult malignancy with operative findings of an inflamed peritoneum that is studded with nodular lesions [4, 5]. We later added steroids to the treatment as lingering suspicion for EGE still remained. Diagnostic dilemma existed for this patient throughout the visit while the result for coccidioidal serology was pending. Eventually the patient was discharged on steroids with outpatient follow-up in the

TABLE 3: Autoimmune laboratory testing.

Parameter	Result
Anti-SCL-70 antibody	Negative
Anti-Smith antibody	Negative
Anti-nRNP antibody	Negative
Anti-dsDNA antibody	Negative
Anti-SSA/Ro antibody	Negative
Anti-SSB/La antibody	Negative
Anti-smooth muscle antibody	Negative
Anti-mitochondrial antibody	Negative
Anti-LKM antibody	Negative
C-ANCA antibody	Negative
P-ANCA antibody	Negative

LKM: liver kidney microsomal antibody; ANCA: anti-nuclear cytoplasmic antibody.

clinic. Soon after discharge, his serology came positive for IgG and IgM antibodies against *Coccidioides immitis*. His steroids were discontinued and treatment was started with 400 mg of fluconazole PO daily. He showed remarkable improvement in the subsequent clinic follow-up after discharge. His ascites has completely resolved and he has started to gain weight with improved weight of 120 pounds at 3 months after discharge.

3. Discussion

Coccidioides species are dimorphic soil-dwelling saprophytes that are predominantly found in the southwestern parts of the United States. In dry seasons these organisms remain dormant in the soil, but when the rains come, they grow into long filamentous molds that can break off and give rise to airborne spores. Inhalation of these airborne spores can cause infection [6].

Of all the individuals who become exposed to *Coccidioides immitis*, only about approximately 40% become symptomatic with the symptoms being mainly limited to the lungs. Only less than 1% develop widespread disseminated infection [7]. The main risk factors for developing the disseminated form of the disease include immunosuppression, HIV infection, pregnancy, skin test anergy, sex (male), and being of Filipino or African ancestry [7, 8]. Peripheral eosinophilia has been proposed to be an indicator of disseminated disease [9]. In fact, it has been suggested that, in a patient with coccidioidomycosis, extreme eosinophilia may be the only indicator of disseminated disease [10]. Typically the extrapulmonary symptoms of disseminated disease appear a few months after the primary infection [11]. The CNS, skin, joints, and bones are the most common sites of extrapulmonary dissemination but almost any site may be infected [7, 8, 12]. Involvement of the abdomen, however, is rare and was first reported in 1939 by Ruddock and Hope [13]. The presentation of IAC is nonspecific and generally imitates other infections or malignancy and the diagnosis mainly relies on tissue examination [4, 5, 14].

IAC most commonly involves the peritoneum, but involvement of liver, spleen, small bowel, appendix, and the adnexa of the uterus has also been reported [3, 14, 15]. Peritoneal coccidioidomycosis can clinically present in a variety of ways ranging from an incidentally found asymptomatic indolent disease to a full-blown acute abdominal process with peritoneal irritation and ascites [3]. Abdominal pain, diarrhea, ileus, and various constitutional symptoms, such as low-grade fever, malaise, nausea, and weight loss (or weight gain from the ascites), may also be present [15]. Diagnosis is based on histopathological examination as well as ascitic fluid or peritoneal tissue cultures [3]. Serologic [16] and laparoscopic [17] examinations have also been reported to provide critical information for making the diagnosis; however, to the best of our knowledge, our report is the first to highlight EA as an important clue to the diagnosis of IAC.

Azole antifungal medications (e.g., fluconazole, ketoconazole, and itraconazole) are considered first line agents in the treatment of various forms of pulmonary as well as disseminated coccidioidal infections [18].

4. Conclusion

Intra-abdominal coccidioidomycosis is very rare even in the endemic areas and can present with eosinophilic ascites as the only apparent clinical manifestation. Healthcare providers need to be aware of this rare presentation to avoid misdiagnosis and unnecessary testing. Azole antifungal medications such as fluconazole are considered first line agents for treatment.

References

[1] B. H. Copeland, O. O. Aramide, S. A. Wehbe, S. M. Fizgerald, and G. Krishnaswamy, "Eosinophilia in a patient with cyclical vomiting: a case report," *Clinical and Molecular Allergy*, vol. 2, no. 1, article 7, 2004.

[2] M.-J. Chen, C.-H. Chu, S.-C. Lin, S.-C. Shih, and T.-E. Wang, "Eosinophilic gastroenteritis: clinical experience with 15 patients," *World Journal of Gastroenterology*, vol. 9, no. 12, pp. 2813–2816, 2003.

[3] P. Phillips and B. Ford, "Peritoneal coccidioidomycosis: case report and review," *Clinical Infectious Diseases*, vol. 30, no. 6, pp. 971–976, 2000.

[4] M. W. Ellis, D. P. Dooley, M. J. Sundborg, L. L. Joiner, and E. R. Kost, "Coccidioidomycosis mimicking ovarian cancer," *Obstetrics and Gynecology*, vol. 104, no. 5, pp. 1177–1179, 2004.

[5] B. A. Eyer, A. Qayyum, A. C. Westphalen, B. M. Yeh, B. N. Joe, and F. V. Coakley, "Peritoneal coccidioidomycosis: a potential CT mimic of peritoneal malignancy," *Abdominal Imaging*, vol. 29, no. 4, pp. 505–506, 2004.

[6] C. Nguyen, B. M. Barker, S. Hoover et al., "Recent advances in our understanding of the environmental, epidemiological, immunological, and clinical dimensions of Coccidioidomycosis," *Clinical Microbiology Reviews*, vol. 26, no. 3, pp. 505–525, 2013.

[7] N. M. Ampel, M. A. Wieden, and J. N. Galgiani, "Coccidioidomycosis: clinical update," *Reviews of Infectious Diseases*, vol. 11, no. 6, pp. 897–911, 1989.

[8] T. M. Chiller, J. N. Galgiani, and D. A. Stevens, "Coccidioidomycosis," *Infectious Disease Clinics of North America*, vol. 17, no. 1, pp. 41–57, 2003.

[9] R. M. Echols, D. L. Palmer, and G. W. Long, "Tissue eosinophilia in human coccidioidomycosis," *Reviews of Infectious Diseases*, vol. 4, no. 3, pp. 656–664, 1982.

[10] W. B. Harley and M. J. Blaser, "Disseminated coccidioidomycosis associated with extreme eosinophilia," *Clinical Infectious Diseases*, vol. 18, no. 4, pp. 627–629, 1994.

[11] C. R. Chung, Y. C. Lee, Y. K. Rhee et al., "Pulmonary coccidioidomycosis with peritoneal involvement mimicking lung cancer with peritoneal carcinomatosis," *American Journal of Respiratory and Critical Care Medicine*, vol. 183, no. 1, pp. 135–136, 2011.

[12] D. A. Stevens, "Coccidioidomycosis," *The New England Journal of Medicine*, vol. 332, no. 16, pp. 1077–1082, 1995.

[13] J. C. Ruddock and R. B. Hope, "Coccidioidal peritonitis: diagnosis by peritoneoscopy," *The Journal of the American Medical Association*, vol. 113, no. 23, pp. 2054–2055, 1939.

[14] J. P. Micha, B. H. Goldstein, P. A. Robinson, M. A. Rettenmaier, and J. V. Brown, "Abdominal/pelvic Coccidioidomycosis," *Gynecologic Oncology*, vol. 96, no. 1, pp. 256–258, 2005.

[15] G. Smith, S. Hoover, R. Sobonya, and S. A. Klotz, "Abdominal and pelvic coccidioidomycosis," *The American Journal of the Medical Sciences*, vol. 341, no. 4, pp. 308–311, 2011.

[16] R. D. Adam, S. P. Elliott, and M. S. Taljanovic, "The spectrum and presentation of disseminated coccidioidomycosis," *The American Journal of Medicine*, vol. 122, no. 8, pp. 770–777, 2009.

[17] P. A. Jamidar, D. R. Campbell, J. L. Fishback, and S. A. Klotz, "Peritoneal coccidioidomycosis associated with human immunodeficiency virus infection," *Gastroenterology*, vol. 102, no. 3, pp. 1054–1058, 1992.

[18] A. Catanzaro, J. N. Galgiani, B. E. Levine et al., "Fluconazole in the treatment of chronic pulmonary and nonmeningeal disseminated coccidioidomycosis," *The American Journal of Medicine*, vol. 98, no. 3, pp. 249–256, 1995.

16

The "Endothelialized Muscularis Mucosae": A Case Report Describing a Large Cavernous Hemangioma at the Terminal Ileum and a New Histologic Clue for Preoperative Diagnosis from Endoscopic Biopsy

Erin K. Purdy-Payne,[1] Jean F. Miner,[2] Brandon Foles,[2] and Tien-Anh N. Tran[3]

[1] *University of Central Florida College of Medicine, 6850 Lake Nona Boulevard, Orlando, FL 32827, USA*
[2] *Department of Surgery, Florida Hospital Orlando, 2415 North Orange Avenue, Suite 400, Orlando, FL 32803, USA*
[3] *Department of Pathology, Florida Hospital Orlando, 601 E. Rollins Street, Orlando, FL 32803, USA*

Correspondence should be addressed to Erin K. Purdy-Payne; erinkpurdy@gmail.com

Academic Editor: Shiro Kikuchi

Cavernous hemangiomas of the gastrointestinal tract are quite rare and, until now, have been difficult to diagnose preoperatively due their nonspecific presentations and imaging features, as well as a lack of histologic description pertaining to small superficial biopsies such as those obtained endoscopically. We report a unique case of a 4 cm transmural cavernous hemangioma in the terminal ileum with literature review and describe a new histologic finding—the "endothelialized muscularis mucosae," which was discovered upon review of the endoscopic biopsy and could potentially facilitate preoperative diagnosis of these lesions from endoscopic biopsies in the future. These lesions have classically required surgical resection in order to make a definitive diagnosis and rule out malignancy, with which they share many historical and radiographic features. Due to their potential to cause bowel obstruction, intussusception, perforation, and hemorrhage, these lesions may ultimately require surgical resection to relieve symptoms or prevent or treat complications—however, surgical planning and patient counseling could be greatly improved by a preoperative diagnosis. Therefore, gastroenterologists, pathologists, and surgeons should be aware of the "endothelialized muscularis mucosae" which can be very helpful in diagnosing GI cavernous hemangiomas from endoscopic biopsies.

1. Introduction

Cavernous hemangiomas of the gastrointestinal tract are quite rare and, until now, difficult to diagnose preoperatively [1] due to a dearth of specific histologic description pertaining to small superficial biopsies such as those obtained endoscopically [2, 3]. We report a unique case of a 4 cm transmural cavernous hemangioma in the terminal ileum with literature review and describe a new histologic finding—the "endothelialized muscularis mucosae," which was discovered upon review of the endoscopic biopsy and could potentially facilitate preoperative diagnosis of these lesions from endoscopic biopsies in the future.

2. Case Description

The patient was a 20-year-old female who presented to the emergency department with a progressive 2-week history of diffuse intermittent abdominal pain, which was aching at rest and sharp upon movement. It was accompanied by nausea for the past two days, with one episode of vomiting. She denied recent changes in her stool but reported passing stool only once per week for the past few years.

The patient also reported a 2-year history of vasovagal syncope, with an increase in presyncopal episodes during the 2-week course of her abdominal pain. These episodes were sometimes associated with heart palpitations, shortness of

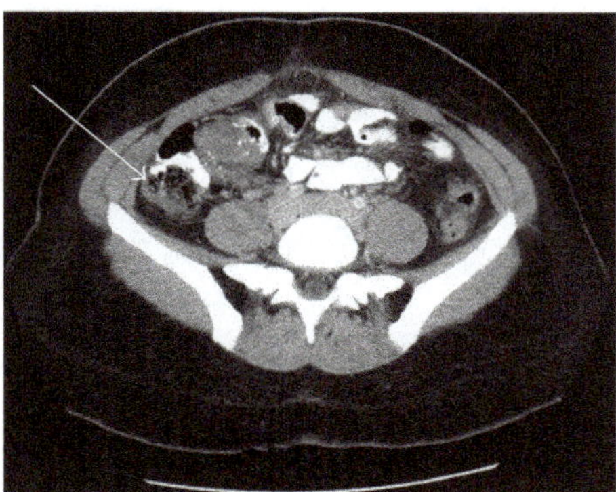

FIGURE 1: Computed tomography without contrast of the abdomen and pelvis was notable for a 4.7 cm mass involving the wall of the terminal ileum, with speckled calcifications, adjacent lymphadenopathy, and a small amount of dense fluid in the pelvis (CT, with arrow).

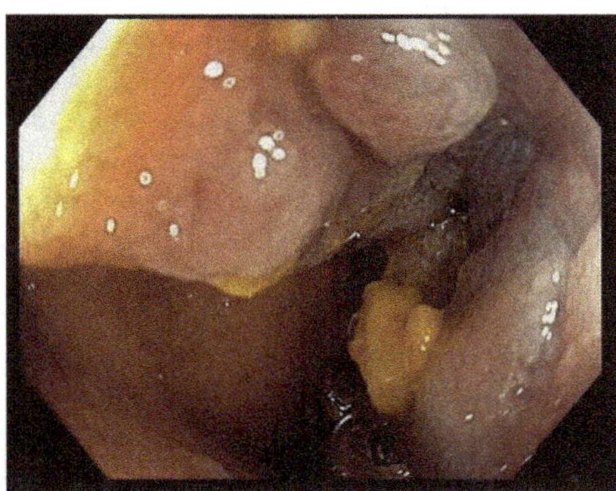

FIGURE 2: On colonoscopy, the luminal surface of the mass was visible through the ileocecal valve and was described as a 4-5 cm friable mass in the terminal ileum (endoscopic view).

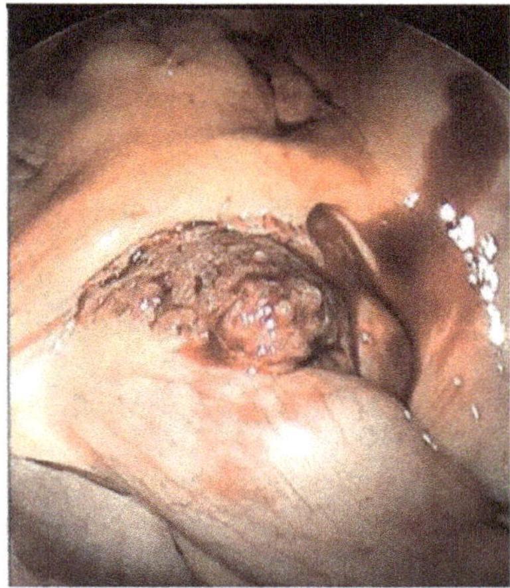

FIGURE 3: Laparoscopy revealed a soft, maroon, cystic mass. It was noted to be friable with scant bleeding and to have a tortuous, dilated blood supply (laparoscopic view).

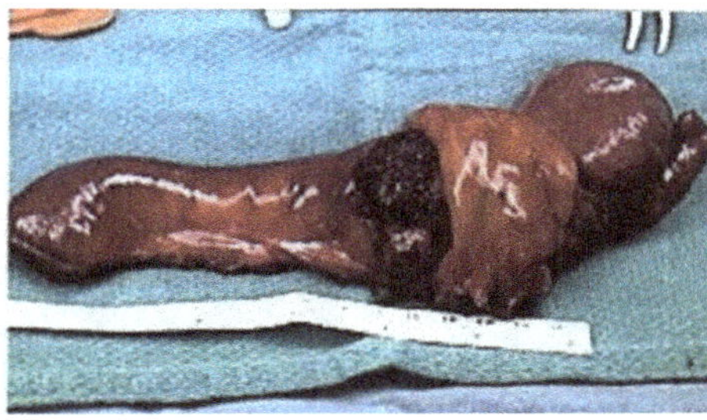

FIGURE 4: The gross resected specimen included an 11 cm segment of terminal ileum and 4 cm portion of cecum, with a 4 × 3.5 × 3 cm dark red, spongy mass at the terminal ileum (gross specimen).

breath, and chest pain, which had previously been diagnosed as anxiety and gastroesophageal reflux disease. The history was otherwise noncontributory.

The patient's vital signs were unremarkable and she was afebrile. There were no masses or tenderness upon abdominal palpation. Initial labs were within normal limits, and screening tests were negative for pregnancy and sexually transmitted infections.

A computed tomography of the abdomen and pelvis without contrast was notable for a 4.7 cm mass involving the wall of the terminal ileum, with speckled calcifications, adjacent lymphadenopathy, and a small amount of dense fluid in the pelvis (Figure 1). No hepatic abnormalities were visualized. Colonoscopy demonstrated a 4-5 cm friable mass in the terminal ileum (Figure 2), and multiple biopsies of this area were taken. The biopsies were originally described as unremarkable small bowel mucosa with preserved villous architecture.

The patient subsequently underwent laparoscopic evaluation and resection of the mass. Upon entry into the abdomen, a small amount of blood was noted to be pooled in dependent locations within the abdomen and pelvis. At the terminal ileum, a soft, maroon, cystic, friable mass associated with scant bleeding and a tortuous, dilated blood supply was noted (Figure 3). A laparoscopic ileocecectomy was completed without any perioperative complications.

The resected specimen was composed of an 11 cm segment of terminal ileum and 4 cm portion of cecum (Figure 4). Gross examination revealed a 4 × 3.5 × 3 cm dark red, spongy mass at the terminal ileum that involved all layers of the small bowel and extended into the attached adipose tissue. Upon opening the bowel, a large amount of blood was noted within the lumen of the terminal ileum. The corresponding mucosal surface of the lesion was seeping fluid blood into the lumen. Histologic examination showed dilated vascular spaces, filled with blood and lined by a layer of flat, benign-appearing endothelial cells. The walls of the vascular channels were composed of smooth muscle and fibrous tissue (Figure 5). Calcifications and calcified phleboliths were observed in the wall and lumen of the vascular lesion. The diagnosis of a cavernous hemangioma was rendered.

Review of the original biopsy revealed a second layer of fibromuscular tissue apposed to the muscularis mucosae of the small bowel mucosa. On the antiluminal side of the intestinal lumen, this second layer of fibromuscular tissue

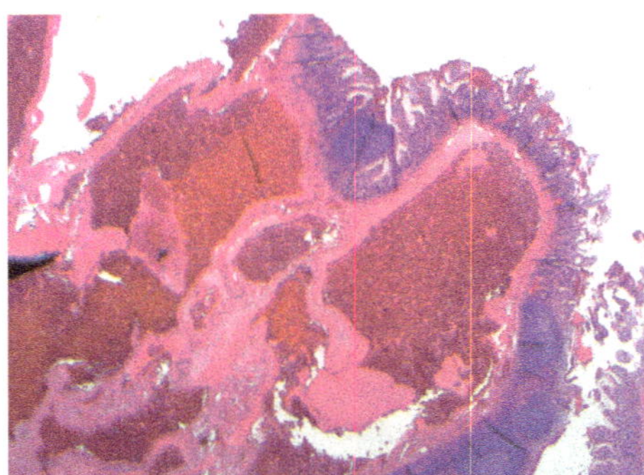

FIGURE 5: Histologic examination of the surgical specimen showed dilated vascular spaces filled with blood and lined by a layer of flat, benign-appearing endothelial cells. The wall of the vascular channels was composed of smooth muscle and fibrous tissue (histology of surgical specimen).

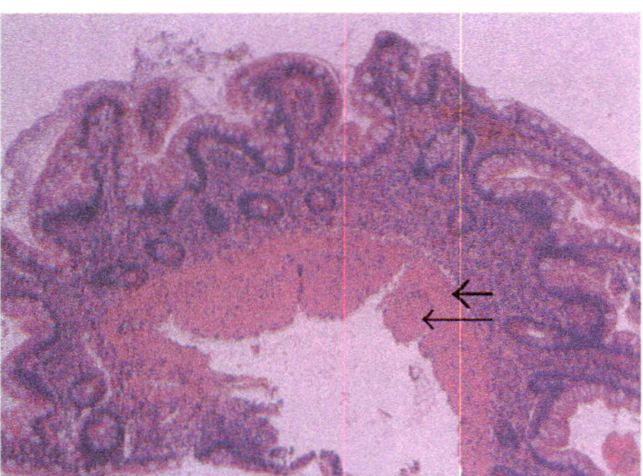

FIGURE 6: Histologic review of the original endoscopic biopsy revealed the so-called "endothelialized muscularis mucosae" characterized by a second layer of fibromuscular tissue (long, fine arrow) apposed to the muscularis mucosae (short, thick arrow) (histology of endoscopic biopsy, with arrows).

was lined by a layer of flat endothelial cells (Figure 6). Immunohistochemical studies with the endothelial markers CD31 and CD34 highlighted the layer of endothelial cells lining one side of the second fibromuscular layer (Figure 7).

3. Discussion

Intestinal hemangiomas are very rare, with multiple histologic variations accounting for a combined incidence of only 0.05% of all gastrointestinal tract (GI) tumors [3]. They are more likely to be found in the jejunum [4], in contrast with most other GI tumors, only 3–6% of which reside in the small bowel [1]. A literature search for cavernous hemangiomas of the terminal ileum revealed only one prior case, which described a 5 cm cavernous hemangioma that was associated with perforation located near the origin of an ileocecal intussusception [3].

Small bowel tumors pose several diagnostic challenges, beginning with their nonspecific symptoms of abdominal pain, nausea, and distension, which could be more easily explained by many prevalent physiologic GI issues. Additionally, many are asymptomatic until later stages. Therefore they are often discovered either incidentally, or after a wide-ranging work-up and a significant delay since the onset of symptoms [1]. Late stage small bowel tumors may present suddenly, with acute intestinal obstruction or frank GI bleeding [1, 5–7], or insidiously, with subacute partial obstruction or chronic anemia secondary to occult GI bleeding [1, 8, 9]. Lesions involving the terminal ileum, such as in our case, may be more likely to present with obstructive symptoms, due to their impediment of this region's intestinal wall motility which is crucial to propulsion of contents through the ileocecal valve [10]. Our patient's dilated terminal ileum and pattern of passing stool only once per week suggest chronic subacute obstruction, likely due to impaired peristalsis at the terminal ileum. Her presenting symptoms of abdominal pain, nausea, and vomiting indicate progression towards a more acute obstruction.

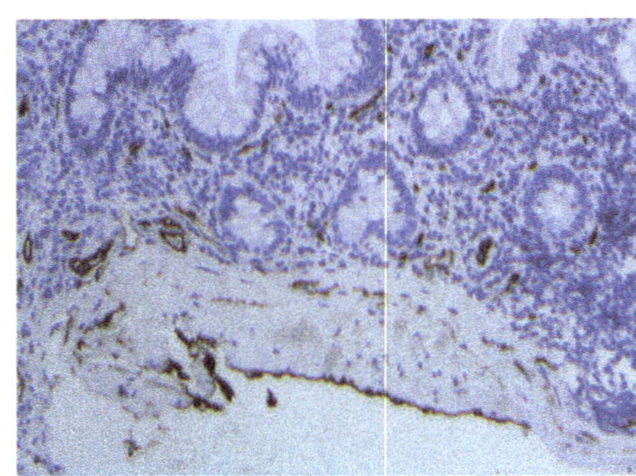

FIGURE 7: Upon immunohistochemical staining of the original endoscopic biopsy specimen, this second layer of smooth muscle/fibrous tissue was also lined on the antiluminal side by a layer of flat endothelial cells, highlighted by the endothelial marker CD34 (immunofluorescence staining of endoscopic biopsy).

Compared to other small bowel tumors, cavernous hemangiomas are more often symptomatic and more likely to present with anemia or bleeding, rarely even causing massive hemorrhaging [4, 6, 11]. With transmural lesions such as in our case, bleeding may occur not only intraluminally but also intra-abdominally [6]. In our patient, the blood noted in the abdominal cavity had likely been causing her sharp abdominal pain secondary to peritoneal irritation. Intestinal hemangiomas have also been associated with complications such as intussusception and perforation [3, 11], or platelet sequestration leading to thrombocytopenia [4]. In some cases, these complications can be life threatening.

Nonspecific features on imaging and limitations in visualization pose additional challenges to preoperative diagnosis of small bowel tumors. Patients who present with abdominal pain or obstructive symptoms are often evaluated by computed tomography (CT), which has a poor detection rate for small bowel tumors and is unlikely to visualize most cavernous hemangiomas [1, 12]. For lesions large enough to visualize, a CT scan can help determine the presence, size, and extension into nearby structures [7] but is usually unhelpful at differentiating the type of lesion [1]. A large cavernous hemangioma may be seen on CT scan as intestinal wall thickening which is persistently enhancing with IV contrast, or which may infiltrate nearby structures such as mesentery or abdominal wall. These features can be misleading and may cause a cavernous hemangioma to be mistaken for a more common tumor such as lymphoma [8]. CT scans can also demonstrate calcifications such as phleboliths, which occur due to vascular thrombosis within the tumor's dilated varicosities [4, 11, 12].

Patients who present with recurrent anemia or GI bleeding due to these lesions are often evaluated by traditional endoscopy, which is unable to reach most of the small bowel, or by capsule endoscopy [1]. When they are visualized on endoscopy, features of a cavernous hemangioma may include a purple or blue color, a nodular gross appearance, and hypervascularity, possibly with friability or visible bleeding [7, 8, 12]. Adjacent features may include mucosal congestion and submucosal dilated varicosities [3, 12]. Other diagnostic modalities, such as radionucleotide imaging or angiography showing hypervascularity, or barium studies demonstrating a nodular luminal defect which is compressible upon air insufflation, may help localize the lesion but cannot render a specific diagnosis [11, 12].

Little has been written in the literature on the histologic findings in biopsies of cavernous hemangiomas of the gastrointestinal tract. Accordingly, even lesions accessible for biopsy have evaded diagnosis due to inconclusive findings [2], and cavernous hemangiomas have almost exclusively required surgical resection for a definitive diagnosis [1, 12]. However, upon review of the original endoscopic biopsy in this case, we observed a second layer of fibromuscular tissue which was tightly apposed to the muscularis mucosae of the small bowel mucosa, with a layer of flat endothelial cells lining the antiluminal side of the second fibromuscular layer. Since duplication of the muscularis mucosae can occur in chronic diseases of the GI tract, immunohistochemical studies with the endothelial markers CD31 and CD34 were particularly helpful in highlighting the flat endothelial cells on the antiluminal side of the second fibromuscular layer. We therefore coined the term "endothelialized muscularis mucosae" to describe this phenomenon. In the future, this histologic sign could potentially aid preoperative diagnosis of GI tract cavernous hemangiomas by serving as a useful diagnostic clue for interpreting small biopsies such as those obtained during endoscopy. Preoperative histologic diagnosis would be helpful in counseling patients on the indications, risks, and benefits of surgery, as well as in planning the operation and the extent of the resection.

While cavernous hemangiomas are benign, they can be locally destructive by way of invading, exerting pressure, or disrupting the physiology of surrounding structures. Due to these factors and the prevalence of complications such as bleeding or bowel obstruction, cavernous hemangiomas require surgical resection more often than other intestinal hemangiomas [4]. Surgery is indicated for a variety of reasons, including to treat or prevent such complications, to relieve symptoms such as abdominal pain, or to rule out malignancy and acquire a diagnosis when the work-up has been nondiagnostic [4, 12]. In this case, all of these factors contributed to the decision for surgical resection, but we believe that surgical planning would have been greatly facilitated by a preoperative knowledge of the diagnosis.

Due to the nonspecific presentation, many patients with GI cavernous hemangiomas will be evaluated with endoscopy at some point, if not early on in their work-up [1]. When these lesions are accessible by traditional endoscopy, they present a problem for the patient and the provider, if the lesion is detected endoscopically but is unable to be diagnosed histologically. The first issue is that an unknown lesion may or may not require resection depending on its histologic diagnosis, but resection is necessary to acquire the histologic diagnosis in the first place. Furthermore, a surgeon in this position must debate whether to perform an excisional biopsy only, subjecting the patient to another abdominal surgery if the histologic diagnosis is malignant, or whether to initially resect a larger portion of the bowel and mesentery, in hopes that the patient will require only one operation to cover the anticipated histologic diagnostic possibilities. At this point in the work-up, either operation may be unnecessary to manage the lesion, depending on the patient's symptoms and the likelihood of complications. For these reasons, we believe our new histologic observation of the "endothelialized muscularis mucosae" has an important role in identifying these cavernous hemangiomas when they are found on endoscopy: establishing the diagnosis of cavernous hemangioma before an operation could save future patients from having a surgical intervention that may be unnecessary or larger than that required for this diagnosis. Additionally, by publishing this histologic finding, we hope that further studies will determine if this clue could be generalized to aid in diagnosis of cavernous hemangiomas from small biopsies in other organs or systems.

4. Conclusion

Small bowel cavernous hemangiomas are extremely rare vascular lesions which present with nonspecific GI symptoms such as abdominal pain and nausea, anemia, and GI bleeding. Complications include bowel obstruction, intussusception, perforation, and hemorrhage. Their size and propensity for bleeding may be affected by comorbid patient conditions which impair venous flow. Diagnostic challenges include nonspecific presentation and features on imaging, inconclusiveness of biopsy, or inaccessibility by endoscopy. Pathologists should be aware of the "endothelialized muscularis mucosae" which can be very helpful in diagnosing GI cavernous hemangiomas, particularly in small biopsies. The ability to acquire a histologic diagnosis preoperatively has important implications in patient counseling and surgical planning. A conservative surgical resection, which may be successfully performed laparoscopically, is recommended in order to relieve symptoms or prevent complications and provide definitive diagnosis when necessary.

References

[1] R. S. Islam, J. A. Leighton, and S. F. Pasha, "Evaluation and management of small-bowel tumors in the era of deep enteroscopy," *Gastrointestinal Endoscopy*, vol. 79, no. 5, pp. 732–740, 2014.

[2] W. T. Parker, J. G. Harper, D. E. Rivera, S. B. Holsten, and T. Bowden, "Mesenteric cavernous hemangioma involving small bowel and appendix: a rare presentation of a vascular tumor," *American Surgeon*, vol. 75, no. 9, pp. 811–816, 2009.

[3] Y. Huang, Q. Zhang, J. Feng, H. Liu, and J. Liu, "Adult intussusception with perforation caused by hemangioma in the distal ileum," *Kaohsiung Journal of Medical Sciences*, vol. 29, no. 10, pp. 582–583, 2013.

[4] F. M. Enziger and S. W. Weiss, *Soft Tissue Tumors*, Mosby-Yearbook, St. Louis, Mo, USA, 3rd edition, 1995.

[5] J. M. Cox, "Cavernous hemangioma (cavernoma) of the ileum," *Journal of the National Medical Association*, vol. 41, no. 6, pp. 259–261, 1949.

[6] J. Santos, J. Ruiz-Tovar, A. López, A. Arroyo, and R. Calpena, "Simultaneous massive low gastrointestinal bleeding and hemoperitoneum caused by a capillary hemangioma in ileocecal valve," *International Journal of Colorectal Disease*, vol. 26, no. 10, pp. 1363–1364, 2011.

[7] J. W. Huh, S. H. Cho, J. H. Lee, and H. R. Kim, "Large cavernous hemangioma in the cecum treated by laparoscopic ileocecal resection," *World Journal of Gastroenterology*, vol. 15, no. 26, pp. 3319–3321, 2009.

[8] A. Guardiola, J. Navajas, J. Valle et al., "Small bowel giant cavernous hemangioma diagnosed by capsule endoscopy," *Revista Española de Enfermedades Digestivas*, vol. 104, no. 5, pp. 277–278, 2012.

[9] M. Sakaguchi, K. Sue, G. Etoh et al., "A case of solitary cavernous hemangioma of the small intestine with recurrent clinical anemic attacks in childhood," *Journal of Pediatric Gastroenterology and Nutrition*, vol. 27, no. 3, pp. 342–343, 1998.

[10] S. F. Phillips, E. M. M. Quigley, D. Kumar, and P. S. Kamath, "Motility of the ileocolonic junction," *Gut*, vol. 29, no. 3, pp. 390–406, 1988.

[11] A. D. Levy, R. M. Abbott, C. A. Rohrmann Jr., A. A. Frazier, and A. Kende, "Gastrointestinal hemangiomas: imaging findings with pathologic correlation in pediatric and adult patients," *American Journal of Roentgenology*, vol. 177, no. 5, pp. 1073–1081, 2001.

[12] A. Corsi, A. Ingegnoli, P. Abelli et al., "Imaging of a small bowel cavernous hemangioma: report of a case with emphasis on the use of computed tomography and enteroclysis," *Acta Bio Medical*, vol. 78, no. 2, pp. 139–143, 2007.

17

Simultaneous Diagnosis of Acute Crohn's Disease and Endometriosis in a Patient Affects HIV

S. Casiraghi,[1] P. Baggi,[1] P. Lanza,[2] A. Bozzola,[3] A. Vinco,[1] V. Villanacci,[3] F. Castelli,[2] and M. Ronconi[1]

[1]*Division of General Surgery, Gardone Val Trompia Hospital, Gardone Val Trompia, Italy*
[2]*Department of Infectious and Tropical Diseases, University of Brescia, Brescia, Italy*
[3]*Institute of Pathology, Brescia Spedali Civili General Hospital, Brescia, Italy*

Correspondence should be addressed to S. Casiraghi; casiraghisilvia@gmail.com

Academic Editor: Warwick S. Selby

This is the case report of a 45-year-old woman affected by HIV, who was hospitalized for diffuse abdominal pain, constipation, and weight loss present for over one month. A colonoscopy showed the presence of a nontransitable stenosis of the ascending colon. A right hemicolectomy was performed. The histological examination reports CD with outbreaks of endometriosis. CD and the HIV infection may coexist in the same individual and it seems that HIV reduces the relapse rate in IBD patients. CD and intestinal endometriosis can also occur simultaneously. The diagnosis is often only made after surgical resection of the diseased segment. These patients were more likely to have stricturing CD but endometriosis does not seem to impact the natural history of CD.

1. Introduction

Crohn's Disease (CD) is a chronic relapsing Inflammatory Bowel Disease (IBD). It is characterized by a transmural granulomatous inflammation which can affect any part of the gastrointestinal tract, most commonly the ileum, colon, or both [1]. The incidence is 6–8% for 100000 and the prevalence is 130–200 per 100000 [2]. It affects both sexes equally, most commonly in the second to fourth decade of life [3].

The etiology may include alterations in the immune system, abnormal cytokine levels, and changes in gut permeability and motility [4]. Clinical signs and symptoms of CD are often subtle and depend on the location and severity of the gastrointestinal involvement as well as inflammatory activity [5].

Endometriosis is defined as the presence of functional endometrial tissue in extrauterine sites and is common in women of reproductive age with an incidence of 5–15% of menstruating women [6]. The reported prevalence of endometriosis is 1–20% in asymptomatic women, 10–25% in infertile patients, and 60–70% in woman with chronic pelvic pain [7].

Endometriosis is distinguished in three different phenotypes: ovarian endometriosis, superficial peritoneal endometriosis, and deep infiltrating endometriosis (DIE). Deep endometriosis was defined arbitrarily as endometriosis infiltrating the peritoneum by >5 mm [7]. DIE includes rectovaginal lesions as well as infiltrative forms that involve structures such as the bowel, ureters, and the bladder. It is the most severe form of the disease with an estimated prevalence of 1% in women of reproductive age and 30–40% of all patients with endometriosis [8].

The clinical presentation can be often nonspecific, by simulating IBD, malignancies, or diverticulitis and can vary from microscopic foci to large space-occupying lesions [8]. Extrapelvic endometriosis affects the GI tract of 5% of women with this condition. The rectosigmoid is the most common site for intestinal endometriosis (70% of all cases) while small bowel involvement, usually confined to the distal ileum, is less frequent (1%–7%) and exclusive localization on the ileum is very rare (1–7%) [9].

2. Case Report

A 45-year-old woman was admitted to our surgical department for the first time in November 2015, suffering from diffuse abdominal pain for over one month. She was also

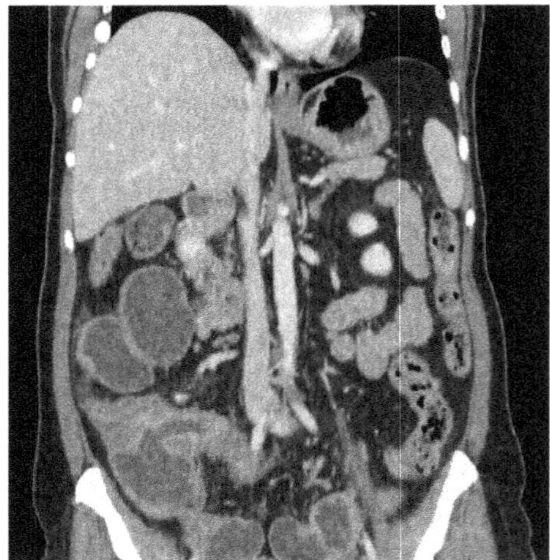

Figure 1

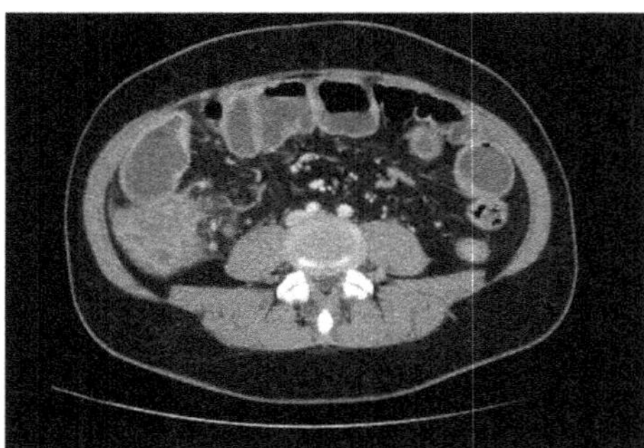

Figure 2

in amenorrhea without any other gynecologic symptoms. From 1988 she took the HAART (Highly Active Antiretroviral Therapy) for HIV infection with regular count of CD4 lymphocytes (last determination of the CD4 lymphocytes was 1005 (25.9%) and HIV viremia was not detectable). She had never been pregnant and had no abdominal surgery in her history. Before the recovery, the patient underwent an outpatient colonoscopy that reported a nontransitable severe stricture of the ascending colon that did not allow the execution of biopsies; the perilesion biopsies did not reveal any morphological specific alteration. During the recovery a CT with contrast medium was performed and a thickening of the wall of the terminal ileum/ascending colon compatible with inflammatory or lymphoproliferative disease was found (Figures 1 and 2). The treatment was only medical with fasting, infusions, antibiotics, and mesalamine (800 mg t.i.d.). One month later, after therapy with mesalamine, another colonoscopy was performed and confirmed the persistence of the stenosis. The patient still suffered severe abdominal pain and vomit. She was admitted to our department, an urgent laparotomy and a right hemicolectomy were performed. Intraoperative mass of the ascending colon occluded the intestinal transit without any adhesions with the other abdominal organs and no signs of endometriosis were found. The postoperative course was regular without complications. She was discharged on the eighth postoperative day. The histological examination on the specimen was "Crohn's Disease with outbreaks of endometriosis." CD10, usually positive in endometriosis, was used for histological diagnosis. The macroscopical appearance of the surgical specimen revealed a stenosis of the terminal ileum at the level of ileocecal valve with accumulation of pills of mesalamine in the distal ileum (Figures 3(a) and 3(b)). The histological evaluation revealed a typical CD with sectorial erosions, ulcerations, and inflammation of the mucosa with multiple lymphoid aggregates in the submucosa, muscularis propria, and serosa together with foci of endometriosis (estrogen and progesteron positive immunostain) (Figures 3(c)–3(h)).

The patient is now incorporated into a multidisciplinary team including Gastroenterologists, Infectious Diseases Specialists, and Gynecologists.

3. Discussion

Our case report talks about two specific correlations, first between CD and HIV infection and second between CD and endometriosis.

Despite several decades of investigation, the etiology and specific pathogenetic mechanism responsible for CD remain poorly defined. T lymphocytes, in particular CD4+, seem to play a key role in regulating mucosal T-cell response to bacterial antigens, which may lead to intestinal inflammation; indeed, there are several reports of CD symptoms which spontaneously improved following the HIV infection and a subsequent decline in CD4+ count [10–13].

Viazis et al. [14] demonstrated that the maintenance of remission was statistically different in patients with IBD infected with HIV compared to a matched control group of IBD patients without HIV. The time to first relapse was longer for IBD-HIV patients, suggesting a protective role of the HIV infection. In particular this could be attributable to the lower CD4+ count, since nonlymphopenic patients without immunosuppression seemed to relapse more often than those with immunosuppression.

A review of 7 cases reports IBD active course or IBD relapse in HIV patients under immunosuppression; on the contrary, some patients who have reconstituted their immune system with HAART can have a silent IBD [15]. In our case, the patient had a high CD4+ count in HAART, like an immunocompetent one; this can justify the active IBD course. On the other hand, IBD and endometriosis are immune mediated chronic inflammatory disorders affecting young women [16]. Both IBD and endometriosis are often in differential diagnosis in women with abdominal pain and a preoperative definite diagnosis is challenging and sometimes impossible [17]. Guadagno et al. investigated the histological correlation between CD and endometriosis and concluded that in women with known endometriosis histological IBD-like lesions, such as crypt distortion and mucosal surface alteration, should be considered as an epiphenomenon of endometriosis, not as a true IBD [18]. A Danish study demonstrated an increased risk of developing IBD among a large cohort of 37661 women with endometriosis and the

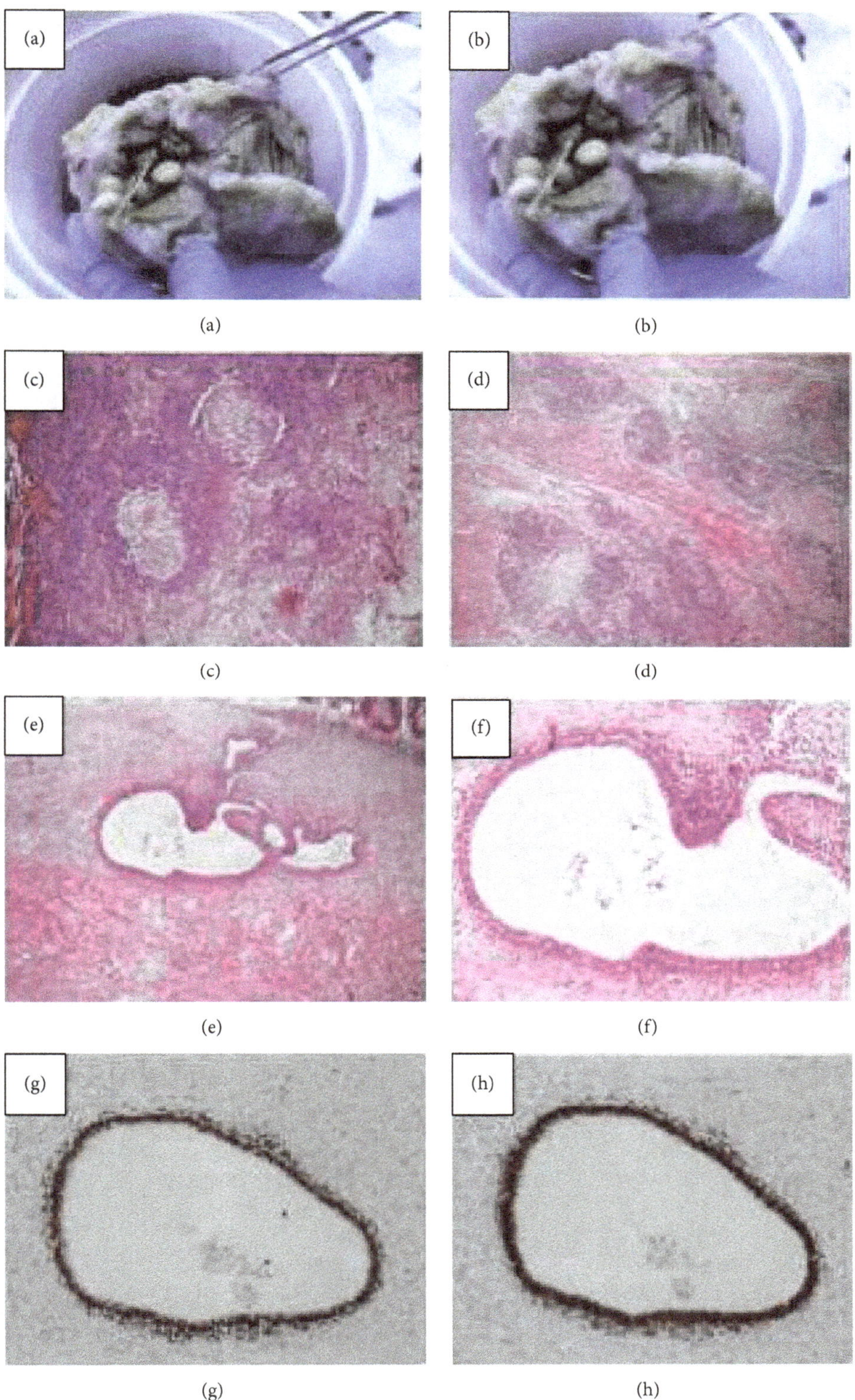

FIGURE 3: ((a), (b)) Macroscopic features of the specimen with the stenotic area and mesalamine pills accumulation. ((c), (d)) CD with typical granuloma ((c) EE 4 HPF) and lymphoid aggregates ((d) EE 10 HPF). ((e)–(h)) Endometriosis focus ((e) EE 4 HPF; (f) EE 10 HPF) and immunohistochemical staining for estrogen ((g) 10 HPF) and progesterone ((h) 10 HPF).

risk was higher in women who had endometriosis verified by surgery [19]. The authors speculated that this association may be explained by shared immunological features between endometriosis and IBD or it may reflect a consequence of endometriosis treatment (in particular the oral contraceptives).

Yantiss et al. [20] reported a large series of 44 surgical cases with intestinal endometriosis; 11 (25%) had luminal strictures secondary to fibrosis and smooth muscle hyperplasia. A total of 19 (42%) had mucosal changes similar to chronic colitis/enteritis as seen in IBD, including villous blunting, branched crypts or crypts distortion, deep lymphoid aggregates and fissures. This study demonstrated that intestinal endometriosis mimics gross and histologic finding of IBD.

Recently, an American study [21] investigated the association and clinical significance of concomitant endometriosis and IBD (51 cases of female IBD patients with endometriosis and 102 controls of female IBD patients without endometriosis). They compared the IBD phenotype and natural history, specifically the use of immunosuppressive and/or biologic therapy and the need for IBD-related surgery, among IBD patient with and without endometriosis. Among endometriosis-CD patients whose endometriosis was surgically verified, there was a higher rate of stricturing disease than CD controls, while there was no difference in natural history of IBD in terms of immunosuppressive therapy and IBD surgery.

In conclusion, the HIV infection seems to have a protective role in the behaviour of the IBD, in particular for the relapse. Endometriosis and IBD can occur simultaneously [22–24] maybe because of the potential mechanisms of disease pathogenesis like immune dysregulation or due to the medical endometriosis therapy (oral contraceptive). The differential diagnosis is difficult for the similar clinical presentation and is often only made after surgical resection of the diseased segment. It seems that CD patients with endometriosis have a high risk to develop structuring CD as in our case report.

References

[1] K. T. Thia, W. J. Sandborn, W. S. Harmsen, A. R. Zinsmeister, and E. V. Loftus Jr., "Risk factors associated with progression to intestinal complications of Crohn's disease in a population-based cohort," *Gastroenterology*, vol. 139, no. 4, pp. 1147–1155, 2010.

[2] M. D. Kappelman, S. L. Rifas-Shiman, K. Kleinman et al., "The Prevalence and Geographic Distribution of Crohn's Disease and Ulcerative Colitis in the United States," *Clinical Gastroenterology and Hepatology*, vol. 5, no. 12, pp. 1424–1429, 2007.

[3] N. A. Molodecky, I. S. Soon, D. M. Rabi et al., "Increasing incidence and prevalence of the inflammatory bowel diseases with time, based on systematic review," *Gastroenterology*, vol. 142, no. 1, pp. 46–54, 2012.

[4] T. Birrenbach and U. Böcker, "Inflammatory bowel disease and smoking. A review of epidemiology, pathophysiology, and therapeutic implications," *Inflammatory Bowel Diseases*, vol. 10, no. 6, pp. 848–859, 2004.

[5] B. A. Hendrickson, R. Gokhale, and J. H. Cho, "Clinical aspects and pathophysiology of inflammatory bowel disease," *Clinical Microbiology Reviews*, vol. 15, no. 1, pp. 79–94, 2002.

[6] D. L. Olive and L. B. Schwartz, "Medical Progress: Endometriosis," *The New England Journal of Medicine*, vol. 328, no. 24, pp. 1759–1769, 1993.

[7] E. A. Pritts and R. N. Taylor, "An evidence-based evaluation of endometriosis-associated infertility," *Endocrinology and Metabolism Clinics of North America*, vol. 32, no. 3, pp. 653–667, 2003.

[8] P. R. Koninckx, A. Ussia, L. Adamyan, A. Wattiez, and J. Donnez, "Deep endometriosis: definition, diagnosis, and treatment," *Fertility and Sterility*, vol. 98, no. 3, pp. 564–571, 2012.

[9] L. C. Kaufman, T. C. Smyrk, M. J. Levy, F. T. Enders, and A. S. Oxentenko, "Symptomatic intestinal endometriosis requiring surgical resection: clinical presentation and preoperative diagnosis," *American Journal of Gastroenterology*, vol. 106, no. 7, pp. 1325–1332, 2011.

[10] A. D. Christ, C. C. Sieber, G. Cathomas, and K. Gyr, "Concomitant active Crohn's disease and the acquired immunodeficiency syndrome," *Scandinavian Journal of Gastroenterology*, vol. 31, no. 7, pp. 733–735, 1996.

[11] B. B. Bernstein, A. Gelb, and R. Tabanda-Lichauco, "Crohn's Ileitis in a Patient with Longstanding HIV Infection," *American Journal of Gastroenterology*, vol. 89, no. 6, pp. 937–939, 1994.

[12] D. R. Sharpstone, A. Duggal, and B. G. Gazzard, "Inflammatory bowel disease in individuals seropositive for the human immunodeficiency virus," *European Journal of Gastroenterology & Hepatology*, vol. 8, no. 6, pp. 575–578, 1996.

[13] E. M. Yoshida, N. H. L. Chan, R. A. Herrick et al., "Human immunodeficiency virus infection, the acquired immunodeficiency syndrome, and inflammatory bowel disease," *Journal of Clinical Gastroenterology*, vol. 23, no. 1, pp. 24–28, 1996.

[14] N. Viazis, J. Vlachogiannakos, O. Georgiou et al., "Course of inflammatory bowel disease in patients infected with human immunodeficiency virus," *Inflammatory Bowel Diseases*, vol. 16, no. 3, pp. 507–511, 2010.

[15] A. Skamnelosa, A. Tatsionib, K. H. Katsanosa, V. Tsianosa, D. Christodouloua, and E. V. Tsianosa, "count remission hypothesis in patients with inflammatory bowel disease and human immunodeficiency virus infection: a systematic review of the literature," *Annals of Gastroenterology*, vol. 28, pp. 337–346, 2015.

[16] L. C. Giudice, "Clinical practice. Endometriosis," *The New England Journal of Medicine*, vol. 362, no. 25, pp. 2389–2398, 2010.

[17] R. Boulton, M. H. Chawla, S. Poole, H. J. F. Hodgson, and I. G. Barrison, "Ileal endometriosis masquerading as Crohn's ileitis," *Journal of Clinical Gastroenterology*, vol. 25, no. 1, pp. 338–342, 1997.

[18] A. Guadagno, F. Grillo, V. G. Vellone et al., "Intestinal Endometriosis: Mimicker of Inflammatory Bowel Disease?" *Digestion*, vol. 92, no. 1, pp. 14–21, 2015.

[19] T. Jess, M. Frisch, K. T. Jørgensen et al., "Increased risk of inflammatory bowel disease in women with endometriosis: a nationwide Danish cohort study," *Gut*, 2011.

[20] R. K. Yantiss, P. B. Clement, and R. H. Young, "Endometriosis of the intestinal tract: a study of 44 cases of a disease that may

cause diverse challenges in clinical and pathologic evaluation," *The American Journal of Surgical Pathology*, vol. 25, no. 4, pp. 445–454, 2001.

[21] K. K. Lee, B. Jharap, E. A. Maser, and J.-F. Colombel, "Impact of Concomitant Endometriosis on Phenotype and Natural History of Inflammatory Bowel Disease," *Inflammatory Bowel Diseases*, vol. 22, no. 1, pp. 159–163, 2016.

[22] M. Craninx, G. D'Haens, K. Cokelaere et al., "Crohn's disease and intestinal endometriosis: An intriguing co-existence," *European Journal of Gastroenterology & Hepatology*, vol. 12, no. 2, pp. 217–221, 2000.

[23] E. Kaemmerer, M. Westerkamp, R. Kasperk, G. Niepmann, A. Scherer, and N. Gassler, "Coincidence of active Crohn's disease and florid endometriosis in the terminal ileum: A case report," *World Journal of Gastroenterology*, vol. 19, no. 27, pp. 4413–4417, 2013.

[24] C. Dong, W. S. Ngu, and S. E. Wakefield, "Endometriosis masquerading as Crohn's disease in a patient with acute small bowel obstruction," *BMJ Case Reports*, article r2014207229, 2015.

Pancreatic Neuroendocrine Tumor in the Setting of Dorsal Agenesis of the Pancreas

Samih Nassif,[1] Cecilia Ponchiardi,[2] and Teviah Sachs[3]

[1] *Boston University School of Medicine, 72 East Concord St., Boston, MA 02118, USA*
[2] *Department of Pathology and Laboratory Medicine, Boston University School of Medicine, 72 East Concord St., Boston, MA 02118, USA*
[3] *Boston University School of Medicine, Moakley Building, 3rd Floor, 830 Harrison Avenue, Boston, MA 02118, USA*

Correspondence should be addressed to Teviah Sachs; teviah.sachs@bmc.org

Academic Editor: Haruhiko Sugimura

Dorsal agenesis of the pancreas (DAP) is an uncommon embryological abnormality where there is absence of the distal pancreas. DAP is mostly asymptomatic, but common presenting symptoms include diabetes mellitus, abdominal pain, pancreatitis, enlarged pancreatic head, and, in a few cases, polysplenia. MRCP and ERCP are the gold standard imaging techniques to demonstrate the absence of the dorsal pancreatic duct. The literature on the association of pancreatic neoplasia and DAP is limited. We present the case of a pancreatic neuroendocrine tumor in a patient with dorsal agenesis of the pancreas, with a review of the related literature.

1. Introduction

Dorsal agenesis of the pancreas (DAP) is an uncommon embryological abnormality where there is absence of the distal pancreas. Here, we present the case of a 48-year-old female who was referred to our surgical oncology clinic for a pancreatic mass and was found to have concurrent DAP. We then discuss the embryology of DAP, as well as the most common clinical presentations of DAP and other established reports of DAP in the literature.

2. Case Report

A 48-year-old female was referred to the surgical oncology clinic for evaluation of a pancreatic mass. This was found incidentally on workup for an endometrial stromal sarcoma, for which she had undergone a total abdominal hysterectomy with bilateral salpingo-oophorectomy. The patient was asymptomatic.

Her past medical history was significant for uterine sarcoma and for venous thromboembolism which led to a pulmonary embolus but was otherwise unremarkable. Her physical exam was unrevealing, as was her serum laboratory evaluation, with normoglycemia, normal hepatobiliary function, normal pancreatic enzymes, and no elevation in carbohydrate antigen 19-9, carbohydrate antigen 125, or carcinoembryonic antigen. CT and MRI imaging (Figure 1) revealed a mass at the neck of the pancreas, measuring 2.9 cm in its largest dimension, as well as the absence of the distal body and tail of the pancreas. The mass closely abutted the confluence of the portal vein and superior mesenteric vein, but there was no invasion. She underwent biopsy of this mass via endoscopic ultrasound which revealed features consistent with a well differentiated neuroendocrine tumor. The tumor was determined to be nonfunctioning given the absence of systemic symptoms and laboratory data to suggest hormone production.

The patient underwent resection of this mass via spleen preserving laparoscopic approach. Intraoperative images confirmed the absence of the distal body and tail of the pancreas (Figure 2). Negative margins were achieved with this resection, and the pancreatic head and uncinate process were preserved, as were the splenic vein and artery. The pancreatic parenchyma was transected using a linear cutting stapler, with a closed staple height of 1.5 mm, and the remnant pancreatic neck was buttressed with an omental patch. A 19 Fr fluted Blake drain was placed at the resection margin at

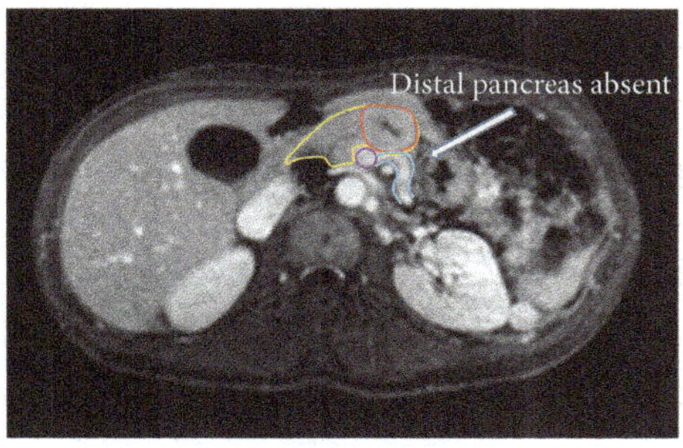

FIGURE 1: Axial image of an MRCP demonstrating the relevant anatomy of the tumor, vessels, and proximal pancreas, with the absence of the dorsal pancreas (white arrow). Outlines represent the pancreatic head and neck (yellow), the pancreatic neuroendocrine tumor (red), the superior mesenteric vein (purple), and the splenic vein (blue).

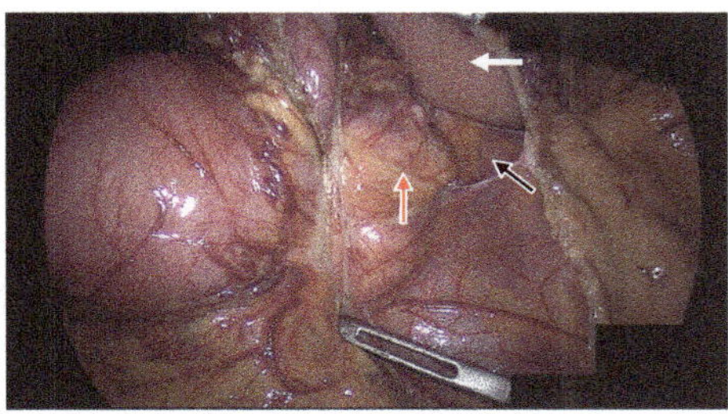

FIGURE 2: Laparoscopic image of the retroperitoneum as seen through a window created in the gastrocolic omentum. The stomach is elevated (white arrow), and the pancreatic neuroendocrine tumor (red arrow) can be seen with the absence of any pancreatic tissue distal to the tumor (black arrow).

the time of surgery. Final pathology revealed a grade 1 well differentiated pancreatic neuroendocrine tumor (Figure 3). Despite our intraoperative efforts to avoid it, the patient's postoperative course was significant for a pancreatic duct leak, which was well controlled by her drain, and she was discharged home on POD 4. Her drain was removed on POD 23. She had no evidence of diabetes or pancreatic insufficiency on follow-up evaluation. Her case was discussed at our multidisciplinary tumor board and no further treatment for this tumor was recommended.

3. Discussion

3.1. Embryology of the Pancreas. During the fourth week of gestation, the dorsal (cranial) and ventral (caudal) buds of the pancreas develop from the endoderm at the junction of the foregut and the midgut. While the dorsal bud develops only into pancreatic tissue (anterior head, body, and tail), the ventral bud also contributed to the liver, gallbladder, bile ducts, and ventral pancreas (posterior neck and head) [1]. The ventral pancreatic duct (duct of Wirsung) and the common bile duct thus share a common entry point to the duodenum at the major papilla. Eventually, the ventral bud rotates clockwise and fuses with the dorsal bud at the seventh week of gestation. At this time, the dorsal pancreatic duct

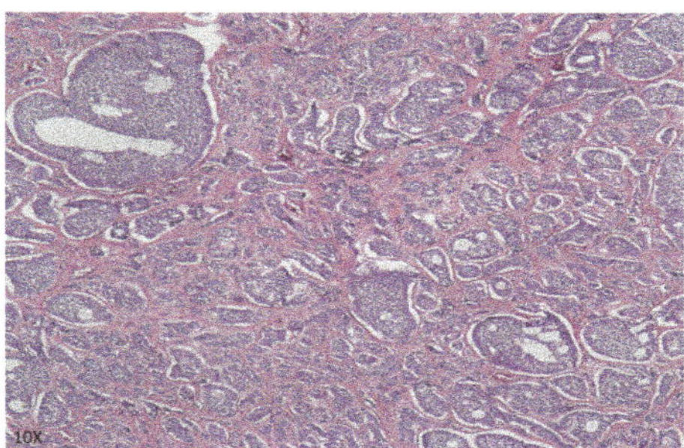

FIGURE 3: Histopathological description of the tumor. It is composed of multiple nests with hyalinized fibrovascular stroma. Tumor cells are relatively uniform with finely granular eosinophilic cytoplasm and centrally located round to oval nucleus with "salt and pepper" chromatin pattern. There were less than 2 mitoses per high-powered field. The tumor was chromogranin positive after immunohistochemical analysis (not shown).

(duct of Santorini) fuses with the ventral pancreatic duct to create the main pancreatic duct [2]. Islets of Langerhans primarily develop in the dorsal pancreas, at week twelve of gestation.

3.2. Dorsal Agenesis. Dorsal agenesis occurs when there is abnormal development of the dorsal pancreatic bud, but there is intact development of the ventral pancreatic bud. Thus, there is absence of the anterior head, body, and the tail of the pancreas with intact formation of the liver, gallbladder, bile ducts, and posterior neck and head of the pancreas. The dorsal pancreatic duct never forms, and pancreatic secretions course from the ventral pancreatic duct into the common bile duct and eventually pass through the major papilla into the second portion of the duodenum.

The first case of dorsal agenesis of the pancreas (DAP) was reported in 1911 as an autopsy finding, and since then there have been relatively few reported cases in the literature [1]. DAP can be complete or partial. In patients with complete DAP, the dorsal duct system and the body and the tail of the pancreas are all missing. However, in partial DAP, the accessory papilla, the terminal end of the main dorsal duct of Santorini, or the pancreatic body is present. Familial DAP has been described in association with other congenital deformities, as well as alone. The molecular basis for DAP is not well defined; however, certain homeobox genes have been associated with DAP in rodent models [10].

DAP can be asymptomatic due to exocrine and endocrine functional reserve in the remaining pancreas. However, given that most of the islets of Langerhans develop in the body and tail of the pancreas, diabetes mellitus can occur [1]. Other common findings in association with DAP include abdominal pain, pancreatitis, enlarged pancreatic head, and, in a few cases, polysplenia [3, 11]. Diagnosis of DAP requires demonstration of the absence of dorsal pancreatic tissue. CT can be useful as an initial study to delineate the size of the pancreas. MRCP and ERCP are the gold standard imaging techniques to demonstrate the absence of the dorsal

Table 1: Cases of pancreatic neoplasia in patients with dorsal agenesis of the pancreas.

Reference	Presenting symptoms	Imaging modality to confirm DAP	Operation	Final tumor histology
Matsusue et al. 1984 [3]	Abdominal pain, weight loss, hyperglycemia	ERCP	Total pancreatectomy	Ductal adenocarcinoma
Nakamura et al. 2001 [4]	None	ERCP	Subtotal pancreatectomy	Solid pseudopapillary tumor
Ulusan et al. 2005 [5]	Abdominal pain, type II diabetes mellitus	CT abdomen and pelvis	Pancreaticoduodenectomy	Solid pseudopapillary tumor
Ulusan et al. 2006 [6]	Abdominal pain, jaundice, hyperglycemia	Unknown	Hepaticojejunostomy	Ductal adenocarcinoma
Rittenhouse et al. 2011 [2]	Abdominal pain, type II diabetes mellitus	ERCP	Pancreaticoduodenectomy	Ductal adenocarcinoma
Rittenhouse et al. 2011 [2]	Abdominal pain, weight loss, type II diabetes mellitus	CT abdomen and pelvis	Pancreaticoduodenectomy	Ductal adenocarcinoma
Rittenhouse et al. 2011 [2]	Elevated liver function tests, asymptomatic	ERCP	Pancreaticoduodenectomy	Ductal adenocarcinoma
Kapoor and Singh 2011 [7]	Painless jaundice, weight loss, cholangitis	Intraoperative pancreatogram	Pancreaticoduodenectomy	Ampullary carcinoma
Sannappa et al. 2014 [8]	Jaundice, weight loss	MRI abdomen	Total pancreatectomy	Periampullary adenocarcinoma
Mistry et al. 2015 [9]	Painless jaundice, type II diabetes mellitus	CT abdomen and pelvis	Pancreaticoduodenectomy	Ampullary carcinoma

pancreatic duct [12]. Treatment of patients with DAP is guided by the symptomatology with which they presented [1].

3.3. Pancreatic Neoplasia and Dorsal Agenesis. The association of pancreatic neoplasia and DAP has not been studied extensively; a PubMed search identified 10 such cases published since 2000 (Table 1) [2–9]. The mechanism of this association is uncertain however. Some theorize that DAP increases the risk of chronic pancreatitis, which in and of itself is a risk factor for pancreatic tumors.

Treatment of pancreatic neoplasia in the setting of DAP does not deviate from current management guidelines [13]. Surgical resection of pancreatic tumors in patients with DAP often requires resection of the remaining pancreatic tissue, with a high rate of insulin dependent diabetes mellitus and exocrine insufficiency. In our case, we were able to preserve the majority of the proximal pancreas, mitigating the risks of postoperative diabetes.

4. Conclusion

We present the case of a pancreatic neuroendocrine tumor in a patient with dorsal agenesis of the pancreas, which, to our knowledge, has not previously been reported in the literature. The patient presented with an asymptomatic, incidentally discovered pancreatic mass at the neck of the pancreas that was resected with negative margins via spleen preserving, laparoscopic approach. This is one of the few cases of pancreatic neoplasia identified in patients with dorsal agenesis of the pancreas (DAP), a rare developmental anomaly where there is absence of the distal pancreas. DAP is most commonly asymptomatic but can present with symptoms of new-onset diabetes mellitus, abdominal pain, or chronic pancreatitis. Because of its silent presentation, there are very few cases of DAP reported in the literature and even fewer cases of DAP with concurrent pancreatic neoplasia.

References

[1] W. J. Schnedl, C. Piswanger-Soelkner, S. J. Wallner et al., "Agenesis of the dorsal pancreas and associated diseases," *Digestive Diseases and Sciences*, vol. 54, no. 3, pp. 481–487, 2009.

[2] D. W. Rittenhouse, E. P. Kennedy, A. A. Mascaro et al., "The novel triad of dorsal agenesis of the pancreas with concurrent pancreatic ductal adenocarcinoma and nonalcoholic chronic calcific pancreatitis: a case series and review of the literature," *Journal of Gastrointestinal Surgery*, vol. 15, no. 9, pp. 1643–1649, 2011.

[3] S. Matsusue, S. Kashihara, and S. Koizumi, "Pancreatectomy for carcinoma of the head of the pancreas associated with multiple anomalies including the preduodenal portal vein," *The Japanese Journal of Surgery*, vol. 14, no. 5, pp. 394–398, 1984.

[4] Y. Nakamura, K. Egami, S. Maeda, M. Hosone, and M. Onda, "Solid and papillary tumor of the pancreas complicating agenesis of the dorsal pancreas," *Journal of Hepato-Biliary-Pancreatic Surgery*, vol. 8, no. 5, pp. 485–489, 2001.

[5] S. Ulusan, N. Bal, O. Kizilkilic et al., "Solid-pseudopapillary tumour of the pancreas associated with dorsal agenesis," *British Journal of Radiology*, vol. 78, no. 929, pp. 441–443, 2005.

[6] S. Ulusan, T. Yakar, Z. Koc, F. Kayaselcuk, and N. Torer, "Adenocarcinoma of the pancreas associated with dorsal agenesis," *Pancreas*, vol. 33, no. 4, pp. 437–439, 2006.

[7] A. Kapoor and R. Singh, "Periampullary carcinoma in a patient with agenesis of dorsal pancreas," *Journal of Surgical Case Reports*, vol. 2011, no. 9, article 4, 2011.

[8] R. M. Sannappa, J. Buragohain, D. Sarma, U. K. Saikia, and B. K. Choudhury, "Agenesis of dorsal pancreas associated with periampullary pancreaticobiliary type adenocarcinoma," *Journal of the Pancreas*, vol. 15, no. 5, pp. 489–492, 2014.

[9] J. H. Mistry, A. Yadav, and S. Nundy, "Ampullary carcinoma in a patient with agenesis of the dorsal pancreas: a case report," *Indian Journal of Surgery*, vol. 77, supplement 1, pp. 32–34, 2015.

[10] M. Martín, J. Gallego-Llamas, V. Ribes et al., "Dorsal pancreas agenesis in retinoic acid-deficient Raldh2 mutant mice," *Developmental Biology*, vol. 284, no. 2, pp. 399–411, 2005.

[11] J. Low, D. Williams, and J. R. Chaganti, "Polysplenia syndrome with agenesis of the dorsal pancreas and preduodenal portal vein presenting with obstructive jaundice—a case report and literature review," *British Journal of Radiology*, vol. 84, no. 1007, pp. e217–e220, 2011.

[12] M. Mohapatra, S. Mishra, P. C. Dalai et al., "Imaging findings in agenesis of the dorsal pancreas. Report of three cases," *Journal of the Pancreas*, vol. 13, no. 1, pp. 108–114, 2012.

[13] N. Toyama, H. Kamiyama, Y. Suminaga, K. Namai, M. Ota, and F. Konishi, "Pancreas head carcinoma with total fat replacement of the dorsal exocrine pancreas," *Journal of Gastroenterology*, vol. 39, no. 1, pp. 76–80, 2004.

Caecal Perforation from Primary Intestinal Tuberculosis in Pregnancy

Soe Lwin,[1] Nina Lau Lee Jing,[2] Haris Suharjono,[2] Mardiana binti Kipli,[1] Tin Moe Nwe,[3] Myat San Yi,[1] and Lucas Luk Tien Wee[2]

[1] *Department of Obstetrics & Gynecology, Faculty of Medicine and Health Sciences, UNIMAS, Kota Samarahan, Malaysia*
[2] *Department of Obstetrics & Gynecology, Sarawak General Hospital, Kuching, Malaysia*
[3] *Department of Basic Health Sciences, Faculty of Medicine and Health Sciences, UNIMAS, Kota Samarahan, Malaysia*

Correspondence should be addressed to Soe Lwin; drslwinmm@gmail.com

Academic Editor: Hideto Kawaratani

The incidence of tuberculosis (TB) is rising worldwide, despite the efficacy of the BCG vaccination. Populations at greatest risk of contracting TB are migrant communities, as well as immunocompromised individuals. The diagnosis of extrapulmonary TB (EPTB) can often present as a diagnostic conundrum, due to its nonspecific and varied presentation, often mimicking inflammatory bowel disease or malignancy. We present a case of caecal TB in pregnancy, which resulted in caecal perforation, a right hemicolectomy, and severe preterm delivery. The aim of this case report is to discuss the diagnosis of extrapulmonary TB, as well as its subsequent management in pregnancy.

1. Introduction

TB remains a global epidemic, with an estimated 10.4 million new cases diagnosed worldwide in 2015. Of these, there was a slight male preponderance, 56% of all new cases, as compared to 34% for women. TB in children contributed to the remaining 10% of new cases. TB mortality rates are alarmingly high and in 2015, approximately 1.8 million deaths were attributable to TB, amongst whom those coinfected with Human Immunodeficiency Virus (HIV) made up a quarter of total deaths [1].

The diagnosis of EPTB can often present as a diagnostic conundrum, due to its nonspecific and varied presentation, often mimicking inflammatory bowel disease or malignancy. Immunocompromised individuals have been found to be more susceptible to EPTB [2] and this may explain its relative predominance in the young female population, as pregnancy is a state of relative immunocompromise.

Abdominal TB accounts for 11% of all EPTBs, with the most common site of involvement being the ileocaecal region [2]. Postulations for the propensity for ileocaecal involvement have included increased physiological stasis and fluid absorption and reduction in digestive activity, as well as the abundance of lymphoid tissue in this region (Peyer's patches) [3].

Symptoms of abdominal TB include chronic abdominal pain, abdominal distension, fever, night sweats, and loss of appetite, as well as rapid and significant weight loss. In diagnosing abdominal TB, a high index of suspicion is required, as the clinical signs are often nonspecific. Pregnancy further confounds clear diagnosis, as pregnancy related abdominal pains such as preterm labour and placental abruption have to be considered. Medical and surgical causes of abdominal pain, such as inflammatory bowel disease, appendicitis, acute pyelonephritis, and colorectal cancer, have to also be excluded.

Diagnostic and treatment modalities, even in pregnancy, are similar to the nonpregnant population.

2. Case Presentation

Patient was 31-year-old female and 15 weeks into her second pregnancy, when she commenced her antenatal care. Her

Body Mass Index (BMI) at booking was only 15.53 kg/m^2, with a booking weight of 36 kg. She had been experiencing intermittent, dull, right-sided abdominal pain that was associated with diarrhea, for 3 months and in this span of time, her weight had decreased markedly by 20 kg. Her primary healthcare provider at the district maternal and child health clinic subsequently treated her for acute gastroenteritis twice in the following weeks, but she experienced no improvement in her symptoms.

At 29 weeks and 6 days of gestation, she was admitted to a district hospital, complaining of acute right-sided abdominal pain that radiated to the right lumbar region. She also complained of dyspnoea and near-syncopal episodes, as well as a reduced effort tolerance the preceding week. She had been compliant to her oral hematinics therapy and denied any history of dysuria, haematuria, haematemesis, or haematochezia. A recent peripheral blood film revealed normochromic, normocytic anaemia, and serum ferritin was normal.

On physical examination, she appeared pale and she was febrile. On palpation, her fundal height corresponded to 30 weeks of gestation. Tenderness and guarding were elicited at the right lumbar region. However, she did not exhibit any signs of preterm contraction and renal punch was negative. Transabdominal scan revealed a singleton fetus, with parameters corresponding to her gestation.

She had hemoglobin of 7.4 g/dl and a white cell count of 15.87×10^9. Broad-spectrum antibiotic was commenced. She was also transfused with 1 pint of packed cells and she was referred to both the obstetrics and surgical teams of a tertiary hospital.

An urgent ultrasound abdomen was arranged, which revealed a heterogeneous collection in the subhepatic region and multiple enlarged mesenteric lymph nodes. A diagnosis of likely perforated appendicitis was made and she underwent an emergency laparotomy.

The intraoperative finding was that of a perforated caecal tumour. The tumour was firm and hard with irregular margins and surface. There was evidence of multiple enlarged mesenteric lymph nodes. A right hemicolectomy was performed. Appendix was normal. She received 3 pints of packed cells transfusion and 4 units of fresh frozen plasma. Postoperatively, she was transferred to the Intensive Care Unit (ICU), where she recovered well and was transferred to the general ward after 2 days. 7 days after surgery, she developed spontaneous preterm contractions and delivered a baby boy of 1.2 kg, at 31 weeks of gestation with Apgar score of 7 in one minutes and 9 in five minutes. The baby was given Bacillus Calmette-Guerin (BCG) vaccination immediately after delivery as routine procedure.

The histopathological examination showed caecal tuberculosis. She was referred to the Infectious Disease (ID) team and started on anti-TB medication. She denied any pulmonary TB contact. Her pulmonary TB work-up including chest X-ray, sputum acid fast bacilli (AFB), and Mantoux test was negative. Screening tests for HIV were negative.

She developed surgical wound breakdown at 14 days postoperatively and secondary suturing was performed. Her baby was initially admitted to the Neonatal Intensive Care Unit (NICU) for extreme prematurity but was subsequently discharged well with good catch-up growth and a negative Tuberculin skin text/Mantoux test. At a subsequent follow-up upon completion of 6 months of anti-TB medications, she had put back most of her weight and her baby was assessed to have achieved age-appropriate developmental milestones.

3. Discussion

EPTB is thought to be a result of reactivation of a prior dormant TB focus. Gastrointestinal TB is the sixth commonest site of extrapulmonary disease [4, 5]. Its occurrence is attributed to four mechanisms: hematological, swallowing of infected sputum in patient with active pulmonary TB, ingestion of contaminated milk or food, and contiguous transcoelomic spread from adjacent organs [6]. The ileocaecal region is affected in 75% of abdominal TB and this can present with perforation, abdominal mass, obstruction, and malabsorption [2, 7–9]. Viscus perforation due to TB is very rare and occurs more commonly in immunosuppressed patients [10]. Pregnancy is a physiological state of relative immunosuppression. Hence, the risk of viscus perforation after contracting abdominal TB in pregnancy may be increased, as was the case in our patient.

Diagnosis abdominal TB is challenging, presenting in a myriad of nonspecific ways, including abdominal pain, weight loss, loss of appetite, fever, diarrhea, constipation, or haematochezia. Diagnostic modalities that may help in the diagnosis of abdominal TB are outlined below.

3.1. Blood Investigations. The full blood count and peripheral blood film may reveal mild anaemia, of the normochromic and normocytic type, as is the case in chronic diseases. A markedly raised erythrocyte sedimentation rate (ESR) portends to the possibility of TB. The white cell count is often normal [2].

3.2. Radiological Investigations. Ultrasound may reveal discrete of conglomerated (matted) lymphadenopathy. Small discrete anechoic areas, representing zones of caseation, may be seen within the nodes [2]. Calcification in healing lesions is seen as discrete reflective lines [2]. Both caseation and calcification are highly reflective of TB, as opposed to a malignant cause of lymphadenopathy.

Computed Tomography scans may be able to distinguish between extraluminal or intraluminal pathology, as well as disease extent.

3.3. Endoscopy/Colonoscopy. Three types of intestinal lesions are commonly seen, ulcerative, stricturous, and hypertrophy. These morphological types may coexist, for example, ulceroconstrictive and ulcerohypertrophic lesions. Crohn's disease typically presents as "skip-lesions," while both sides of the ileocaecal valve are commonly involved in ileocaecal TB, leading to incompetence of the valve. A finding of ileocaecal valve incompetence may thus help distinguish tuberculosis from Crohn's disease [2].

It is important to distinguish between Crohn's disease and TB, as steroid therapy instituted for Crohn's disease could have disastrous effects on a patient who has EPTB instead.

3.4. Ultrasound Guided Fine Needle Aspiration Cytology (FNAC)/Biopsy. FNAC may be useful in guiding to a diagnosis of EPTB. Tissue biopsy specimens are typically more helpful in diagnosing EPTB. Features such as granulomatous inflammation, with epithelioid macrophages, Langhans' giant cells, and lymphocytes, accompanied by characteristic caseation necrosis typify TB infection [2]. However, these features are not pathognomonic for TB and a culture (Ziehl-Neelsen stain for acid fast mycobacterium) is required to establish a laboratory diagnosis of EPTB [2, 10].

3.5. Laparoscopy. Laparoscopic findings can be classified into 3 categories: thickened peritoneum with military yellowish white tubercles, only thickened peritoneum, and fibroadhesive pattern. Visual diagnosis and histological diagnosis made on the basis of typical granuloma are comparable, to the experienced eye [2].

3.6. Others. Molecular genetics is at the forefront of modern day medicine and a variety of molecular diagnostic tools have been found to be effective in diagnosis EPTB as well. These include Quanti FERON-TB gold (QFT-G), Nucleic Acid Amplification (NAA) assays for Mycobacterium TB DNA, and Polymerase Chain Reaction (PCR) [2, 10].

4. Management

4.1. Anti-TB Drugs. As with pulmonary TB, the first line of treatment for EPTB is anti-TB medications. Multidrug therapy, including at least 2 of isoniazid, rifampicin, and ethambutol, are considered to be effective in preventing drug-resistant TB [2, 10]. A 6-month course of therapy, including an initial intensive phase, followed by a continuation phase eliminates most of the residual bacilli and reduces the risk of treatment failure and TB recurrence [10]. Directly Observed Treatment, Short Course (DOTS) has also proven to be very effective in ensuring treatment compliance and reducing drug-resistant TB.

4.2. Surgery. In most cases of EPTB, medical treatment is curative. Surgery is usually reserved for patients who have developed complications, including perforations, fistulas, massive bleeding, obstruction, or those not responding to medical therapy [2]. The vast majority of patients exhibit rapid symptom improvement, within 2 weeks of anti-TB treatment. Laparotomy may thus be considered, if a patient with EPTB does not appear to respond to treatment beyond this time.

4.3. In Pregnancy. A high index of suspicion is required in at-risk populations, such as ethnic minorities, migrant communities, and immunocompromised individuals. Tuberculin skin testing is a valuable screening test in pregnancy and should be carried out if latent TB is suspected. Imaging modalities such as chest X-ray with shielding, CT scan, or ultrasound can be performed as necessary [10].

Pregnancy does not affect the course of TB. However, any delay in diagnosis and treatment could result in catastrophic repercussions to mother and baby, such as the resultant viscus perforations and severe preterm delivery as seen in our case described or even mortality. Intrauterine growth restriction and vertical transmission have also been described [10]. Coinfection with HIV increases maternal mortality rates [10].

First-line antituberculous drugs such as isoniazid, rifampicin, and ethambutol can be used safely in pregnancy and while breastfeeding.

EPTB is an important diagnosis to be considered in high risk women with a nonspecific presentation of abdominal pain and chronic constitutional symptoms, as in our case. Diagnostic delay can lead to unnecessary maternal and fetal morbidity and mortality [11].

In our case described, a pregnant lady presenting with chronic constitutional symptoms should have been thoroughly investigated for possible causes, at primary contact, with referral to the obstetrics and medical teams for specialist care.

Normochromic normocytic anaemia, which does not respond to oral iron therapy, warrants further investigations to look for chronic blood loss, chronic disease, and malignancy. With an earlier referral, a biopsy might have sufficed, with consequent medical anti-TB therapy commenced. Viscus perforation may have been avoided, with resultant less morbidity for both mother and baby.

5. Conclusion

Tuberculosis remains an important cause of mortality and severe morbidity in the world, despite the availability of sound Bacillus Calmette-Guerin (BCG) vaccination programmes in most countries. It is often difficult to differentiate EPTB from Crohn's disease or malignancy. In populations where TB is endemic or in marginalized communities such as migrant populations, a high index of suspicion is crucial in diagnosing and appropriately managing EPTB.

Increased vigilance should be afforded to the pregnant population presenting with constitutional symptoms such as drastic weight loss or chronic malaise and night sweats. Early specialist consult should be sought and a thorough investigation made, bearing in mind the possibility of TB in at-risk populations. With early multidisciplinary team involvement and the commencement of appropriate treatment, medical cure rates and prognosis is excellent for patients with EPTB in pregnancy.

Abbreviations

AFB: Acid fast bacilli
BCG: Bacillus Calmette-Guerin
EPTB: Extrapulmonary tuberculosis
ID: Infectious Disease
TB: Tuberculosis.

Consent

Written informed consent was obtained from the patient for publication of this case report and any accompanying images.

References

[1] *Global Tuberculosis Report*, World Health Organization, 2016.

[2] V. K. Kapoor, R. Pravin, and G. Pravir, "Abdominal tuberculosis," *Journal of The Association of Physicians of India*, vol. 64, February 2016.

[3] A. Michalopoulos, V. N. Papadopoulos, S. Panidis, T. S. Papavramidis, A. Chiotis, and G. Basdanis, "Cecal obstruction due to primary intestinal tuberculosis: A case series," *Journal of Medical Case Reports*, vol. 5, article no. 128, 2011.

[4] S. T. Ved Bhushan, M. A. Mulla, and V. Kumar, "Ruptured appendix in tuberculous abdomen," *Biological System*, vol. 4, no. 1, pp. 1–6, 2015.

[5] F. F. Paustian, "Tuberculosis of the intestine," in *Gastroenterology*, H. L. Bockus, Ed., vol. 311, W.B. Saunders Co., Philadelphia, Pa, USA, 2nd edition, 1964.

[6] A. Nisar, H. Muhammad, and I. Muhammad, "Tuberculosis as a cause of small bowel obstruction in adults," *Gomal Journal of Medical Sciences*, vol. 9, article 233, no. 2, 2011.

[7] S. K. Bhansali, "Abdominal tuberculosis. Experiences with 300 cases," *American Journal of Gastroenterology*, vol. 67, pp. 324–337, 1977.

[8] A. Prakash, "Ulcero-constrictive tuberculosis of the bowel," *International Surgery*, vol. 63, pp. 23–29, 1978.

[9] J. R. Hoon, M. B. Dockerty, and J. Pemberton, "Ileocaecal tuberculosis including a comparison of this disease with non-specific regional enterocolitis and non- caseous tuberculated enterocolitis," *International Abstracts of Surgery*, vol. 91, pp. 417–440, 1950.

[10] A. Mahendru et al., "Review Diagnosis and Management of tuberculosis in pregnancy," *The Obstetrician & Gynaecologist*, vol. 12, no. 3, 2011.

[11] N. Kangeyan, S. N. E. Webster, A. Sanyal et al., "Tuberculosis in pregnancy - diagnostic dilemma," *Open Journal of Obstetrics and Gynecology*, vol. 2, pp. 174-175, 2012.

20

An Unusual Case of Pancreatic Metastasis from Squamous Cell Carcinoma of the Lung Diagnosed by EUS-Guided Fine Needle Biopsy

Takuya Ishikawa,[1,2] Yoshiki Hirooka,[3] Carolin J. Teman,[4] Hidemi Goto,[2] and Paul J. Belletrutti[1]

[1]*Division of Gastroenterology and Hepatology, Department of Medicine, University of Calgary, Calgary, AB, Canada*
[2]*Department of Gastroenterology, Nagoya University Graduate School of Medicine, Nagoya, Japan*
[3]*Department of Endoscopy, Nagoya University Hospital, Nagoya, Japan*
[4]*Division of Anatomic Pathology and Cytopathology, Department of Pathology and Laboratory Medicine, University of Calgary, Calgary, AB, Canada*

Correspondence should be addressed to Paul J. Belletrutti; pjbellet@ucalgary.ca

Academic Editor: Vladimir Schraibman

We report a case of a 70-year-old man who presented with abdominal pain and weight loss, with initial imaging showing simultaneous mass lesions in the pancreas and lungs along with extensive lymphadenopathy in the thorax up to the left supraclavicular region. Core biopsies of the left supraclavicular lymph node showed squamous cell carcinoma, which required differentiation between secondary and primary pancreatic neoplasms. Endoscopic ultrasound-guided sampling using a novel fine needle biopsy system was key to making a definite histological diagnosis and determining the best treatment plan.

1. Introduction

Metastatic tumors in the pancreas are uncommon, and most cases are difficult to distinguish from a primary pancreatic cancer. Accurate identification of isolated pancreatic metastases is critical in determining the best surgical and/or medical management [1]. Although lung cancer can metastasize to the pancreas, the frequency ranges according to the histological subtype, and the incidence of pancreas involvement with squamous cell carcinoma is reported as 1.1% of all pancreatic metastases [2]. Here we report a case of histologically certified metastatic squamous cell carcinoma involving the pancreas from a primary lung cancer, definitively diagnosed with endoscopic ultrasound-guided fine needle biopsy (EUS-FNB).

2. Case Report

A 70-year-old man presented with a three-month history of progressive abdominal pain and weight loss. His past medical history was unremarkable including no prior history of malignancy. On examination by his primary physician, he was alert and without jaundice or scleral icterus. He had mild epigastric tenderness on abdominal examination, and there were palpable lymph nodes in the left supraclavicular fossa. The remainder of his examination was unremarkable. Laboratory test results were all within normal limits including common blood cell counts, liver chemistries, and serum lipase. Transabdominal ultrasound showed a large distal pancreatic mass. CT scanning revealed a 3.8 cm hypodense mass in the pancreatic body with lymphadenopathy in the left supraclavicular region. It also showed a 3 cm lung mass posterior to the left main stem bronchus (Figure 1). Percutaneous biopsy of one of the left supraclavicular lymph nodes revealed squamous cell carcinoma. The patient was referred to our institution for a tissue diagnosis via endoscopic ultrasound (EUS) of the mediastinal mass and to determine the origin of the pancreas mass. Endoscopically there was no abnormality

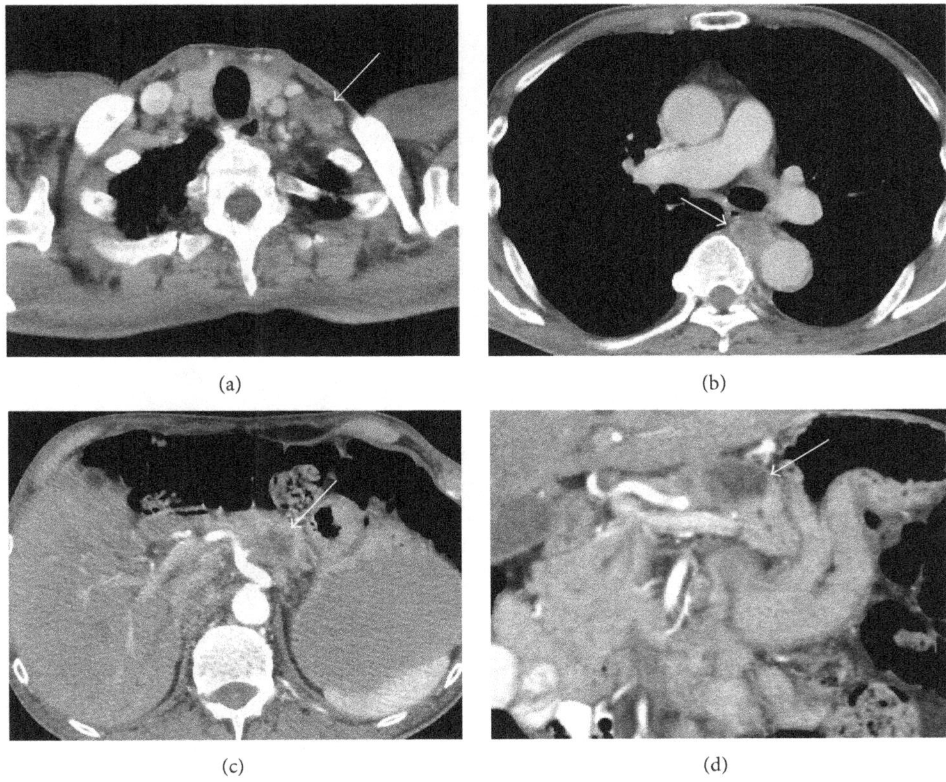

FIGURE 1: Computed tomography. (a) A conglomerate of lymph nodes in the left supraclavicular fossa measuring 3 cm (arrow). (b) A 2 cm left mid lung mass posterior to the left main stem bronchus (arrow). (c and d) A 3.8 cm hypodense mass in the pancreatic body with associated ill-defined soft tissue inseparable from the distal celiac axis and its branches (arrow).

in the esophagus or the laryngopharynx. EUS using a linear-array echoendoscope (PENTAX EG-3870UTK) revealed two well-defined hypoechoic lesions with similar echotexture firstly in the mediastinum posterior to the left main stem bronchus and secondly in the pancreatic body. EUS-FNB of these two lesions was performed (Figure 2) with a 25-gauge needle using a novel fine needle biopsy system (Beacon SharkCore, Medtronic Corp., Boston, USA). Histopathological examination of both of the specimens revealed a carcinoma morphologically similar to the supraclavicular lymph node biopsy. Immunostains performed on both specimens showed positivity for CK5/6 and p63 (Figures 3 and 4). The patient was thus diagnosed with a metastatic squamous cell carcinoma involving the pancreas from a primary lung cancer. Palliative chemotherapy was planned for the patient.

3. Discussion

Clinically apparent pancreatic metastases, while infrequent, are not rare, accounting for up to 3% of solid pancreatic lesions [3]. Although lung cancer is the second most common primary malignancy that metastasizes to the pancreas (next to renal cell carcinoma), the frequency ranges according to the histological subtype [4], and squamous cell carcinoma is extremely rare. The most frequent type is small cell carcinoma with a pancreatic metastasis incidence of 10%, followed by adenocarcinoma (2.4%), large cell carcinoma (1.9%), and finally squamous cell carcinoma with an incidence of only 1.1% [2].

These metastatic lesions are usually asymptomatic or the symptoms are nonspecific. In many cases, the metastatic lesions are discovered incidentally and are mistaken for primary pancreatic tumors. There are no radiological findings that are pathognomonic of pancreatic metastases. On EUS evaluation, it is reported that metastatic lesions are more likely to have well-defined borders compared with primary pancreatic cancer, but, otherwise, EUS features cannot distinguish between the two groups [5]. Therefore, pathological confirmation of pancreatic tumors is the best method for the diagnosis of pancreatic metastases.

The usefulness of EUS-guided tissue sampling in the diagnosis of pancreatic metastases has previously been reported [1, 5–7]. However, some of the metastatic tumors to the pancreas (e.g., esophageal and non-SCLC metastases) cannot be definitively confirmed by cytomorphology alone [5], and obtaining optimal histological samples is highly desirable to improve diagnostic accuracy and certainty. Tissue specimens for histological examination can provide the opportunity to immunostain the tissue, further increasing differential diagnostic capabilities for suspected metastatic lesions. Several new "core" FNA needles have been developed, and one such needle, SharkCore, is attracting attention now.

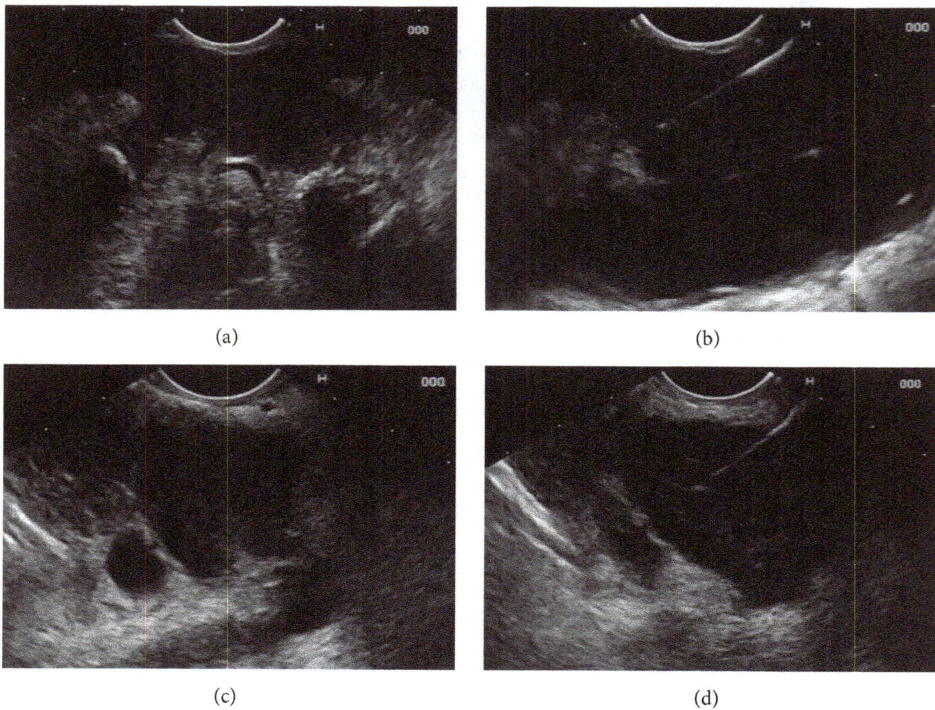

Figure 2: (a) Endoscopic ultrasound (EUS) demonstrating a 3 cm hypoechoic mass in the left lung. (b) EUS-guided fine needle biopsy (FNB) of the left lung nodule with a 25-gauge needle. (c) EUS demonstrating a 3.8 cm hypoechoic mass in the pancreatic body abutting the splenic artery. It shows the same internal echotexture as the lesion in the mediastinum. (d) EUS-FNB of the pancreatic mass with a 25-gauge needle.

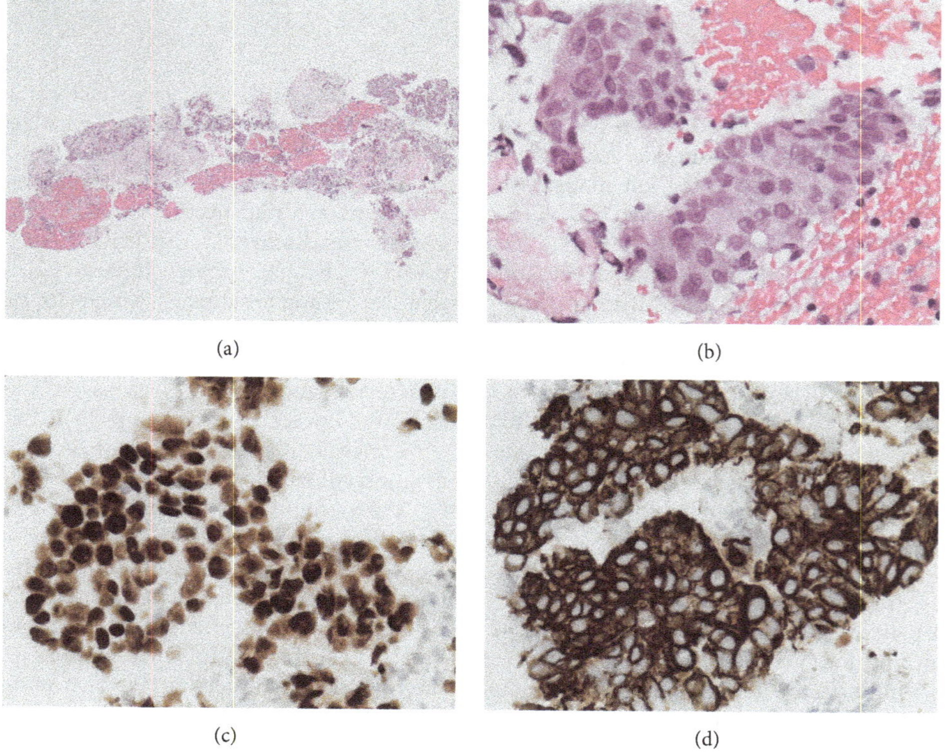

Figure 3: (a) Hematoxylin and eosin staining of a specimen obtained from lung mass with EUS-guided fine needle biopsy. (b) Small core biopsy fragments show invasive carcinoma with clusters and cords of cells that show squamous morphology. (c and d) Immunostains showed that the neoplastic cells express p63 (c) and CK 5/6 (d).

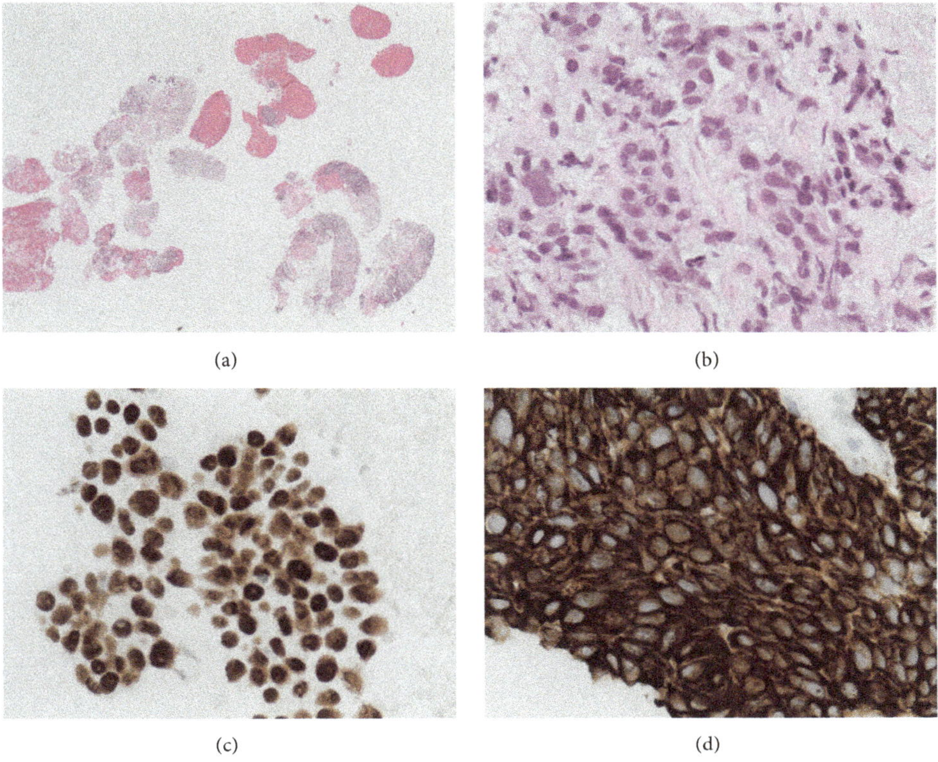

FIGURE 4: (a) Hematoxylin and eosin staining of a specimen obtained from pancreatic mass with EUS-guided fine needle biopsy. (b) Biopsy fragments show invasive carcinoma morphologically similar to the carcinoma identified in the supraclavicular lymph node and the mediastinal mass. (c and d) Immunostains show that the neoplastic cells express p63 (c) and CK 5/6 (d).

Kandel et al. [8] demonstrated that histological cores were obtained from 95% of the FNB samples compared with 59% of the FNA samples in a total of 156 patients, and the histology yield was significantly higher using the SharkCore needle compared with the EUS-FNA needle ($P = 0.01$). Additionally, a large North American multicenter study of the SharkCore needle was recently reported [9]. In this study, a total of 250 lesions were biopsied in 226 patients, and the overall pathologic diagnostic rate was 88% with a median number of 2 passes. In the present case, the core needle made it possible to obtain adequate histological specimens enabling multiple immunostains to be performed leading to the correct diagnosis and allowing appropriate clinical management to be started without the need for additional time-consuming diagnostic procedures.

In conclusion, although pancreatic metastases from squamous cell carcinoma of the lung are unusual, differentiation from primary pancreatic neoplasms is important. EUS-FNB can allow for a definite histological diagnosis and determination of the most appropriate treatment plan.

References

[1] I. I. El Hajj, J. K. Leblanc, S. Sherman et al., "Endoscopic ultrasound-guided biopsy of pancreatic metastases: a large single-center experience," *Pancreas*, vol. 42, no. 3, pp. 524–530, 2013.

[2] C. Garcia Vidal, E. Carrillo, and B. Barreiro, "Solitary metastasis to the pancreas in a patient with lung cancer," *Archivos de Bronconeumologia*, vol. 39, no. 12, Article ID 601, 2003.

[3] J. C. Ardengh, C. V. Lopes, L. F. de Lima et al., "Diagnosis of pancreatic tumors by endoscopic ultrasound-guided fine-needle aspiration," *World Journal of Gastroenterology*, vol. 13, no. 22, pp. 3112–3116, 2007.

[4] N. Liratzopoulos, E. I. Efremidou, M. S. Papageorgiou, K. Romanidis, G. J. Minopoulos, and K. J. Manolas, "Extrahepatic biliary obstruction due to a solitary pancreatic metastasis of squamous cell lung carcinoma. Case report," *Journal of Gastrointestinal and Liver Diseases*, vol. 15, no. 1, pp. 73–75, 2006.

[5] J. DeWitt, P. Jowell, J. LeBlanc et al., "EUS-guided FNA of pancreatic metastases: a multicenter experience," *Gastrointestinal Endoscopy*, vol. 61, no. 6, pp. 689–696, 2005.

[6] M. Sekulic, K. Amin, T. Mettler, L. K. Miller, S. Mallery, and J. R. Stewart, "Pancreatic involvement by metastasizing neoplasms as determined by endoscopic ultrasound-guided fine needle aspiration: a clinicopathologic characterization," *Diagnostic Cytopathology*, vol. 45, no. 5, pp. 418–425, 2017.

[7] R. Pannala, K. M. Hallberg-Wallace, A. L. Smith et al., "Endoscopic ultrasound-guided fine needle aspiration cytology of metastatic renal cell carcinoma to the pancreas: a multi-center experience," *CytoJournal*, vol. 13, no. 1, pp. 13–24, 2016.

[8] P. Kandel, G. Tranesh, A. Nassar et al., "EUS-guided fine needle biopsy sampling using a novel fork-tip needle: a case-control study," *Gastrointestinal Endoscopy*, vol. 84, no. 6, pp. 1034–1039, 2016.

[9] C. J. DiMaio, J. M. Kolb, P. C. Benias et al., "Initial experience with a novel EUS-guided core biopsy needle (SharkCore): results of a large North American multicenter study," *Endoscopy International Open*, vol. 4, no. 9, pp. E974-E979, 2016.

Diarrhea as a Presenting Symptom of Disseminated Toxoplasmosis

Matthew Glover, Zhouwen Tang, Robert Sealock, and Shilpa Jain

Baylor College of Medicine, Houston, TX, USA

Correspondence should be addressed to Shilpa Jain; shilpaj@bcm.edu

Academic Editor: Hideto Kawaratani

Disseminated toxoplasmosis is uncommon in both immunocompetent and immunocompromised hosts with gastrointestinal involvement being rarely described. We report a case of disseminated gastrointestinal toxoplasmosis in an immunocompromised man who presented with one month of diarrhea and abdominal pain. Imaging showed thickening of the ascending colon and cecum. Esophagogastroduodenoscopy and colonoscopy biopsies revealed *Toxoplasma gondii*, confirmed by immunostain. Symptoms completely resolved following treatment with pyrimethamine, sulfadiazine, and leucovorin. This case highlights the importance of including toxoplasmosis in the differential diagnosis of any immunocompromised individual presenting with gastrointestinal symptoms.

1. Introduction

Gastrointestinal toxoplasmosis is a rare manifestation of a relatively common disease. Disseminated *Toxoplasma gondii* must be considered in the differential diagnosis of any immunocompromised individual presenting with nonspecific gastrointestinal symptoms, particularly if from or traveling from a region with high *T. gondii* seropositivity. A biopsy is necessary for definitive diagnosis.

2. Case Report

A 54-year-old man who recently immigrated from El-Salvador with a past medical history of Human Immunodeficiency Virus (HIV) presented with one-month progressive diarrhea, abdominal pain, subjective fevers, and 30-pound weight loss. There were no neurologic complaints. He was immunocompromised with an absolute CD4 count of 6 cells/μL after being off antiretroviral therapy for the past 10 years. He had been working full time as a car mechanic and reported having multiple indoor pet cats throughout his life. The patient was cachectic and frail appearing but with an otherwise unremarkable physical exam. Laboratory showed a HIV viral load of >130,000 copies/mL with *Toxoplasma* IgG > 700 IU/mL. Laboratory was unremarkable otherwise with *Toxoplasma* IgM < 3 AU/mL, no fecal ova or parasites observed, negative cryptococcal antigen, negative enteric cultures, and a nonreactive rapid plasma reagin. CT of the chest, abdomen, and pelvis demonstrated diffuse circumferential colonic wall thickening with prominent mesenteric lymph nodes (Figure 1). Bidirectional endoscopy was performed with esophagogastroduodenoscopy showing large ulcerations in the gastric cardia and fundus. Severe inflammation and ulcerations in the right colon and cecum were noted on colonoscopy (Figure 2). Biopsies were taken from both the gastric and colonic ulcerations. Histologic examination revealed markedly active gastritis and colitis with ulceration and ischemic changes (Figure 3). Many free tachyzoites and encysted forms were identified in the lamina propria as well as the cytoplasm of epithelial, endothelial, and smooth muscle cells (Figures 3, 4, and 5). Immunohistochemistry (polyclonal rabbit anti-*Toxoplasma*, 1:200; Dako Corporation, Carpinteria, Calif) confirmed the diagnosis of toxoplasmosis (Figure 5). Follow-up CT head demonstrated a 1.6 cm peripherally enhancing lesion consistent with toxoplasmosis. There was subtle surrounding vasogenic edema without midline shift. The patient was diagnosed

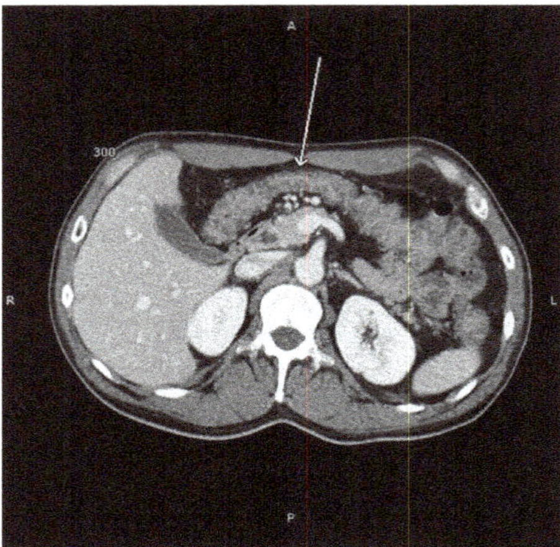

FIGURE 1: Abdominal computed tomography showing diffuse circumferential thickening of the colonic wall. The arrows refer to circumferential thickening of the transverse colon.

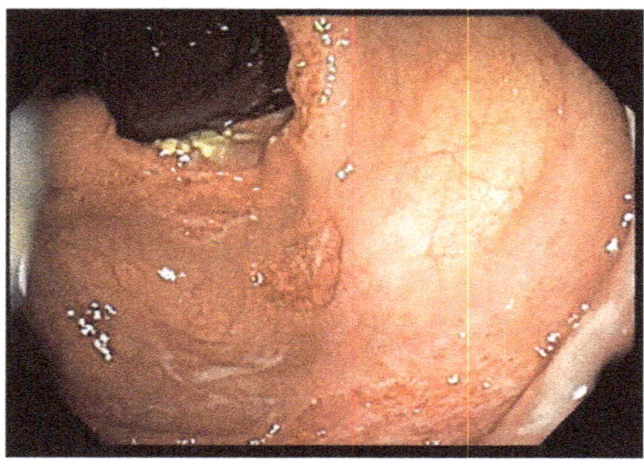

FIGURE 2: Colonoscopy with ulcerations in the cecum and ascending colon.

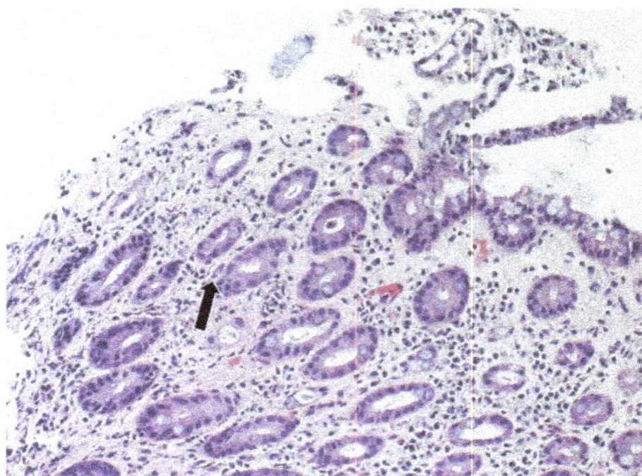

FIGURE 3: Colonic ulcer biopsy demonstrating ischemic morphology with hyalinization of the lamina propria and atrophic crypts. Small cystic forms are evident. The arrows refer to toxoplasmosis cyst present within the colonic ulcer biopsy.

with disseminated toxoplasmosis and treatment was initiated with pyrimethamine, sulfadiazine, and leucovorin with subsequent resolution of his gastrointestinal and intracranial toxoplasmosis.

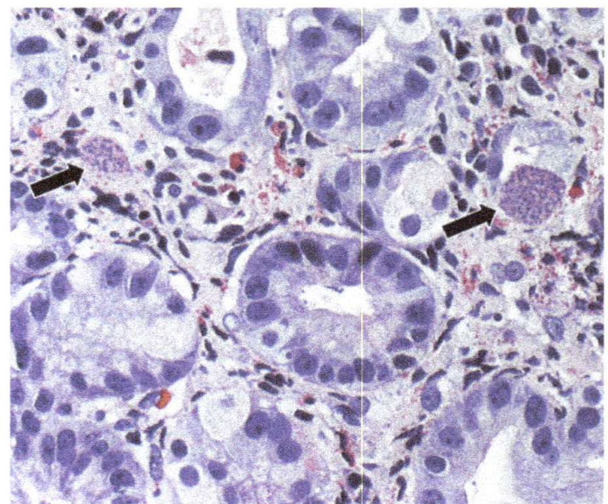

FIGURE 4: Gastric biopsy specimen showing large cystic forms present in the glandular epithelium and stroma within a background of eosinophils. The arrows refer to toxoplasmosis cyst present within the gastric biopsy.

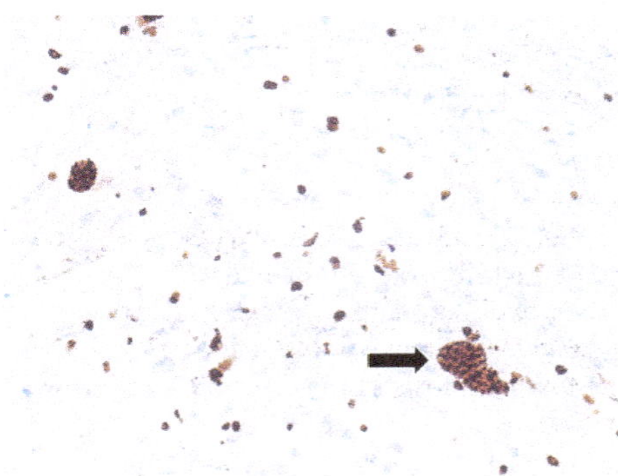

FIGURE 5: Pathologic specimen with confirmation of *T. gondii* by immunohistochemistry. Cystic forms are present alongside dispersed tachyzoites. The arrows refer to toxoplasmosis cyst highlighted by immunohistochemistry.

3. Discussion

T. gondii is an obligate intracellular parasite with felines serving as the definitive host. *T. gondii* can take several forms including oocysts containing sporozoites, tachyzoites, and bradyzoites contained within tissue cysts. Oral ingestion is the primary route of adult infection through consumption of either raw meat containing cysts or water contaminated with the oocysts of infected cat feces [1]. Primary infection is asymptomatic in the vast majority of immunocompetent patients [2]. Infection becomes latent in the form of tissue cysts and reactivation is rare. In immunocompromised individuals however, reactivation of latent infection is the most common cause of symptomatic toxoplasmosis. Patients with Acquired Immunodeficiency Syndrome (AIDS) and a CD4 count < 100 cells/μL who are *T. gondii* seropositive without prophylaxis have a 30% chance of developing reactivated toxoplasmosis [3]. The most common site of reactivation is the central nervous system followed by the eye, myocardium, skeletal muscle, lungs, bone marrow, and peripheral blood [2, 4]. Extracranial toxoplasmosis occurs in less than 2% of all immunocompromised individuals with reactivation [5, 6].

Although the gastrointestinal tract serves as the most common port of entry into the adult human, gastrointestinal manifestations of toxoplasmosis are rare, occurring in only 6–20% of patients with disseminated disease (defined as affecting >1 organ system) [1, 4, 7–9]. The reason for this paradoxical sparing remains unclear. Antemortem diagnosis is rare with only a handful of cases ever described [10]. When gastrointestinal toxoplasmosis has been identified, the most common underlying risk factor has been severe immunosuppression, with a CD4 count < 60 cells/μL [4, 5, 11]. Previous studies have found between 6.5% and 9.7% of all AIDS patients to have evidence of gastrointestinal toxoplasmosis at time of autopsy [9, 12]. Disseminated toxoplasmosis is often difficult to diagnose due to its nonspecific symptoms and requisite immunohistochemical techniques. For this reason, gastrointestinal toxoplasmosis is often identified postmortem leading to a likely underestimation of its prevalence [13]. Symptoms of gastrointestinal toxoplasmosis include diarrhea, abdominal pain, nausea, vomiting, anorexia, and ascites [14]. Complete or partial involvement of the gastrointestinal tract may be present [15]. If toxoplasmosis is suspected, biopsies are necessary as disseminated toxoplasmosis is almost invariably fatal if left untreated [11, 16]. The most common endoscopic findings of gastrointestinal toxoplasmosis are thickened gastric folds, ulcerative lesions, and nonspecific inflammation [4, 14, 17, 18].

Primary infection with *T. gondii* initially gives an IgM immune response which is followed by a *T. gondii* specific IgG response. These IgG antibodies last for life, resulting in lifelong seropositivity [19]. Seropositivity rates vary with geography and age with older individuals and those living in tropical climates more likely to be seropositive [1, 20]. With particular relevance to this case report, one study in El-Salvador found a 97% seropositivity rate by the 6th decade of life with an overall population seropositivity of 59% [21]. This is in stark contrast with a 12.4% overall seropositivity rate in the United States [22]. Although it remains impossible to say whether this particular case was primary versus reactivated toxoplasmosis, given the patients age, immigration history, and immunocompromised state, it is likely he was *T. gondii* seropositive at time of immigration arguing for reactivation over primary infection.

Unfortunately, data on treatment of extracerebral toxoplasmosis remains lacking. At current, disseminated treatment consists of the standard regimens typically used for cerebral toxoplasmosis. In all patients with diagnosed extracranial toxoplasmosis, even in the absence of neurologic symptoms, occult intracranial toxoplasmosis must be ruled out as up to 41% may have central nervous system involvement [5].

In summary, gastrointestinal toxoplasmosis is a rare manifestation of a relatively common disease. As demonstrated by this case report, disseminated *T. gondii* must be considered in the differential diagnosis of any immunocompromised individual presenting with nonspecific gastrointestinal symptoms, particularly if from or traveling from a region with high *T. gondii* seropositivity. A biopsy is necessary for definitive diagnosis.

Consent

Informed consent was obtained for this case report and can be provided upon request.

Disclosure

Zhouwen Tang is now an advanced endoscopy fellow at UT Southwestern Medical Center, Dallas, TX, United States.

Authors' Contributions

Matthew Glover wrote the manuscript and is the article guarantor. Zhouwen Tang and Robert Sealock revised and edited the manuscript and provided endoscopic imaging. Shilpa Jain revised and edited the manuscript and provided pathologic imaging.

References

[1] J. G. Montoya and O. Liesenfeld, "Toxoplasmosis," *The Lancet*, vol. 363, no. 9425, pp. 1965–1976, 2004.

[2] J. G. Montoya, "Laboratory diagnosis of Toxoplasma gondii infection and toxoplasmosis," *Journal of Infectious Diseases*, vol. 185, no. 1, pp. S73–S82, 2002.

[3] R. T. Gandhi, "Toxoplasmosis in HIV-infected patients," in *UpToDate*, T. W. Post, Ed., Waltham, MA, USA, 2016.

[4] M. Merzianu, S. M. Gorelick, V. Paje, D. P. Kotler, and C. Sian, "Gastric toxoplasmosis as the presentation of acquired immunodeficiency syndrome," *Archives of Pathology & Laboratory Medicine*, vol. 129, no. 4, pp. e87–90, 2005.

[5] C. Rabaud, T. May, C. Amiel et al., "Extracerebral toxoplasmosis in patients infected with HIV: a french national survey," *Medicine (Baltimore)*, vol. 73, no. 6, pp. 306–314, 1994.

[6] F. Belanger, F. Derouin, L. Grangeot-Keros, and L. Meyer, "Incidence and risk factors of toxoplasmosis in a cohort of human immunodeficiency virus-infected patients: 1988-1995," *Clinical Infectious Diseases*, vol. 28, no. 3, pp. 575–581, 1999.

[7] L. W. Garcia, R. B. Hemphill, W. A. Marasco, and P. S. Ciano, "Acquired immunodeficiency syndrome with disseminated toxoplasmosis presenting as an acute pulmonary and gastrointestinal illness," *Archives of Pathology and Laboratory Medicine*, vol. 115, no. 5, pp. 459–463, 1991.

[8] T. H. Gleason and W. B. Hamlin, "Disseminated toxoplasmosis in the compromised host: a report of five cases," *Archives of Internal Medicine*, vol. 134, no. 6, pp. 1059–1062, 1974.

[9] G. Jautzke, M. Sell, U. Thalmann et al., "Extracerebral toxoplasmosis in AIDS: histological and immunohistological findings based on 80 autopsy cases," *Pathology Research and Practice*, vol. 189, no. 4, pp. 428–436, 1993.

[10] P. A. Mackowiak, M. Asmal, R. E. Factor, and R. P. Walensky, "An HIV-infected man with an upset stomach," *Clinical Infectious Diseases*, vol. 47, no. 7, pp. 979-980, 2008.

[11] S. L. Williams and E. C. Burton, "Disseminated toxoplasmosis in a patient with undiagnosed AIDS," *Proceedings (Baylor University Medical Center)*, vol. 22, no. 1, pp. 20–22, 2009.

[12] L. C. Guimarães, A. C. A. L. Silva, A. M. R. Micheletti, E. N. M. Moura, M. L. Silva-Vergara, and S. J. Adad, "Morphological changes in the digestive system of 93 human immunodeficiency virus positive patients: An autopsy study," *Revista do Instituto de Medicina Tropical de Sao Paulo*, vol. 54, no. 2, pp. 89–93, 2012.

[13] P. Hofman, E. Bernard, J. F. Michiels, A. Thyss, Y. Le Fichoux, and R. Loubiere, "Extracerebral toxoplasmosis in the acquired immunodeficiency syndrome (AIDS)," *Pathology Research and Practice*, vol. 189, no. 8, pp. 894–901, 1993.

[14] M. Ganji, A. Tan, M. I. Maitar, C. M. Weldon-Linne, E. Weisenberg, and D. P. Rhone, "Gastric toxoplasmosis in a patient with acquired immunodeficiency syndrome: a case report and review of the literature," *Archives of Pathology and Laboratory Medicine*, vol. 127, no. 6, pp. 732–734, 2003.

[15] M. Tahmasbi, S. Al Diffalha, C. M. Strosberg, R. Sandin, and M. Ghayouri, "Duodenal toxoplasmosis in a bone marrow transplant patient: a rare case report," *Human Pathology: Case Reports*, 2015.

[16] M. Yang and D. Perez, "Disseminated toxoplasmosis as a cause of diarrhea," *Southern Medical Journal*, vol. 88, no. 8, pp. 860-861, 1995.

[17] L. Alpert, M. Miller, E. Alpert, R. Satin, E. Lamoureux, and L. Trudel, "Gastric toxoplasmosis in acquired immunodeficiency syndrome: Antemortem diagnosis with histopathologic characterization," *Gastroenterology*, vol. 110, no. 1, pp. 258–264, 1996.

[18] D. Lowe, R. Hessler, J. Lee, R. Schade, and A. Chaudhary, "Toxoplasma colitis in a patient with acquired immune deficiency syndrome," *Gastrointestinal Endoscopy*, vol. 63, no. 2, pp. 341-342, 2006.

[19] T. Yohanes, S. Debalke, and E. Zemene, "Latent toxoplasma gondii infection and associated risk factors among HIV-infected individuals at Arba Minch Hospital, south Ethiopia," *AIDS Research and Treatment*, vol. 2014, Article ID 652941, 2014.

[20] H. Akuffo, E. Linder, M. Wahlgren, and I. Ljungström, *Parasites of the Colder Climates*, CRC Press, 2002.

[21] J. S. Remington, B. Efron, E. Cavanaugh, H. J. Simon, and A. Trejos, "Studies on toxoplasmosis in El Savador prevalence and incidence of toxoplasmosis as measured by the Sabin-Feldman dye test," *Transactions of the Royal Society of Tropical Medicine and Hygiene*, vol. 64, no. 2, pp. 252–267, 1970.

[22] J. L. Jones, D. Kruszon-Moran, H. N. Rivera, C. Price, and P. P. Wilkins, "Toxoplasma gondii seroprevalence in the United States 2009-2010 and comparison with the past two decades," *American Journal of Tropical Medicine and Hygiene*, vol. 90, no. 6, pp. 1135–1139, 2014.

22

Magnifying Endoscopic Features of Follicular Lymphoma Involving the Stomach: A Report of Two Cases

Masaya Iwamuro,[1,2] Katsuyoshi Takata,[3] Seiji Kawano,[1] Nobuharu Fujii,[4] Yoshiro Kawahara,[5] Tadashi Yoshino,[3] and Hiroyuki Okada[1]

[1]*Department of Gastroenterology and Hepatology, Okayama University Graduate School of Medicine, Dentistry, and Pharmaceutical Sciences, Okayama 700-8558, Japan*
[2]*Department of General Medicine, Okayama University Graduate School of Medicine, Dentistry, and Pharmaceutical Sciences, Okayama 700-8558, Japan*
[3]*Department of Pathology, Okayama University Graduate School of Medicine, Dentistry, and Pharmaceutical Sciences, Okayama 700-8558, Japan*
[4]*Department of Hematology and Oncology, Okayama University Hospital, Okayama 700-8558, Japan*
[5]*Department of Endoscopy, Okayama University Hospital, Okayama 700-8558, Japan*

Correspondence should be addressed to Masaya Iwamuro; iwamuromasaya@yahoo.co.jp

Academic Editor: Hirotada Akiho

A 70-year-old woman presented with follicular lymphoma involving the stomach, duodenum, jejunum, bone, and lymph nodes. Esophagogastroduodenoscopy revealed multiple depressed lesions in the stomach. Examination with magnifying endoscopy showed branched abnormal vessels along with gastric pits, which were irregularly shaped but were preserved. The second case was a 45-year-old man diagnosed with stage II_1 follicular lymphoma with duodenal, ileal, and colorectal involvement, as well as lymphadenopathy of the mesenteric lymph nodes. Esophagogastroduodenoscopy performed six years after the diagnosis revealed multiple erosions in the gastric body and angle. Magnifying endoscopic observation with narrow-band imaging showed that the gastric pits were only partially preserved and were destroyed in most of the stomach. Branched abnormal vessels were also seen. Pathological features were consistent with follicular lymphoma in both cases. The structural differences reported between the two cases appear to reflect distinct pathologies. Disappearance of gastric pits in the latter case seems to result from loss of epithelial cells, probably due to chronic inflammation. In both cases, branched abnormal vasculature was observed. These two cases suggest that magnified observations of abnormal branched microvasculature may facilitate endoscopic detection and recognition of the extent of gastric involvement in patients with follicular lymphoma.

1. Introduction

Follicular lymphoma is the second most frequent subtype of lymphoid malignancies observed in western countries. In patients with follicular lymphoma, the gastrointestinal tract can be primarily or secondarily involved [1]. Most gastrointestinal involvement of follicular lymphoma is found in the small intestine, especially in the duodenum [2–4], whereas gastric involvement is less frequent. Therefore, the macroscopic and microscopic features of follicular lymphoma involving the stomach have not been fully revealed to date.

Recently we experienced two cases of systemic follicular lymphoma involving the stomach. This paper focuses on the pathologic and endoscopic features of gastric lesions of follicular lymphoma. We also speculate on the pathophysiological processes behind the microstructural findings in both presented cases.

2. Case Report

2.1. Case 1. A 70-year-old woman underwent a screening esophagogastroduodenoscopy at her family clinic during

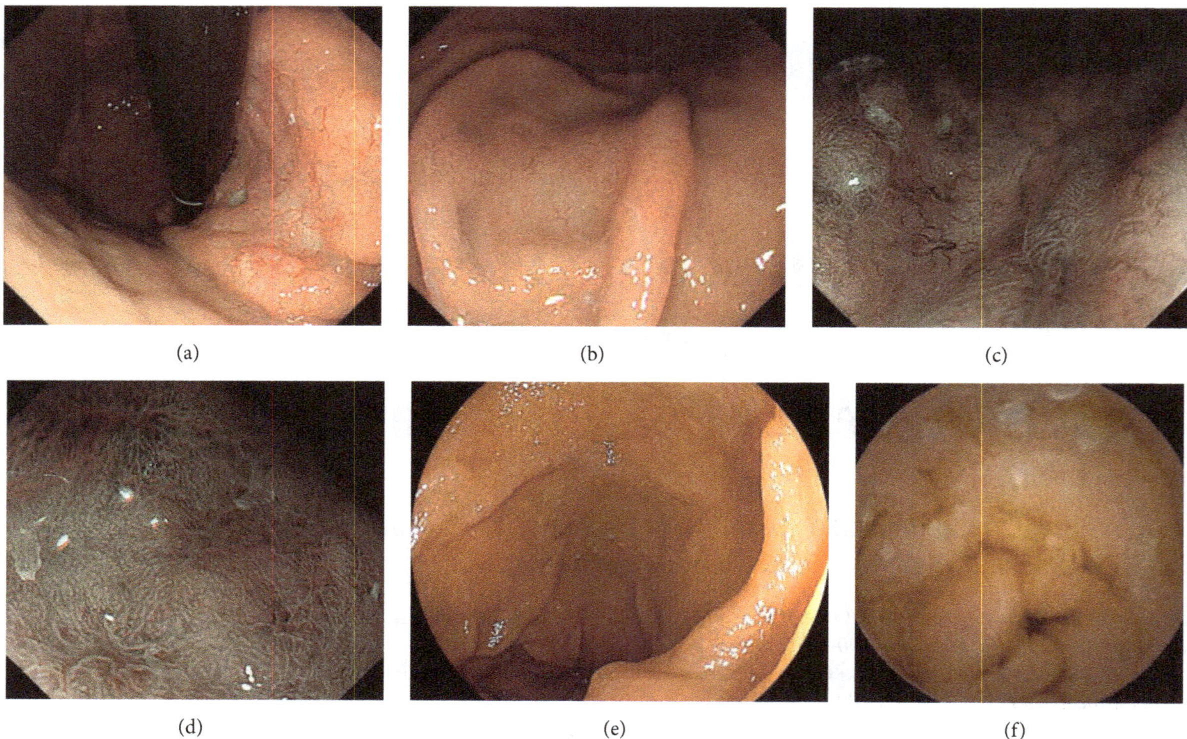

FIGURE 1: Endoscopic images from case 1. Slightly depressed lesions with thickened peripheral folds were seen in the upper (a) and lower gastric bodies (b). Branched abnormal vessels (c) and irregularly shaped gastric pits (c, d) were observed by using magnifying endoscopy with narrow-band imaging. In the duodenum, multiple whitish depositions were detected (e). Video capsule enteroscopy showed whitish granules in the jejunum (f).

a routine medical checkup, and a slightly depressed area was found in the gastric corpus. The patient was referred to Okayama University Hospital for further investigation and treatment. Esophagogastroduodenoscopy (GIF-H260Z; Olympus, Tokyo) showed slightly depressed lesions with thickened peripheral folds in the upper (Figure 1(a)) and lower gastric body (Figure 1(b)). Magnifying endoscopic observation with narrow-band imaging revealed branched abnormal vessels (Figure 1(c)). The gastric pits in the lesions were found to be irregular (Figures 1(c) and 1(d)), and the appearance of the gastric pits was denser than that of the peripheral intact mucosa. No absence or destruction of gastric pits was observed. In addition, multiple whitish depositions were identified in the duodenum (Figure 1(e)). The patient had tested negative for *Helicobacter pylori* infection. Biopsy samples from the peripheral intact mucosa had no neoplastic cells, whereas samples from the gastric lesions showed dense, diffuse infiltration of small- to medium-sized lymphoma cells (Figure 2). Lymphoepithelial lesions were absent. Immunohistochemistry analysis showed that the lymphoma cells were positive for CD20, CD10, and BCL2, while they were negative for CD3. The antibodies used to analyze the case were as follows (clone, dilutions): CD20 (L26, 1 : 200), CD10 (56C6, 1 : 50), BCL2 (3.1, 1 : 200), and CD3 (PS-1, 1 : 50). Positivity was determined when 30% or more lymphoma cells were positive for their antibodies. Fluorescence in situ hybridization analysis revealed that translocation t(14;18)(q32;q21) was present in the gastric lymphoma

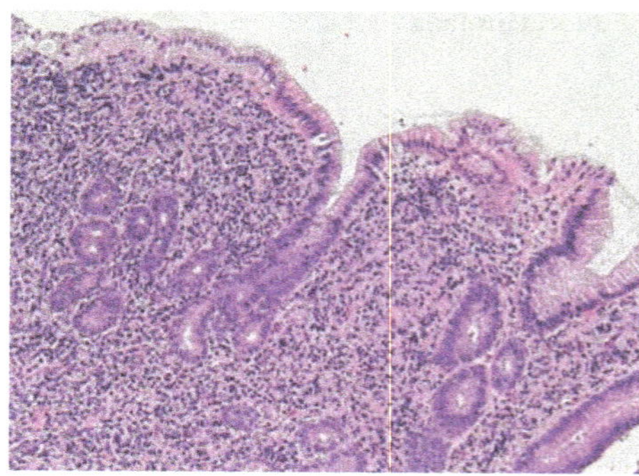

FIGURE 2: Histological image of stomach tissue biopsies from case 1. Dense, diffuse infiltration of small to medium-sized lymphoma cells was observed (hematoxylin and eosin staining, ×40). Lymphoepithelial lesions were absent.

cells. Pathological features were consistent with follicular lymphoma. Biopsy specimens obtained from the duodenum showed small- to medium-sized neoplastic lymphoid cells forming lymphoid structures. These pathological findings are representative of duodenal follicular lymphomas [3].

Video capsule enteroscopy showed whitish granules in the jejunum (Figure 1(f)). Computed tomography (CT) and positron emission tomography revealed involvement of multiple lymph nodes around the stomach, aorta, mesentery, and rectum. A bone marrow aspirate and biopsy revealed

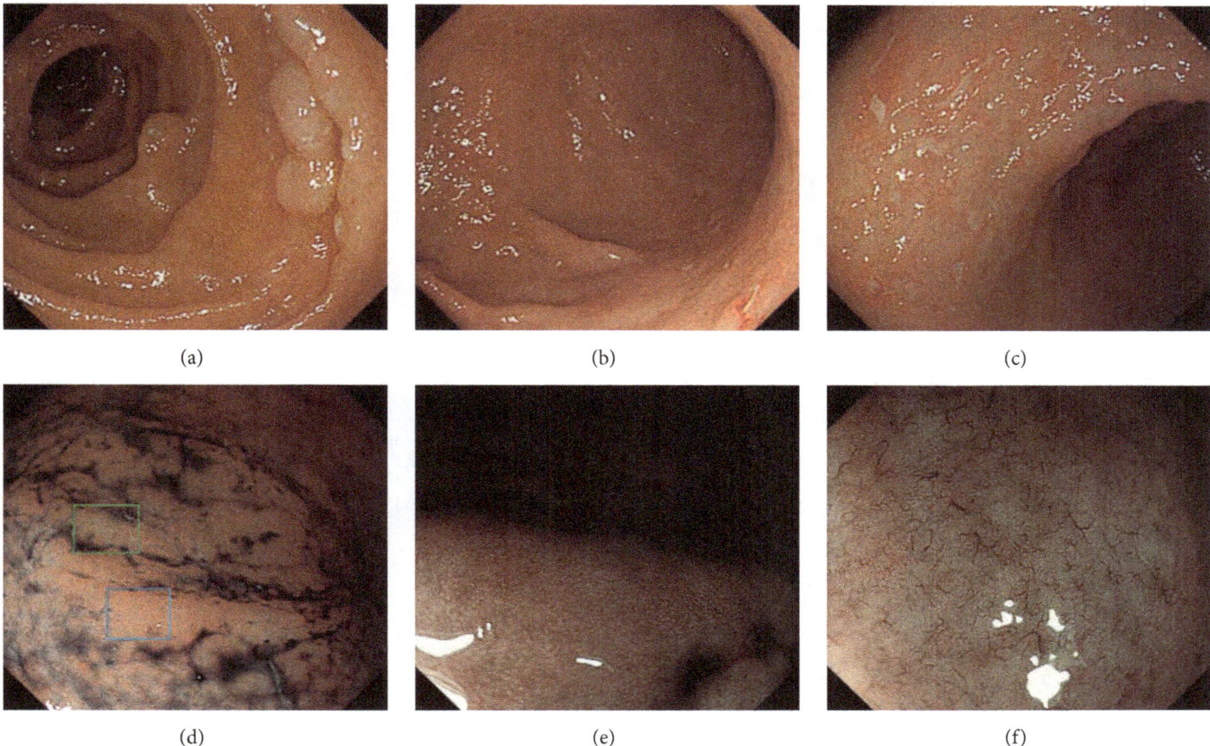

FIGURE 3: Endoscopic images from case 2. Esophagogastroduodenoscopy revealed multiple whitish depositions in the duodenum (a). In the stomach, multiple erosions in the body and angle were observed (b, c). There were no erosions in the greater curvature of the gastric body (d). Magnifying endoscopic observation with narrow-band imaging of the gastric body ((d), blue square) showed that the gastric pits were only partially preserved (e). Imaging a second area ((d), green square) showed destruction of gastric pits and branched abnormal vessels (f).

infiltration of the neoplastic cells into the bone marrow. Consequently, we diagnosed the case as systemic follicular lymphoma involving the stomach, duodenum, jejunum, intraabdominal lymph nodes, and bone marrow. The clinical stage was classified as stage IV.

2.2. Case 2. A 45-year-old man was diagnosed with stage II_1 follicular lymphoma with duodenal, ileal, colorectal involvement and lymphadenopathy of the mesenteric lymph nodes. Lymphoma progression with axillary and inguinal lymph node swelling was noted one year later, but the patient was kept under active surveillance (i.e., watch and wait). Two years after the initial diagnosis, gastric involvement was diagnosed. Esophagogastroduodenoscopy performed six years after the diagnosis revealed whitish depositions in the duodenum (Figure 3(a)). Multiple erosions in the gastric body and angle were also observed (Figures 3(b) and 3(c)). No erosions were observed in the greater curvature of the gastric body (Figure 3(d)). However, magnifying endoscopic observations using narrow-band imaging showed that the gastric pits were only partially preserved (Figure 3(e)), whereas they were heavily destroyed for the most part (Figure 3(f)). Branched abnormal vessels were also seen in areas where the gastric pits were absent. *Helicobacter pylori* titer was negative in this patient. Biopsy samples from the gastric lesions showed a diffuse infiltration of small- to medium-sized lymphoma cells, in addition to the existence of granulation tissue and lymphoid follicle (Figures 4(a), 4(b), and 4(c)). Immunohistochemistry confirmed the diagnosis of gastric follicular lymphoma, with staining positive for CD20 (Figure 4(d)), CD10 (Figure 4(e)), and BCL2 (Figure 4(f)). Staining for CD3 expression was negative (Figure 4(g)) in the neoplastic lymphoid cells. Pathological analysis found that epithelial cells were preserved in biopsy samples taken from the gastric mucosa where intact gastric pits were observed (Figures 4(a) and 4(b)). In contrast, epithelial cell loss was observed in biopsy samples taken from areas with damaged or absent gastric pits (Figure 4(c)). Esophagogastroduodenoscopy performed eight years after the initial diagnosis revealed an increased number of gastric erosions and spontaneous bleeding from the gastric mucosa (Figure 5). Because lymphoma progression was prominent in the stomach, rituximab monotherapy was initiated to prevent gastric bleeding.

3. Discussion

Lymphoma derived gastric lesions present with diverse endoscopic features, varying from mass-forming tumors to diffuse infiltrating lesions or superficial mucosal changes [5]. Moreover, formation of multiple lesions in the stomach is frequently observed in lymphomas [6]. Since most cases presenting with gastric lymphoma are extranodal marginal-zone lymphoma of mucosa-associated lymphoid tissue (MALT lymphoma) or diffuse large B-cell lymphoma [7], only a few

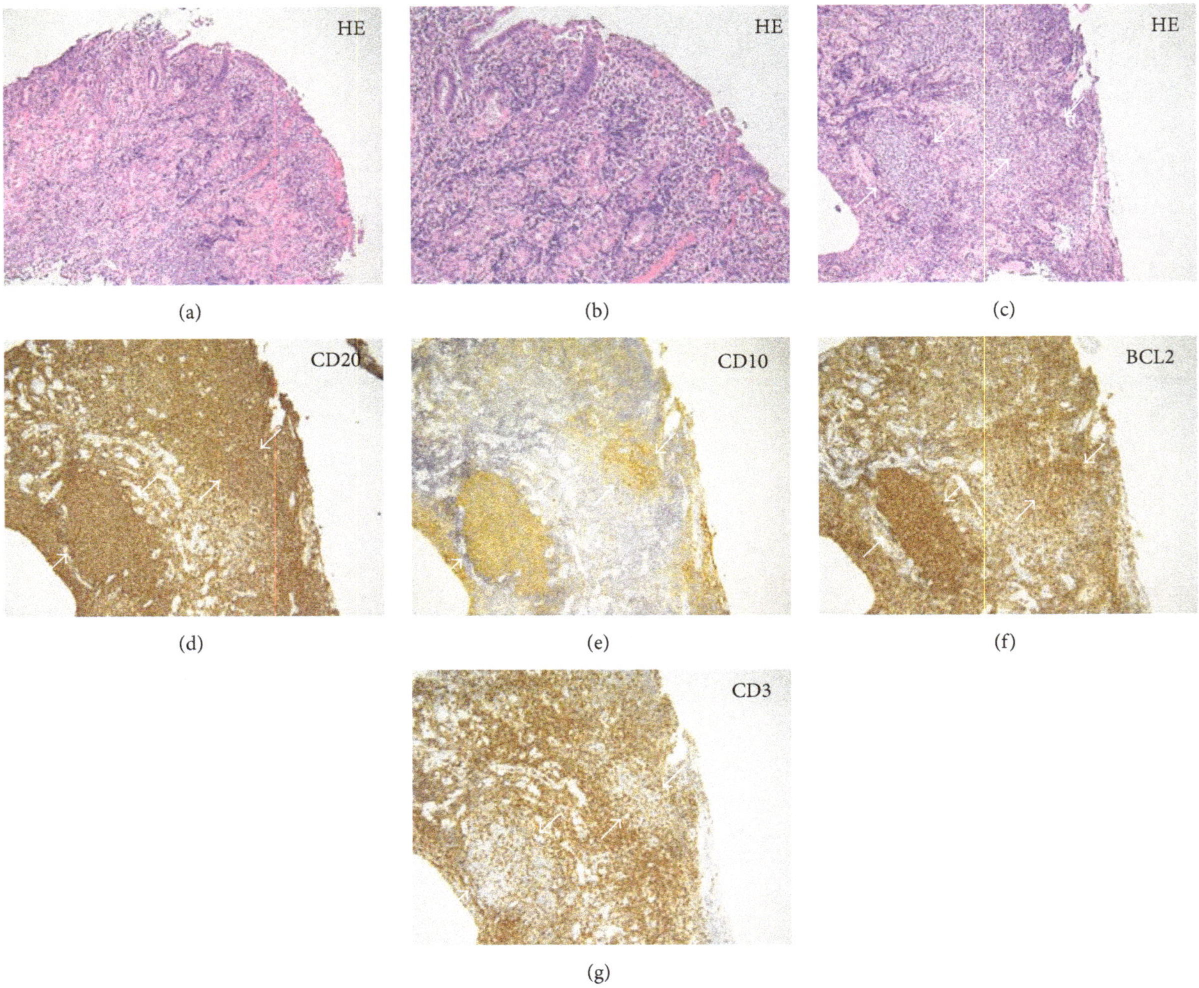

FIGURE 4: Histological images of stomach tissue biopsies from case 2. Dense, diffuse infiltration of small- to medium-sized lymphoma cells was observed, in addition to the existence of granulation tissues, with preserved epithelial cells, from biopsy samples taken from the gastric mucosa where intact pits were observed (hematoxylin and eosin staining, (a) ×20, (b) ×40). An image from biopsy samples taken from where damaged gastric pits were observed shows lymphoma infiltration, but with loss of epithelial cells ((c), hematoxylin and eosin staining, ×20). Neoplastic lymphoid follicles are shown (arrows). Lymphoma cells were positive for CD20 ((d), ×20), CD10 ((e), ×20), and BCL2 ((f), ×20) and negative for CD3 ((g), ×20).

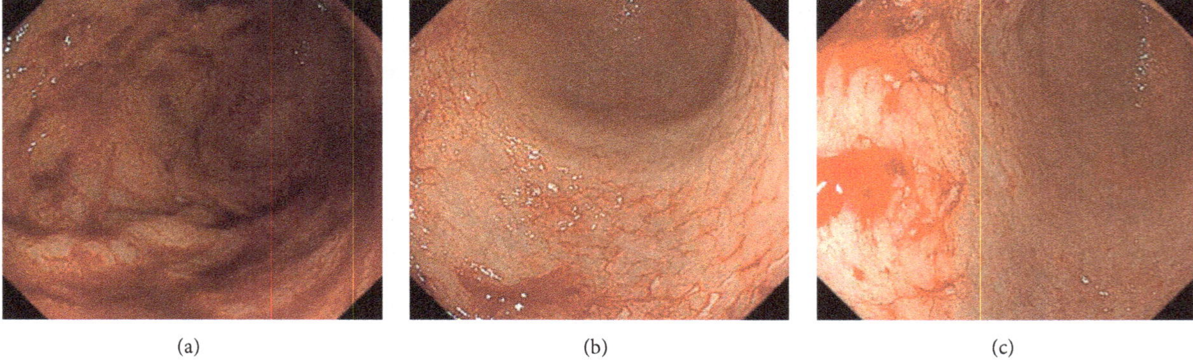

(a) (b) (c)

FIGURE 5: Esophagogastroduodenoscopy performed eight years after the initial diagnosis. Spontaneous bleeding from the gastric mucosa was observed.

articles describing gastric lesions from follicular lymphoma have been reported. In cases of gastrointestinal follicular lymphoma, involvement of the duodenum is a predominant feature [2, 8]. Recent reports have revealed a high proportion of cases ranging from 66.7% to 100%, with extensive involvement of the jejunum and/or ileum [3, 9–14]. Meanwhile, involvement of the stomach is infrequent in follicular lymphoma. A previous report by Takata et al. described observation of duodenal lesions in 111/125 cases (88.8%), jejunal lesions in 50/125 cases (40.0%), and ileal lesions in 28/125 cases (22.4%), while gastric lesions were found in only 2/125 cases (1.6%) [3]. Macroscopic features described for gastric lesions of follicular lymphoma include shallow depressed lesions [15], thickened rugae exhibiting a slight redness [16], elevated nodular lesions [17], mucosal inflammation and ulceration [18], multiple small ulcerations [19], and a submucosal tumor-like lesion [20, 21]. Based on the varied descriptions used to describe follicular lymphoma, no specific macroscopic features have been identified in association with the gastric lesions.

Although gastric involvement is infrequent in follicular lymphoma patients, it is important to evaluate the gastric mucosa during both the initial evaluation and the follow-up period as part of a thorough diagnostic examination. During the initial diagnostic workup of follicular lymphoma patients, determination of the extent of disease present is recommended for stage I and II patients who are being considered for radiotherapy as a curative treatment. Staging in these patients is important since disease relapse tends to occur outside the involved field of radiation [22]. Even though case 2 did not have any gastric involvement at the initial staging, it is possible for gastric lesions to emerge during the follow-up period. Case 2 required initiation of rituximab monotherapy to prevent gastric bleeding, since spontaneous bleeding from gastric mucosa occurred secondary to the gastric follicular lymphoma lesions.

To the best of our knowledge, magnifying endoscopic features observed in gastric involvement of follicular lymphoma have not been reported to date. As described above, involvement of the stomach is more frequent in MALT lymphoma, which has been a well-recognized entity among lymphomas involving the stomach since first described by Isaacson and Wright in 1983 [23]. Typical magnifying endoscopic features of MALT lymphoma include the appearance of abnormal vessels and the destruction of gastric pits [24, 25]. Ono et al. investigated 11 cases of gastric MALT lymphoma and using magnified endoscopy observed the two aforementioned features in all cases [24, 26]. Moreover, after achieving a complete response of MALT lymphoma, by *Helicobacter pylori* eradication, abnormal vessels were no longer detected and gastric pits reemerged, though those pits were irregularly patterned and had a different form and a different density from those in the adjacent intact mucosa. Consequently, unusual-shaped vasculature, a nonstructural pattern, and destruction of gastric pits appear to be specific for untreated gastric MALT lymphomas.

In both of the present cases, magnifying endoscopic observations with narrow-band imaging showed abnormal branched vessels. As described above, branched microvasculature observed in our cases was similar to the reported features in cases of MALT lymphoma [24]. Moreover, such branched vessels can be seen in *H. pylori*-associated chronic gastritis and diffuse type of gastric cancer [24, 27]. Therefore, distinguishing gastric follicular lymphoma from other lymphoma subtypes and other gastric diseases seems difficult or impossible by considering this feature alone. However, despite the limitations associated with magnified endoscopic observation, we consider that understanding magnifying endoscopic features of gastric follicular lymphoma lesions will aid endoscopists for the following reasons. First, magnifying endoscopy may aid in the determination of appropriate biopsy sites. In case 1, biopsy samples from the depressed lesion with abnormal branched vessels showed lymphoma cells, whereas samples from the peripheral mucosa had no neoplastic cells [26]. Second, detection of gastric involvement may alter treatment strategy in patients with follicular lymphoma. For example, rituximab monotherapy was initiated in case 2 to prevent gastric mucosa bleeding after esophagogastroduodenoscopy confirmed progressive gastric involvement. Although subsequent further investigation will be required, magnified endoscopic observations and recognition of abnormal branched microvasculature may facilitate detecting gastric involvement in patients with follicular lymphoma.

In case 1, the gastric pits were found in an irregular pattern but were nonetheless intact. In contrast, case 2 exhibited diffuse destruction of gastric pits with only limited sections showing intact pit structure. We speculate that the structural differences between the two cases reflect distinct pathologies. The destruction of gastric pits observed by endoscopy in case 2 seems to result from the loss of epithelial cells (Figure 4(c)). On the other hand, in case 1 the gastric pits though irregular seem to have been preserved along with the epithelial cells. The presence of granulation tissue in case 2 suggests that chronic inflammation caused by follicular lymphoma cell infiltration led to damage of the gastric epithelial cells, finally resulting in the destruction of pit structure. Since our interpretation is based on the observations derived from only two cases, further investigation will be required to reveal the pathological and endoscopic features of gastric follicular lymphoma. Nonetheless, it is likely that gastric pits are not uniformly affected and may be intact or destroyed, unlike MALT lymphoma cases.

In conclusion, we treated two patients with follicular lymphoma involving the stomach. Abnormal branched microvessels were observed in both cases, whereas gastric pits were preserved in one patient and destroyed in the other. Although appropriate pathological assessment with immunohistological analysis of biopsy samples is essential for definitive diagnosis, magnified endoscopy of microvascular structures and gastric pits may be useful in alerting physicians to the potential for lymphoma lesions in the stomach.

References

[1] M. Dreyling, M. Ghielmini, R. Marcus, G. Salles, and U. Vitolo, "ESMO Guidelines Working Group: newly diagnosed and relapsed follicular lymphoma: ESMO Clinical Practice Guidelines for diagnosis, treatment and followup," *Annals of Oncology*, vol. 22, supplement 6, pp. i59–i63, 2011.

[2] N. L. Harris, S. H. Swerdlow, E. S. Jaffe et al., "Follicular lymphoma," in *WHO Classification of Tumours of Haematopoietic and Lymphoid Tissues*, S. H. Swerdlow, E. Campo, N. L. Harris et al., Eds., pp. 220–226, IARC, Lyon, France, 2008.

[3] K. Takata, H. Okada, N. Ohmiya et al., "Primary gastrointestinal follicular lymphoma involving the duodenal second portion is a distinct entity: a multicenter, retrospective analysis in Japan," *Cancer Science*, vol. 102, no. 8, pp. 1532–1536, 2011.

[4] T. Yoshino, K. Miyake, K. Ichimura et al., "Increased incidence of follicular lymphoma in the duodenum," *American Journal of Surgical Pathology*, vol. 24, no. 5, pp. 688–693, 2000.

[5] S. Nakamura, T. Yao, K. Aoyagi, M. Iida, M. Fujishima, and M. Tsuneyoshi, "*Helicobacter pylori* and primary gastric lymphoma. A histopathologic and immunohistochemical analysis of 237 patients," *Cancer*, vol. 79, no. 1, pp. 3–11, 1997.

[6] H. Isomoto, K. Matsushima, T. Hayashi et al., "Endocytoscopic findings of lymphomas of the stomach," *BMC Gastroenterology*, vol. 13, article 174, 2013.

[7] T. Terada, "Gastrointestinal malignant lymphoma: a pathologic study of 37 cases in a single Japanese institution," *American Journal of Blood Research*, vol. 2, no. 3, pp. 194–200, 2012.

[8] S. Yamamoto, H. Nakase, K. Yamashita et al., "Gastrointestinal follicular lymphoma: review of the literature," *Journal of Gastroenterology*, vol. 45, no. 4, pp. 370–388, 2010.

[9] A.-I. Schmatz, B. Streubel, E. Kretschmer-Chott et al., "Primary follicular lymphoma of the duodenum is a distinct mucosal/submucosal variant of follicular lymphoma: a retrospective study of 63 cases," *Journal of Clinical Oncology*, vol. 29, no. 11, pp. 1445–1451, 2011.

[10] T. Akamatsu, Y. Kaneko, H. Ota, H. Miyabayashi, N. Arakura, and E. Tanaka, "Usefulness of double balloon enteroscopy and video capsule endoscopy for the diagnosis and management of primary follicular lymphoma of the gastrointestinal tract in its early stages," *Digestive Endoscopy*, vol. 22, no. 1, pp. 33–38, 2010.

[11] N. Higuchi, Y. Sumida, K. Nakamura et al., "Impact of double-balloon endoscopy on the diagnosis of jejunoileal involvement in primary intestinal follicular lymphomas: a case series," *Endoscopy*, vol. 41, no. 2, pp. 175–178, 2009.

[12] M. Kodama, Y. Kitadai, T. Shishido et al., "Primary follicular lymphoma of the gastrointestinal tract: A retrospective case series," *Endoscopy*, vol. 40, no. 4, pp. 343–346, 2008.

[13] S. Nakamura, T. Matsumoto, J. Umeno et al., "Endoscopic features of intestinal follicular lymphoma: the value of double-balloon enteroscopy," *Endoscopy*, vol. 39, supplement 1, pp. E26–E27, 2007.

[14] M. Iwamuro, H. Okada, S. Kawano et al., "A multicenter survey of enteroscopy for the diagnosis of intestinal follicular lymphoma," *Oncology Letters*, vol. 10, no. 1, pp. 131–136, 2015.

[15] M. Iwamuro, A. Imagawa, N. Kobayashi et al., "Synchronous adenocarcinoma and follicular lymphoma of the stomach," *Internal Medicine*, vol. 52, no. 8, pp. 907–912, 2013.

[16] M. Iwamuro, H. Okada, K. Takata et al., "Diagnostic role of 18F-fluorodeoxyglucose positron emission tomography for follicular lymphoma with gastrointestinal involvement," *World Journal of Gastroenterology*, vol. 18, no. 44, pp. 6427–6436, 2012.

[17] M. Kanda, K. Ohshima, J. Suzumiya et al., "Follicular lymphoma of the stomach: immunohistochemical and molecular genetic studies," *Journal of Gastroenterology*, vol. 38, no. 6, pp. 584–587, 2003.

[18] A. Tzankov, A. Hittmair, H.-K. Müller-Hermelink, T. Rüdiger, and S. Dirnhofer, "Primary gastric follicular lymphoma with parafollicular monocytoid B-cells and lymphoepithelial lesions, mimicking extranodal marginal zone lymphoma of MALT," *Virchows Archiv*, vol. 441, no. 6, pp. 614–617, 2002.

[19] H. Matsumoto, K. Haruma, and T. Akiyama, "An unusual case of multiple small ulcerations throughout the GI tract," *Gastroenterology*, vol. 141, no. 5, pp. e11–e12, 2011.

[20] D. Norimura, E. Fukuda, T. Yamao et al., "Primary gastric follicular lymphoma manifesting as a submucosal tumor-like lesion," *Digestive Endoscopy*, vol. 24, no. 5, p. 389, 2012.

[21] M. Iwamuro, H. Okada, K. Takata et al., "Diagnostic accuracy of endoscopic biopsies for the diagnosis of gastrointestinal follicular lymphoma: a clinicopathologic study of 48 patients," *Annals of Diagnostic Pathology*, vol. 18, no. 2, pp. 99–103, 2014.

[22] A. Wirth, M. Foo, J. F. Seymour, M. P. Macmanus, and R. J. Hicks, "Impact of [^{18}f] fluorodeoxyglucose positron emission tomography on staging and management of early-stage follicular non-hodgkin lymphoma," *International Journal of Radiation Oncology, Biology, Physics*, vol. 71, no. 1, pp. 213–219, 2008.

[23] P. Isaacson and D. H. Wright, "Malignant lymphoma of mucosa-associated lymphoid tissue. A distinctive type of B-cell lymphoma," *Cancer*, vol. 52, no. 8, pp. 1410–1416, 1983.

[24] S. Ono, M. Kato, Y. Ono et al., "Characteristics of magnified endoscopic images of gastric extranodal marginal zone B-cell lymphoma of the mucosa-associated lymphoid tissue, including changes after treatment," *Gastrointestinal Endoscopy*, vol. 68, no. 4, pp. 624–631, 2008.

[25] K. Nonaka, K. Ohata, N. Matsuhashi et al., "Is narrow-band imaging useful for histological evaluation of gastric mucosa-associated lymphoid tissue lymphoma after treatment?" *Digestive Endoscopy*, vol. 26, no. 3, pp. 358–364, 2014.

[26] S. Ono, M. Kato, Y. Ono et al., "Target biopsy using magnifying endoscopy in clinical management of gastric mucosa-associated lymphoid tissue lymphoma," *Journal of Gastroenterology and Hepatology (Australia)*, vol. 26, no. 7, pp. 1133–1138, 2011.

[27] S. Hayashi, J. Imamura, K. Kimura, S. Saeki, and T. Hishima, "Endoscopic features of lymphoid follicles in Helicobacter pylori -associated chronic gastritis," *Digestive Endoscopy*, vol. 27, no. 1, pp. 53–60, 2015.

23

Laparoscopic Resection of Pancreatic Tail Solid Pseudopapillary Tumour in a Young Male

W. G. P. Kanchana,[1] R. A. A. Shaminda,[1] K. B. Galketiya,[1] V. Pinto,[2] D. Walisinghe,[3] S. Wijetunge,[3] and R. Heendeniya[1]

[1]*Department of Surgery, Teaching Hospital Peradeniya, Peradeniya, Sri Lanka*
[2]*Department of Anaesthesiology, Teaching Hospital Peradeniya, Peradeniya, Sri Lanka*
[3]*Department of Pathology, Teaching Hospital Peradeniya, Peradeniya, Sri Lanka*

Correspondence should be addressed to W. G. P. Kanchana; pulasthi@live.com

Academic Editor: Shiro Kikuchi

Background. Solid Pseudopapillary Tumours of the pancreas are a rare entity and more commonly seen in women than in men. These tumours have typically reached large sizes when clinically detected. *Case Description.* A 21-year-old male was found to have a left hypochondrial mass on physical examination following a trivial soft tissue injury. Contrast-enhanced computed topography (CT) of the abdomen showed a 10.3 × 7.6 × 10.3 cm size arising from the body and the tail of the pancreas. He underwent laparoscopic resection of distal pancreatic tumour en bloc with spleen. Large tumour was noted originating from the body and tail of the pancreas with dilated veins surrounding the tumour. Histology revealed a clear cell variant of solid pseudopapillary neoplasm with steatotic pattern. Resection margin was free of tumour. *Discussion.* Several studies have shown significant short term advantages using laparoscopic approach compared to open surgery, in terms of lower blood loss, resumption of oral intake, and hospital stay. This case and few other case reports published in world literature have shown that laparoscopic approach is safe and oncologically adequate.

1. Introduction

Solid Pseudopapillary Tumours of the pancreas are a rare entity and more commonly seen in women than in men (ratio 9 : 1) [1]. There are few case reports published in world literature, where mean age at description is around 30 years [2, 3]. Most of the patients have nonspecific symptoms or tumour found at examination following trauma or gynaecological/obstetric examinations. These tumours have typically reached large sizes when clinically detected.

2. Case

A 21-year-old male was found to have a left hypochondrial mass on physical examination following a trivial soft tissue injury. Ultrasound scan revealed a large retroperitoneal mass in the pancreatic tail region with a mild splenomegaly. No other abnormality was noted in the ultrasound scan. Contrast-enhanced computed topography (CT) of the abdomen showed a 10.3 × 7.6 × 10.3 cm size heterogeneous mass with mild contrast enhancement arising from the body and the tail of the pancreas with no calcifications (Figure 1). Multiple vascular channels were seen around the lesion. Splenic vein was compressed and displaced by the mass with enlargement of the spleen. Mass effect had displaced the left kidney posteriorly. All other intra-abdominal viscera were normal. All haematological investigations were normal.

He underwent laparoscopic resection of distal pancreatic tumour en bloc with spleen. Patient was operated on in right lateral position with head-up tilt using five ports. Figure 2 shows the ports arrangement. Large tumour was noted originating from the body and tail of the pancreas with dilated veins surrounding the tumour. Patient also had a large spleen and an enlarged liver. Dissection was performed using ultrasound dissector and bipolar diathermy. Splenic artery divided between clips and splenic vein was ligated and clipped before

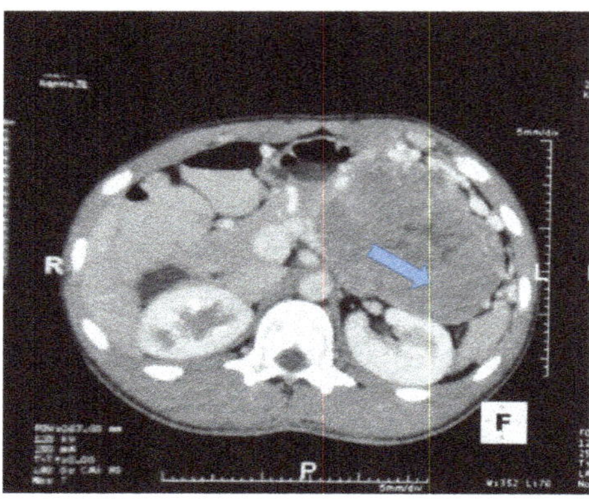

FIGURE 1: CT image demonstrating presence of a heterogeneous well-demarcated mass arising from the body and tail of the pancreas (marked with a blue arrow) and extending towards the splenic hilum.

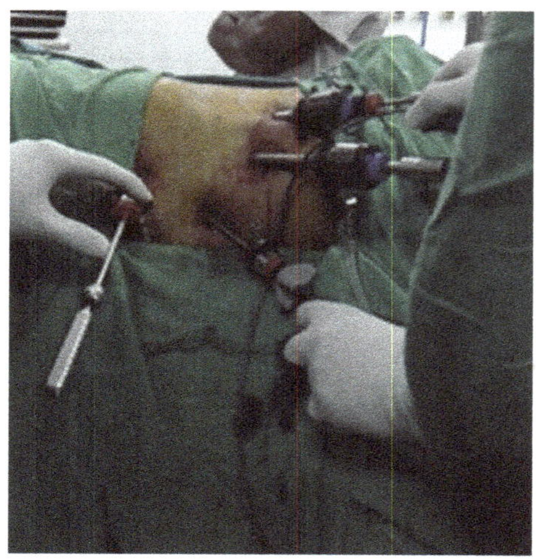

FIGURE 2: Patient operated on in right lateral position with head-up tilt using ports arranged as in this image.

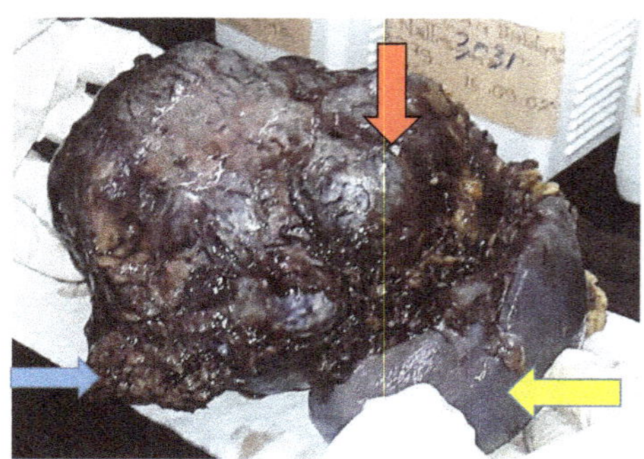

FIGURE 3: Macroscopic appearance of distal pancreatectomy with splenectomy specimen containing well-demarcated lobulated mass (red arrow), part of body of pancreas (blue arrow), and spleen (yellow arrow).

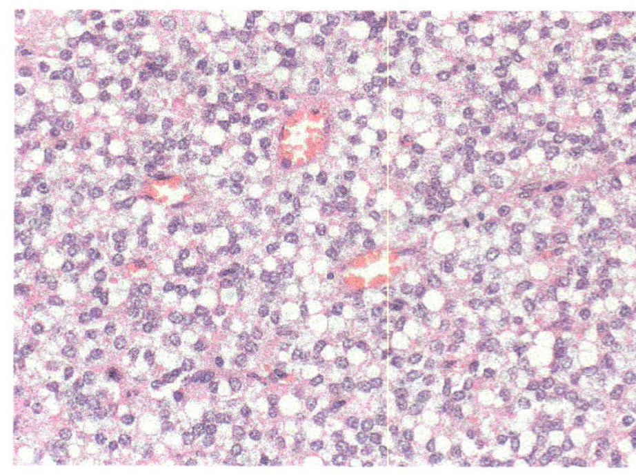

FIGURE 4: Haematoxylin and eosin stained section showing sheets of polygonal cells displaying bland nuclei and a thin rim of eosinophilic cytoplasm containing sharp vacuolations. Occasional mitotic figures are present (×400).

dividing. Pancreas was divided just distal to the portal vein using bipolar diathermy and ultrasound dissector. The specimen (Figure 3) was delivered in a bag through a 7.5 cm incision.

Postoperative period was uneventful and he was discharged on 4th postoperative day.

Histology revealed a tumour predominantly composed of sheets of round to polygonal cells containing sharp cytoplasmic vacuolations and bland nuclei. The eosinophilic cytoplasm was seen as a rim in the periphery. Very occasional mitotic figures were present (Figure 4). The focal pseudopapillae formation was also evident with vascular cores lined by neoplastic cells (Figure 5). The stroma was highly vascular (Figure 6). There were thick fibrous septae and focal hyalinization in the stroma. Cystic and haemorrhagic foci were present. Cholesterol clefts surrounded by a giant cell reaction were also noted. Thin fibrous capsule was noted encircling the tumour (Figure 7). Multiple foci of partial capsular infiltration were also noted (Figure 8). However, the adjacent pancreatic tissue was not infiltrated by the tumour.

Final diagnosis of a clear cell variant of solid pseudopapillary neoplasm with a steatotic pattern was made. Patient was referred to the oncologist for follow-up.

3. Discussion

Line of cellular differentiation of Solid Pseudopapillary Tumours remains unknown [1]. These are solid tumours that undergo cystic degeneration upon growth. Microscopically these show solid nests of cells with abundant small blood vessels. Cells which are distant to blood vessels degenerate leaving a cuff of tissue surrounding blood vessels forming a characteristic pseudopapillary architecture [1]. They can also show microscopic infiltrative growth pattern.

Even though they exhibit an indolent natural history, they are considered biologically malignant. Ten percent to fifteen percent of the cases have metastases (mainly to liver and peritoneum) [4]. Even the patients with metastatic disease survive decades without many symptoms. Current practice in resectable lesions is to offer en bloc resection with clear margins, since this gives the best chance for cure. Even for

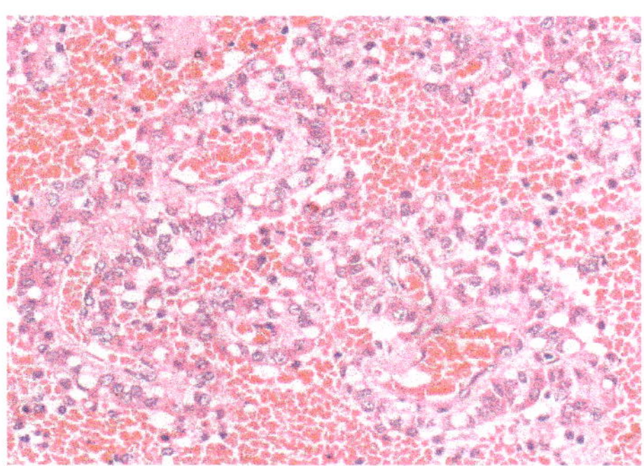

FIGURE 5: Haematoxylin and eosin stained sections revealing foci of pseudopapillae and rosettes with vascular cores lined by neoplastic cells (×400).

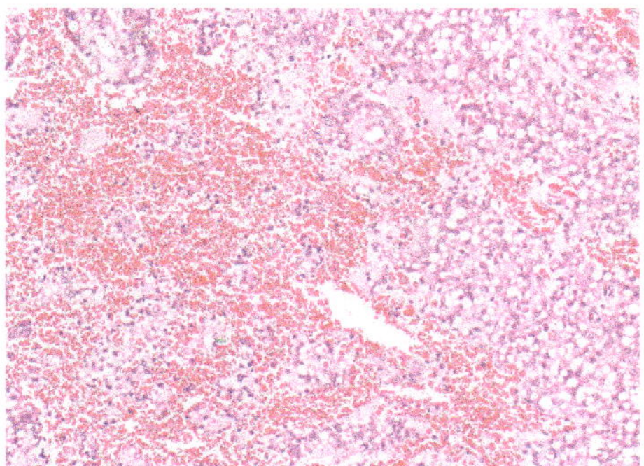

FIGURE 6: Haematoxylin and eosin stained sections displaying highly vascular and haemorrhagic stroma. Loosely cohesive cellular clusters are seen scattered within the stroma (×400).

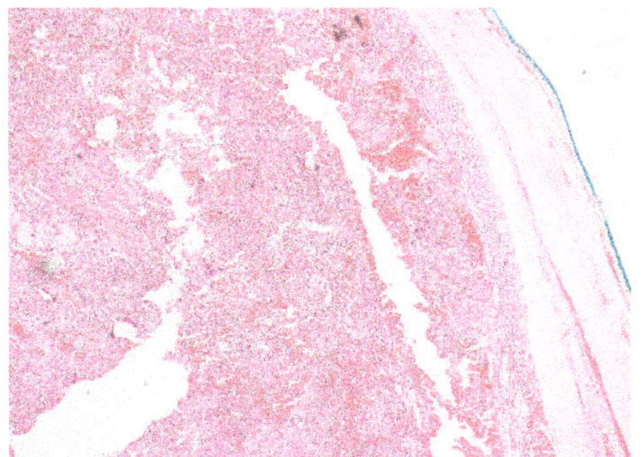

FIGURE 7: Haematoxylin and eosin stained section showing thin fibrous capsule encircling the tumour (×200).

metastatic disease, aggressive resection has shown to yield long term survival [5–8].

A retrospective study done by Zhang et al. has shown significant short term advantages using laparoscopic approach compared to open surgery, in terms of lower blood loss, resumption of oral intake, and hospital stay [9]. This report and few other studies have shown that laparoscopic approach is safe and oncologically adequate [10, 11]. We have published the first laparoscopic distal pancreatectomy in Sri Lanka in 2013 for a Solid Pseudopapillary Tumour in a young female [12].

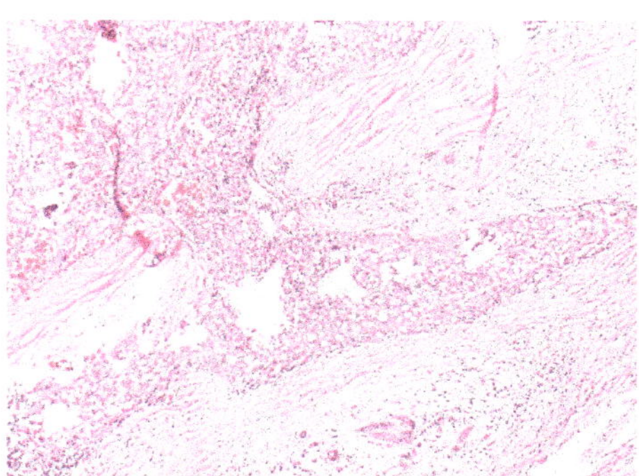

FIGURE 8: Haematoxylin and eosin stained section showing focus of partial capsular infiltration by the tumour (×100).

Even though splenic preservation is possible in some, in this patient as the tumour was large and abutting on the splenic hilum, distal pancreatectomy was performed en bloc with spleen for better oncological clearance.

Consent

Written and informed consent was taken from the patient regarding publication of this case report.

References

[1] D. S. Klimstra and N. V. Adsay, "Solid pseudopapillary neoplasm. Tumors of the pancreas and ampulla of Vater," in *Surgical Pathology of the GI Tract, Liver, Biliary Tract and Pancreas*, R. D. Odze and J. R. Goldblum, Eds., pp. 909–960, Elsevier, Philadelphia, Pa, USA, 2nd edition, 2009, http://www.sciencedirect.com/science/book/9781416040590.

[2] K. Nishihara, M. Nagoshi, M. Tsuneyoshi, K. Yamaguchi, and I. Hayashi, "Papillary cystic tumors of the pancreas: assessment of their malignant potential," *Cancer*, vol. 71, no. 1, pp. 82–92, 1993.

[3] M. J. Zinner, M. S. Shurbaji, and J. L. Cameron, "Solid and papillary epithelial neoplasms of the pancreas," *Surgery*, vol. 108, pp. 475–480, 1990.

[4] G. Kloppel, R. H. Hurban, D. S. Klimstra et al., "Solid-pseudopapillary neoplasm of the pancreas," in *WHO Classification of Tumors of the Digestive System*, p. 327, IARC, Lyon, France, 4th edition, 2010.

[5] K. Y. Lam, C. Y. Lo, and S. T. Fan, "Pancreatic solid-cysticpapillary tumor: clinicopathologic features in eight patients from Hong Kong and review of the literature," *World Journal of Surgery*, vol. 23, no. 10, pp. 1045–1050, 1999.

[6] R. C. G. Martin, D. S. Klimstra, M. F. Brennan, and K. C. Conlon, "Solid-pseudopapillary tumor of the pancreas: a surgical enigma?" *Annals of Surgical Oncology*, vol. 9, no. 1, pp. 35–40, 2002.

[7] J. M. Butte, M. F. Brennan, M. Gönen et al., "Solid pseudopapillary tumors of the pancreas. Clinical features, surgical

outcomes, and long-term survival in 45 consecutive patients from a single center," *Journal of Gastrointestinal Surgery*, vol. 15, no. 2, pp. 350–357, 2011.

[8] T. Morikawa, T. Onogawa, S. Maeda, T. Takadate, K. Shirasaki, and H. E. Yoshida, "Solid psudopapillary neoplasms of the pancreas: an 18-year experience at a single Japanese institution," *Surgery Today*, vol. 41, no. 1, pp. 91–96, 2012.

[9] R.-C. Zhang, J.-F. Yan, X.-W. Xu, K. Chen, H. Ajoodhea, and Y.-P. Mou, "Laparoscopic vs open distal pancreatectomy for solid pseudopapillary tumor of the pancreas," *World Journal of Gastroenterology*, vol. 19, no. 37, pp. 6272–6277, 2013.

[10] R. O. Giovanardi, H. J. Giovanardi, M. R. Ali, and G. Giovanardi, "Laparoscopic pancreatic resection without advanced laparoscopic devices," *Hepato-Gastroenterology*, vol. 60, no. 125, pp. 1206–1210, 2013.

[11] T. Ikeda, S. Yoshiya, T. Toshima et al., "Laparoscopic distal pancreatectomy preserving the spleen and splenic vessels for benign and low-grade malignant pancreatic neoplasm," *Fukuoka Igaku Zasshi*, vol. 104, no. 3, pp. 54–63, 2013.

[12] K. B. Galketiya, V. Pinto, N. Rathnathunga, W. M. M. P. B. Wanasinghe, and S. P. M. Peiris, "Laparoscopic distal pancreatectomy: a Sri Lankan experience," *The Sri Lanka Journal of Surgery*, vol. 31, no. 1, pp. 22–23, 2013.

Obstructive Giant Inflammatory Polyposis: Is It Related to the Severity or the Duration of the Inflammatory Bowel Disease? Two Case Reports

Antoine Abou Rached,[1] **Jowana Saba**,[1] **Leila El Masri**,[1] **Mary Nakhoul**,[1] **and Carla Razzouk**[2]

[1] *Lebanese University, School of Medicine, Lebanon*
[2] *Saint-Joseph University, School of Medicine, Lebanon*

Correspondence should be addressed to Antoine Abou Rached; abourachedantoine@gmail.com

Academic Editor: Chia-Tung Shun

We report two cases of giant inflammatory polyposis (GIP) with totally different presentation and evolution. The first patient had two giant pseudopolyps after one year of the diagnosis of UC. The second patient had one obstructive giant pseudopolyp secondary to CD at the level of the transverse colon, being totally asymptomatic years before the presentation. GIP is a rare complication of inflammatory bowel disease (IBD). It consists of numerous filiform polyps that look like a "mass of worms" or a "fungating" mass. Surgical resection is inevitable when GIP presents with obstructive symptoms.

1. Introduction

Giant inflammatory polyposis (GIP) is a rare complication of inflammatory bowel disease (IBD) [1]. It occurs more frequently in ulcerative colitis (UC) than in Crohn's disease (CD) [2–4]. We report here two cases of obstructive GIP with totally different presentation and evolution. The first patient had two giant pseudopolyps after one year of the diagnosis of UC. The second patient had one obstructive giant pseudopolyp secondary to CD at the level of the transverse colon, being totally asymptomatic years before the presentation.

2. Case Report

2.1. Case 1. A 20-year-old male presented with worsening bloody diarrhea of 4 months' duration associated with cramping abdominal pain and weight loss of 4 Kg. On admission, he was hemodynamically stable. Physical examination showed mild tenderness to deep palpation in the left lower quadrant. Laboratory tests were consistent with anemia (hemoglobin = 10.5 mg/dl, hematocrit = 33.5%), thrombocytosis (platelets = 568000/mm^3), low iron level (iron = 25mg/dl), and normal C-reactive protein (CRP). Stool analysis, ova and parasite test, *Clostridium difficile* toxin assay, and stool culture were negative. Colonoscopy revealed left-sided colitis with marked erythema, absent vascular pattern, and friability erosions (Mayo score 2). Biopsies showed chronic active colitis consistent with UC. Based on the clinical presentation and laboratory, endoscopic, and pathologic findings, the patient was diagnosed with moderate left-sided UC and was started on oral and topical 5-aminosalicylic acid (5-ASA) without any response to treatment: bloody diarrhea (more than 5 bowel movement per day), severe abdominal pain, low grade fever, and additional weight loss in addition to severe anemia (hemoglobin = 7.3g/dl) and high CRP with negative stool tests. High dose steroids therapy was started with marked improvement. Steroid tapering caused recurrence of symptoms and anemia at 20mg prednisone per day. Relying on the findings above, the patient had left-sided UC and is

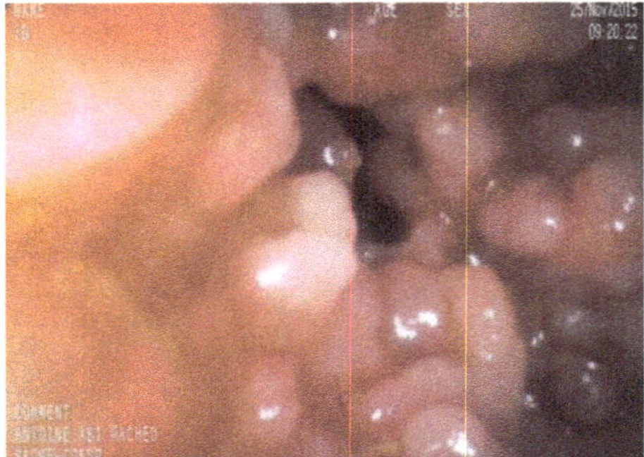

Figure 1: GIP of left colon.

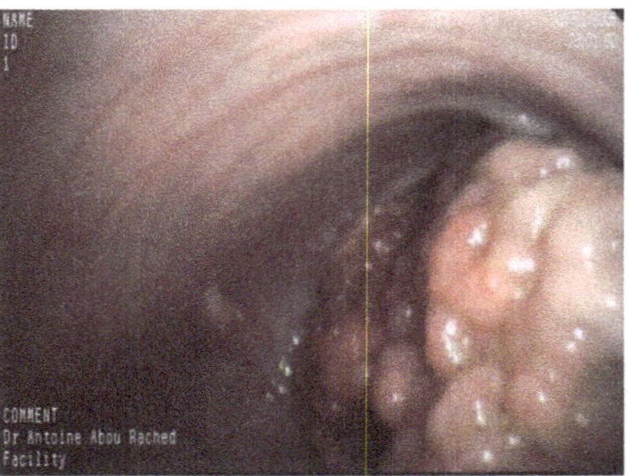

Figure 2: Obstructive GIP of the splenic flexure.

steroid-dependent, so Infliximab 5mg/kg was initiated at 0, 2, and 6 weeks, then every 8 weeks without any improvement after 4 months of treatment with persistent bloody diarrhea and severe iron deficiency anemia. Repeated colonoscopy showed severe inflammatory mucosa with deep ulcerations and pseudopolyps formation at the splenic flexure and the distal part of the left colon, separated by healed mucosa. Biopsies from the pathologic area revealed severe chronic active colitis consistent with inflammatory bowel disease/UC without any evidence of cytomegalovirus inclusions. Given the lack of response to Infliximab and the worsening endoscopic findings, resistance to therapy was suspected. Additional laboratory tests showed low Infliximab through level with high antibodies level to Infliximab. The patient was switched to combination therapy with Adalimumab 160mg at week 0, 80mg at week 2, and 40mg every other week plus Azathioprine 2.5mg/Kg with only partial response: improvement of diarrhea but persistence of severe nocturnal colicky abdominal pain. Adalimumab trough level was very low with the absence of anti-drug antibodies. So, Adalimumab was increased to 40mg per week. Two months later, he continued to have severe colicky abdominal pain and distension with weight loss. New colonoscopy revealed complete mucosal healing and a giant pseudopolyp in the left colon and another obstructive one at the level of the splenic flexure (Figures 1 and 2). Biopsies were consistent with chronic inflammation with architectural distortion and cryptic abscess. Abdominal CT scan confirmed the presence of two giant pseudopolyps with evidence of obstruction at the splenic flexure (Figures 3 and 4). The patient had total colectomy (Figure 5) with ileoanal anastomosis and J pouch.

2.2. Case 2. A 71-year-old male, previously healthy, was seen for the first time in May 2011 for diarrhea and rectal bleed. His physical examination was unremarkable. Laboratory tests were within normal range. Ileocolonoscopy showed mucosal inflammation and ulcerations over a segment of 7cm at the level of transverse colon. Biopsies were in favor of chronic active colitis. The patient was treated as colonic IBD and was started on Mesalamine 4g per day but he was lost to follow-up. Four years later, he was seen again in January 2015 for the same previously described symptoms. He stated that he took Mesalamine for 6 months and stopped by his own after marked improvement and he was asymptomatic since

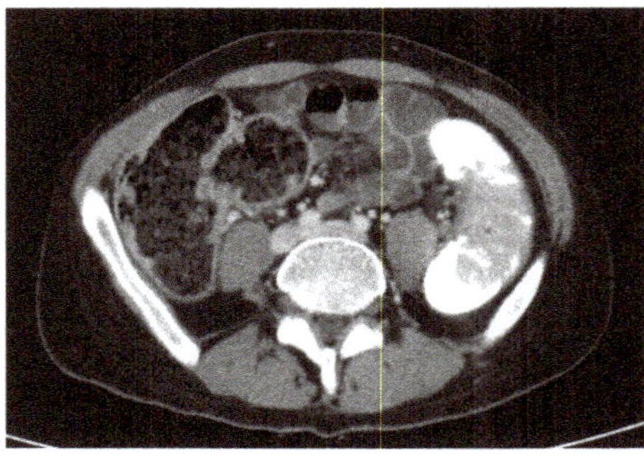

Figure 3: Abdominal CT scan showing GIP the left colon.

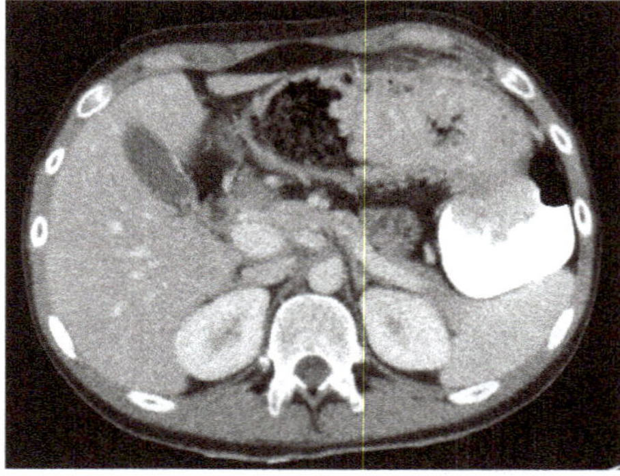

Figure 4: Abdominal CT scan showing obstructive GIP of the splenic flexure.

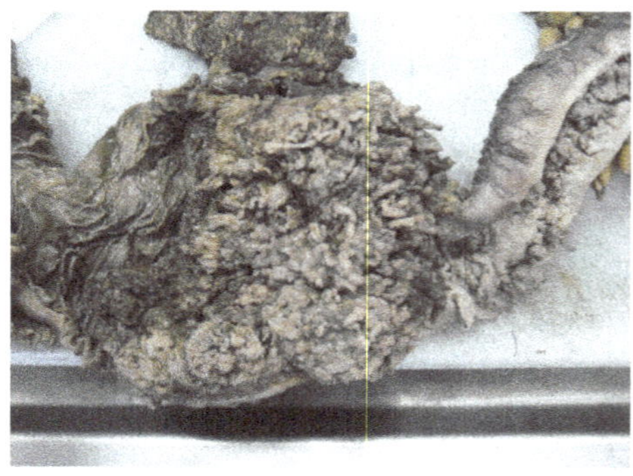

Figure 5: Surgical resection of GIP.

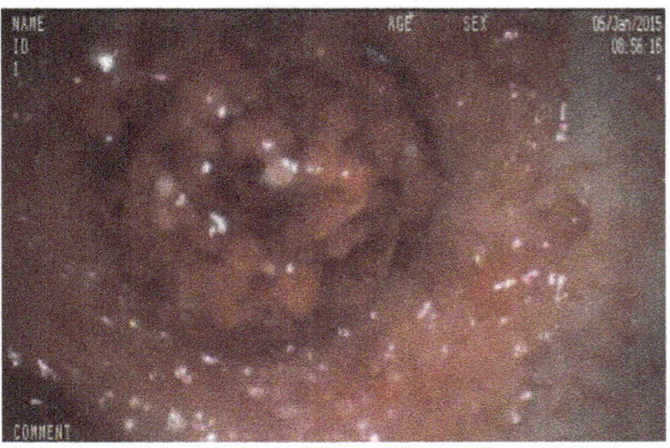

FIGURE 6: GIP of the transverse colon.

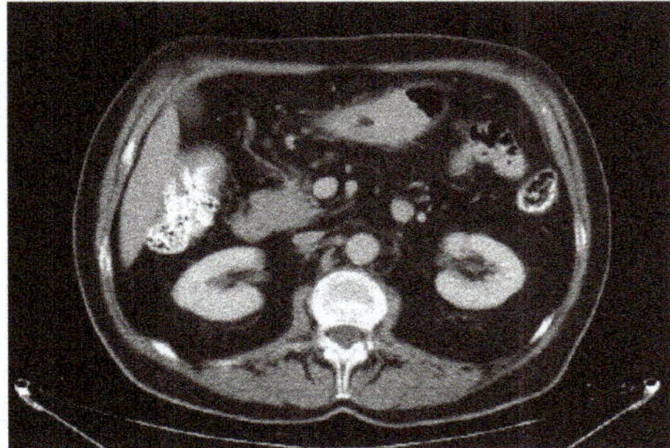

FIGURE 7: Abdominal CT scan showing stenotic GIP.

then until the reappearance of symptoms associated with abdominal pain few days prior to the presentation. Physical examination and lab tests were normal. Colonoscopy revealed an obstructive giant pseudopolyp (Figure 6) at the level of the transverse colon; biopsies showed chronic inflammation with architectural distortion and granulation tissue formation. Abdominal CT scan confirmed the presence of giant pseudopolyp (Figure 7). The patient was treated with segmental colonic resection and the surgical pathologic report was CD. The final diagnosis was colonic CD complicated by an obstructive giant pseudopolyp.

3. Discussion

We present two cases of obstructive GIP that developed in two different patients: one with UC and the other with CD. The development of GIP may be related to the severity of the disease in the patient with UC and to the duration of the disease in the patient with CD. In the first case, the patient had UC with severe inflammatory disease leading to the development of two GIP formations, one of them being totally obstructive. In the second, the patient had a quiescent Crohn's colitis disease causing obstructive GIP 5 years after the diagnosis.

GIP is defined by the presence of large polyps that are more than 1.5cm [1, 2]. It consists of numerous filiform polyps that look like a "mass of worms" or a "fungating" mass. It is an uncommon manifestation of inflammatory bowel disease [1], and its presence might be correlated with the severity and the duration of the disease [3]. It occurs most commonly in the transverse colon, followed by the sigmoid and descending colon, the cecum, and the splenic and hepatic flexure [5]. It is associated twice as often in UC compared to CD [2–4]. Yada S et al. reported that the time from the diagnosis of UC to GIP formation ranges from 3 to 276 months [6].

GIP pathogenesis results from repeated peristalsis and fecal stream causing enlarged mucosal tags [5]. Others propose that GIP is formed when inflamed colonic mucosa heals in a polypoid configuration during the regenerative phase, and this happens when ulcerated mucosa becomes surrounded by granulation tissue [3, 4].

The histopathological features include inflammatory infiltrates overlying the muscularis mucosae, deep fissure-like ulcers, chronic mucosal inflammation with lymphoid hyperplasia, and nerve hyperplasia in the surrounding mucosa [6–11].

In a systematic review of literature, Maggs et al. identified 81 GIP formations in 78 patients with IBD. In those with ulcerative colitis, the majority (70%) had extensive colitis and none had proctitis. GIP formations were located throughout the colon although the majority was in the transverse and descending colon [3].

GIP can produce symptoms similar to IBD, such as bloating, diarrhea, discomfort, rectal bleed, abdominal pain, and palpable abdominal mass [3, 12]. 15% were complicated with obstruction and subobstruction and 3% with intussusception of mechanical etiology due to the large size [3]. Others rare complications were noted like protein-losing enteropathy, bleeding, and iron deficiency anemia [13].

GIP is clinically, endoscopically, and radiologically similar to neoplastic lesions and is frequently mistaken for one another [14–19]. The differential diagnosis of GIP includes villous adenoma, dysplasia associated lesion or mass, polypoid carcinoma, lymphoma, and colitis cystica profunda [14–16]. There has only been one reported case of an occult carcinoma arising in a patient who was diagnosed with localized GIP [9]. The incidence of malignancy in a patient with UC is 3–5%, indicating that the risk of malignancy is equal in a patient having UC with or without GIP [9].

Surgical resection is inevitable when GIP presents with obstructive symptoms such as luminal obliterations and/or intussusceptions or they cannot be removed by polypectomy. Extension, chronicity, and acute complications make total coloproctectomy with ileoanal anastomosis the most reasonable therapeutic choice. Some have performed local excision of the pseudopolyp in a bowel-sparing method [20].

In conclusion, we report here two rare cases of GIP associated with UC and CD. The first patient had a dramatic evolution of his UC with the development of two GIP formations within one year of the diagnosis of IBD, one of them being totally obstructive at the splenic flexure, the least common site of GIP. The second patient had CD was totally asymptomatic prior to the development of obstructive GIP.

References

[1] M. R. Sheikholeslami, R. F. Schaefer, and P. Mukunyadzi, "Diffuse giant inflammatory polyposis: a challenging clinicopathologic diagnosis," *Archives of Pathology & Laboratory Medicine*, vol. 128, no. 11, pp. 1286–1288, 2004.

[2] G. Syal and Budhraja V., "Recurrent Obstructive Giant Inflammatory Polyposis of the Colon," *ACG Case Reports Journal*, vol. 3, no. 4, p. e89, 2016.

[3] J. R. L. Maggs, L. C. Browning, B. F. Warren, and S. P. L. Travis, "Obstructing giant post-inflammatory polyposis in ulcerative colitis: Case report and review of the literature," *Journal of Crohn's and Colitis*, vol. 2, no. 2, pp. 170–180, 2008.

[4] Y. S. Choi, J. P. Suh, I. T. Lee et al., "Regression of giant pseudopolyps in inflammatory bowel disease," *Journal of Crohn's and Colitis*, vol. 6, no. 2, pp. 240–243, 2012.

[5] M. Nagashima, Y. Sugishita, A. Moriyama et al., "Tumor-like growth of giant inflammatory polyposis in a patient with ulcerative colitis," *Case Reports in Gastroenterology*, vol. 7, no. 2, pp. 352–357, 2013.

[6] S. Yada, T. Matsumoto, T. Kudo et al., "Colonic obstruction due to giant inflammatory polyposis in a patient with ulcerative colitis," *Journal of Gastroenterology*, vol. 40, no. 5, pp. 536–539, 2005.

[7] C. Rozenbajgier, P. Ruck, H. Jenss, and E. Kaiserling, "Filiform polyposis: A case report describing clinical, morphological, and immunohistochemical findings," *The Clinical Investigator*, vol. 70, no. 6, pp. 520–528, 1992.

[8] K. J. Bauknecht, G. Grosse, J. Kleinert, A. Lachmann, and F. Niedobitek, "Filiform polyposis of the colon in chronic inflammatory bowel disease (so-called giant inflammatory polyps)," *Zeitschrift für Gastroenterologie*, vol. 38, no. 10, pp. 845–854, 2000.

[9] N. Okayama, M. Itoh, Y. Yokoyama et al., "Total obliteration of colonic lumen by localized giant inflammatory polyposis in ulcerative colitis: report of a Japanese case," *Internal Medicine*, vol. 35, no. 1, pp. 24–29, 1996.

[10] D. P. Hurlstone, "Large-bowel obstruction secondary to localized rectal giant pseudopolyposis complicating ulcerative colitis: First reported case," *Endoscopy*, vol. 34, no. 12, p. 1025, 2002.

[11] M. Tanaka, H. Saito, T. Kusumi et al., "Spatial distribution and histogenesis of colorectal Paneth cell metaplasia in idiopathic inflammatory bowel disease," *Journal of Gastroenterology and Hepatology*, vol. 16, no. 12, pp. 1353–1359, 2001.

[12] J. D. Fitterer, L. G. Cromwell, and J. E. Sims, "Colonic obstruction by giant pseudopolyposis," *Gastroenterology*, vol. 72, no. 1, pp. 153–156, 1977.

[13] R. Anderson, I. T. Kaariainen, and S. B. Hanauer, "Protein-losing enteropathy and massive pulmonary embolism in a patient with giant inflammatory polyposis and quiescent ulcerative colitis," *American Journal of Medicine*, vol. 101, no. 3, pp. 323–325, 1996.

[14] J. Munchar, H. A. Rahman, and M. M. Zawawi, "Localized giant pseudopolyposis in ulcerative colitis," *European Journal of Gastroenterology & Hepatology*, vol. 13, no. 11, pp. 1385–1387, 2001.

[15] B. Ooi, J. J. Tjandra, J. S. Pedersen, and P. S. Bhathal, "Giant pseudopolyposis in inflammatory bowel disease," *ANZ Journal of Surgery*, vol. 70, no. 5, pp. 389–393, 2000.

[16] H. R. Hinrichs and H. Goldman, "Localized Giant Pseudopolyps of the Colon," *Journal of the American Medical Association*, vol. 205, no. 4, pp. 248-249, 1968.

[17] C. J. Ferguson, T. W. Balfour, and C. J. H. Padfield, "Localized giant pseudopolyposis of the colon in ulcerative colitis - Report of a case," *Diseases of the Colon & Rectum*, vol. 30, no. 10, pp. 802–804, 1987.

[18] S. Katz, R. F. Rosfnberg, and I. Katzka, "Giant pseudopolyps in crohn's colitis: a nonoperative approach," *American Journal of Gastroenterology*, vol. 76, no. 3, pp. 267–271, 1981.

[19] R. S. Fishman, C. R. Fleming, and D. H. Stephens, "Roentgenographic simulation of colonic cancer by benign masses in Crohn's colitis," *Mayo Clinic Proceedings*, vol. 53, no. 7, pp. 447–449, 1978.

[20] T. S. Maldonado, B. Firoozi, D. Stone, and K. Hiotis, "Colocolonic intussusception of a giant pseudopolyp in a patient with ulcerative colitis: A case report and review of the literature," *Inflammatory Bowel Diseases*, vol. 10, no. 1, pp. 41–44, 2004.

25

Adverse Effects of Proton Pump Inhibitors on Platelet Count: A Case Report and Review of the Literature

Subhajit Mukherjee,[1] Tanima Jana,[1] and Jen-Jung Pan[2]

[1]*Division of Gastroenterology, Hepatology and Nutrition, Department of Internal Medicine, The University of Texas Health Science Center, Houston, TX 77030, USA*
[2]*Division of Gastroenterology and Hepatology, Department of Medicine, University of Arizona College of Medicine, Tucson, AZ 85724, USA*

Correspondence should be addressed to Subhajit Mukherjee; drsubhajit@gmail.com

Academic Editor: Chia-Tung Shun

Proton pump inhibitors (PPIs) are the most effective and preferred class of drugs used to treat peptic ulcer disease, gastroesophageal reflux disease, and other diseases associated with increased production of gastric acid. PPIs in general have an excellent long-term safety profile and are well-tolerated. However, studies have shown some adverse reactions (e.g., osteoporosis, *Clostridium difficile*-associated diarrhea, Vitamin B12 and iron deficiency, and acute interstitial nephritis) on long-term PPI use. Thrombocytopenia attributed to use of PPIs has been described in a few case reports and a retrospective study. In this case report, we describe a case of PPI-induced thrombocytopenia. In our patient, thrombocytopenia immediately developed after the initiation of PPI on two separate occasions and resolved after its discontinuation. The strong association found in our case implies the potential role of PPI in causing this rare but serious adverse reaction. Based on this case report and the observation from other studies, a PPI-induced adverse event should be considered as a possible etiology for new-onset idiopathic thrombocytopenia.

1. Introduction

Proton pump inhibitors (PPIs) are the most commonly used class of drugs for the treatment of gastric acid-related disorders [1]. PPIs inhibit gastric acid production by inhibiting the gastric parietal cell hydrogen potassium ATPase, which is needed for the final step of acid secretion [1, 2]. PPIs are the most potent inhibitor of this enzyme currently available and hence their therapeutic role in the treatment of acid-related disorders is well-established [1, 2]. Conditions in which PPIs are more effective and commonly used include peptic ulcer disease, gastroesophageal reflux disease (GERD), Zollinger-Ellison syndrome, eradication of *Helicobacter pylori* infection, treatment of bleeding gastro-duodenal ulcers and esophageal strictures, and the maintenance therapy for Barrett's esophagus [3–12].

Omeprazole was the first PPI used in clinical practice (in the late 1980s). Since then, several other PPIs have become available [13]. Although the different types of PPIs differ with regard to their pharmacokinetic profile, bioavailability, and route of excretion, their clinical effectiveness is very similar [1, 14]. In fact, findings from various clinical trials have been unsuccessful in selecting one type of PPI over another based on their therapeutic efficacy and cost-effectiveness [14, 15]. PPIs in general are very safe drugs, especially if they are used for short-term purposes, but recent literature has shown concern with their long-term use [16]. Some of the adverse sequelae of long-term PPI use include osteoporosis with increased risk of bone fractures, *Clostridium difficile*-associated diarrhea, pneumonia, hypomagnesemia, Vitamin B12 deficiency, iron deficiency, acute interstitial nephritis, hypergastrinemia, and chronic atrophic gastritis [17–25]. The Food and Drug Administration (FDA) has raised safety concerns regarding long-term PPI use mainly for osteoporosis, *Clostridium difficile*-associated diarrhea, and hypomagnesemia. However, in their 2008 guidelines for GERD management, the American Gastroenterological Association (AGA) did not recommend any routine safety monitoring in patients on long-term PPI, due to insufficient evidence for these adverse events [16]. In fact, none of the gastroenterology societies have recommended any surveillance for potential adverse risks in long-term PPI users.

Short-term adverse events of PPIs are rare. Only a few case reports have shown an increased incidence of rebound gastrointestinal symptoms and community-acquired pneumonia after short-term PPI use [26, 27]. While nine case reports and one retrospective study have demonstrated that PPIs may cause thrombocytopenia, another large retrospective study failed to show any increased incidence of thrombocytopenia after PPI use [28–38].

In this report, we describe a case of life-threatening thrombocytopenia after PPI use. In our patient, the thrombocytopenia occurred after the initiation of PPI and resolved after its discontinuation. The causality of PPI with regard to thrombocytopenia in this particular case was further strengthened by the observation of another episode of thrombocytopenia when the PPI was reintroduced. Complete recovery of the platelet count only occurred when the PPI was stopped and, hence, the PPI was subsequently listed as a drug allergy for this patient.

2. Case

A 35-year-old Hispanic female was admitted for worsening upper abdominal pain, nausea, and vomiting. She had a past medical history of heartburn which was being treated with PPI. She was initially seen in the emergency department for worsening epigastric abdominal pain and was discharged home on daily omeprazole. She returned to her primary care clinic 2 months later complaining of similar symptoms while being on omeprazole. Since omeprazole was not effective, she was switched to esomeprazole. Two months later, she visited her home country of El Salvador and was evaluated for abdominal pain. Due to her persistent symptoms, cholecystectomy was performed, without much relief of her symptoms. Patient reported that she was unable to take the initially prescribed esomeprazole secondary to financial issues and was not on any acid-suppressing medications in the previous 2 months. Upper endoscopy was then performed and it showed multiple gastric ulcers. She was then started on pantoprazole. After returning to the United States, she continued to have pain and started taking nonsteroidal anti-inflammatory drugs (NSAIDs) for relief. Subsequently, she visited her primary care office with worsening of her pain associated with nausea and vomiting. During this clinic visit, she was switched to dexlansoprazole and was asked to come to the emergency department if she continued to have symptoms. She returned to the emergency department the next day for further evaluation of her worsening symptoms. On initial evaluation in the emergency department, she was afebrile and had stable hemodynamics. She endorsed severe abdominal pain and a 30-pound weight loss over the last year, but denied any hematemesis, melena, or hematochezia. Laboratory evaluation revealed white blood cell count of 26.5 $\times 10^3/mm^3$, hemoglobin 13.8 g/dl, and platelet count of 116 $\times 10^3/mm^3$. On review of laboratory data, patient's last platelet count checked 6 months priorly was normal ($264 \times 10^3/mm^3$) and had been obtained before the patient was started on a PPI for the first time. No other laboratory tests had been obtained until this recent emergency department visit. Therefore, the effect of PPI on the platelet count for the next 6 months after initiation of therapy was not available to us. Chemistry panel, liver function, urinalysis, and blood/urine cultures were negative. CT imaging of the abdomen and pelvis showed diffuse steatosis but was otherwise normal.

Gastroenterology was consulted and due to refractory abdominal pain, weight loss, and NSAID use, an upper endoscope was recommended. Additionally, intravenous esomeprazole twice daily was started. Her platelet count continued to drop, falling to $72 \times 10^3/mm^3$ the next day and to $12 \times 10^3/mm^3$ the day after. Hematology was consulted for the rapid drop in platelet count and the etiology was thought to be secondary to drug-induced thrombocytopenia, infection, or idiopathic thrombocytopenic purpura. Of note, the patient did not have any history of bleeding or clotting disorders. Additionally, there was no evidence of hemolysis on the peripheral blood smear and the patient was not coagulopathic. On review of medications, since there were no other drugs (except for one prophylactic dose of heparin) that could be attributed to thrombocytopenia, it was recommended to hold the PPI. The PPI was then stopped, and platelet count recovered to $99 \times 10^3/mm^3$ within two days. Upper endoscope performed at that time revealed nonspecific gastritis. Biopsies were found to be negative for *Helicobacter pylori* infection. Due to the spontaneously improved platelet count, antibodies to heparin-platelet factor 4 complex were not checked to rule out heparin-induced thrombocytopenia. Since our patient's platelet count normalized after stopping PPI, this current episode of thrombocytopenia was deemed likely secondary to PPI use.

Our patient was subsequently discharged home, but continued to have persistent epigastric pain. She tried a H2 (histamine 2) receptor antagonist with minimal symptom relief. She was next seen in the Gastroenterology Clinic. At this time, the platelet count was $135 \times 10^3/mm^3$. During this visit, the question of whether patient's thrombocytopenia was truly related to PPI use was revisited, given that heparin-induced thrombocytopenia was not ruled out. Since a PPI was warranted due to her persistent symptoms, the decision was made to restart dexlansoprazole with close follow-up. She ultimately got readmitted to the hospital 7 days later for persistent epigastric pain (while on PPI). This time the platelet count was found to have decreased further to 43 $\times 10^3/mm^3$. The platelet count continued to drop, similar to her prior admission while on PPI, with the lowest count being $10 \times 10^3/mm^3$. PPI was held because of prior concern for PPI-induced thrombocytopenia. On this admission, our patient did not receive any heparin products and peripheral blood smear was not consistent with hemolysis. She did not receive any medications known to cause thrombocytopenia. Platelet count improved to $50 \times 10^3/mm^3$ while off PPI and she was discharged home. Patient's symptoms improved on H2 antagonist, sucralfate, and pain control with morphine. On this admission, PPIs were listed as a drug allergy and documented in the patient's medical record. She was seen in

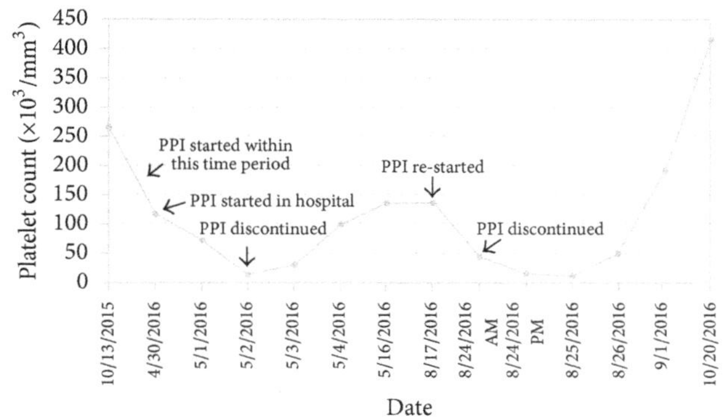

FIGURE 1: Platelet count trend of the patient. Thrombocytopenia developed after starting PPI for the first time and later on when it was restarted. Platelet count recovered after PPI was discontinued on both occasions (x-axis: actual date; y-axis: platelet count in $10^3/mm^3$).

the Gastroenterology Clinic after hospital discharge and it was noted that her symptoms were partially controlled on H2 antagonist, sucralfate, and scopolamine (which she received from her home country for control of nausea). Platelet count ultimately improved to $415 \times 10^3/mm^3$. A complete pictorial description of our patient's platelet count is shown in Figure 1.

3. Discussion

PPIs are an important class of medications for long-term use in patients suffering from GERD and Barrett's esophagus [8, 11]. They are also important for the treatment of peptic ulcers, especially in acute settings when patients present with upper gastrointestinal bleeding [12]. Generally, PPIs are very safe medications, but a few case reports have implicated their role in causing thrombocytopenia [28, 33]. This side effect of PPIs should be taken seriously, as the drop in the platelet count in our patient was very severe, and this side effect poses significant consequences such as life-threatening bleeding.

Drug-induced thrombocytopenia is a diagnosis of exclusion and its incidence is less than 1% in the general population for nonheparin drug products [39]. In our patient, the temporal relationship of the drop in platelet count with the introduction of PPI, along with the subsequent revival of the count upon its withdrawal, was sufficient to implicate PPI use as the reason for the thrombocytopenia. A reasonable first step in the evaluation and diagnosis of drug-induced thrombocytopenia is to discontinue the offending drug and look for the normalization of platelet counts. However, *in vitro* testing for the detection of drug-dependent antibodies provides a direct analytical method to diagnose this condition. This test can be used as an adjunct to clinical findings in making a diagnosis of drug-induced thrombocytopenia and also for drug surveillance [40].

Previous case reports have shown similar effects of PPI-induced thrombocytopenia for several types of PPI (e.g., pantoprazole, lansoprazole, and omeprazole). In all cases, platelet count dropped the very next day after starting PPI. The first case of pantoprazole-induced thrombocytopenia was reported by Watson et al. [28]. Subsequently, other authors have also documented a similar effect after pantoprazole administration [29–31, 34]. In keeping with these observations of pantoprazole-induced thrombocytopenia, Binnetoğlu et al. in a retrospective study of 35 patients demonstrated significant thrombocytopenia after pantoprazole infusion [33]. However, Dotan et al., in a retrospective study of 468 hospitalized patients, failed to demonstrate increased incidence of thrombocytopenia after pantoprazole use [32].

A small number of case reports have demonstrated thrombocytopenia with different types of PPI. While Zlabek and Anderson and Ogoshi et al. documented evidence of thrombocytopenia after oral intake of lansoprazole, Hayashibara and Rudelli et al. described similar effects of thrombocytopenia with omeprazole use [35–38]. Finally, Ranzino et al. reported a case of thrombocytopenia after coadministration of esomeprazole and hydantoin, but a direct causal relationship of esomeprazole use and thrombocytopenia was not established in their study [41].

In our case, both esomeprazole and dexlansoprazole caused thrombocytopenia, so it is likely that this effect is not drug-specific, but is rather a class effect. Additionally, both intravenous and oral use of PPI caused similar effects in dropping platelet counts, with platelet counts decreasing as low as $10 \times 10^3/mm^3$. Hematology work-up including examination of a peripheral smear was also done, excluding other causes of thrombocytopenia.

Based on the findings from these case reports and from our observation, it appears that PPIs can cause thrombocytopenia. However, the mechanism of action is unknown. Future research should be focused on discovering how this class of drugs, which primarily works by inhibiting hydrogen potassium ATPase, can cause thrombocytopenia. Irrespective of the mechanism, we should exercise caution when prescribing PPIs for long-term use and monitor patient's platelet counts carefully while on PPIs.

References

[1] M. M. Wolfe and G. Sachs, "Acid suppression: Optimizing therapy for gastroduodenal ulcer healing, gastroesophageal reflux disease, and stress-related erosive syndrome," *Gastroenterology*, vol. 118, no. 2, pp. S9–S31, 2000.

[2] M. M. Wolfe, L. S. Welage, and G. Sachs, "Proton pump inhibitors and gastric acid secretion," *American Journal of Gastroenterology*, vol. 96, no. 12, pp. 3467-3468, 2001.

[3] S. Holt and C. W. Howden, "Omeprazole - Overview and opinion," *Digestive Diseases and Sciences*, vol. 36, no. 4, pp. 385–393, 1991.

[4] T. Poynard, M. Lemaire, and H. Agostini, "Meta-analysis of randomized clinical trials comparing lansoprazole with ranitidine or famotidine in the treatment of acute duodenal ulcer," *European Journal of Gastroenterology & Hepatology*, vol. 7, no. 7, pp. 661–665, 1995.

[5] R. T. Jensen and D. L. Fraker, "Zollinger-Ellison Syndrome: Advances in Treatment of Gastric Hypersecretion and the Gastrinoma," *Journal of the American Medical Association*, vol. 271, no. 18, pp. 1429–1435, 1994.

[6] D. C. Metz, G. M. Comer, E. Soffer et al., "Three-year oral pantoprazole administration is effective for patients with Zollinger-Ellison syndrome and other hypersecretory conditions," *Alimentary Pharmacology & Therapeutics*, vol. 23, no. 3, pp. 437–444, 2006.

[7] A. Tamura, K. Murakami, and J. Kadota, "Prevalence and independent factors for gastroduodenal ulcers/erosions in asymptomatic patients taking low-dose aspirin and gastroprotective agents: the OITA-GF study," *QJM: An International Journal of Medicine*, vol. 104, no. 2, pp. 133–139, 2011.

[8] P. J. Kahrilas, C. W. Howden, and N. Hughes, "Response of regurgitation to proton pump inhibitor therapy in clinical trials of gastroesophageal reflux disease," *American Journal of Gastroenterology*, vol. 106, no. 8, pp. 1419–1426, 2011.

[9] W. D. Chey and B. C. Y. Wong, "American College of Gastroenterology guideline on the management of Helicobacter pylori infection," *American Journal of Gastroenterology*, vol. 102, no. 8, pp. 1808–1825, 2007.

[10] R. D. Marks, J. E. Richter, J. Rizzo et al., "Omeprazole versus H2-receptor antagonists in treating patients with peptic stricture and esophagitis," *Gastroenterology*, vol. 106, no. 4, pp. 907–915, 1994.

[11] F. Kastelein, M. C. W. Spaander, E. W. Steyerberg et al., "Proton pump inhibitors reduce the risk of neoplastic progression in patients with barrett's esophagus," *Clinical Gastroenterology and Hepatology*, vol. 11, no. 4, pp. 382–388, 2013.

[12] J. Y. Lau, J. J. Sung, K. K. Lee et al., "Effect of Intravenous Omeprazole on Recurrent Bleeding after Endoscopic Treatment of Bleeding Peptic Ulcers," *The New England Journal of Medicine*, vol. 343, no. 5, pp. 310–316, 2000.

[13] B. T. Vanderhoff and R. M. Tahboub, "Proton pump inhibitors: An update," *American Family Physician*, vol. 66, no. 2, pp. 273–280, 2002.

[14] M. S. McDonagh, S. Carson, and S. Thakurta, "Drug class review: proton pump inhibitors," Update 5, http://www.ohsu.edu/drugeffectiveness/reports/final.cfm.

[15] N. Vakil and M. B. Fennerty, "Systematic review: Direct comparative trials of the efficacy of proton pump inhibitors in the management of gastro-oesophageal reflux disease and peptic ulcer disease," *Alimentary Pharmacology & Therapeutics*, vol. 18, no. 6, pp. 559–568, 2003.

[16] P. J. Kahrilas, N. J. Shaheen, and M. F. Vaezi, "American Gastroenterological Association Institute Technical Review on the Management of Gastroesophageal Reflux Disease," *Gastroenterology*, vol. 135, no. 4, pp. 1392–1413, 2008.

[17] Y.-X. Yang, J. D. Lewis, S. Epstein, and D. C. Metz, "Long-term proton pump inhibitor therapy and risk of hip fracture," *Journal of the American Medical Association*, vol. 296, no. 24, pp. 2947–2953, 2006.

[18] S. Janarthanan, I. Ditah, D. G. Adler, and M. N. Ehrinpreis, "Clostridium difficile-associated diarrhea and proton pump inhibitor therapy: a meta-analysis," *American Journal of Gastroenterology*, vol. 107, no. 7, pp. 1001–1010, 2012.

[19] R. J. F. Laheij, M. C. J. M. Sturkenboom, R.-J. Hassing, J. Dieleman, B. H. C. Stricker, and J. B. M. J. Jansen, "Risk of community-acquired pneumonia and use of gastric acid-suppressive drugs," *Journal of the American Medical Association*, vol. 292, no. 16, pp. 1955–1960, 2004.

[20] M. W. Hess, J. G. J. Hoenderop, R. J. M. Bindels, and J. P. H. Drenth, "Systematic review: hypomagnesaemia induced by proton pump inhibition," *Alimentary Pharmacology & Therapeutics*, vol. 36, no. 5, pp. 405–413, 2012.

[21] J. R. Lam, J. L. Schneider, W. Zhao, and D. A. Corley, "Proton pump inhibitor and histamine 2 receptor antagonist use and vitamin B12 deficiency," *Journal of the American Medical Association*, vol. 310, no. 22, pp. 2435–2442, 2013.

[22] K. E. McColl, "Effect of Proton Pump Inhibitors on Vitamins and Iron," *American Journal of Gastroenterology*, vol. 104, no. S2, pp. S5–S9, 2009.

[23] K. Sampathkumar, R. Ramalingam, A. Prabakar, and A. Abraham, "Acute interstitial nephritis due to proton pump inhibitors," *Indian Journal of Nephrology*, vol. 23, no. 4, pp. 304–307, 2013.

[24] J. W. Freston, "Omeprazole, hypergastrinemia, and gastric carcinoid tumors," *Annals of Internal Medicine*, vol. 121, no. 3, pp. 232-233, 1994.

[25] E. J. Kuipers, "Proton pump inhibitors and gastric neoplasia," *Gut*, vol. 55, no. 9, pp. 1217–1221, 2006.

[26] C. Reimer, B. Søndergaard, L. Hilsted, and P. Bytzer, "Proton-pump inhibitor therapy induces acid-related symptoms in healthy volunteers after withdrawal of therapy," *Gastroenterology*, vol. 137, no. 1, pp. 80.e1–87.e1, 2009.

[27] J. J. Heidelbaugh, A. H. Kim, R. Chang, and P. C. Walker, "Overutilization of proton-pump inhibitors: what the clinician needs to know," *Therapeutic Advances in Gastroenterology*, vol. 5, no. 4, pp. 219–232, 2012.

[28] T. D. Watson, J. E. Stark, and K. S. Vesta, "Pantoprazole-induced thrombocytopenia," *Annals of Pharmacotherapy*, vol. 40, no. 4, pp. 758–761, 2006.

[29] U. Korkmaz, A. Alcelik, M. Eroglu, A. N. Korkmaz, and G. Aktas, "Pantoprazole-induced thrombocytopenia in a patient with upper gastrointestinal bleeding," *Blood Coagulation & Fibrinolysis*, vol. 24, no. 3, pp. 352-353, 2013.

[30] J. L. Miller, A. K. Gormley, and P. N. Johnson, "Pantoprazole-induced thrombocytopenia," *The Indian Journal of Pediatrics*, vol. 76, no. 12, pp. 1278-1279, 2009.

[31] A. Kallam, A. Singla, and P. Silberstein, "Proton pump induced thrombocytopenia: A case report and review of literature," *Platelets*, vol. 26, no. 6, pp. 598–601, 2015.

[32] E. Dotan, R. Katz, J. Bratcher et al., "The prevalence and pantoprozole associated thrombocytopenia in a community hospital," *Expert Opinion on Pharmacotherapy*, vol. 8, no. 13, pp. 2025–2028, 2007.

[33] E. Binnetoğlu, E. Akbal, H. Şen et al., "Pantoprazole-induced thrombocytopenia in patients with upper gastrointestinal bleeding," *Platelets*, vol. 26, no. 1, pp. 10–12, 2015.

[34] A. Tafi, "Thrombocytopenia as a side effect of pantoprazole," *The Turkish Journal of Gastroenterology*, vol. 24, no. 3, pp. 295-296, 2013.

[35] J. A. Zlabek and C. G. Anderson, "Lansoprazole-induced thrombocytopenia," *Annals of Pharmacotherapy*, vol. 36, no. 5, pp. 809–811, 2002.

[36] K. Ogoshi, T. Kato, S. Saito, M. Niwa, and H. Watanabe, "Clinical study of AG-1749 (lansoprazole): Effects on serum gastrin levels and gastric mucosal ECL cell density," *Yakuri to Chiryo*, vol. 19, pp. 933–946, 1991.

[37] T. Hayashibara, "Hemolytic anemia and thrombocytopenia associated with anti-omeprazole antibody," *Rinsho Ketsueki*, vol. 39, pp. 447–452, 1998.

[38] A. Rudelli, I. Leduc, C. Traulle et al., "Thrombopenia following treatment with omeprazole," *Presse Medicale*, vol. 22, no. 20, p. 966, 1993.

[39] S. D. Zondor, J. N. George, and P. J. Medina, "Treatment of drug-induced thrombocytopenia," *Expert Opinion on Drug Safety*, vol. 1, no. 2, pp. 173–180, 2002.

[40] B. R. Curtis, "Non-chemotherapy drug-induced neutropenia: key points to manage the challenges," *Hematology. American Society of Hematology. Education Program*, vol. 1, pp. 187–193, 2017.

[41] A. M. Ranzino, K. R. Sorrells, and S. M. Manor, "Possible acute thrombocytopenia post esomeprazole and hydantoin coadministration," *Journal of Pharmacy Practice*, vol. 23, no. 2, pp. 140–143, 2010.

Giant Inflammatory Fibroid Polyp of the Hepatic Flexure of Colon Presenting with an Acute Abdomen

Ashish Lal Shrestha and Pradita Shrestha

Department of General Surgery, United Mission Hospital, Tansen, Palpa, Nepal

Correspondence should be addressed to Ashish Lal Shrestha; butchgrunty@yahoo.com

Academic Editor: Yoshihiro Moriwaki

Background. Inflammatory Fibroid Polyp (IFP) of the colon is an exceedingly rare condition. Since 1952 till now only 32 cases have been reported worldwide of which only 5 were giant (>4 cm) polyps mostly found in the caecum (15 cases) with only 3 in the descending colon. *Case Presentation.* A 36-year-old female with no previous illness presented to the emergency unit with an acute onset pain over the right hypochondrium for 3 days associated with intermittent fever and anorexia. As she had evidence of localized peritonitis she underwent a diagnostic laparoscopy and subsequently an exploratory laparotomy. A mass measuring 8 × 7 × 5 cm arising from the hepatic flexure of colon was noted. Right hemicolectomy with ileotransverse anastomosis was performed. The mass was subsequently reported to be IFP. *Conclusion.* IFP is a very rare condition with clinical presentation depending upon its size and location. Definitive diagnosis is possible with histopathological examination of tissue aided by immunohistochemical studies. Surgical resection has been the most common method of treatment especially for large and giant colonic IFPs owing to challenges in terms of diagnosis and technical difficulties associated with endoscopic methods.

1. Introduction

The first case of IFP was described by Konjetzny in 1920 as "Polypoid Fibroma" [1]. In 1949, Vanek made a report of 6 cases of gastric lesions which he referred to as gastric submucosal granuloma with eosinophilic infiltration [2]. The term Inflammatory Fibroid Polyp was introduced by Helwig and Ranier in 1953 [3]. The etiology and pathogenesis are not well known [4, 5].

The presentation of IFP varies and because of its rarity the correct preoperative diagnosis is often difficult and delayed. We report an interesting, rare case of IFP of the hepatic flexure of colon in an adult female. Its clinical presentation, investigative findings, and management are discussed and relevant literatures are reviewed. The rarities of this case are the atypical site of its occurrence and acuteness of its presentation.

2. Case Presentation

A 36-year-old female with no previous illness presented with an acute onset pain over the right hypochondrium for 3 days associated with intermittent fever and anorexia. Physical examination revealed a tender and guarded right upper abdomen. Hematological and biochemical tests were normal. Abdominal radiographs were unremarkable. Abdominal sonography revealed a double walled solid mass in the right upper abdomen very close to the liver and bilateral ovarian cysts. In view of patient's general condition and lack of facilities, CT scan and Colonoscopy could not be done. With differential diagnoses of ruptured hydatid cyst, duodenal ulcer perforation, acute acalculous cholecystitis, and an ulcerated GIST (Gastrointestinal Stromal Tumour) an emergency diagnostic laparoscopy followed by midline laparotomy was performed. At diagnostic laparoscopy purulent and fibrinous reaction in the subhepatic region was noted based on which decision to proceed further was made. At laparotomy, a mass measuring 8 × 7 × 5 cm arising from the hepatic flexure of colon was noted as shown in Figure 1. Right hemicolectomy with ileotransverse anastomosis was performed.

Histopathologically, gross examination confirmed the operative findings and the cut section revealed an obvious bulge in the serosa caused by the mass that seemed to involve

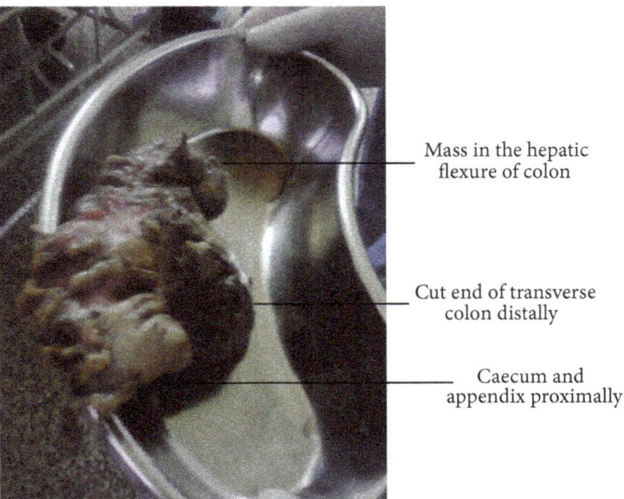

FIGURE 1: Intraoperative appearance of Inflammatory Fibroid Polyp arising from the hepatic flexure of colon. Caecum and appendix can be seen proximally and cut section of transverse colon can be seen distally.

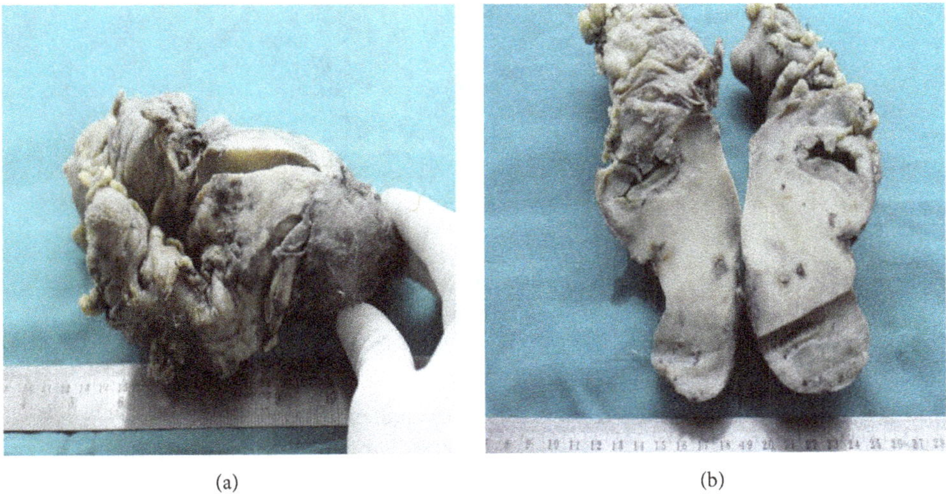

(a) (b)

FIGURE 2: (a) Gross appearance before cutting it open. (b) Gross appearance after longitudinally opening the specimen.

the full thickness of bowel wall, besides its glary myxoid appearance as shown in Figure 2.

Microscopically, there was an intact mucosal lining and the mass was located in the submucosa spreading up to the serosa. There was low cellularity with proliferation of spindle-to-stellate shaped cells in a myxoid-to-pink hyalinized background. The stellate cells had plump nuclei and conspicuous nucleoli. The intervening vascularity was prominent with associated moderate mixed inflammatory infiltrates with large number of eosinophils. The serosal aspect showed necrosis with collections of acute inflammatory exudates. There was no evidence of cellular atypia, pleomorphism, or increased mitotic activity as shown in Figure 3(a). The features were in favor of IFP with a differential diagnosis of GIST.

Immunohistochemical staining was found negative for CD34, CK PAN, and CD117 as shown in Figures 3(b) and 3(c) and hence the diagnosis of IFP was confirmed.

The patient had an uneventful recovery and was discharged on the 10th postoperative day. At one-year follow-up, she remained symptom-free.

3. Discussion

IFPs are rare benign mesenchymal gastrointestinal tumours [5, 6]. Also referred to as Vanek's tumour, these tumours do not have a specific age or gender predilection [7]. Ranging from few millimeters to several centimeters (giant > 4 cm), these often clinically mimic malignancy and are treated radically. With newer advancements in endoscopic surgery, these are now treatable with less invasive procedures except when the presentation is that of an acute abdomen [5].

Regarded by many as reactive tumours of nonneoplastic origin until 2008, the neoplastic nature of IFPs became evident after the detection of activating PDGFRA mutations [4].

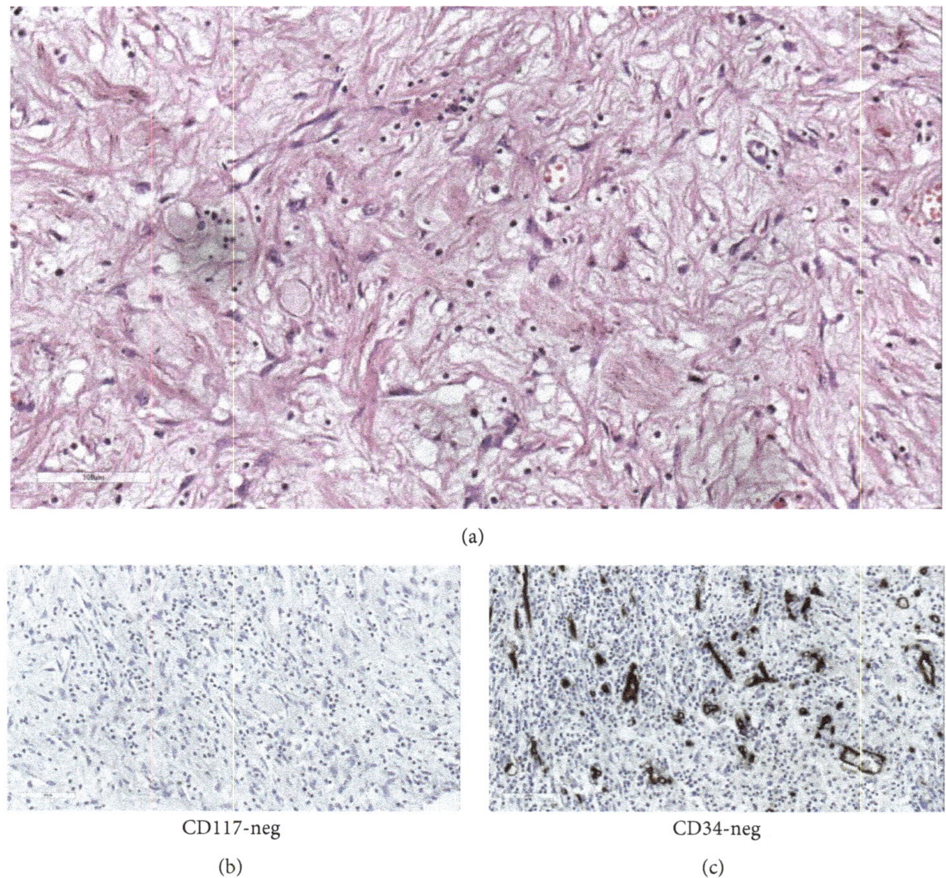

(a)

(b)

(c)

FIGURE 3: (a) Microscopic appearance of IFP (Eosin/Hematoxylin stain). (b) Immunohistochemical staining negative for CD34. (c) Immunohistochemical staining negative for CD117.

IFPs are found mostly in the stomach (70%) and the small intestine (20%). Colonic IFPs are exceedingly rare and most commonly located in proximal colon, especially in the caecum. They can be sessile or pedunculated and usually contain blood vessels, fibroblasts, and an edematous stroma rich in eosinophils [5, 6].

Clinical presentation depends on size and location generally. With enlargement they can cause abdominal pain, hematochezia, anemia, weight loss, diarrhea, and intussusceptions [5]. Definitive diagnosis is possible with histopathological examination of tissue. Using immunohistochemical studies, spindle cells that are generally positive for CD34 and negative for S-100 protein, P53, C-kit, and Bcl-2 can be differentiated from GIST [5, 8].

An extensive search in PubMed, Medline, and Google in reference to colonic IFPs showed that from 1952 till now only 32 cases have been reported worldwide of which only 5 were giant (>4 cm) polyps mostly found in the caecum (15 cases) with only 3 in the descending colon.

Treatment approach was surgical in 20 (58%) while endoscopic resection was done in only 8 (23%). There was no reported recurrence in the colon [5].

Surgical resection has been the most common method of treatment specially for large and giant colonic IFPs owing to challenges in terms of diagnosis and technical difficulties associated with endoscopic methods such as limited view due to large size, morphology (sessile or pedunculated), and location (flexural or sharp curve) and concerns regarding completion of procedure, recurrence, and cure.

In a setup like ours where the presentation was of an acute abdomen and the possibility of CT scan and Colonoscopy was remote, we opted for an open resection. However, provided that latest technology exists, it will be worthwhile attempting the least invasive methods.

4. Conclusion

In conclusion, Inflammatory Fibroid Polyp of the colon is an uncommon presentation of an uncommon diagnosis. The clinical and radiological picture may mimic carcinoma and definitive diagnosis may be possible with histopathological evaluation aided with immunohistochemical analysis. Once resected with negative margins, IFP does not require further treatment and has a good clinical outcome. Therefore, awareness of the clinical presentation and good pathological expertise are important adjuncts in the diagnosis. Surgery is the mainstay of treatment in the acute presentation.

Abbreviations

IFP: Inflammatory Fibroid Polyp
CT: Computed Tomography
GIST: Gastrointestinal Stromal Tumour.

Consent

Written informed consent was obtained from the patient for publication of this case report and accompanying images.

Authors' Contributions

Ashish Lal Shrestha participated in the conception and design of the report and wrote the paper and Pradita Shrestha analyzed the report. Both have been involved in the diagnosis, surgical management, and follow-up of the patient. Both authors read and approved the final paper. Both the authors were involved in planning, analysis of the case, and writing of the paper.

Acknowledgments

The authors would like to thank the ward staff of the hospital for providing support and helping in management of the patient.

References

[1] G. E. Konjetzny, "Uber magenfibrome," *Beitrage zur Klinischen Chirurgie*, vol. 119, pp. 53–61, 1920.

[2] J. Vanek, "Gastric submucosal granuloma with eosinophilic infiltration," *The American Journal of Pathology*, vol. 25, no. 3, pp. 397–411, 1949.

[3] E. B. Helwig and A. Ranier, "Inflammatory fibroid polyps of the stomach," *Surgery, Gynecology & Obstetrics*, vol. 96, no. 3, pp. 335–367, 1953.

[4] H.-U. Schildhaus, T. Caviar, E. Binot, R. Büttner, E. Wardelmann, and S. Merkelbach-Bruse, "Inflammatory fibroid polyps harbour mutations in the platelet-derived growth factor receptor alpha (PDGFRA) gene," *The Journal of Pathology*, vol. 216, no. 2, pp. 176–182, 2008.

[5] A. Kayyali, A. Toumeh, U. Ahmad, L. E. De Las Casas, and A. Nawras, "Giant inflammatory fibroid polyp of the descending colon treated with endoscopic resection," *ACG Case Reports Journal*, vol. 1, no. 1, pp. 36–39, 2013.

[6] S. Hirasaki, M. Matsubara, F. Ikeda, H. Taniguchi, and S. Suzuki, "Inflammatory fibroid polyp occurring in the transverse colon diagnosed by endoscopic biopsy," *World Journal of Gastroenterology*, vol. 13, no. 27, pp. 3765–3766, 2007.

[7] S. Akbulut, "Intussusception due to inflammatory fibroid polyp: a case report and comprehensive literature review," *World Journal of Gastroenterology*, vol. 18, no. 40, pp. 5745–5752, 2012.

[8] R. Birla and K. Mahawar, "Inflammatory fibroid polyp: a review," *Gastroenterology Today*, vol. 18, no. 2, 2008.

Spontaneous Resolution of Symptomatic Hepatic Sarcoidosis

Viva Nguyen[1] **Henry N. Ngo,**[2,3] **and Hamza H. Awad**[4]

[1] *Mercer University School of Medicine, Columbus, GA, USA*
[2] *Department of Internal Medicine, St. Francis Columbus Clinic, Columbus, GA, USA*
[3] *Department of Internal Medicine, Mercer University School of Medicine, Columbus, GA, USA*
[4] *Department of Community Medicine, Department of Internal Medicine, Mercer University School of Medicine, Macon, GA, USA*

Correspondence should be addressed to Viva Nguyen; vbnguyen8@gmail.com

Academic Editor: Hideto Kawaratani

Sarcoidosis is an inflammatory process of unknown etiology, characterized by noncaseating granulomas. Isolated extrapulmonary disease is rare. We present a case of a 60-year-old woman with chronically elevated alkaline phosphatase. Upon obtaining a liver biopsy, granulomatous hepatitis was observed, suggestive of sarcoidosis. No particular treatment was initiated, and 3 years following the onset of elevated alkaline phosphatase, her levels decreased spontaneously.

1. Introduction

Sarcoidosis is an inflammatory process of unknown etiology, characterized by noncaseating granulomas. The disease can affect multiple organs of the body, including the liver. Hepatic involvement is common with 50% to 60% of patients having granulomas on liver biopsy, but the majority of patients are asymptomatic [1]. Despite the possible presence of granulomas on biopsy, abnormal liver enzymes, or radiological imaging indicative of disease, most patients do not exhibit any signs or symptoms [2]. In the United States, hepatic sarcoidosis is approximately twice as common among African-Americans compared to Caucasians [3]. Health professionals need to be aware of the possible diagnosis of isolated granulomatous hepatitis due to sarcoidosis. Hepatic sarcoidosis can be resolved without treatment, unlike other organs, such as the lungs. The aim of this case report is to demonstrate that liver involvement in sarcoidosis can be symptomatic. In spite of the abdominal pain and weight loss exhibited by this patient in this case, spontaneous resolution of liver hepatitis required no treatment.

2. Case Report

A 60-year-old African American female was following up for her chronically elevated alkaline phosphatase levels. She had a history of hypertension, hyperlipidemia, type 2 diabetes mellitus, allergic rhinitis, and chronic lower back pain. Patient has a family history of arthritis, cardiovascular disease, and diabetes mellitus; she denies ever using alcohol or tobacco.

With the onset of elevated alkaline phosphatase level and vague abdominal pain in 2013, an abdominal ultrasound performed in December showed hepatic steatosis. Viral serologies for hepatitis during 2013 were negative, as a gastrointestinal consult was required to determine the need for a liver biopsy. A liver biopsy was subsequently performed, which showed focal mixed micro and macrovesicular steatosis. Portal tracts showed minimal focal chronic inflammation, no significant fibrosis, and no iron deposition.

The vague abdominal pain that she was experiencing waxed and waned for two years. Additionally, the patient experienced some vague chest pain and dyspnea that prompted an echocardiogram in February of 2015, which demonstrated a left ventricle ejection fraction of 44%. Consequently, a left heart catheterization in the following month showed no significant coronary disease with a dilated left ventricle with an ejection fraction of 50%. A 2-year follow-up in July of 2015 showed suspicious cirrhosis by Computed Tomography (CT) scan (Figure 1), possibly due to granulomatous changes and chronic inflammation. A CT scan was determined to be necessary for our patient because

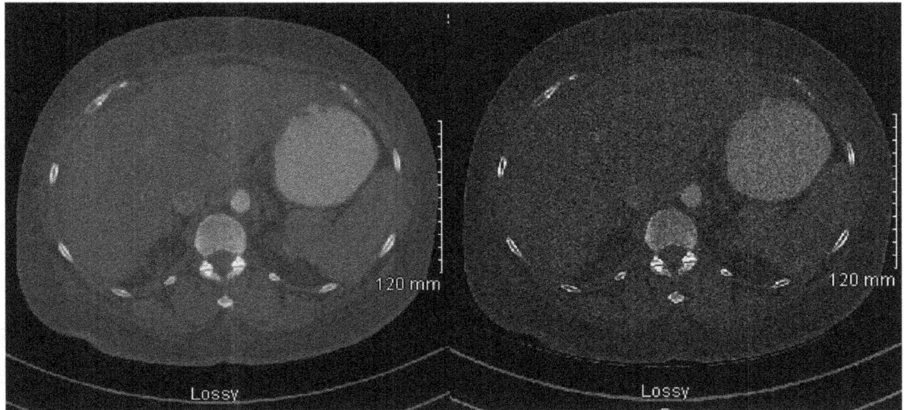

FIGURE 1: Abdominal Computed Tomography (CT), 2015.

TABLE 1: Laboratory values at subsequent follow-ups.

Laboratory	November 2016	March 2017	June 2017	Normal Value
WBC	5.8	5.5	6.3	3.0-11.0 K/μL
RBC	5.30	5.30	4.61	4.20-5.40 M/μL
Glucose:	366	402	245	65-99 mg/dL
Calcium:	9.9	9.9	9.1	8.6-10.3 mg/dL
Total Protein:	8.6	8.2	6.8	6.0-8.3 g/dL
Albumin:	3.4	4.0	3.6	3.5-5.7 g/dL
Total bilirubin:	1.8	1.0	0.5	0.3-1.0 mg/dL
Alkaline Phosphatase:	510	338	226	34-104 IU/L
AST:	42	34	20	13-39 IU/L
ALT:	32	30	16	7-52 IU/L
Magnesium:	1.4			1.9-2.7 mg/dL
Hemoglobin A1c:		13.0%	9.7%	4.0-6.0%

of rising alkaline phosphatase without other explainable etiologies, in addition to the patient's appetite suppression and vague abdominal pains. Patient's weight during this time was 207 lbs (93.89 kg) and was advised to diet and exercise. After 4 months of continuous symptoms, especially with abdominal pain, a laparoscopic cholecystectomy was performed with a liver biopsy that showed subsequent granulomatous changes in September of 2015. The liver biopsy showed coalescing periportal nonnecrotizing epithelioid granulomas with associated multinucleated giant cells and chronic inflammation. The chronic and patchy inflammation is representative of the granulomatous hepatitis, despite not having elevated transaminases. The granulomatous changes suggested possible sarcoidosis (Figure 2). The liver biopsy was not histologically suggestive of nonalcoholic steatohepatitis, with no steatosis noted. Chest X-ray at that time showed no significant findings.

Inflammatory bowel disease (IBD) was not explored in the patient because she never had clinical signs on past or present examinations, denying any symptoms of IBD including alternating bowel habits, predominant constipation, or diarrhea. Laboratory studies 2 years and 6 months since the onset, at the end of 2015 showed negative antinuclear antibodies (ANA), negative rheumatoid arthritis factor, negative cyclic citrullinated peptide (CCP) antibodies (IgG/IgA), elevated C-reactive protein of 8.9 mg/L, normal complement C3/C4, elevated B-type natriuretic peptide 688.6 pg/mL, and negative mitochondrial (M2) antibody. Subsequent office visits and additional laboratory results are shown in Table 1.

Additionally, patient experienced peak weight loss with a weight of 154 lbs. (69.85 kg) in 2016. During this time period, an echocardiogram showed a decreased ejection fraction of 26%. This result and a history of having ventricular tachycardia resulted in the patient having an automated implantable cardioverter-defibrillator (ICD) placed.

Urinalysis in June 2017 showed RBC 0-5/hpf, WBC 0-5/hpf, bacteria 2+, and moderate calcium oxalate crystals. Additionally, patient's weight increased in 2017 to 190 lbs. (86.18 kg).

3. Discussion

Sarcoidosis can affect many different organ systems, leading to long term or severe disease if left untreated with up to 7% risk of death [4]. The spectrum of liver disease in sarcoidosis is broad. The majority have hepatic granulomas on liver

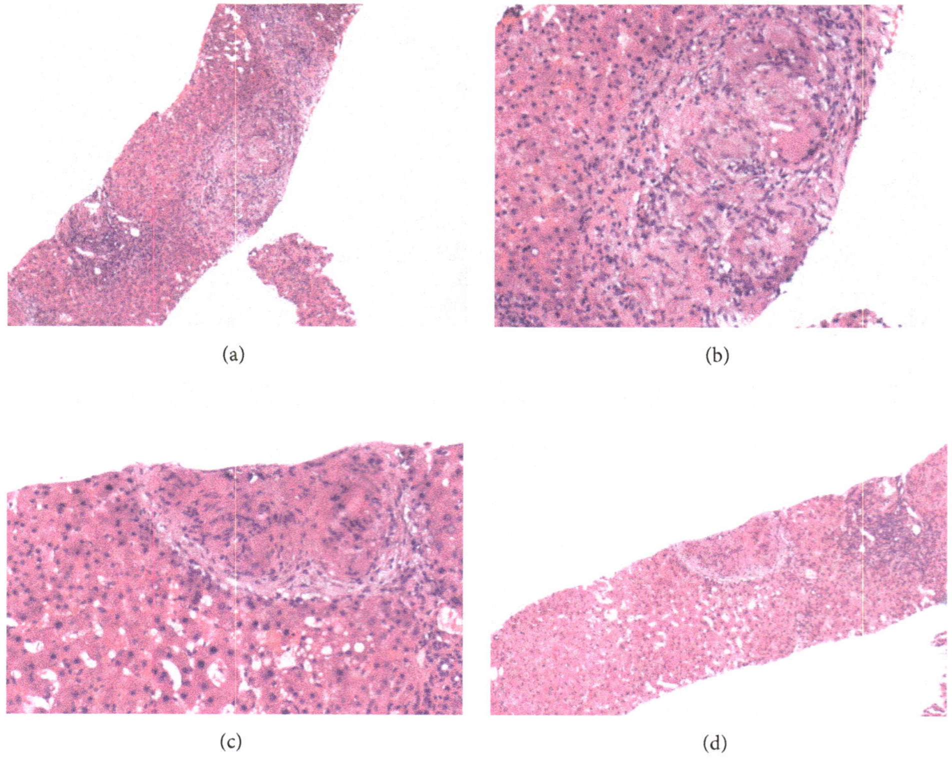

(a) (b) (c) (d)

FIGURE 2: Liver biopsy, 2015. (a) Liver, H+E, 40x, low power view showing liver parenchyma with focal replacement by noncaseating granulomas. (b) Liver, H+E, 200X, high power view demonstrating noncaseating granulomas and giant cells. (c) Liver, H+E, 200X, high power view demonstrating noncaseating granulomas and giant cell. (d) Liver, H+E, 40x, low power view demonstrating noncaseating granuloma (center).

biopsy, while some have elevated serum liver enzymes and hepatomegaly. Serum aminotransferases can rise up to 70% in those with hepatic sarcoidosis, but the degree of increase in serum alkaline phosphatase is greater, relative to the liver transaminases [5]. Hepatomegaly is seen in 5% to 15% and cirrhosis develops in 6% of patients with hepatic sarcoidosis [1, 5]. However, the evidence of organ dysfunction is rare. Therefore, the diagnosis of sarcoidosis with liver involvement can be difficult with asymptomatic patients or those with mild symptoms.

Elevations in alkaline phosphatase, as seen in our patient, and/or gamma glutamyltranspeptidase are indications of liver and biliary involvement. Alkaline phosphatase can rise up to 10-fold the upper limit of normal. While elevated alkaline phosphatase is specific to any disease or condition, the patient's medication was excluded as a cause, as alkaline phosphatase remained high despite adjustment and elimination of the medications. With our patient, the alarming factor was the consistently elevated alkaline phosphatase with weight loss. Aminotransferases elevations tend to be milder and less frequent compared to the alkaline phosphatase [1]. With our patient, after her laparoscopic cholecystectomy, one would expect her liver enzymes to decrease. However, her alkaline phosphatase levels remained highly elevated. The ongoing weight loss, fortunately, seemed to have helped her with her uncontrolled diabetes, as indicated by the decline in hemoglobin A1c from 13.0% to 9.7%. Angiotensin converting enzyme (ACE) levels were not obtained because of the insensitivity of the test and was determined to be unhelpful in the diagnosis of sarcoidosis.

Radiological studies, such as ultrasonography or Computed Tomography, may show hepatomegaly or hypoattenuated nodules in the liver. These nodules may be confused with liver metastasis or other granulomatous diseases [6]. Our patient's CT in 2015 initially showed possible cirrhosis with granulomatous changes in a span of 3 months since the onset of major symptoms. No hepatomegaly was noted during that time.

Liver biopsy should be considered if the diagnosis is uncertain, as was done with our patient. Moderate to severe liver-test abnormalities indicate a need for liver biopsy [7, 8]. Histopathological examination is a definitive tool; however, liver biopsy is not histologically suggestive of nonalcoholic steatohepatitis. In sarcoidosis, noncaseating and epithelioid granulomas are seen in the periportal and the portal regions of the liver. Sarcoid epithelioid granulomas are characterized by macrophages that form giant cells surrounded by fibrin rings. In some cases, granulomas may be due to hepatitis C or prior exposure to interferon therapy for hepatitis C. Other causes of granulomatous lesions in the liver, such as tuberculosis, fungal infections, primary biliary cholangitis, Hodgkin disease, and drug toxicity, should be considered before making a diagnosis of sarcoidosis.

Therapeutic regimen for hepatic sarcoidosis remains undefined. Observation alone is sufficient for patients with asymptomatic liver disease or isolated mild elevations of serum liver enzymes. Hepatomegaly alone is not an indication for treatment. In some asymptomatic patients, abnormal serum liver tests can resolve spontaneously or remain stable for many years. With the weight loss and decrease in appetite, the concern became whether or not to initiate any treatment. What if the patient was particularly thin and experienced these weight losses? Would that have changed the management? Our patient demonstrated spontaneous improvement in her alkaline phosphatase levels, along with her aminotransferases. The time frame of approximately 1.5 years demonstrated the gradual decline in the alkaline phosphatase levels and improvement of symptoms. One could predict that her alkaline phosphatase levels should continue to improve, despite not being on any particular treatment for the sarcoidosis.

Death of patients with sarcoidosis usually occurs from severe pulmonary, cardiac, and central nervous system disease, rather than hepatic involvement [9]. Chronic hepatic sarcoidosis may lead to portal hypertension and cirrhosis. When managing treatment of sarcoidosis, consultations with specialists are important due to the multiorgan effect of the disease, especially with the pulmonary and central nervous system. The need to start systemic glucocorticoids was considered, but after weighing the risks and benefits, the patient opted to observe and wait with a watchful eye on possible complications.

The plan for our patient will be to continue monitoring her liver functions, as well as monitoring her pulmonary, cardiac, and central nervous systems with the appropriate specialist, for any developments. Our patient had systolic heart failure and tachyarrhythmia that required an ICD. Cardiac sarcoidosis can manifest as heart blocks, arrhythmias, and heart failure. While findings of the echocardiogram did not suggest cardiac involvement, further cardiac work-up in the form of cardiac magnetic resonance (CMR) imaging, nuclear imaging, cardiac metaiodobenzylguanidine (MIBG) imaging, or endomyocardial biopsy might be warranted for confirmation of cardiac sarcoidosis, bearing in mind the limitations of these modalities based on their sensitivity, specificity, availability, and local expertise.

References

[1] M. Judson, "Extrapulmonary Sarcoidosis," *Seminars in Respiratory and Critical Care Medicine*, vol. 28, no. 1, pp. 083–101, 2007.

[2] R. P. Baughman, A. S. Teirstein, M. A. Judson et al., "Clinical characteristics of patients in a case control study of sarcoidosis," *American Journal of Respiratory and Critical Care Medicine*, vol. 164, no. 10, pp. 1885–1889, 2001.

[3] Y. C. Cozier, J. S. Berman, J. R. Palmer, D. A. Boggs, D. M. Serlin, and L. Rosenberg, "Sarcoidosis in Black Women in the United States," *CHEST*, vol. 139, no. 1, pp. 144–150, 2011.

[4] M. S. Wijsenbeek and D. A. Culver, "Treatment of Sarcoidosis," *Clinics in Chest Medicine*, vol. 36, no. 4, pp. 751–767, 2015.

[5] K. Devaney, Z. D. Goodman, M. S. Epstein, H. J. Zimmerman, and K. G. Ishak, "Hepatic sarcoidosis. Clinicopathologic features in 100 patients," *The American Journal of Surgical Pathology*, vol. 17, no. 12, Article ID 8238735, pp. 1272–1280, 1993, http://europepmc.org/abstract/MED/8238735.

[6] F. Ufuk and D. Herek, "CT of hepatic sarcoidosis: small nodular lesions simulating metastatic disease," *Polish Journal of Radiology*, vol. 80, pp. 945–954, 2015.

[7] J. P. Cremers, M. Drent, R. P. Baughman, P. A. Wijnen, and G. H. Koek, "Therapeutic approach of hepatic sarcoidosis," *Current Opinion in Pulmonary Medicine*, vol. 18, no. 5, pp. 472–482, 2012.

[8] U. Syed, H. Alkhawam, M. Bakhit, R. A. C. Companioni, and A. Walfish, "Hepatic sarcoidosis: Pathogenesis, clinical context, and treatment options," *Scandinavian Journal of Gastroenterology*, vol. 51, no. 9, pp. 1025–1030, 2016.

[9] X. Hu, E. M. Carmona, E. S. Yi, P. A. Pellikka, and J. Ryu, "Causes of death in patients with chronic sarcoidosis," *Sarcoidosis Vasc Diffuse Lung Dis*, vol. 33, no. 3, pp. 275–280, 2016.

28

Recurrent Enterolithiasis Small Bowel Obstruction: A Case Seldom Described

Ashish Lal Shrestha and Pradita Shrestha

Department of General Surgery, United Mission Hospital, Tansen, Palpa, Nepal

Correspondence should be addressed to Ashish Lal Shrestha; butchgrunty@yahoo.com

Academic Editor: Warwick S. Selby

Background. Enterolithiasis of the small bowel is a rare phenomenon in humans although it has been frequently described in equines. Primary enteroliths have been described including those occurring secondary to conditions like Crohn's disease, small bowel diverticula, tuberculous or postoperative strictures, and blind loops but those occurring in an otherwise normal gut are exceedingly rare. Of even greater rarity is a recurrent small bowel enterolith presenting with obstruction. This may be the first report of such kind. *Case Presentation.* A 70-year-old man undergoing treatment for stable alcoholic liver disease presented to the emergency with gradually progressive diffuse abdominal pain associated with vomiting and constipation for 7 days. He had gaseous abdominal distention but was not obstipated. He had a history of 2 laparotomies in the past for small bowel obstruction secondary to enterolith impaction. He was initially managed conservatively but since there was no significant clinical improvement, he underwent an exploratory laparotomy. A recurrent enterolith 5×5 cm in size was found impacted in the mid ileum with multiple dense serosal adhesions and bands. Adhesiolysis and enterotomy with removal of enterolith were performed. *Conclusion.* Recurrent enterolithiasis of the small bowel is a rare phenomenon and may present with recurrent obstruction. Definitive preoperative diagnosis is not always possible and a high index of suspicion is required to avoid table misdiagnosis. Surgery is the mainstay of treatment once conservative measures fail. Laparoscopic methods may help in diagnosis and avoid possibility of a subsequent adhesive bowel obstruction but are associated with technical challenges.

1. Introduction

The term "enterolith" is applied to the calculi that form within the intestinal lumen. Though common in equine population, these are cases of rarity in humans. The first reported case was that by Chomelin J in 1710 in Historie de l'Academie Royal in an autopsy report with a duodenal diverticulum [1]. Pfahler and Stamm are credited for the first radiologic description of alimentary stone in 1915 [1].

Gut hypomotility or stasis is thought to be the causal factor for this, the usual contents being inspissated fecal matter, calcium phosphates, magnesium, bacteria, epithelial debris, and unconjugated choleic acid with little or no cholesterol [1–4].

We report an interesting case of a rare recurrent small bowel enterolithiasis presenting with recurrent obstruction. Its clinical presentations, investigative findings, and management are discussed and relevant literatures are reviewed. The rarity of this case is the unusual mode of presentation of an unusual disease.

2. Case Presentation

A 70-year-old man previously being treated for stable alcoholic liver disease presented with gradually progressive diffuse abdominal pain associated with vomiting and constipation for 7 days. Physical examination revealed gaseous abdominal distention without tenderness or mass. He had a history of 2 laparotomies in the past both for small bowel obstruction secondary to enterolith impaction that had failed to resolve with conservative measures.

The finding on first operation 3 years ago was that of a 3×5 cm obstructing enterolith in the ileum 20 cm proximal to the ileocaecal junction. This was removed through an enterotomy and the affected segment of ileum was resected with

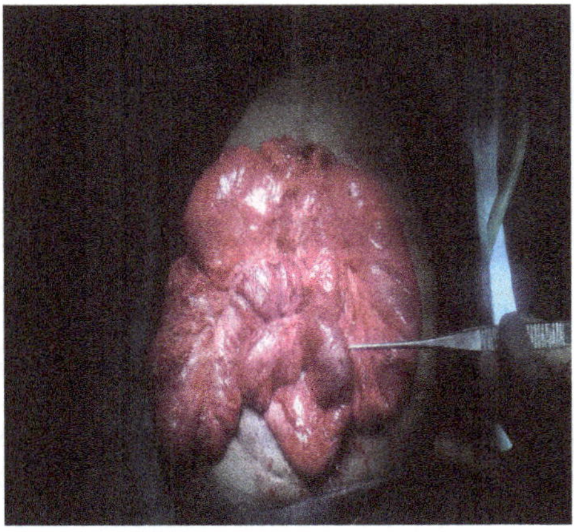

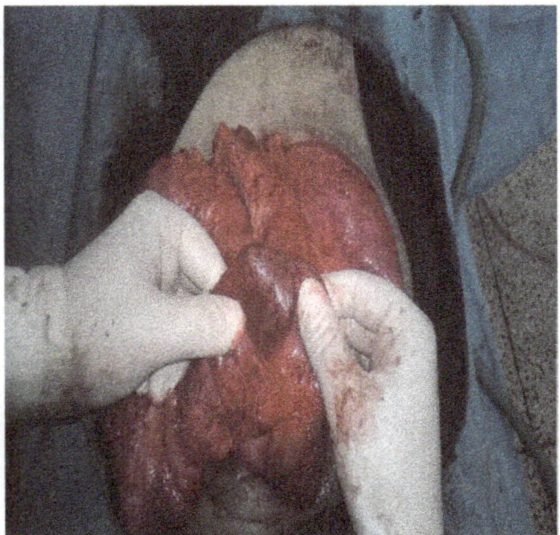

Figure 1: Intraoperative appearance of enterolith impacted in the mid ileum prior to enterotomy with multiple dense adhesions and bands.

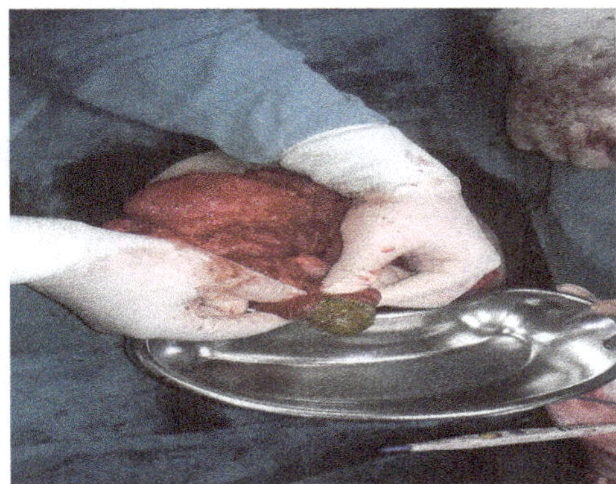

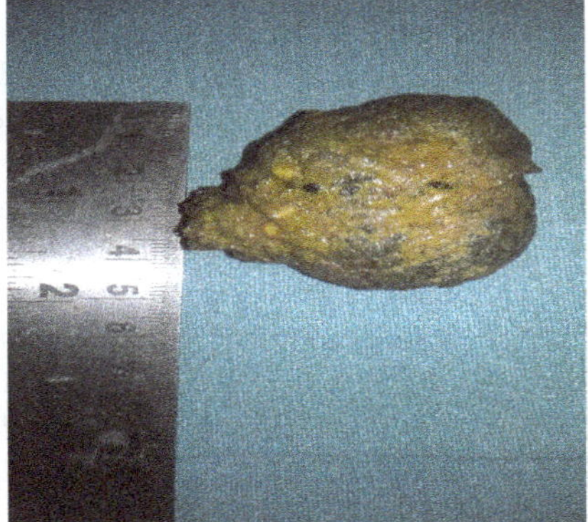

Figure 2: Intraoperative appearance of enterolith impacted in the mid ileum following enterotomy.

primary end to end anastomosis. There were no diverticula or any other inciting factors identified. The histopathology of the resected small bowel was reported to have no specific findings.

Following this, he presented 2 years later with similar symptoms. On second operation the findings were again similar to that of the first operation with an impacted enterolith in the mid ileum along with minimal adhesions. He underwent enterotomy and removal of the enterolith. Following the second operation he was asymptomatic till this presentation.

At the current presentation, his hematological and biochemical workup was normal and abdominal radiographs were inconclusive. USG revealed a normal study.

He was initially managed conservatively in lines of adhesive bowel obstruction.

In view of patient's general condition and lack of facilities, CT scan and endoscopy could not be done.

After a mild initial symptomatic improvement, he developed gradual and progressive abdominal distention with pain and obstipation. Suspecting adhesive obstruction and keeping in mind the possibility of a recurrent enterolith bowel obstruction, he was taken for an exploratory laparotomy. On table findings were those of a recurrent enterolith 5 × 5 cm in size impacted in the mid ileum with multiple dense serosal adhesions and bands as shown in Figures 1 and 2. Apart from this no other abnormal findings were identified.

The enterolith was disimpacted through an ileal enterotomy followed by primary closure of the enterotomy.

The enterolith was not sent for biochemical analysis considering that it may not contribute to additional information from management point of view.

His subsequent postoperative course was stormy and developed burst abdomen on 8th postoperative day that required mass closure. But following this he showed gradual and steady improvement. After a total stay of 6 weeks, he was discharged in a stable state and had improved on follow-up visit at 3 months. At follow-up he was advised to avoid high roughage diet and consume stool softeners on PRN basis thinking that this would help him avoid another similar episode.

3. Discussion

In 1947, Grettve classified enteroliths into primary and secondary types based on their source: primary-inside the bowel and secondary-outside the bowel (associated organs like gall bladder) [1, 5].

Primary enteroliths can occur secondary to conditions like Crohn's disease, small bowel diverticula, tuberculous or postoperative strictures, and blind loops [2, 6–8]. But enterolith occurring in an otherwise normal gut is rarely described and even rarer is recurrent enterolith causing small bowel obstruction [4]. In fact, this may be the first report of a recurrent enterolith. An extensive search in PubMed, Medline, and Google in reference to recurrent enterolithiasis did not show any case reports from 1950 till now.

In 1960, Atwell and Pollock further classified primary enteroliths into true and false based on the chemical analysis of stone composition and their location [1, 2].

The true types are uncommon and formed by the precipitation of alimentary chime while the false types result from the agglutination of indigestible foreign materials like seeds, bone, vegetable material (phytobezoar), hair (trichobezoar), and so forth [2].

Specific preoperative radiological diagnosis of enteroliths is difficult even with water soluble contrast study combined with a cross sectional imaging like CT [4]. Plain radiographs may suggest the probable level of obstruction but may not reveal specific shadows, making it a diagnostic surprise on table. Probably owing to low calcium content in these stones, they are rarely picked up in plain X-rays [9, 10]; on the other hand findings like pneumobilia on the same could suggest gallstone ileus that must be supported with findings of biliary abnormalities on ultrasonography [11].

Definitive treatment is surgical [1]. The consensus management policy at laparotomy is to first attempt manual lysis of the calculus without enterotomy and then milking the smaller parts into proximal colon allowing exit via rectum [1, 12]. If this is not possible, enterotomy removal from a proximal less edematous portion can be done [1, 6]. Bowel resection and anastomosis are usually done if there is a coexistent severe inflammation, perforation, necrotic bowel diverticulosis, or long segment or multiple strictures causing enterolithiasis [1, 2].

The options of minimally invasive techniques may be explored especially if preoperative diagnosis can be made, in order to avoid future adhesions if recurrent enteroliths can be kept in mind as a distant possibility.

4. Conclusion

In conclusion, recurrent small bowel enterolithiasis with obstruction is an uncommon presentation of a rare diagnosis. The clinical and radiological picture may not always lead to a definitive diagnosis preoperatively and many a time this may be possible only on table. An accurate preoperative diagnosis requires a high index of clinical suspicion. Once conservative measures fail, surgical treatment remains the mainstay of management.

Abbreviations

CT: Computed tomography
USG: Ultrasonography of the abdomen and pelvis
PRN: Pro re nata (as and when required).

Consent

Written informed consent was obtained from the patient for publication of this case report and accompanying images.

Authors' Contributions

Ashish Lal Shrestha participated in the conception and design of the report and wrote the paper and Pradita Shrestha analyzed the report. Both have been involved in the diagnosis, surgical management, and follow-up of the patient. Both authors read and approved the final paper. Both the authors were involved in planning, analysis of the case, and writing of the paper.

Acknowledgments

The authors would like to thank the ward staff of the hospital for providing support and helping in management of the patient.

References

[1] G. E. Gurvits and G. Lan, "Enterolithiasis," *World Journal of Gastroenterology*, vol. 20, no. 47, pp. 17819-29, 2014.

[2] A. Perathoner, P. Kogler, C. Denecke, J. Pratschke, R. Kafka-Ritsch, and M. Zitt, "Enterolithiasis-associated ileus in Crohn's disease," *World Journal of Gastroenterology*, vol. 18, no. 42, pp. 6160–6163, 2012.

[3] K. Shetty and A. Sridhar, "An unusual presentation of enterolithiasis," *J Gastrointest Liver Dis JGLD*, vol. 20, no. 4 article 348, p. 348, 2011.

[4] B. Kirshtein, Z. H. Perry, J. Klein, L. Laufer, and N. Sion-Vardi, "Giant enterolith in ileal diverticulum following ileoplastic bladder augmentation," *International Journal of Surgery Case Reports*, vol. 4, no. 4, pp. 385–387, 2013.

[5] S. Grettve, "A contribution to the knowledge of primary true concrements in the small bowel," *Acta Chirurgica Scandinavica*, vol. 95, no. 5, pp. 387–410, 1947.

[6] D. Mishra, S. Singh, and M. Juneja, "Enterolithiasis: an uncommon finding in abdominal tuberculosis," *Indian Journal of Pediatrics*, vol. 76, no. 10, pp. 1049-1050, 2009.

[7] B. Chaudhery, P. A. Newman, and M. D. Kelly, "Small bowel obstruction and perforation secondary to primary enterolithiasis in a patient with jejunal diverticulosis," *BMJ Case Reports*, vol. 2014, 2014.

[8] R. L. Wroblewski and R. P. Sticca, "Images in clinical medicine. Primary small-bowel enterolithiasis," *New England Journal of Medicine*, vol. 359, no. 12 article 1271, 2008.

[9] A. Brettner and E. J. Euphrat, "Radiological significance of primary enterolithiasis," *Radiology*, vol. 94, no. 2, pp. 283–288, 1970.

[10] M. L. Paige, G. G. Ghahremani, and J. J. Brosnan, "Laminated radiopaque enteroliths: diagnostic clues to intestinal pathology,"

American Journal of Gastroenterology, vol. 82, no. 5, pp. 432–437, 1987.

[11] F. Lassandro, N. Gagliardi, M. Scuderi, A. Pinto, G. Gatta, and R. Mazzeo, "Gallstone ileus analysis of radiological findings in 27 patients," *European Journal of Radiology*, vol. 50, no. 1, pp. 23–29, 2004.

[12] U. Gadhia, D. Raju, and R. Kapoor, "Large enterolith in a Meckels diverticulum causing perforation and bowel obstruction: an interesting case with review of literature," *Indian Journal of Surgery*, vol. 75, supplement 1, pp. 177–179, 2013.

A Single Mass Forming Colonic Primary Mantle Cell Lymphoma

Fady Daniel,[1] Hazem I. Assi,[2] Walid Karaoui,[1] Jean El Cheikh,[2] Sami Bannoura,[3] and Samer Nassif[3]

[1]*Division of Gastroenterology, Department of Internal Medicine, American University of Beirut Medical Center, P.O. Box 11-0236, Riad El Solh, Beirut 110-72020, Lebanon*
[2]*Division of Hematology & Oncology, Department of Internal Medicine, American University of Beirut Medical Center, P.O. Box 11-0236, Riad El Solh, Beirut 110-72020, Lebanon*
[3]*Pathology and Laboratory Medicine Department, American University of Beirut Medical Center, P.O. Box 11-0236, Riad El Solh, Beirut 110-72020, Lebanon*

Correspondence should be addressed to Fady Daniel; fd21@aub.edu.lb

Academic Editor: Yoshiro Kawahara

Mantle cell lymphoma (MCL) is a subtype of non-Hodgkin's lymphoma (NHL) comprising around 7% of adult NHL. It is characterized by a chromosomal translocation t(11:14) and overexpression of Cyclin D1. The incidence of secondary gastrointestinal tract involvement in MCL ranges from 10 to 28% in various series. However primary gastrointestinal MCL is very rare, accounting for only 1 to 4% of primary gastrointestinal lymphomas. The most common endoscopic feature of primary intestinal MCL is multiple lymphomatous polyposis. In rare cases it presents as protruded lesions or superficial lesions. Single colonic mass presentation is an extremely infrequent presentation. MCL has an aggressive course with quick progression, and most cases are discovered in the advanced stages. Colonic biopsies with histologic examination and specific immunohistochemical staining are the gold standard for a proper diagnosis. We report a case of a single mass forming mantle cell lymphoma of the ascending colon in a 57-year-old female patient with unusual colonoscopic and radiologic features and describe the therapy the patient received, thereby adding to the spectrum of clinical presentations of this aggressive lymphoproliferative disorder.

1. Introduction

Mantle cell lymphoma (MCL) is a small B-cell non-Hodgkin's lymphoma and is recognized as an aggressive B-cell lymphoma derived from a subset of naive pregerminal center cells with a propensity to involve extranodal sites. The gastrointestinal tract is the most common extranodal site involved by lymphoma, accounting for 5–20% of all cases of extranodal involvement [1]. Despite the high rate of secondary colonic involvement by MCL, primary gastrointestinal (GI) lymphomas are infrequently reported, accounting for only about 1–4% of all gastrointestinal malignancies [2]. The neoplastic cells are believed to originate from the mantle zone of the lymphoid follicles within the intestinal mucosa [3]. The molecular signature of MCL is an overexpression of the cyclin-D1 (CCND1) gene as a result of the chromosomal translocation t(11;14) that juxtaposes the protooncogene CCND1 to the immunoglobulin heavy-chain promoter [4]. As a result of this mutation, the lymphoma cells are usually immunohistochemically positive for cyclin-D1 and aberrantly coexpress CD5. Around 49% of MCL patients have gastroduodenal involvement, and specifically 38% to 62% have colorectal involvement [5, 6]. The difficulty in the diagnosis of primary GI lymphoma arises in part from the nonspecific and often benign gross endoscopic appearance. Of note, the most common endoscopic presentation of MCL is lymphomatous polyposis. In rare cases its presents as protruded lesions or superficial lesions [7]. MCL has an aggressive course with quick progression and most cases are discovered in the advanced stages. Primary MCL of the colon is a rare entity and its presentation as a single mass forming tumor is extremely unusual. We report a case of a single mass forming mantle cell lymphoma of the ascending colon in a 57-year-old female patient with unusual colonoscopic and radiologic features and describe the therapy the patient received.

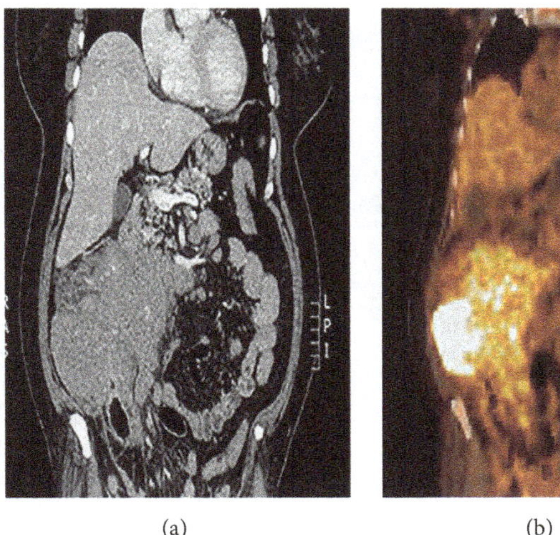

(a) (b)

FIGURE 1: PET-CT scan image.

2. Case Presentation

A 57-year-old woman with a history of hypertension and type 2 diabetes mellitus presented to our clinic with abdominal pain of 2 months duration, unintentional weight loss of 5 kg, night sweats, and fatigue. Abdominal physical examination revealed a palpable mass on the right side involving the right upper and lower quadrants at the level of the right colonic area. No organomegaly or palpable lymph nodes were noted. Her complete blood count was remarkable only for microcytic anemia, while chemistry studies including liver function tests and tumor markers (CEA, CA 19-9) were within normal limits. An abdominal CT scan showed a large soft tissue lesion arising from the wall of the ascending colon, with surrounding soft tissue deposits and enlarged pericolonic lymph nodes (Figure 1). Gastroscopy was normal with no evidence of gastritis or duodenal villous atrophy on corresponding biopsies. However, colonoscopy demonstrated a large fungating, ulcerated, and obstructing mass at the level of the ascending colon (Figure 2). The mass involved circumferentially the colonic wall with narrowing of the lumen, thereby preventing access to the terminal ileum. Additionally, the mass was friable and easily bleeding at scope contact. The remaining colonic segments were normal.

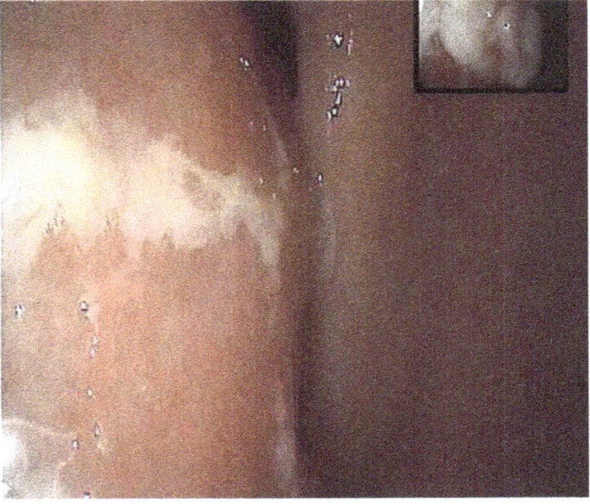

FIGURE 2: Endoscopic picture showing the colonic mass.

Biopsies were taken from the mass and showed lamina propria expansion by a diffuse population of medium-sized lymphocytes with mild to moderate nuclear irregularity and mildly increased mitotic activity (Figure 3). On immunohistochemical staining, the atypical lymphoid infiltrate was diffusely positive for CD20 and CD79s with coexpression of CD5, CD43, cyclin-D1, and BCL-2 and negative for CD3, CD10, CD23, and BCL-6. Proliferation index Ki-67 was around 40–50% (Figure 3). The morphologic and immunohistochemical findings were consistent with a mantle cell lymphoma.

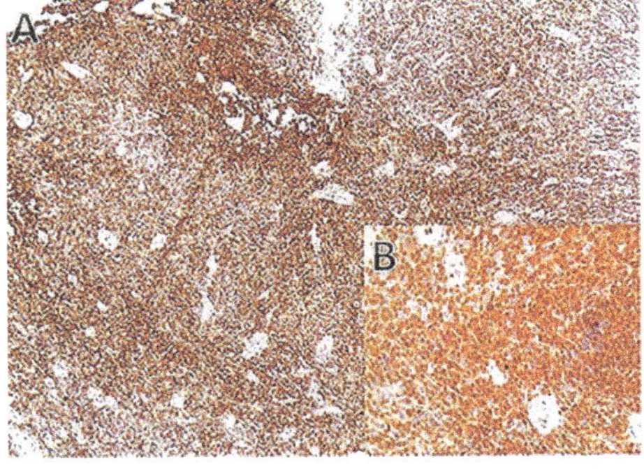

FIGURE 3: Immunohistochemical staining showing a diffuse CD20 positive B-cells ((A), 40x) coexpressing cyclin-D1 (B) (20x).

Subsequently, staging radiologic studies were performed. Abdominal CT scan with intravenous contrast administration disclosed an enhancing solid mass replacing the entire right colonic area, with corresponding mesenteric blood vessels encasement. Positron Emission Tomography PET-CT scan showed hypermetabolic large right colonic mass with adjacent retroperitoneal, mesenteric lymph nodes, peritoneal deposits, and heterogeneous bone marrow uptake. Since no uptake was noted in the small bowel, balloon enteroscopy was not preformed. Additionally, a bone marrow core biopsy showed marrow involvement by MCL.

In view of the above findings, the patient's stage was determined as IV E as per the Ann Arbor classification. She was treated by induction chemotherapy alternating R-CHOP/R-DHAP for a total of 3 cycles of each protocol. A very good response was achieved, and the patient subsequently underwent conditioning with high dose chemotherapy (BEAM) followed by autologous stem cell transplantation (ASCT). Her overall treatment was well tolerated except for fatigue and grade 2 mucositis as well as febrile neutropenia. Evaluations after ASCT with a PET-CT scan on day 100 and day 180 showed a continuous complete remission. However, the patient refused colonoscopy after completion of chemotherapy.

3. Discussion

Mantle cell lymphoma is a subtype of non-Hodgkin's lymphoma (NHL) comprising around 7% of adult NHL [4]. It is characterized by a chromosomal translocation t(11:14) and overexpression of Cyclin D1 [4]. MCL commonly presents with advanced-stage disease, with about 80% of patients showing involvement of extranodal sites at presentation, including the bone marrow, spleen, Waldeyer's ring, and gastrointestinal tract [8].

Gastrointestinal tract involvement is recognized occasionally as being the presenting sign of lymphoproliferative disorders, and early recognition is important for staging, prognosis, and selection of appropriate treatment. Of note, the incidence of secondary gastrointestinal tract involvement in MCL ranges from 10 to 28% in various series [5]. At endoscopy, MCL in the intestines commonly manifests as numerous, small, spherical, or hemispherical polyps, a finding termed multiple lymphomatous polyposis (MLP) [2]. MLP can involve segments of the small intestine and large intestine, and the morphologic and immunohistochemical features of MCL presenting as MLP are similar to those of nodal MCL [9]. However primary gastrointestinal MCL is very rare accounting for only 1 to 4% of primary gastrointestinal lymphomas, and there is insufficient data to describe this rare entity [10]. The most common endoscopic feature of primary intestinal MCL is multiple lymphomatous polyposis [7]. Less commonly it presents as a single protruded lesion in the colon [7]. Ghimire et al. described seven cases of primary gastrointestinal lymphoma over a period of 11 years. Of these, three cases had colonic involvement with a diffuse morphology, one case showed gastric and colonic involvement, and one also showed rectal involvement [2]. In addition, Chung et al. described a series of seven cases of MCL over a period of 6 years. The majority of patients in their series were elderly and six out of seven cases had multiple polypoidal lesions ranging from 0.1 to 4 cm with central ulcerations. Additionally, diffuse polyposis was seen uniformly in their series, and polyposis was predominantly seen in the rectum and ascending colon, rather than in other sections of the colon [11]. Systemic chemotherapy usually consists of Cyclophosphamide, Adriamycin, Vincristine, and Prednisone plus Rituximab (R-CHOP) [5]. Dasappa et al. treated five patients with CHOP chemotherapy. Only one patient achieved complete remission and remained disease-free for 21 months before being lost to follow-up. The remaining four patients had inadequate response to CHOP chemotherapy with a median survival of 6 months [12]. Our patient was unusual in that she presented with a single large mass involving the right colon with luminal obstruction, with sparring of the remaining colonic segments. She received chemotherapy, followed by ASCT. Due to known poor survival in MCL and low response rate to systemic chemotherapy, we used an aggressive regimen alternating R-CHOP/R-DHAP followed by ASCT [13]. Seven months after transplant, the patient was still disease-free.

In summary, we described the case of primary colonic mantle cell lymphoma with an unusual presentation, thereby adding to the spectrum of clinical manifestations of this aggressive lymphoproliferative disorder. Although a rare entity, primary colonic lymphomas should be included in the differential diagnosis of single colonic lesions. Awareness of such occurrences is necessary and might help refine diagnostic methods for gastrointestinal lymphoproliferative disorders.

Authors' Contributions

Fady Daniel, Hazem I. Assi, and Walid Karaoui equally contributed to this work.

References

[1] C. Freeman, J. W. Berg, and S. J. Cutler, "Occurrence and prognosis of extranodal lymphomas," *Cancer*, vol. 29, no. 1, pp. 252–260, 1972.

[2] P. Ghimire, G.-Y. Wu, and L. Zhu, "Primary gastrointestinal lymphoma," *World Journal of Gastroenterology*, vol. 17, no. 6, pp. 697–707, 2011.

[3] M. Fraga, E. Lloret, L. Sanchez-Verde et al., "Mucosal mantle cell (centrocytic) lymphomas," *Histopathology*, vol. 26, no. 5, pp. 413–422, 1995.

[4] V. X. Nguyen, B. D. Nguyen, G. De Petris, and C. C. Nguyen, "Gastrointestinal: gastrointestinal involvement of mantle cell lymphoma," *Journal of Gastroenterology and Hepatology*, vol. 27, no. 3, pp. 617–617, 2012.

[5] J. E. Romaguera, L. J. Medeiros, F. B. Hagemeister et al., "Frequency of gastrointestinal involvement and its clinical significance in mantle cell lymphoma," *Cancer*, vol. 97, no. 3, pp. 586–591, 2003.

[6] A. Salar, N. Juanpere, B. Bellosillo et al., "Gastrointestinal involvement in mantle cell lymphoma: a prospective clinic, endoscopic, and pathologic study," *The American Journal of Surgical Pathology*, vol. 30, no. 10, pp. 1274–1280, 2006.

[7] M. Esmadi, D. S. Ahmad, D. J. Duff, and H. T. Hammad, "Mantle cell lymphoma of the colon," *Endoscopy*, vol. 46, no. 1, pp. E126–E127, 2014.

[8] A. G. Neto, G. Oroszi, P. Protiva, M. Rose, N. Shafi, and R. Torres, "Colonic in situ mantle cell lymphoma," *Annals of Diagnostic Pathology*, vol. 16, no. 6, pp. 508–514, 2012.

[9] P. M. Banks, J. Chan, M. L. Cleary et al., "Mantle cell lymphoma: a proposal for unification of morphologic, immunologic, and molecular data," *The American Journal of Surgical Pathology*, vol. 16, no. 7, pp. 637–640, 1992.

[10] S. Gurbuxani and J. Anastasi, "What to do when you suspect gastrointestinal lymphoma: a pathologist's perspective," *Clinical Gastroenterology and Hepatology*, vol. 5, no. 4, pp. 417–421, 2007.

[11] H.-H. Chung, Y. H. Kim, J. H. Kim et al., "Imaging findings of mantle cell lymphoma involving gastrointestinal tract," *Yonsei Medical Journal*, vol. 44, no. 1, pp. 49–57, 2003.

[12] L. Dasappa, M. C. Suresh Babu, N. T. Sirsath et al., "Primary gastrointestinal mantle cell lymphoma: A Retrospective Study," *Journal of Gastrointestinal Cancer*, vol. 45, no. 4, pp. 481–486, 2014.

[13] R. Delarue, C. Haioun, V. Ribrag et al., "CHOP and DHAP plus rituximab followed by autologous stem cell transplantation in mantle cell lymphoma: a phase 2 study from the Groupe d'Etude des Lymphomes de l'Adulte," *Blood*, vol. 121, no. 1, pp. 48–53, 2013.

30

Breast Cancer Metastasis to the Stomach That Was Diagnosed after Endoscopic Submucosal Dissection

Masahide Kita,[1] Masashi Furukawa,[2] Masaya Iwamuro,[1] Keisuke Hori,[1] Yoshiro Kawahara,[3] Naruto Taira,[2] Tomohiro Nogami,[2] Tadahiko Shien,[2] Takehiro Tanaka,[4] Hiroyoshi Doihara,[2] and Hiroyuki Okada[1]

[1] *Department of Gastroenterology and Hepatology, Okayama University Graduate School of Medicine, Dentistry, and Pharmaceutical Sciences, Okayama, Japan*
[2] *Department of Breast and Endocrine Surgery, Okayama University Hospital, Okayama, Japan*
[3] *Department of Endoscopy, Okayama University Hospital, Okayama, Japan*
[4] *Department of Pathology, Okayama University Hospital, Okayama, Japan*

Correspondence should be addressed to Masaya Iwamuro; iwamuromasaya@yahoo.co.jp

Academic Editor: Gregory Kouraklis

A 52-year-old woman presented with stage IIB primary breast cancer (cT2N1M0), which was treated using neoadjuvant chemotherapy (epirubicin, cyclophosphamide, and paclitaxel). However, the tumor persisted in patchy areas; therefore, we performed modified radical mastectomy and axillary lymph node dissection. Routine endoscopy at 8 months revealed a depressed lesion on the gastric angle's greater curvature, and histology revealed signet ring cell proliferation. We performed endoscopic submucosal dissection for gastric cancer, although immunohistochemistry revealed that the tumor was positive for estrogen receptor, mammaglobin, and gross cystic disease fluid protein-15 (E-cadherin-negative). Therefore, we revised the diagnosis to gastric metastasis from the breast cancer.

1. Introduction

Breast cancer can metastasize to local or distant locations, and the common locations for extramammary metastasis are the bones, lungs, liver, soft tissues, and adrenal glands [1, 2]. However, breast cancer metastasis to the gastrointestinal tract is uncommon, and the diagnosis of gastrointestinal metastasis or carcinomatosis can be complicated by its infrequency and its morphological resemblance to primary gastrointestinal neoplasms [1, 3].

Herein we report a patient with breast cancer who underwent radical mastectomy and developed a gastric lesion 8 months later. The gastric lesion was initially diagnosed as primary gastric cancer, based on the endoscopic features and histopathological findings. However, histological reassessment of an endoscopically resected specimen ultimately allowed us to reach the correct diagnosis of gastric metastasis from the primary breast cancer. This case highlights the importance of considering gastric metastasis of breast cancer as a differential diagnosis in patients who present with a gastric lesion and a history of breast cancer.

2. Case Presentation

A 52-year-old woman was diagnosed with stage IIB primary breast cancer in the left breast (cT2N1M0). On immunohistochemical examination, the tumor was positive for estrogen receptor (ER) but was borderline (2+) for human epidermal growth factor receptor 2 (HER2) expression. Fluorescence *in situ* hybridization revealed that the tumor cells were negative for *HER2* amplification. The patient was treated via neoadjuvant chemotherapy with epirubicin and cyclophosphamide, followed by paclitaxel. After the chemotherapy, computed tomography and magnetic resonance imaging revealed that the tumor was still present in patchy areas. Therefore, we performed modified radical mastectomy and axillary lymph

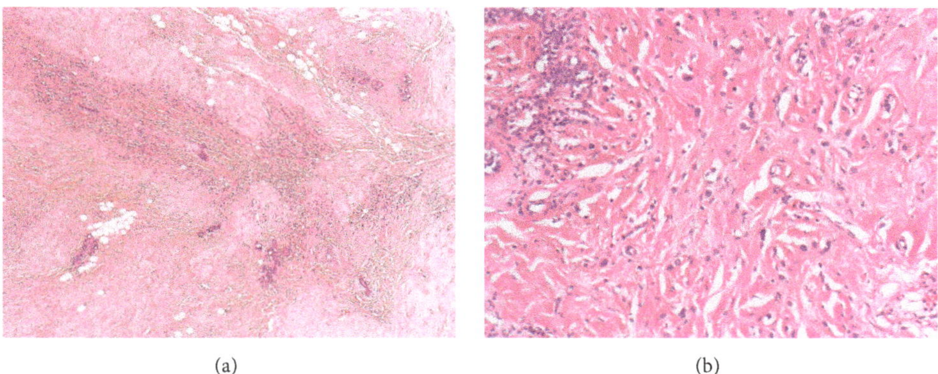

(a) (b)

FIGURE 1: Histological analysis of the left breast. The initial diagnosis was scirrhous carcinoma, because the tumor cells were associated with a dense connective tissue in the stroma. The diagnosis was later revised to invasive lobular carcinoma.

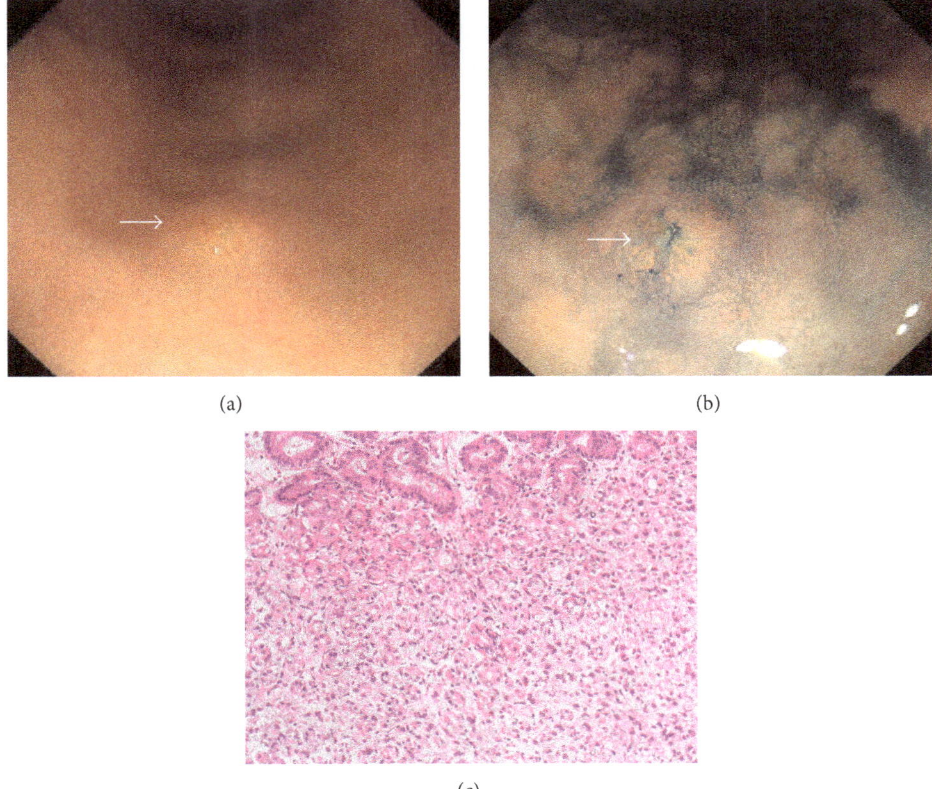

(a) (b)

(c)

FIGURE 2: Esophagogastroduodenoscopy reveals a 0-IIc lesion with a size of 4 mm on the greater curvature of the gastric angle.

node dissection for the left breast cancer. Histological analysis revealed that most of the mammary tissue was hyalinized, due to the effect of the neoadjuvant chemotherapy, and only a few viable carcinoma cells were present. The postsurgical histological diagnosis was scirrhous carcinoma of the left breast that had metastasized to seven lymph nodes in the axillary region (Figure 1). The cancer cells were positive for ER, partially positive for progesterone receptor (PgR), and negative for HER2 expression (1+). Therefore, we started tamoxifen therapy after the surgery, with radiation (50 Gy) of the entire affected area.

At 8 months after the surgery, the patient underwent esophagogastroduodenoscopy for a general health check-up. The endoscopic examination revealed a slightly depressed lesion with a size of 4 mm on the greater curvature of the gastric angle (Figures 2(a) and 2(b)). Histological evaluation of a biopsy specimen revealed proliferation of signet ring cells in the proper mucosal layer of the stomach (Figure 2(c)). Destruction of the fundic glands by the cancer cells was also observed, although atypical cells were absent from the epithelium. Therefore, based on a diagnosis of primary gastric cancer, endoscopic submucosal dissection was performed.

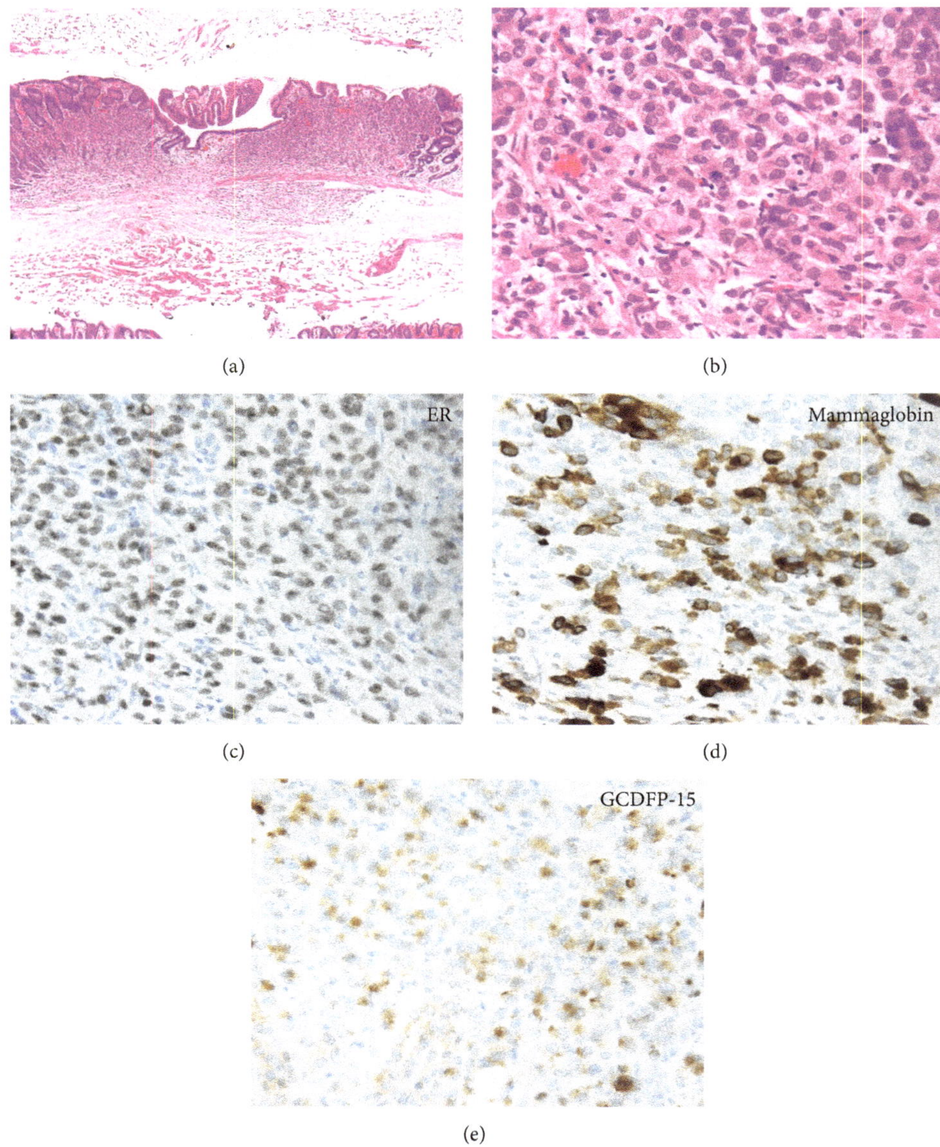

(a) (b) (c) (d) (e)

FIGURE 3: Histopathology of the tumor, which was localized within the mucosal layer to the submucosal layer.

Histopathological examination of the resected specimen revealed that the tumor cells were confined to the mucosal and submucosal layers (Figures 3(a) and 3(b)). Immunostaining revealed that the tumor cells were positive for ER (Figure 3(c)), mammaglobin (Figure 3(d)), and gross cystic disease fluid protein-15 (GCDFP-15) (Figure 3(e)) and were negative for E-cadherin. Therefore, the diagnosis was revised to gastric metastasis from the primary breast cancer. The type of the primary breast cancer was also revised to invasive lobular carcinoma (rather than scirrhous carcinoma), based on the morphological and immunophenotypic characteristics of the gastric cancer cells. Although the primary breast cancer was initially misdiagnosed as scirrhous carcinoma because the tumor cells were associated with a dense connective tissue in the stroma, replacement of tumor cells with connective tissue was likely caused by the neoadjuvant chemotherapy.

The endoscopic submucosal dissection appeared to have completed removing the metastatic tumor, and esophagogastroduodenoscopy, computed tomography, and bone scintigraphy were used to confirm that there were no other metastases throughout the patient's body. The patient was subsequently treated with anastrozole, although we detected multiple metastatic tumors at 40 months after the endoscopic treatment. These tumors were located in the gastric body (Figure 4, arrows), and local recurrence was documented in the endoscopically treated area.

3. Discussion

It is uncommon for the gastrointestinal tract to be the first site for breast cancer metastasis, as McLemore et al. found that only 41 of 12,001 patients with breast cancer (0.3%) exhibited

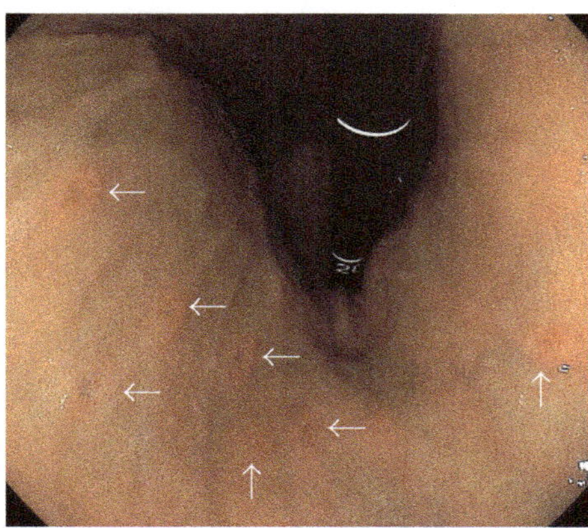

FIGURE 4: Multiple recurrence was documented at 40 months after the endoscopic treatment.

metastasis in the gastrointestinal tract [1]. Diffuse infiltration into the stomach wall is a representative form of gastric metastasis from breast cancers, which is referred to as the linitis plastica type [4–6]. This type of metastasis is generally visualized via radiography as a rigid and thickened gastric wall, and the macroscopic features can include enlarged mucosal folds, erosions, and/or polypoid lesions [5, 7, 8]. However, metastasis from a breast tumor can also appear as a localized lesion in the stomach, which can mimic early-stage gastric cancers, and present as flat elevated, erosive, ulcerative, or polypoid lesions [3, 7–9].

Invasive ductal carcinoma is the most common type among all patients with breast cancer. However, invasive ductal carcinoma is less frequent among metastatic tumors in the gastrointestinal tract, and invasive lobular carcinoma is the predominant type. Taal et al. have reported 51 patients with gastric metastases from breast carcinoma, which included lobular breast carcinoma (n = 36; 70.6%), ductal carcinoma (n = 10; 19.6%), and other types (n = 5; 9.8%) [10]. McLemore et al. have also reported that 73 patients with 81 breast cancers experienced gastrointestinal metastasis [1] and that 44 of the breast cancers (54.3%) were invasive lobular carcinoma. Interestingly, metastatic tumors from invasive lobular breast cancer occasionally exhibit signet ring cells in the pathological findings, which we also observed in the present case. This issue may mislead clinicians and pathologists and potentially result in a misdiagnosis of primary gastric cancer [11].

To reach an accurate diagnosis, immunostaining is recommended to differentiate between primary gastric cancer and breast cancer metastasis to the stomach [3, 5]. Immunostaining for ER and PgR has been reported to be useful for diagnosing metastatic tumors from breast cancer, although 32% and 12% of primary gastric cancer cases are positive for ER and PgR, respectively. Moreover, metastases from breast carcinoma may exhibit negative ER and PgR staining, even if the primary breast cancer is positive for ER and PgR [5, 12]. Therefore, immunostaining for ER and PgR may not be able to definitively differentiate between breast cancer metastases and primary gastric cancers. Immunostaining for mammaglobin and GCDFP-15 may be more practical for identifying breast cancers, because these markers are sensitive and specific for cells that originate from the mammary glands. Therefore, staining for ER, PgR, mammaglobin, and GCDFP-15 may provide more definitive information that can be used to reach the correct diagnosis.

In the present case, the gastric tumor was initially diagnosed as a primary gastric cancer, based on its macroscopic and histopathological features, which included a signet cell-like appearance. Unfortunately, the final diagnosis of a metastatic tumor from breast cancer was only made after pathological evaluation of an endoscopically resected specimen. Thus, cautious evaluation of the gastric epithelium in the biopsied specimen might have provided a diagnostic clue that could have indicated more exhaustive immunostaining for breast cancer markers. Therefore, the possibility of gastric metastasis from breast cancer should be considered if a patient presents with a gastric lesion and a history of breast cancer. Moreover, it is vital to distinguish between breast cancer metastasis to the stomach and primary gastric cancer, because treatment for the metastatic tumor usually involves systemic therapy, rather than a local treatment (e.g., surgical resection) for gastric lesions.

In summary, we experienced a case of invasive lobular breast carcinoma with a metastatic gastric tumor. However, the endoscopic and histopathological features of the metastatic gastric lesion were very similar to those of primary gastric cancer. Therefore, despite the low prevalence of gastric metastasis, physicians should consider the possibility of gastrointestinal metastasis when gastrointestinal tumors are identified in patients with a history of breast cancer.

References

[1] E. C. McLemore, B. A. Pockaj, C. Reynolds et al., "Breast cancer: presentation and intervention in women with gastrointestinal metastasis and carcinomatosis," *Annals of Surgical Oncology*, vol. 12, no. 11, pp. 886–894, 2005.

[2] N. Cifuentes and J. W. Pickren, "Metastases from carcinoma of mammary gland: an autopsy study," *Journal of Surgical Oncology*, vol. 11, no. 3, pp. 193–205, 1979.

[3] W. K. Eo, "Breast cancer metastasis to the stomach resembling early gastric cancer," *Cancer Research and Treatment*, vol. 40, no. 4, pp. 207–210, 2008.

[4] O. Saphir and M. L. Parker, "Metastasis of primary carcinoma of the breast," *Archives of Surgery*, vol. 42, no. 6, p. 1003, 1941.

[5] K. Koike, K. Kitahara, M. Higaki, M. Urata, F. Yamazaki, and H. Noshiro, "Clinicopathological features of gastric metastasis from breast cancer in three cases," *Breast Cancer*, vol. 21, no. 5, pp. 629–634, 2014.

[6] W. J. Cormier, T. A. Gaffey, J. M. Welch, J. S. Welch, and J. H. Edmonson, "Linitis plastica caused by metastatic lobular carcinoma of the breast," *Mayo Clinic Proceedings*, vol. 55, no. 12, pp. 747–753, 1980.

[7] T. Reiman and C. A. Butts, "Upper gastrointestinal bleeding as a metastatic manifestation of breast cancer: a case report and

review of the literature," *Canadian Journal of Gastroenterology*, vol. 15, no. 1, pp. 67–71, 2001.

[8] F. L. Dumoulin and R. Sen Gupta, "Breast cancer metastasis to the stomach resembling small benign gastric polyps," *Gastrointestinal Endoscopy*, vol. 69, no. 1, pp. 174–175, 2009.

[9] G. E. Jones, D. C. Strauss, M. J. Forshaw, H. Deere, U. Mahedeva, and R. C. Mason, "Breast cancer metastasis to the stomach may mimic primary gastric cancer: report of two cases and review of literature," *World Journal of Surgical Oncology*, vol. 5, article 75, 2007.

[10] B. G. Taal, H. Peterse, and H. Boot, "Clinical presentation, endoscopic features, and treatment of gastric metastases from breast carcinoma," *Cancer*, vol. 89, no. 11, pp. 2214–2221, 2000.

[11] T. Kudo, T. Matsumoto, S. Nakamura et al., "Solitary minute metastasis from breast cancer mimicking primary intramucosal gastric signet-cell cancer," *Gastrointestinal Endoscopy*, vol. 62, no. 1, pp. 139–140, 2005.

[12] R. E. Schwarz, D. S. Klimstra, and A. D. M. Turnbull, "Metastatic breast cancer masquerading as gastrointestinal primary," *American Journal of Gastroenterology*, vol. 93, no. 1, pp. 111–114, 1998.

31

An Atypical Presentation of Sporadic Jejunal Burkitt's Lymphoma

Pratik Naik,[1] James Wang,[2] Michael J. Brazeau,[1] and Domingo Rosario[3]

[1] *Department of Internal Medicine, William Beaumont Army Medical Center (WBAMC), 5005 North Piedras Street, El Paso, TX 79920, USA*
[2] *Division of Gastroenterology, Department of Internal Medicine, William Beaumont Army Medical Center (WBAMC), 5005 North Piedras Street, El Paso, TX 79920, USA*
[3] *Department of Pathology, William Beaumont Army Medical Center (WBAMC), 5005 North Piedras Street, El Paso, TX 79920, USA*

Correspondence should be addressed to Pratik Naik; pratik_naik@ymail.com

Academic Editor: R. J. L. F. Loffeld

Burkitt's lymphoma is a very aggressive type of B-cell NHL with replication approaching 100%. Primary gastrointestinal lymphoma is rare. In our case, a 24-year-old male initially presented with symptomatic anemia. He was initially evaluated with colonoscopy and EGD, both of which were unremarkable. A capsule endoscopy was then performed to further evaluate his significant anemia which revealed friable inflamed ulcerated mass in the jejunum. A push enteroscopy was then performed to obtain tissue from the jejunal mass. Biopsy results and immunohistochemical stains were consistent with Burkitt's lymphoma. PET/CT scan revealed only jejunal involvement. Treatment consisted of bowel resection prior to chemotherapy due to concern for perforation with chemotherapy. Patient achieved complete remission after the treatment.

1. Introduction

Primary gastrointestinal (GI) non-Hodgkin's lymphoma (NHL) is rare, and it is the most common extranodal lymphoma site. NHL most occurs in the stomach followed by ileum and ileocecum [1]. Diffuse B-cell Lymphoma is the most common type of GI lymphoma occurring in all of GI tract [1]. Only 2% of sporadic GI malignancies occur in the small intestine [2]. Primary sporadic jejunal Burkitt's lymphoma (BL) is extremely rare. There are no specific symptoms of GI NHL and diagnosis remains difficult. Initial presentation with obstruction and perforation has been documented in the past in all types of NHL [3]. Lymphomas can present as multiple ulcerated lesions mimicking inflammatory bowel disease and most specifically Crohn's disease if the small bowel is primarily involved [4]. Our case is unique in that the initial presentation was misleading due to iron deficiency anemia with questionable ulcerated mass in jejunum, which was suggestive of Crohn's disease.

2. Case Report

A 24-year-old US Army soldier was found to be anemic on routine blood work while he was in Kuwait. He was referred to gastroenterology for further evaluation. A colonoscopy and an esophagogastroduodenoscopy (EGD) performed in Kuwait were unremarkable. One month later, he started experiencing weakness, dyspnea, reduced exercise tolerance, dizziness, and lightheadedness. At that time, he was not experiencing any diarrhea, abdominal pain, night sweats, melena, or hematochezia. After further evaluation, the patient was found to be severely anemic with hemoglobin of 5.6 g/dL, MCV of 77 fL, iron saturation < 2%, and ferritin of 2.0 ng/mL. He received 4 units of PRBCs in Kuwait. The patient was immediately medically evacuated to Fort Bliss, TX, for further evaluation and treatment of his anemia. A colonoscopy and EGD were repeated with normal findings. Due to concern for obscure GI bleed, a capsule endoscopy was performed, which showed a 10 cm long questionable

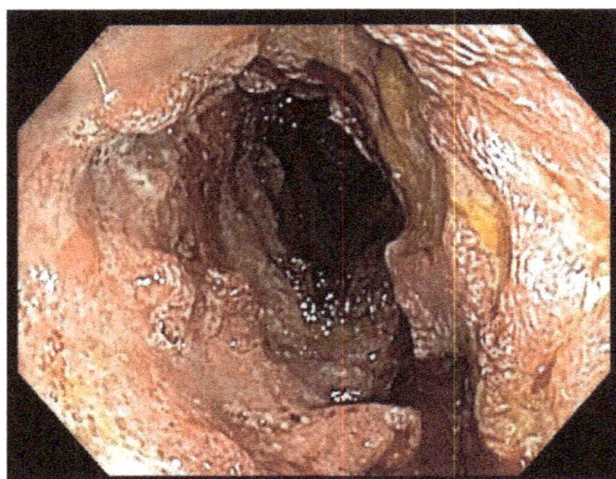

Figure 1: A push enteroscopy shows a 10 cm long, friable, ulcerated mass in the 3rd part of the jejunum.

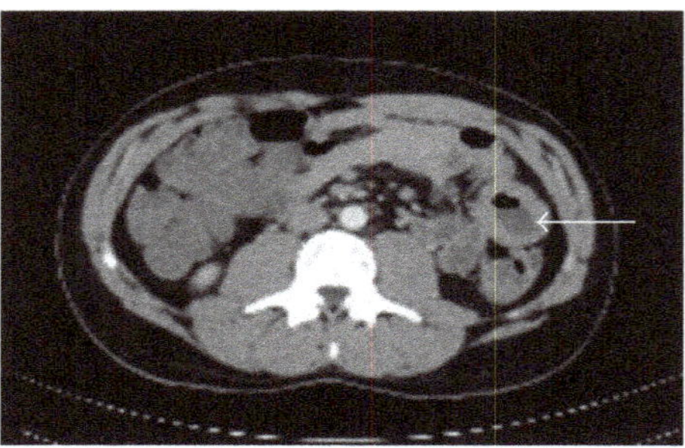

Figure 2: A computed tomography (CT) of abdomen shows lumen thickening with narrowing in distal jejunum (arrow).

jejunal lesion. A push enteroscopy was performed and a biopsy was taken from a friable, ulcerated mass in the 3rd part of the jejunum (Figure 1). A computed tomography (CT) of abdomen was also obtained which showed lumen thickening with narrowing in distal jejunal area (Figure 2). At this point, his presentation was suggestive of Crohn's disease. The initial pathology report was notable for a malignant process and was positive for CD20 (Figure 3(b)) and CD 79a immunohistochemical stains. Further immunostaining revealed a Ki-67 proliferative fraction approaching 100%, reflecting a very rapidly growing neoplasm (Figure 3(d)). Other staining types were notable for CD10 and BCL6 positivity and negative for MUM1, BCL2, CD44, CD5, Cyclin D1, c-Myc (Figure 3(c)), and TdT. He was also screened for anti-HIV antibody and anti-EBV IgM and IgG, which were seronegative. His other evaluations consisted of a positron emission tomography (PET) scan with avid uptake localized to the jejunum only (Figure 4) and a bone marrow biopsy without evidence of lymphoma involvement. He was given a diagnosis of BL, Stage 1EB (WHO classification). Treatment consisted of prophylactic bowel resection followed by adjuvant chemotherapy (CODOX-M/IVAC). Patient achieved complete remission after the treatment.

3. Conclusion/Discussion

Burkitt's lymphoma is a very aggressive type of B-cell NHL with replication approaching 100%. BL has three clinical forms: endemic, sporadic, and immunodeficiency-associated. The sporadic variant is seen in the US and Western Europe. Sporadic type BL comprises 30% of pediatric lymphomas and less than 1% of adult non-Hodgkin lymphomas in the US [5]. The GI tract is the predominant site of extranodal lymphoma involvement. Primary gastrointestinal lymphoma is rare usually secondary to the widespread nodal diseases constituting only about 1%–4% of all gastrointestinal malignancies [1]. These lymphomas have been described in ileum, stomach, cecum and/or mesentery, kidney, testis, ovary, breast, bone marrow, and CNS. BL is mostly seen in pediatric population, and it is associated with Epstein-Barr virus (EBV) and HIV/AIDS patients [1].

The presentation and symptoms of lymphomas of the small intestine are nonspecific and can be misleading. BL can present as GI bleeding, bowel obstruction, intussusceptions, colicky abdominal pain, nausea, vomiting, and weight loss. GI lymphomas can mimic acute appendicitis and Crohn's disease [5]. Primary BL in the jejunum has been reported in literature with initial presentation of obstruction and perforation [3]. Primary intestine lymphomas with multiple ulcers can have similar presentation to Crohn's disease. Classically Crohn's disease involves the terminal ileum and ileocecal valve with multiple small punctiform, rounded nodules, or superficial erosions known as aphthoid lesions. Over a period of time, the erosions become confluent and give rise to larger longitudinal ulcers, known as serpiginous ulcers [6]. Bowel wall thickening with luminal narrowing can be seen on CT abdomen in Crohn's disease [7], as was also seen in our patient. There is an increased risk of lymphomas with chronic inflammatory disease such as rheumatoid arthritis, Hashimoto's thyroiditis, and Sjogren's syndromes [8]. Prior large population cohort studies have demonstrated no increased risk of B-cell lymphomas in inflammatory bowel disease and risk of NHL is similar to general population [9, 10].

Tissue biopsies are critical for diagnosis. Criteria for diagnosis BL include immunohistochemical stains CD 20 (+), CD10 (+), BCL-6 (+), and BCL-2 (−) and a proliferative fraction >95% as per WHO classification [11]. c-Myc gene translocation can be present; however, 10–15% BL can be c-Myc negative [12]. In our case, the patient had all the criteria for BL as per WHO classification but was negative for c-Myc loci, which makes our case more unique. Double hit lymphomas or B-cell lymphomas, unclassifiable with intermediate features between diffuse large B-cell lymphoma (DLBCL) and BL, usually will show variably strong positivity for BCL-2 and larger more pleomorphic nuclei instead of medium-sized nuclei. Both of these features (i.e., pleomorphic nuclei and BCL2 positivity) were absent in the current case, making the diagnosis of BL more likely. Also, DLBCL usually shows a Ki-67 proliferation rate of about 65–70% (the current case is essentially 100%). In addition, CD44 is most likely to be expressed in CD10+ positive DLBCL and it was negative in the current case, further supporting the diagnosis of BL [13].

Radiological findings of small intestinal lymphoma are nonspecific and biopsy is required for definitive diagnosis. BL usually presents as a bulky mass in the right lower

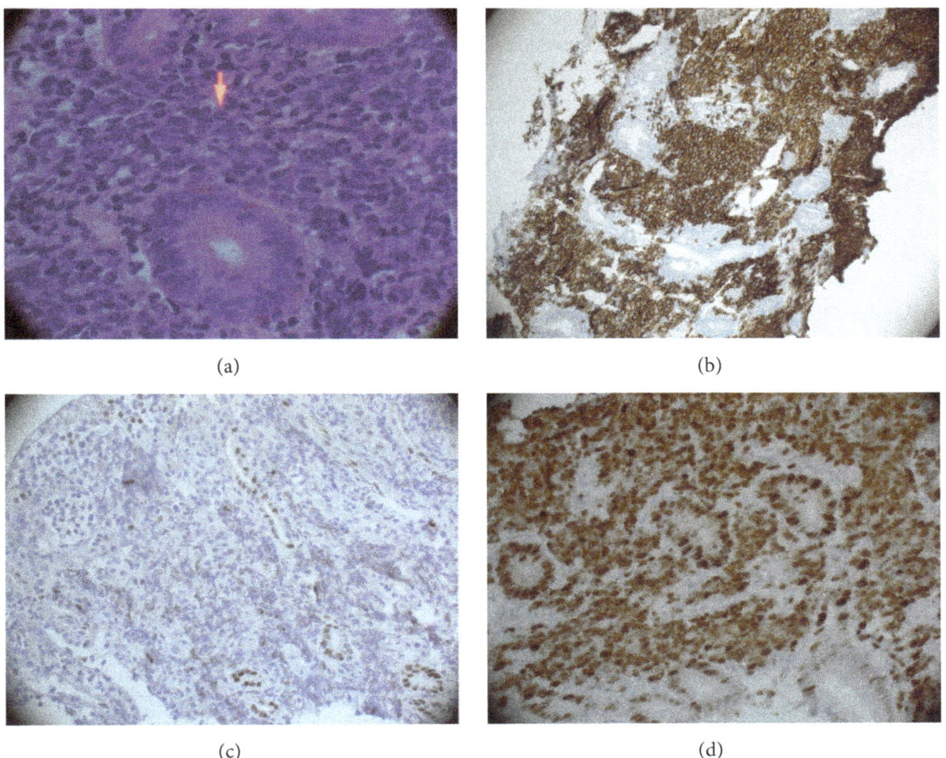

FIGURE 3: (a) High power (400x), H&E (hematoxylin and eosin), medium to large lymphoid cells invading the lamina propria featuring multiple nucleoli (arrow) consistent with high grade lymphoma (Burkitt's lymphoma shows multiple nucleoli). (b) CD20 highlights lamina propria atypical lymphoid infiltrate, consistent with high grade B-cell lymphoma. (c) Negative staining for MYC immunohistochemical stain. (d) 100% nuclear positivity for Ki-67, consistent with high proliferation rate.

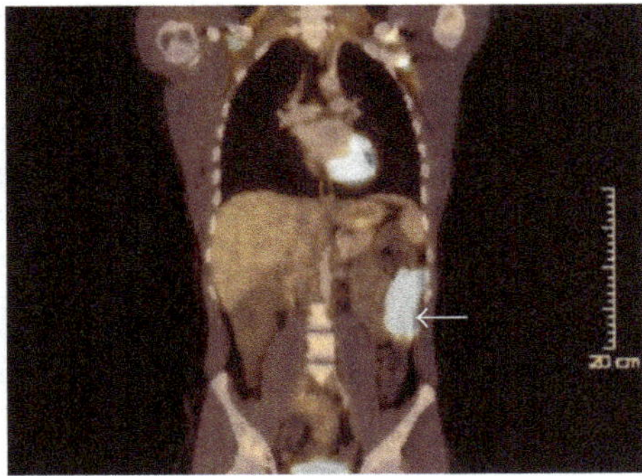

FIGURE 4: PET scan shows FDG avid small bowel segment with circumferential thickening (arrow) with no evidence of distant disease.

quadrant on a CT scan [1]. Evaluation and diagnosis of small bowel lymphomas have been more effective with the use of capsule endoscopy and double-balloon technique of push-and-pull enteroscopy. Initial evaluation such as biopsies and other interventions can be performed using a double-balloon enteroscopy which can potentially limit need for surgeries [1]. In our case, we were able to identify the jejunal lesion on a capsule endoscopy. Staging is usually done by a PET scan and/or a CT scan of chest, abdomen, and pelvis. Bone marrow or CNS involvement portends poor prognosis.

BL is a rapidly growing tumor and prophylactic surgery can be considered if a high risk of perforation or other complications are suspected. The role of elective surgery in the management of intestinal lymphoma is not well defined. In a retrospective study, 9% (92 of 1062) of the patients with primary GI lymphomas developed perforation, of which 55% occurred after chemotherapy. The risk of perforation was higher with aggressive B-cell lymphomas such as DLBCL and BL compared to indolent B-cell lymphomas. DLBCL was the most common lymphoma (59%) and small intestine was the most common site (59%) associated with perforation [14]. A recent systemic review noted overall survival benefit with surgery and no reported increased postoperative morbidity or mortality [15]. Other prior studies also reported better outcomes and event-free survival with surgical resection followed by chemotherapy [16, 17]. Prospective studies are needed to further define benefits of resection before chemotherapy but it is a reasonable approach for localized intestinal lymphomas. However, there have been no reports of cure with resection alone and aggressive early chemotherapy is required even after a surgical resection.

Short term multiregimen chemotherapy such as CALGB 10002, CODOX-M/IVAC, EPOCH, and HyperCVAD with rituximab is highly effective with a complete remission rate up to 90% [2, 18]. In a small study involving 19 HIV-free patients, the use of a less toxic dose adjusted EPOCH (etoposide, prednisone, vincristine, cyclophosphamide, and adriamycin) plus rituximab (DA-REPOCH) led to an event-free survival of 96% and an overall survival of 100% [19].

Disclosure

The views expressed in this presentation are those of the authors and do not reflect the official policy of the Department of the Army, Department of Defense, or US Government. This case has been previously presented as a podium presentation at American College of Physicians/Far Northwest Region Oral Clinical Vignette Competition, Texas Tech University Health Sciences Center, Paul L. Foster School of Medicine, El Paso.

Acknowledgments

The authors would like to thank Dr. Warren Alexander, M.D. (Division of Hematology & Oncology, WBAMC), for helping and coordinating care for the patient. Also, they would like to thank Larissa A. Schmersal, Ph.D. (Senior Research Reviewer/IRB Administrator Department of Clinical Investigation, WBAMC), for providing writing assistance.

References

[1] P. Ghimire, G.-Y. Wu, and L. Zhu, "Primary gastrointestinal lymphoma," *World Journal of Gastroenterology*, vol. 17, no. 6, pp. 697–707, 2011.

[2] A. Samaiya, S. V. S. Deo, S. Thulkar et al., "An unusual presentation of a malignant jejunal tumor and a different management strategy," *World Journal of Surgical Oncology*, vol. 3, p. 3, 2005.

[3] S. F. Shah, M. T. Abdullah, S. H. Waqar, I. A. Khan, Z. I. Malik, and M. A Zahid, "Burkitt's lymphoma of the jejunum: a rare gastrointestinal tumor," *Annals of Pakistan Institute of Medical Sciences*, vol. 9, no. 3, pp. 52–54, 2013.

[4] S.-T. Pan, C.-H. Wei, M.-C. Yang, and S.-S. Chuang, "Primary jejunal diffuse large b-cell lymphoma with multiple skip ulcers and perforation mimicking Crohn's disease," *The Open Pathology Journal*, vol. 6, no. 1, pp. 17–20, 2012.

[5] G. Erkan, M. Çoban, A. Çalıskan et al., "A Burkitt's lymphoma case mimicking Crohn's disease: a case report," *Case Reports in Medicine*, vol. 2011, Article ID 685273, 4 pages, 2011.

[6] K. Geboes, "Histopathology of crohn's disease and ulcerative colitis," in *Inflammatory Bowel Diseases*, J. Satsangi and L. R. Sutherland, Eds., pp. 255–276, Churchill-Livingstone, New York, NY, USA, 4th edition, 2003.

[7] K. M. Horton, F. M. Corl, and E. K. Fishman, "CT evaluation of the colon: inflammatory disease," *Radiographics*, vol. 20, no. 2, pp. 399–418, 2000.

[8] K. E. Smedby, E. Baecklund, and J. Askling, "Malignant lymphomas in autoimmunity and inflammation: a review of risks, risk factors, and lymphoma characteristics," *Cancer Epidemiology Biomarkers and Prevention*, vol. 15, no. 11, pp. 2069–2077, 2006.

[9] J. D. Lewis, W. B. Bilker, C. Brensinger, J. J. Deren, D. J. Vaughn, and B. L. Strom, "Inflammatory bowel disease is not associated with an increased risk of lymphoma," *Gastroenterology*, vol. 121, no. 5, pp. 1080–1087, 2001.

[10] C. A. Siegel, "Risk of lymphoma in inflammatory bowel disease," *Gastroenterology and Hepatology*, vol. 5, no. 11, pp. 784–790, 2009.

[11] L. M. Morton, S. S. Wang, S. S. Devesa, P. Hartge, D. D. Weisenburger, and M. S. Linet, "Lymphoma incidence patterns by WHO subtype in the United States, 1992–2001," *Blood*, vol. 107, no. 1, pp. 265–276, 2006.

[12] A. Onnis, G. de Falco, G. Antonicelli et al., "Alteration of microRNAs regulated by c-Myc in Burkitt Lymphoma," *PLoS ONE*, vol. 5, no. 9, article e12960, 2010.

[13] R. R. Miles, M. Raphael, K. McCarthy et al., "Pediatric diffuse large B-cell lymphoma demonstrates a high proliferation index, frequent c-Myc protein expression, and a high incidence of germinal center subtype: report of the French-American-British (FAB) International Study Group," *Pediatric Blood & Cancer*, vol. 51, no. 3, pp. 369–374, 2008.

[14] R. Vaidya, T. M. Habermann, J. H. Donohue et al., "Bowel perforation in intestinal lymphoma: incidence and clinical features," *Annals of Oncology*, vol. 24, no. 9, pp. 2439–2443, 2013.

[15] A. L. Lightner, E. Shannon, M. M. Gibbons, and M. M. Russell, "Primary gastrointestinal non-Hodgkin's lymphoma of the small and large intestines: a systematic review," *Journal of Gastrointestinal Surgery*, vol. 20, no. 4, pp. 827–839, 2016.

[16] P. L. Zinzani, M. Magagnoli, G. Pagliani et al., "Primary intestinal lymphoma: clinical and therapeutic features of 32 patients," *Haematologica*, vol. 82, no. 3, pp. 305–308, 1997.

[17] E. M. Ibrahim, A. A. Ezzat, A. N. El-Weshi et al., "Primary intestinal diffuse large B-cell non-Hodgkin's lymphoma: clinical features, management, and prognosis of 66 patients," *Annals of Oncology*, vol. 12, no. 1, pp. 53–58, 2001.

[18] S. R. Nayak, G. B. Rao, S. S. Yerraguntla, and S. Bodepudi, "Jejunal perforation: a rare presentation of burkitt's lymphoma—successful management," *Case Reports in Oncological Medicine*, vol. 2014, Article ID 538359, 4 pages, 2014.

[19] K. Dunleavy, S. Pittaluga, M. Shovlin et al., "Low-intensity therapy in adults with burkitt's lymphoma," *The New England Journal of Medicine*, vol. 369, no. 20, pp. 1915–1925, 2013.

Dental Impaction in the Cecum: Case Report and Review of Gastrointestinal Foreign Body Impactions

Mouhanna Abu Ghanimeh,[1] Omar Abughanimeh,[2] Sakher Albadarin,[3] Osama Kaddourah,[2] and John H. Helzberg[4,5]

[1] *Henry Ford Health System, 2799 W Grand Blvd, Gastroenterology K-7 Room E-744, Detroit, MI 48202, USA*
[2] *University of Missouri-Kansas City, School of Medicine, Internal Medicine-Graduate Medical Education, 2411 Holmes Street, M2-302, Kansas City, MO 64108, USA*
[3] *Saint Luke's Hospital of Kansas City, Division of Gastroenterology, Mid-America Gastro-Intestinal Consultants, 4401 Wornall Rd, Kansas City, MO 64111, USA*
[4] *University of Missouri of Kansas City/School of Medicine, 2411 Holmes Street, Kansas City, MO 64108, USA*
[5] *Saint Luke's Hospital of Kansas City, 4401 Wornall Rd, Kansas City, MO 64111, USA*

Correspondence should be addressed to Mouhanna Abu Ghanimeh; mouhannaka87@yahoo.com

Academic Editor: Özlem Yönem

Approximately 20% of the adult population in the United States wears dentures. Foreign body ingestions, including dentures, are not uncommon. Although the majority of all ingested foreign bodies pass spontaneously through the gastrointestinal tract, impaction may occur, especially with physiologic constrictions, angulations, or stenosis. The esophagus is the most common site of impaction, whereas colonic impaction is extremely uncommon. We present a case of an 84-year-old male who was referred to the gastroenterology clinic for denture impaction, which lasted for two weeks. The patient had already failed to pass the denture following conservative treatment with laxatives, and repeated abdominal imaging showed the dental plate in the cecum. Colonoscopy was performed three weeks after the ingestion of his dentures, and tripod forceps were used to dislodge the end of the dental plate and ultimately remove it. The patient was asymptomatic for the entire period.

1. Introduction

Foreign body ingestion is not uncommon. It is more common in children and males [1–7]. In addition, certain factors increase the risk of foreign body ingestion, including extreme age, edentulism, maxillofacial trauma, psychoneurological deficit, and impaired sensorium [1, 8, 9]. Approximately 80% of all ingested foreign bodies, including dentures, pass spontaneously through the gastrointestinal tract [3, 4]. However, impaction with physiologic constrictions, angulations. or stenosis is possible [10–12]. The esophagus is the most common site of impaction. In contrast, impaction in the small and large bowel is far less common [5, 9, 10]. The clinical presentation of foreign body impaction depends on the site of impaction and the presence of complications. Three management modalities have been described for foreign body ingestion and impaction: observation (wait and watch), endoscopy. and surgery [1]. Perforation, penetration of adjacent organs, bleeding, and obstruction are reported complications that warrant urgent surgical intervention [13–16]. Fortunately, less than 1% of all cases require surgery [17].

2. Case Summary

An 84-year-old male was referred to the gastroenterology clinic due to colonic foreign body impaction. The patient reported that while eating a nectarine two weeks prior to his clinic visit, he believed that he had inadvertently swallowed his partial denture. The patient was asymptomatic.

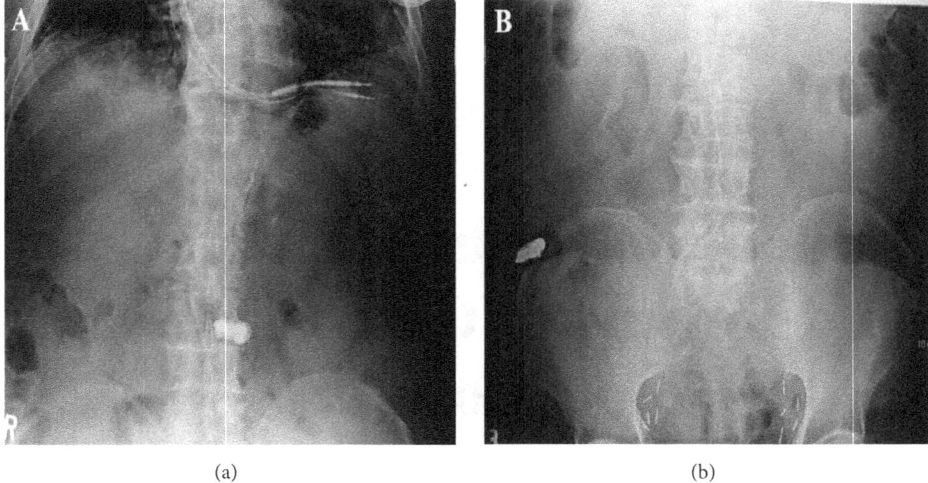

(a) (b)

FIGURE 1: (a) The first abdominal radiograph demonstrating the dental plate in the mid abdomen. (b) The second abdominal radiography demonstrating the dental plate in the right lower quadrant and likely in the cecum.

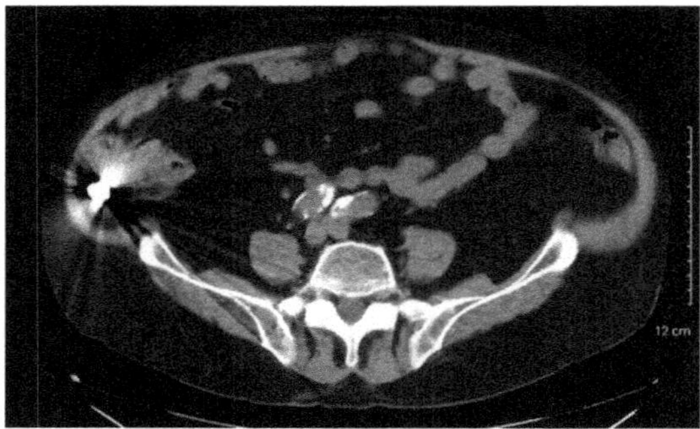

FIGURE 2: A CT abdomen and pelvis without contrast demonstrating the dental bridge persistently in the base of the cecum.

Prior to his referral to the gastroenterology clinic, the patient's primary care physician had managed him conservatively with laxatives and obtained two abdominal radiographs to document the possible passage of the denture. The first radiograph showed the dental plate in the mid abdomen [Figure 1(a)]. The second radiograph revealed that the dental plate was in the right lower quadrant and likely in the cecum [Figure 1(b)].

A CT scan of the abdomen and pelvis was obtained to determine the exact location of the dental plate (cecum or terminal ileum) and showed it at the base of the cecum [Figure 2].

As the patient failed to pass the denture following conservative management with laxatives, the decision was made to attempt endoscopic removal. Colonoscopy was performed three weeks after the ingestion and showed that the dental plate had embedded in the cecal wall by a wire. The appearance was that of a face with smiling teeth. Tripod forceps were used to dislodge the end of the dental plate. It was then removed without difficulty or complication (Figures 3(a)–3(c)).

3. Discussion

Dentures are medical prostheses that are used to improve the mastication, articulation, and even self-esteem of people with poor dental or oral conditions. [1] Approximately 20% of the adult population in the United States wears dentures [1]. Denture ingestion is considered to be a multidisciplinary problem [1]. Gastroenterologists have an important role in its diagnosis and management; however, dentists, surgeons, and otolaryngologists play a crucial role in some cases.

Foreign body ingestion, including dentures, is not uncommon. The type of foreign body as well as the clinical presentation can differ between children and adults [2]. Whereas the peak incidence of foreign body ingestion is between 6 months and 6 years [3], it is less frequent among adults and varies across populations [1]. Although nonbony food bolus is the most common in Western countries [4], in Asia, chicken and fish bones are more frequent [5]. Foreign body ingestion is slightly more common in males than females, with a ratio of 1.5 : 1 [6, 7]. Known risk factors of foreign body ingestion include extreme age [1], edentulism [8], maxillofacial trauma [9], psychoneurological deficit, and

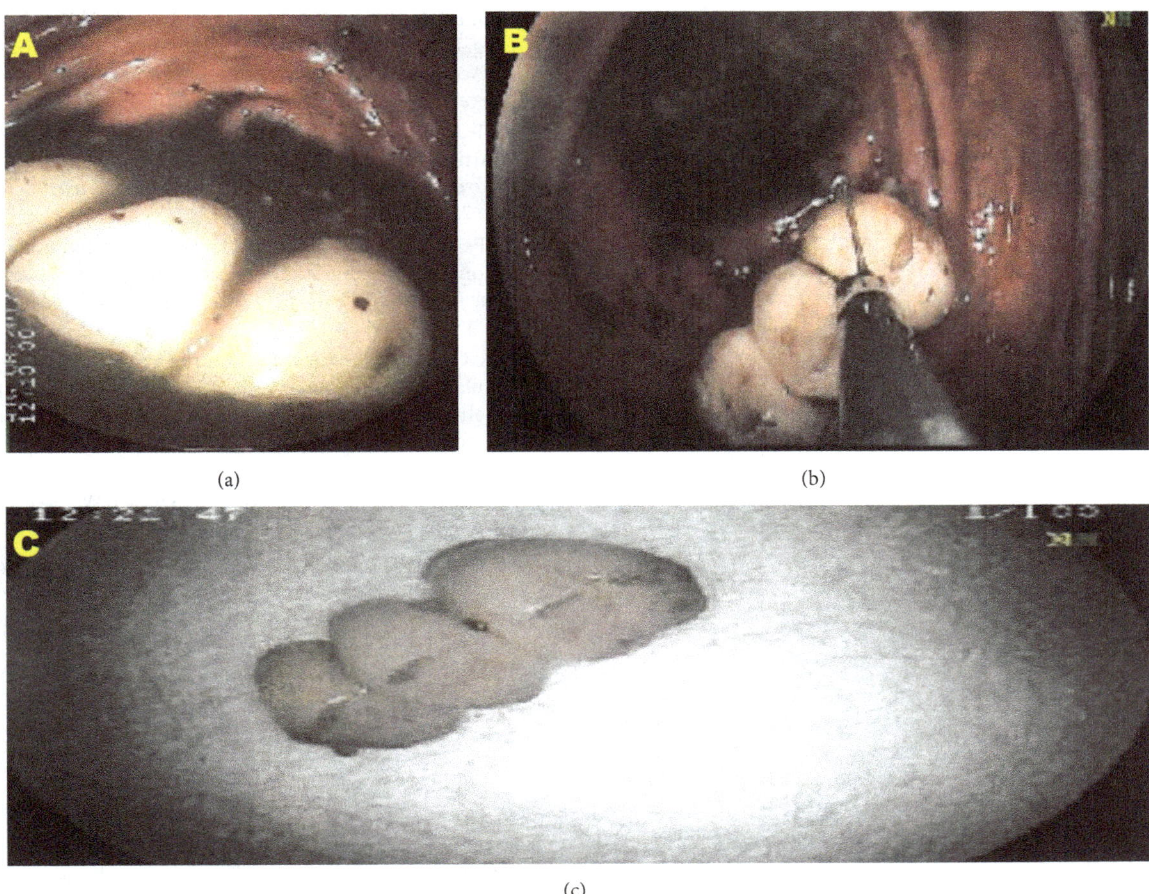

FIGURE 3: (a) Dental plate impacted in the cecum. (b) A colonoscopy forceps was used to grasp the end of the dental plate and to extract it. (c) The dental plate after extraction.

acute disorders of consciousness such as cerebrovascular accidents, alcohol intoxication, drug overdose, or general anesthesia [8].

Approximately 80% of all ingested foreign bodies pass spontaneously through the entire gastrointestinal tract [3, 4]. However, there is still significant morbidity and mortality associated with foreign body impaction [7]. Foreign body impaction usually occurs with physiologic constrictions, angulations, or stenosis of the gastrointestinal tract [11, 12]. The esophagus is the most common site of impaction, accounting for up to 70% of cases [5, 10]. Foreign body impaction in the small intestine is rare, and almost all reported cases occur in the terminal ileum [18, 19]. Finally, impaction in the large bowel is even less common, given its larger diameter compared to other areas of the gastrointestinal tract [9]. Thus, if any foreign body passes through the ileocecal valve, it generally passes through the colon without difficulty, unless there is a pathological stenosis or stricture such as with cancer.

The clinical presentation of foreign body impactions depends on the site of impaction and the presence of complications. Reported symptoms include dysphagia, odynophagia, chest pain, abdominal pain, or nausea/vomiting [20]. Additionally, surgical complications have been reported, including perforation, penetration of adjacent organs, bleeding, and obstruction [13–16].

Three management modalities have been described for foreign body ingestion and impaction: observation (wait and watch), endoscopy, and surgery [1]. Observation is possible when objects are small and do not provoke trauma to the gastrointestinal tract and the location is distal to the ligament of Treitz at the time of presentation [1]. In general, this strategy is more commonly used for uncomplicated lower gastrointestinal tract foreign bodies [1]. Endoscopy is the preferred modality for uncomplicated impaction, especially in the upper gastrointestinal tract [10]. Surgical intervention is warranted in complicated cases, regardless of the site of impaction [1]. Less than 1% of all cases require surgery [17].

Consent

The patient has provided permission to publish these features of his case, and the identity of the patient has been protected.

Disclosure

The case's abstract was accepted for poster presentation in the American College of Gastroenterology (ACG) 2016 Annual Scientific Meeting. The abstract was published in a special supplement of the American Journal of Gastroenterology (AJG).

Authors' Contributions

All authors contributed to the manuscript. Mouhanna Abu Ghanimeh, Omar Abughanimeh, and Osama Kaddourah wrote the manuscript. Sakher Albadarin edited the initial manuscript draft and provided endoscopy images. John H. Helzberg reviewed, edited, and approved the final manuscript.

References

[1] M. Gachabayov, M. Isaev, L. Orujova, E. Isaev, E. Yaskin, and D. Neronov, "Swallowed dentures: two cases and a review," *Annals of Medicine and Surgery*, vol. 4, no. 4, pp. 407–413, 2015.

[2] M. Bekkerman, A. H. Sachdev, J. Andrade, Y. Twersky, and S. Iqbal, "Endoscopic Management of Foreign Bodies in the Gastrointestinal Tract: A Review of the Literature," *Gastroenterology Research and Practice*, vol. 2016, pp. 1–6, 2016.

[3] W. Cheng and P. K. H. Tam, "Foreign-body ingestion in children: experience with 1,265 cases," *Journal of Pediatric Surgery*, vol. 34, no. 10, pp. 1472–1476, 1999.

[4] W. A. Webb, "Management of foreign bodies of the upper gastrointestinal tract: update," *Gastrointestinal Endoscopy*, vol. 41, no. 1, pp. 39–51, 1995.

[5] P. Nandi and G. B. Ong, "Foreign body in the esophagus: review of 2394 cases," *British Journal of Surgery*, vol. 65, no. 1, pp. 5–9, 1978.

[6] V. Tumay, O. S. Guner, M. Meric, O. Isik, and A. Zorluoglu, "Endoscopic Removal of Duodenal Perforating Fishbone - A Case Report," *Chirurgia (Bucharest, Romania : 1990)*, vol. 110, no. 5, pp. 471–473, 2015.

[7] C.-C. Yao, I.-T. Wu, and L.-S. Lu, "Endoscopic management of foreign bodies in the upper gastrointestinal tract of adults," *BioMed Research International*, vol. 2015, Article ID 658602, 6 pages, 2015.

[8] T. Toshima, M. Morita, N. Sadanaga et al., "Surgical removal of a denture with sharp clasps impacted in the cervicothoracic esophagus: report of three cases," *Surgery Today*, vol. 41, no. 9, pp. 1275–1279, 2011.

[9] E. D. Hodges, T. M. Durham, and R. T. Stanley, "Management of aspiration and swallowing incidents: a review of the literature and report of a case," *ASDC J Dent Child*, vol. 59, no. 6, pp. 413–419, 1992.

[10] S. N. Bandyopadhyay, S. Das, S. K. Das, and A. Mandal, "Impacted dentures in the oesophagus," *The Journal of Laryngology & Otology*, vol. 128, no. 5, pp. 468–474, 2014.

[11] G. G. Ginsberg, "Management of ingested foreign objects and food bolus impactions," *Gastrointestinal Endoscopy*, vol. 41, no. 1, pp. 33–38, 1995.

[12] S. Khadda, A. K. Yadav, A. Ali, A. Parmar, H. Beniwal, and A. Nagar, "A rare Case Report of Sigmoid Colon Perforation Due to Accidental Swallowing of Partial Denture," *Indian Journal of Surgery*, vol. 77, no. 2, pp. 152–154, 2015.

[13] R. F. Candia-De La Rosa, R. Candia-García, and M. C. Pérez-Martínez, "Intestinal obstruction by a foreign body in a patient with colon adenocarcinoma. A case report," *Cirugía y Cirujanos*, vol. 78, no. 1, pp. 87–91, 2010.

[14] B. Peison, B. Benisch, and E. Lim, "Perforation of the sigmoid colon following ingestion of a dental plate.," *New Jersey medicine : the journal of the Medical Society of New Jersey*, vol. 92, no. 7, pp. 452-453, 1995.

[15] V. I. Odigie, L. M. Yusufu, P. Abur et al., "Broncho-oesophageal fistula (BOF) secondary to missing partial denture in an alcoholic in a low resource country," *Oman Medical Journal*, vol. 26, no. 1, pp. 50–52, 2011.

[16] G. Jüngling, V. Wiessner, and C. Gebhardt, "Enterocolic fistula due to foreign body perforation. Dtsch Med Wochenschr," *Dtsch Med Wochenschr*, vol. 119, no. 3, pp. 63–66, 1994.

[17] S. O. Ikenberry, T. L. Jue, and M. A. Anderson, "Management of ingested foreign bodies and food impactions," *Gastrointestinal Endoscopy*, vol. 73, no. 6, pp. 1085–1091, 2011.

[18] F. Rashid, J. Simpson, G. Ananthakrishnan, and G. M. Tierney, "Swallowed dental bridge causing ileal perforation: a case report," *Cases Journal*, vol. 1, no. 1, p. 392, 2008.

[19] J. Bunni and F. Youssef, "Swallowed dental bridge perforating the terminal ileum," *Southern Medical Journal*, vol. 103, no. 6, pp. 593-594, 2010.

[20] S. Hachimi-Idrissi, L. Corne, and Y. Vandenplas, "Management of ingested foreign bodies in childhood: our experience and review of the literature," *European Journal of Emergency Medicine*, vol. 5, no. 3, pp. 319–323, 1998.

Splenic Trauma during Colonoscopy: The Role of Intra-Abdominal Adhesions

Chukwunonso Chime, Charbel Ishak, Kishore Kumar, Venkata Kella, and Sridhar Chilimuri

Bronx Care Hospital Health System, Affiliate of Icahn School of Medicine at Mount Sinai, New York, NY, USA

Correspondence should be addressed to Chukwunonso Chime; cchime@bronxleb.org

Academic Editor: Olga I. Giouleme

Splenic rupture following colonoscopy is rare, first reported in 1974, with incidence of 1–21/100,000. It is critical to anticipate splenic trauma during colonoscopy as one of the causes of abdominal pain after colonoscopy especially when located in the left upper quadrant or left shoulder. Postoperative adhesions is a predisposing factor for splenic injury, and management is either operative or nonoperative, based on hemodynamic stability and/or extravasation which can be seen on contrast-enhanced CT scan of the abdomen. We present a case of a splenic rupture after colonoscopy in a patient with splenocolic adhesions, requiring splenectomy as definite treatment.

1. Introduction

Colonoscopy is a reliable and widely used procedure for the diagnosis and management of colorectal disorders, but it is not without its risks, with the commonest being bleeding and perforation, with estimated incidences of 1.8–2.5% and 0.34–2.14%, respectively [1]. Splenic rupture is a very rare complication following colonoscopy, with 103 cases published until the end of 2012 [1]. It has an incidence of 1–21/100,000 with the first case reported in 1974 [2]. These patients are mainly female (71.5%) and have a mean age of 63 years as well as a previous history of abdominal surgery (50.8–65%) [1]. It is essential to identify this complication and to treat it as soon as possible, due to the elevated morbidity and mortality [3, 4]. We present a case of a splenic rupture after screening colonoscopy resulting in splenectomy.

2. Case Report

51-year-old female presented to our emergency room with abdominal pain, one day after a routine screening colonoscopy done in an outside facility. Patient had colonoscopy done in the morning of the previous day and by evening she noticed a sharp left upper quadrant abdominal pain with radiation to the left shoulder, which is aggravated by respiration. Her medical history is remarkable for hypertension, diabetes, and obstructive sleep apnea. She had colonoscopy in 2009 for iron deficiency anemia and hysterectomy done in 2010. In the emergency room, she had a blood pressure of 124/67 mmhg and pulse rate of 75 bpm; respiratory rate was within normal limits. Her laboratory results revealed hemoglobin of 11.9 g/dl, white cell count of 11.1 k/ul ml, platelets of 221 k/ul ml, INR of 1.0, BUN of 14 mg/dl, and creatinine of 0.7 mg/dl. Physical examination revealed no abdominal distension, but tenderness of the left upper and lower quadrants, guarding but no rebound. Chest radiograph did not reveal any pneumothorax or air under diaphragm. Computerized tomography (CT) of the abdomen revealed a 4 × 7 cm perisplenic/subcapsular hematoma with an area of active bleeding along the subcapsular region and possible splenocolic adhesions (see Figures 1(a)–1(d)). She was admitted under the care of the surgical service and managed conservatively for 4 days, during which she received 2 packed red cells for drop in hemoglobin. On day four of admission, she was deemed to have failed conservative management evidenced by continued drop in hemoglobin despite transfusion, tachycardia, and a repeat CT of the abdomen demonstrating increasing size of splenic hematoma with perisplenic, perihepatic, and pelvic hemorrhagic ascites. Patient was then

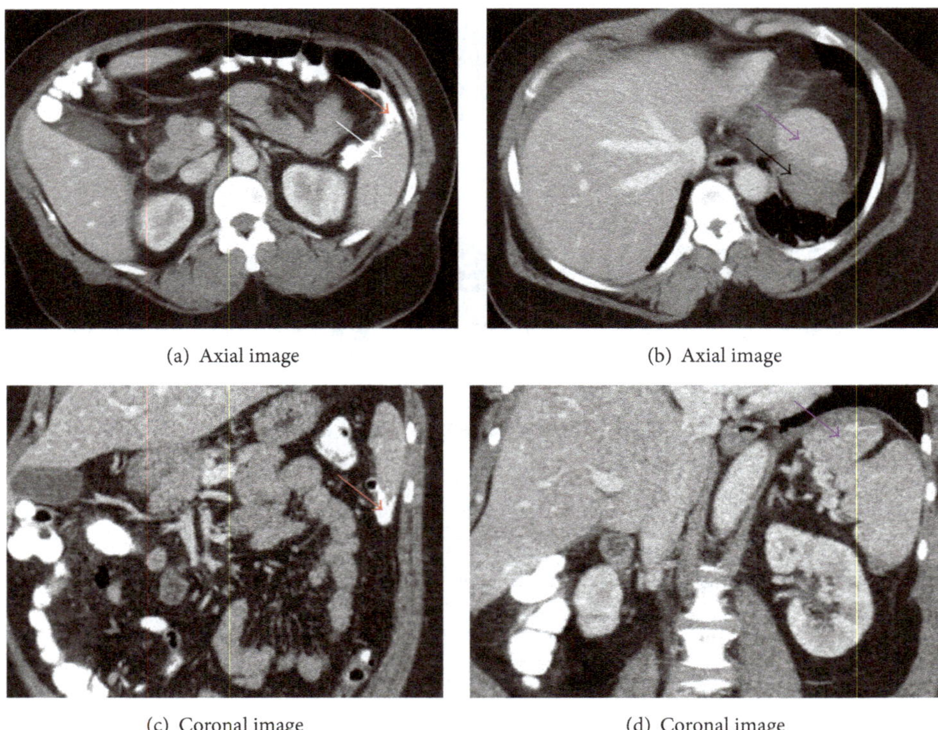

(a) Axial image (b) Axial image

(c) Coronal image (d) Coronal image

FIGURE 1: CT, 05/05/17: perisplenic and subcapsular hematoma (black arrow) along the dome of the spleen, with an area of active bleeding along the superior subcapsular region (purple arrows) with no clear fat plane separation between the colonic splenic flexure and the lower portion of the spleen (white arrows) and contrast tracking irregularly along diverticula/splenocolic adhesions and splenocolic ligament (red arrows).

taken to the operating room for laparoscopic splenectomy. On the fourth postoperative day with updated vaccination and uneventful recovery, she was discharged home.

3. Discussion

Colonoscopy is the procedure most related to iatrogenic splenic injury; however, it is infrequent to have splenic injury as a complication of colonoscopy [5]. Predisposing factors for splenic trauma include splenomegaly, adhesions related to previous operations, anticoagulant use, smoking, inflammatory bowel disease, difficult colonoscopy, intention to rush during the procedure, and insufficient visualization due to inadequate bowel cleansing [6]. In addition, during colonoscopy, maneuvers such as hooking the splenic flexure to straighten left colon, applying external pressure on the left hypochondrium, slide by advancement, and alpha maneuver, can be risk factors for splenic injury [7]. Left lateral position can be considered a protective factor; it reduces the excessive traction of the splenocolic ligament or possible adhesions, as the spleen and the splenic angle of the colon approximate in the left side [8].

Symptoms in most cases begin in the first 24 hours after colonoscopy [8] but may be rarely delayed and it must be kept in mind that symptoms can present after several days [9]. The first and second most common symptoms are left upper quadrant pain with prevalence of 93% and left shoulder pain in 88%, respectively; the latter is caused by diaphragmatic irritation, related to distention of splenic capsule following bleeding [6]. Similar symptoms presenting within 24 hours of colonoscopy prompted our patient for her emergency room visit.

Diagnosis can be challenging as abdominal discomfort is common after colonoscopy due to trapped air in the colon leading to misdiagnoses of some cases of mild splenic rupture [1, 8]. Although computerized tomography is highly sensitive, suspecting this complication is the best way to assist in the early diagnosis [10]. Contrast-enhanced CT scan of the abdomen is the gold standard for diagnosis as it can describe the splenic injury grading in accordance with the American Association for the Surgery of Trauma (AAST) [11]. According to Corcillo et al., ultrasound (conventional and contrast-enhanced) provides a good alternative in patients with contraindications to CT contrast agents and in hemodynamically compromised patients (focused assessment with sonography for trauma (FAST)) [12].

Therapeutic options available for treatment include conservative management, surgery, or embolization of the splenic artery [12] depending on type of injury and hemodynamic stability. In hemodynamically unstable patients with ongoing bleeding, splenectomy is a common treatment option [1, 12]. Failure rate in patients initially treated conservatively and eventually requiring a splenectomy or embolization

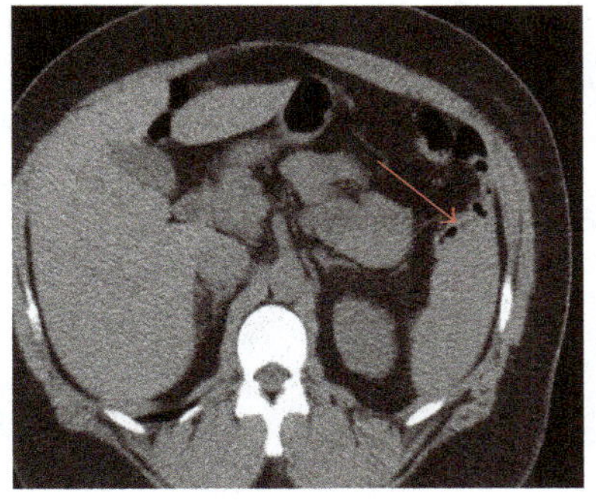
(a) Axial image

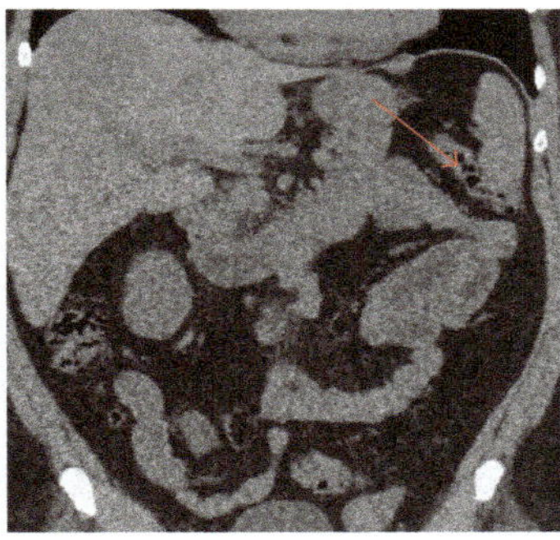
(b) Coronal image

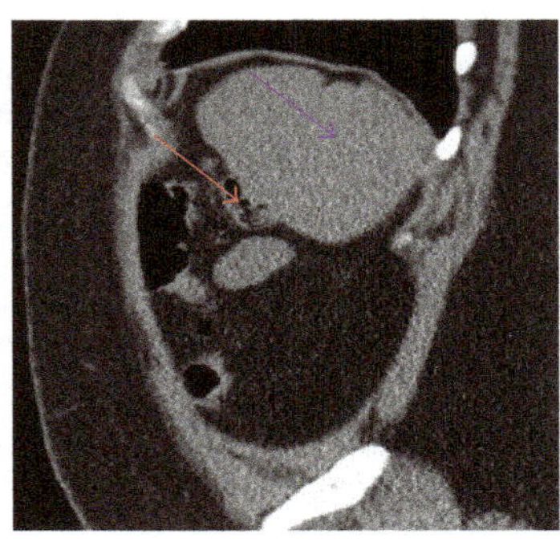
(c) Sagittal image

FIGURE 2: CT, 06/06/12: diverticula abutting the splenic capsule of the lower pole (red arrows) with splenomegaly (purple arrow).

can be up to 44% [12]. Our patient was initially managed conservatively, but she continued to bleed as evidenced by further drop in hemoglobin and imaging evidence of the same. Options of embolization versus surgery were considered and we decided that splenectomy would lead to a more favorable outcome given her instability.

Given the important immune functions of the spleen, it is imperative not to overlook the importance of vaccination against encapsulated organisms in these patients, as they are prone to overwhelming sepsis from the organisms. According to Hammerquist et al., in nonemergent cases, vaccination against encapsulated organisms should be attempted ideally 2 weeks before surgery; however, during emergency splenectomy, vaccination should be performed until 2 weeks postoperatively [13, 14].

We suggest that the presence of possible splenocolic adhesions, as evidenced by colonic diverticula abutting on splenic capsule, seen on abdominal imaging done before index elective colonoscopy (see Figures 2(a)–2(c)), would have contributed to her risk of splenic trauma during the colonoscopy. Laparotomy with splenectomy was decided as patient had progression of hemoperitoneum and hemodynamic instability.

4. Conclusion

Splenic trauma during colonoscopy is quite a rare occurrence, but anticipating it as one of the causes of abdominal pain after colonoscopy is critical especially when located in the left upper quadrant or left shoulder. Multiple risk factors have been described in literature; a few may have culminated in splenic trauma in our patient during index colonoscopy, notably splenocolic adhesions, and splenomegaly. The gold standard diagnostic examination is the contrast-enhanced CT scan of the abdomen; other diagnostic options include ultrasound (conventional and contrast-enhanced). Management of splenic injury may be one of 3 therapeutic options: conservative, surgery, or embolization of the splenic artery, based on patient's hemodynamics and ongoing extravasation.

References

[1] G. Piccolo, M. Di Vita, A. Cavallaro et al., "Presentation and management of splenic injury after colonoscopy: a systematic review," *Surgical Laparoscopy Endoscopy & Percutaneous Techniques*, vol. 24, no. 2, pp. 95–102, 2014.

[2] J. F. Ha and D. Minchin, "Splenic injury in colonoscopy: a review," *International Journal of Surgery*, vol. 7, no. 5, pp. 424–427, 2009.

[3] M. J. Garcia, R. C. Gonzalez, B. M. Rivas, M. G. Ruiz, and M. R. Tirado, "Splenic rupture after colorectal cancer screening," *Revista Espanola de Enfermedades Digestivas: Organo Oficial de la Sociedad Espanola de Patologia Digestiva*, vol. 107, no. 11, pp. 705-706, 2015.

[4] A. H. De Tejada, L. Giménez-Alvira, E. Van Den Brule et al., "Severe splenic rupture after colorectal endoscopic submucosal dissection," *World Journal of Gastroenterology*, vol. 20, no. 28, pp. 9618–9620, 2014.

[5] A. S. Kamath, C. W. Iqbal, M. G. Sarr et al., "Colonoscopic splenic injuries: incidence and management," *Journal of Gastrointestinal Surgery*, vol. 13, no. 12, pp. 2136–2140, 2009.

[6] K. V. Rao, G. D. Beri, M. J. Sterling, and G. Salen, "Splenic injury as a complication of colonoscopy: a case series," *American Journal of Gastroenterology*, vol. 104, no. 6, pp. 1604-1605, 2009.

[7] C. Zandonà, S. Turrina, N. Pasin, and D. De Leo, "Medico-legal considerations in a case of splenic injury that occurred during colonoscopy," *Journal of Forensic and Legal Medicine*, vol. 19, no. 4, pp. 229–233, 2012.

[8] S. Abunnaja, L. Panait, J. A. Palesty, and S. Macaron, "Laparoscopic splenectomy for traumatic splenic injury after screening colonoscopy," *Case Reports in Gastroenterology*, vol. 6, no. 3, pp. 624–628, 2012.

[9] S. J. Fishback, P. J. Pickhardt, S. Bhalla, C. O. Menias, R. G. Congdon, and M. MacAri, "Delayed presentation of splenic rupture following colonoscopy: clinical and CT findings," *Emergency Radiology*, vol. 18, no. 6, pp. 539–544, 2011.

[10] M. Sarhan, A. Ramcharan, and S. Ponnapalli, "Splenic injury after elective colonoscopy," *Journal of the Society of Laparoendoscopic Surgeons*, vol. 13, no. 4, pp. 616–619, 2009.

[11] T. J. Esposito, G. Tinkoff, J. Reed et al., "American Association for the Surgery of Trauma Organ Injury Scale (OIS): past, present, and future," *Journal of Trauma and Acute Care Surgery*, vol. 74, no. 4, pp. 1163–1174, 2013.

[12] A. Corcillo, S. Aellen, T. Zingg, P. Bize, N. Demartines, and A. Denys, "Endovascular treatment of active splenic bleeding after colonoscopy: a systematic review of the literature," *CardioVascular and Interventional Radiology*, vol. 36, no. 5, pp. 1270–1279, 2013.

[13] R. J. Hammerquist, K. A. Messerschmidt, A. A. Pottebaum, and T. R. Hellwig, "Vaccinations in asplenic adults," *American Journal of Health-System Pharmacy*, vol. 73, no. 9, pp. e220–e228, 2016.

[14] G. P. Kealey, V. Dhungel, M. J. Wideroff et al., "Patient education and recall regarding postsplenectomy immunizations," *Journal of Surgical Research*, vol. 199, no. 2, pp. 580–585, 2015.

Organizing Pneumonia in a Patient with Quiescent Crohn's Disease

Satoshi Tanida,[1] Masaya Takemura,[2] Tsutomu Mizoshita,[1] Keiji Ozeki,[1] Takahito Katano,[1] Takaya Shimura,[1] Yoshinori Mori,[1] Eiji Kubota,[1] Hiromi Kataoka,[1] Takeshi Kamiya,[1] and Takashi Joh[1]

[1]*Department of Gastroenterology and Metabolism, Nagoya City University Graduate School of Medical Sciences, Nagoya, Aichi Prefecture 467-8601, Japan*
[2]*Department of Respiratory Medicine, Allergy and Clinical Immunology, Nagoya City University Graduate School of Medical Sciences, Nagoya, Aichi Prefecture 467-8601, Japan*

Correspondence should be addressed to Satoshi Tanida; stanida@med.nagoya-cu.ac.jp

Academic Editor: Daniel C. Damin

A 64-year-old man with Crohn's disease (CD) was admitted to our hospital due to moderate risk of pneumonia while receiving scheduled adalimumab maintenance therapy. Symptoms remained virtually unchanged following administration of antibiotics. A final diagnosis of organizing pneumonia (OP) was made based on findings of intra-alveolar buds of granulation tissue and fibrous thickening of the alveolar walls on pathological examination and patchy consolidations and ground glass opacities on computed tomography. Immediate administration of prednisolone provided rapid, sustained improvement. Although a rare complication, OP is a pulmonary manifestation that requires attention in CD patients.

1. Introduction

Inflammatory bowel diseases (IBDs), such as ulcerative colitis (UC) and Crohn's disease (CD), often affect the entire digestive system and organs, but extraintestinal manifestations account for approximately 21–41% of IBD cases [1, 2]. Noninfectious pulmonary diseases associated with CD are uncommon. These associations are generally considered to arise from extraintestinal manifestations of the disease itself and adverse effects to therapeutic drugs prescribed to ameliorate inflammation [3].

Organizing pneumonia (OP) is a particular form of pneumonia presenting as diffuse interstitial lung disease that affects the distal bronchioles, respiratory bronchioles, alveolar ducts, and alveolar walls [4–6]. OP appearing with CD is extremely rare. Only a single report has described non-resolving pneumonia in 3 CD patients receiving immunosuppressive agents: 2 patients had pneumonia presenting as noncaseating granuloma with accompanying giant cells and 1 patient had OP [7]. Here, we report a rare case of OP in a CD patient who had been in remission after receiving 5-aminosalicylic acid and adalimumab (ADA).

2. Case Report

This patient was a 64-year-old man who had previously undergone partial ileal resection due to intestinal obstruction and partial peritonitis at the age of 30. He had since been admitted to other hospitals because of repeated temporary obstructions at the anastomotic site. At the age of 62, the patient was referred to our hospital with recurrent severe abdominal pain and exacerbation of CD. The patient had no history of lung disease, occupational exposures, or extraintestinal manifestations and no family history of CD. Physical examination revealed the following: body temperature, 39.2°C; hemoglobin oxygen saturation as measured by pulse oximetry, 99%; and blood pressure, 100/66 mmHg.

A small bowel series showed longitudinal ulcers and strictures at the ileal anastomotic site. Colonoscopy and pathological examination of a biopsied ulcer specimen showed

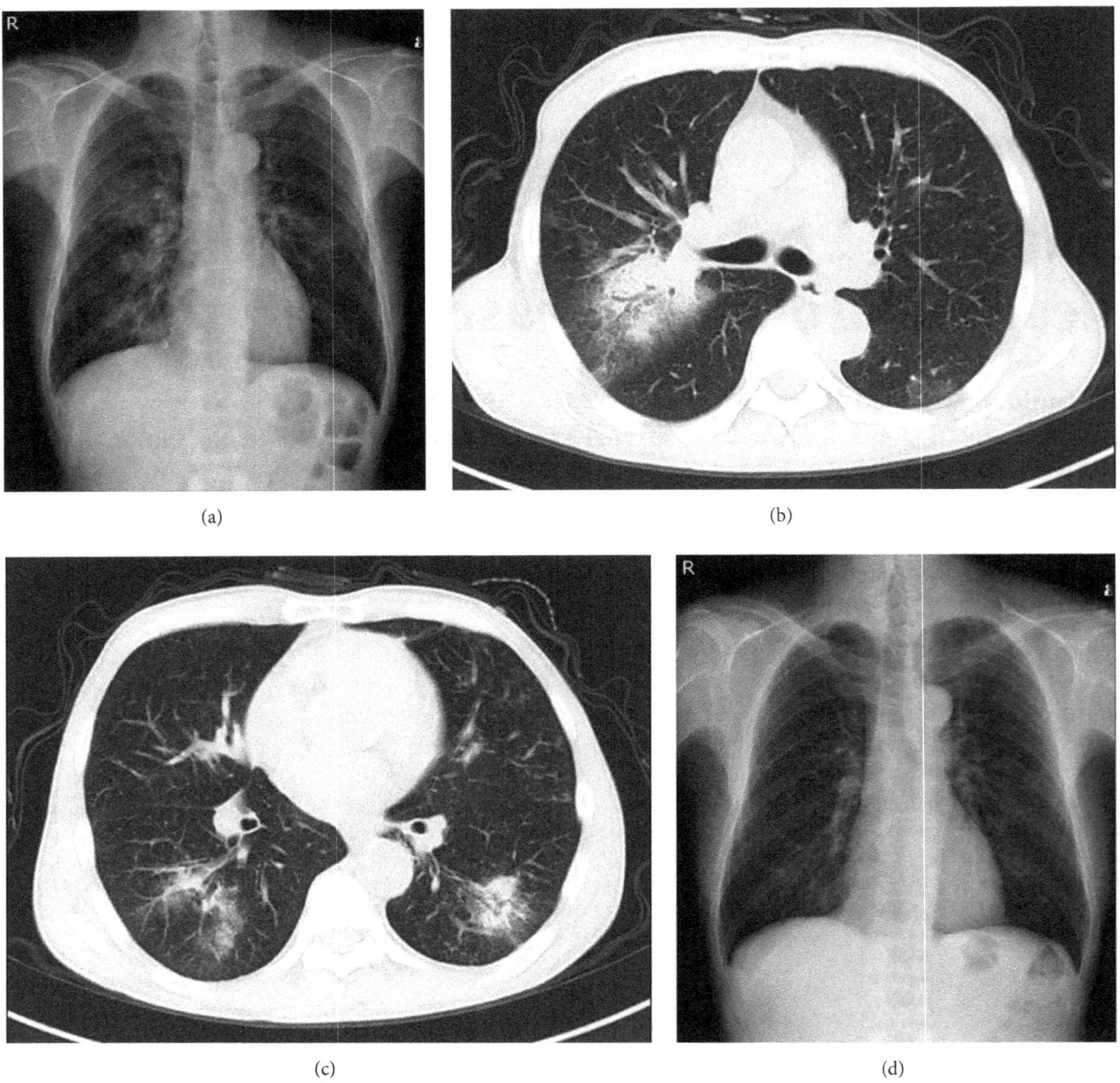

(a) (b) (c) (d)

Figure 1: (a) Chest radiograph shows patchy bilateral consolidation in the middle lobe and bilateral lower lobes. (b, c) Chest computed tomography reveals patchy consolidation, ground glass opacities, and small nodular opacities in the middle (b) and bilateral lower lobes (c). (d) Follow-up chest radiograph after 3 weeks shows resolution of abnormal findings.

moderate to severe inflammatory cell infiltrates with some epithelioid granulomas in the lamina muscularis mucosae and submucosa. Based on these findings, CD was initially diagnosed. ADA induction therapy was then initiated at 160/80/40 mg every other week [8] and afforded complete remission. Two years later, the patient was admitted to our hospital due to rapid exacerbation of productive cough, accompanied by fever of up to 39.2°C, and findings on chest radiography of patchy bilateral consolidation and ground glass opacities (Figure 1(a)). Laboratory investigations showed the following: white blood cell count, 13,800/μL; red blood cell count, 386 $\times$ $10^4/\mu$L; hemoglobin, 10.7 g/dL; total protein, 5.3 g/dL; albumin, 2.1 mg/dL; aspartate aminotransferase, 58 IU/L; alanine aminotransferase, 34 IU/L; C-reactive protein, 22.2 mg/dL. Low albuminemia was due to severe inflammation and loss of appetite. Negative results were obtained from tests for influenza virus types A and B, *Aspergillus* antigen, (1→3)-β-D-glucan, QuantiFERON, and cytomegalovirus antigenemia C-7HRP. Sputum cultures isolated *Streptococcus pneumoniae* and α-hemolytic streptococcal species (Table 1). Chest computed tomography (CT) revealed patchy consolidations, ground glass opacities, and small nodular opacities, predominantly in the middle, lingula, and bilateral lower lobes (Figures 1(b) and 1(c)). Based

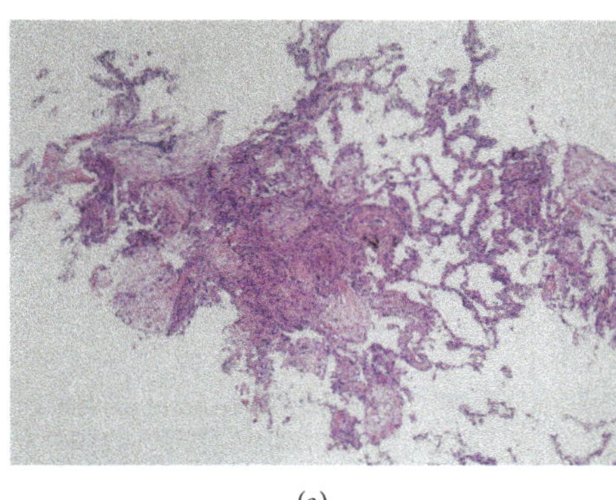
(a)

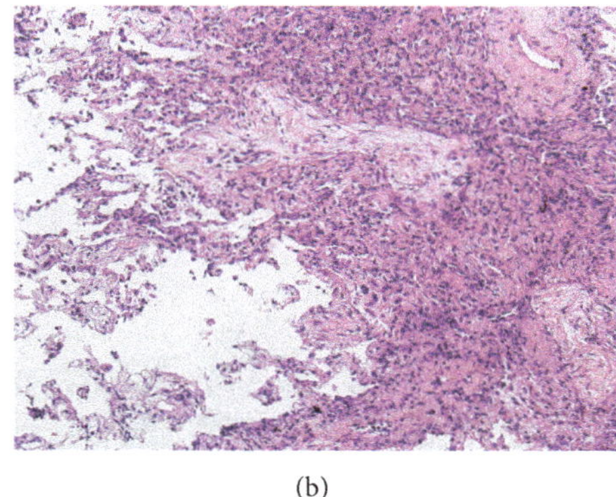
(b)

FIGURE 2: Pathologic examinations of transbronchial lung biopsy specimen with hematoxylin and eosin stain ((a) ×40 and (b) ×100) show intra-alveolar buds of granulation tissue and fibrous thickening of the alveolar wall.

TABLE 1: Laboratory findings on admission.

		Normal range
Hematology		
WBC	13600/μL	3,600–9,600/μL
RBC	$386 \times 10^4/\mu$L	$400–552 \times 10^4/\mu$L
Hb	10.7 g/dL	13.2–17.2 g/dL
PLT	$193 \times 10^3/\mu$L	$148–339 \times 10^3/\mu$L
Serum biochemistry		
TP	5.3 g/dL	6.7–8.3 g/dL
Alb	2.1 g/dL	4.0–5.0 g/dL
AST	58 U/L	13–33 U/L
ALT	34 U/L	6–30 U/L
LDH	303 U/L	214–466 U/L
BUN	19.2 mg/dL	8–22 mg/dL
Cre	0.9 mg/dL	0.6–1.1 mg/dL
Na	138 mmol/L	138–146 mmol/L
K	4.4 mmol/L	3.6–4.9 mmol/L
Cl	99 mmol/L	99–109 mmol/L
CRP	22.2 mg/dL	≤0.30 mg/dL
Serologic tests		
Influenza virus types A and B	Negative	
Antigenemia (C-7HRP)	Negative	
Aspergillus antigen	Negative	
(1→3)-β-D-glucan	Negative	
QuantiFERON	Negative	
Sputum culture	*Streptococcus pneumoniae*, α-hemolytic streptococcal species	

on these findings, we considered a diagnosis of bacterial pneumonia due to streptococcal species. Despite antibiotic treatment with intravenous piperacillin-tazobactam and meropenem and supportive care for 14 days, respiratory symptoms remained unimproved and radiographic findings gradually deteriorated. A transbronchial lung biopsy from a right lung lesion showed fibrous thickening of the alveolar wall and intra-alveolar buds of granulation tissue associated with fibroblasts (Figure 2). Based on these findings, a final diagnosis of OP associated with CD was made though postinfectious OP could not be completely ruled out. Upon starting prednisolone at a dose of 30 mg/day, dramatic clinical improvement was observed and complete radiographic clearing of the lung infiltrates was confirmed within 3 weeks (Figure 1(d)). The prednisolone dose was gradually tapered to 1 mg/day (Figure 3). The patient has remained well for a year.

3. Discussion

CD often shows extraintestinal manifestations such as uveitis and ankylosing spondylitis [9]. On the other hand, primary lung involvement is rare and reportedly includes bronchiolitis obliterans organizing pneumonia (BOOP), pulmonary interstitial emphysema, desquamative interstitial pneumonia, nonspecific interstitial pneumonia, fibrosing alveolitis, and eosinophilic pneumonitis [2, 3]. Lung involvement can also be secondary to the drug used to treat CD [10]. OP is the most commonly reported parenchymal manifestation of IBD, particularly UC [11]. In this type of idiopathic diffuse interstitial lung disease, granulation tissue obstructs the alveolar ducts and alveolar spaces and chronic inflammation arise in the adjacent alveoli [5, 6]. Pulmonary interstitial emphysema is characterized by air trapping outside the normal air passages and inside the connective tissue of the peribronchovascular sheaths, interlobular septa, and visceral pleura; this disease entity is more frequent in premature infants who require mechanical ventilation for severe lung disease [12]. Desquamative interstitial pneumonia is a chronic lung inflammation characterized by mononuclear cell infiltration of the airspaces. It occurs almost exclusively in current or former cigarette smokers [13]. Fibrosing alveolitis is characterized by inflammation and thickening of the alveolar walls and usually occurs in individuals over the age of 40 years [14]. Eosinophilic pneumonitis is a disease characterized by accumulation of eosinophils in bronchoalveolar lavage and lung tissue [15]. In the present case, the final diagnosis of OP associated with CD was made based on the pathological and CT findings and the clinical course [16–18]. However,

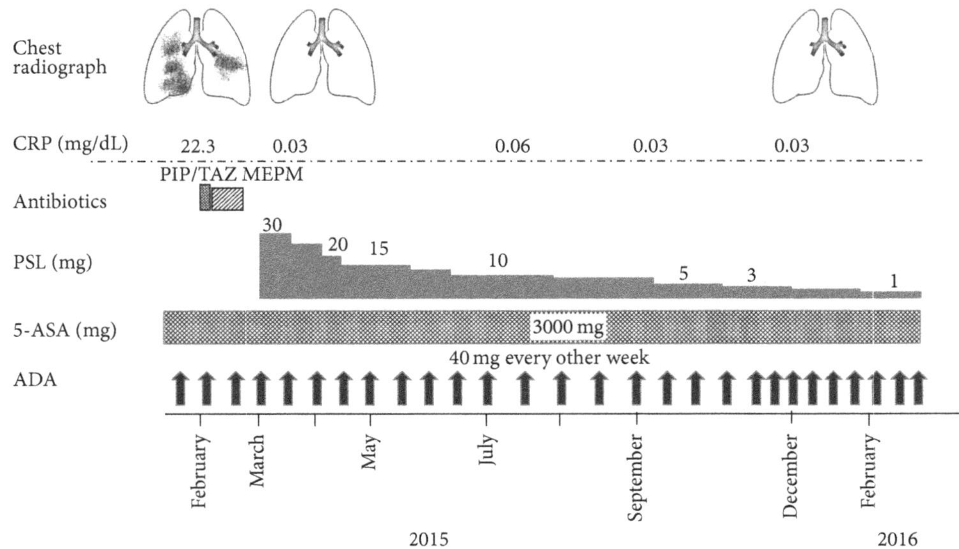

FIGURE 3: The clinical course of the patient, a 64-year-old man with Crohn's disease. Progressive pulmonary symptoms and manifestations were seen during scheduled ADA maintenance therapy. Treatment with prednisolone induced rapid, sustained improvements. CRP: C-reactive protein; PIP/TAZ: piperacillin/tazobactam; MEPM: meropenem; PSL: prednisolone; 5-ASA: 5-aminosalicylic acid; ADA: adalimumab.

in terms of the clinical features, postpneumonic OP and secondary OP, these are actually fairly similar. Differentiating postpneumonic OP from secondary OP based on the radiographic findings was difficult. We initially diagnosed acute bacterial pneumonia due to streptococcal species based on the rapid development after disease onset and the positive result of sputum cultures for *Streptococcus pneumoniae* and α-hemolytic streptococcal species. Despite the use of wide-spectrum antibiotics, respiratory symptoms persisted and findings on chest radiography gradually deteriorated. In general, in the early period of postpneumonic OP, antibiotics therapies are partially effective and yield some degree of improvement in symptoms and radiological findings [19, 20]. Based on the above, we concluded that secondary OP was more likely than postpneumonic OP.

Lung disease is known to sporadically occur after long-term use of 5-aminosalicylic acid [21] and anti-tumor necrosis factor (TNF)-α antibodies [22, 23]. Consensus is currently lacking regarding a definitive approach to diagnosing drug-induced lung disease. In a few cases, drug-induced lung disease can show a clinical course and radiographic findings like OP [24, 25]. In the present case, at disease onset, the patient was immediately given prednisolone, which provided rapid and sustained improvement. The prednisolone was subsequently tapered while ADA and mesalazine were continued. As a result, the patient has remained well without recurrence of OP. These results suggest that this lung disorder was unlikely to present a drug-induced lung disease and was instead more likely to be OP associated with CD.

For patients with progressive symptoms of cryptogenic organizing pneumonia (COP) and diffuse radiographic changes, initial therapy with oral glucocorticoids is recommended for promising clinical outcomes [26, 27]. However, one case has been described in which initial treatment with glucocorticoids led to poor outcome, whereas a dramatic response to infliximab was seen. In the present case with OP occurring with CD in clinical remission, we selected prednisolone therapy because we considered that TNF-α was unlikely to have played a pivotal role in the development of OP and because the patient had received ADA treatment. Interestingly, OP cases have not been known to be associated with the disease activity of IBD [2, 11, 28].

In conclusion, although OP is a rare complication, due vigilance is required regarding the occurrence of pulmonary symptoms and manifestations in CD and IBD patients.

Authors' Contributions

Satoshi Tanida and Masaya Takemura contributed equally to this work.

References

[1] J. B. Kirsner and R. G. Shorter, "Recent developments in 'nonspecific' inflammatory bowel disease. (First of two parts)," *The New England Journal of Medicine*, vol. 306, no. 13, pp. 775–785, 1982.

[2] P. Camus, F. Piard, T. Ashcroft, A. A. Gal, and T. V. Colby, "The lung in inflammatory bowel disease," *Medicine*, vol. 72, no. 3, pp. 151–183, 1993.

[3] H. Black, M. Mendoza, and S. Murin, "Thoracic manifestations of inflammatory bowel disease," *Chest*, vol. 131, no. 2, pp. 524–532, 2007.

[4] J.-F. Cordier, "Cryptogenic organising pneumonia," *European Respiratory Journal*, vol. 28, no. 2, pp. 422–446, 2006.

[5] G. R. Epler, "Bronchiolitis obliterans organizing pneumonia," *Archives of Internal Medicine*, vol. 161, no. 2, pp. 158–164, 2001.

[6] G. R. Epler, T. V. Colby, T. C. McLoud, C. B. Carrington, and E. A. Gaensler, "Bronchiolitis obliterans organizing pneumonia," *The New England Journal of Medicine*, vol. 312, no. 3, pp. 152–158, 1985.

[7] S. Krishnan, A. Banquet, L. Newman, U. Katta, A. Patil, and A. J. Dozor, "Lung lesions in children with Crohn's disease presenting as nonresolving pneumonias and response to infliximab therapy," *Pediatrics*, vol. 117, no. 4, pp. 1440–1443, 2006.

[8] J. F. Colombel, P. J. Rutgeerts, W. J. Sandborn et al., "Adalimumab induces deep remission in patients with Crohn's disease," *Clinical Gastroenterology and Hepatology*, vol. 12, no. 3, pp. 414–422.e5, 2014.

[9] S. R. Vavricka, L. Brun, P. Ballabeni et al., "Frequency and risk factors for extraintestinal manifestations in the Swiss inflammatory bowel disease cohort," *The American Journal of Gastroenterology*, vol. 106, no. 1, pp. 110–119, 2011.

[10] J. D. Reid, B. Bressler, and J. English, "A case of adalimumab-induced pneumonitis in a 45-year-old man with Crohn's disease," *Canadian Respiratory Journal*, vol. 18, no. 5, pp. 262–264, 2011.

[11] B. Basseri, P. Enayati, A. Marchevsky, and K. A. Papadakis, "Pulmonary manifestations of inflammatory bowel disease: case presentations and review," *Journal of Crohn's and Colitis*, vol. 4, no. 4, pp. 390–397, 2010.

[12] S. M. Hart, M. McNair, H. R. Gamsu, and J. F. Price, "Pulmonary interstitial emphysema in very low birthweight infants," *Archives of Disease in Childhood*, vol. 58, no. 8, pp. 612–615, 1983.

[13] L. E. Heyneman, S. Ward, D. A. Lynch, M. Remy-Jardin, T. Johkoh, and N. L. Müller, "Respiratory bronchiolitis, respiratory bronchiolitis-associated interstitial lung disease, and desquamative interstitial pneumonia: different entities or part of the spectrum of the same disease process?" *American Journal of Roentgenology*, vol. 173, no. 6, pp. 1617–1622, 1999.

[14] J. M. Fellrath and R. M. du Bois, "Idiopathic pulmonary fibrosis/cryptogenic fibrosing alveolitis," *Clinical and Experimental Medicine*, vol. 3, no. 2, pp. 65–83, 2003.

[15] M. Naughton, J. Fahy, and M. X. FitzGerald, "Chronic eosinophilic pneumonia. A long-term follow-up of 12 patients," *Chest*, vol. 103, no. 1, pp. 162–165, 1993.

[16] A.-L. A. Katzenstein, J. L. Myers, W. D. Prophet, L. S. Corley III, and M. S. Shin, "Bronchiolitis obliterans and usual interstitial pneumonia. A comparative clinicopathologic study," *American Journal of Surgical Pathology*, vol. 10, no. 6, pp. 373–381, 1986.

[17] J. W. Lee, K. S. Lee, H. Y. Lee et al., "Cryptogenic organizing pneumonia: serial high-resolution CT findings in 22 patients," *American Journal of Roentgenology*, vol. 195, no. 4, pp. 916–922, 2010.

[18] I. M. Faria, G. Zanetti, M. M. Barreto et al., "Organizing pneumonia: chest HRCT findings," *Jornal Brasileiro de Pneumologia*, vol. 41, no. 3, pp. 231–237, 2015.

[19] H. Zhou, W. Gu, and C. Li, "Post-infectious organizing pneumonia: an indistinguishable and easily misdiagnosed organizing pneumonia," *Clinical Laboratory*, vol. 61, no. 11, pp. 1755–1761, 2015.

[20] D. H. Akbar and O. S. Alamoudi, "Bronchiolitis obliterans organizing pneumonia associated with *Pseudomonas aeruginosa* infection," *Saudi Medical Journal*, vol. 21, no. 11, pp. 1081–1084, 2000.

[21] R. H. Moseley, K. W. Barwick, K. Dobuler, and V. A. DeLuca Jr., "Sulfasalazine-induced pulmonary disease," *Digestive Diseases and Sciences*, vol. 30, no. 9, pp. 901–904, 1985.

[22] R. Perez-Alvarez, M. Perez-de-Lis, C. Diaz-Lagares et al., "Interstitial lung disease induced or exacerbated by TNF-targeted therapies: analysis of 122 cases," *Seminars in Arthritis and Rheumatism*, vol. 41, no. 2, pp. 256–264, 2011.

[23] R. Caccaro, E. Savarino, R. D'Incà, and G. C. Sturniolo, "Noninfectious interstitial lung disease during infliximab therapy: case report and literature review," *World Journal of Gastroenterology*, vol. 19, no. 32, pp. 5377–5380, 2013.

[24] S. Sen, C. Peltz, K. Jordan, and T. J. Boes, "Infliximab-induced nonspecific interstitial pneumonia," *The American Journal of the Medical Sciences*, vol. 344, no. 1, pp. 75–78, 2012.

[25] P. Camus, The Drug-Induced Respiratory Disease, http://www.pneumotox.com/.

[26] G. R. Epler, "Heterogeneity of bronchiolitis obliterans organizing pneumonia," *Current Opinion in Pulmonary Medicine*, vol. 4, no. 2, pp. 93–97, 1998.

[27] J.-F. Cordier, "Organising pneumonia," *Thorax*, vol. 55, no. 4, pp. 318–328, 2000.

[28] P. Gil-Simón, J. Barrio Andrés, R. Atienza Sánchez, L. Julián Gómez, C. López Represa, and A. Caro-Patón, "Bronchiolitis obliterans organizing pneumonia and Crohn's disease," *Revista Espanola de Enfermedades Digestivas*, vol. 100, no. 3, pp. 175–177, 2008.

35

Endoscopic Resection of a Pedunculated Brunner's Gland Hamartoma of the Duodenum

Masaya Iwamuro,[1,2] Takehiro Tanaka,[3] Satoko Ando,[1] Tatsuhiro Gotoda,[1] Hiromitsu Kanzaki,[1] Seiji Kawano,[1] Yoshiro Kawahara,[4] and Hiroyuki Okada[1]

[1] *Department of Gastroenterology and Hepatology, Okayama University Graduate School of Medicine, Dentistry, and Pharmaceutical Sciences, 2-5-1 Shikata-cho, Kita-ku, Okayama 700-8558, Japan*
[2] *Department of General Medicine, Okayama University Graduate School of Medicine, Dentistry, and Pharmaceutical Sciences, 2-5-1 Shikata-cho, Kita-ku, Okayama 700-8558, Japan*
[3] *Department of Pathology, Okayama University Hospital, Okayama 700-8558, Japan*
[4] *Department of Endoscopy, Okayama University Hospital, Okayama 700-8558, Japan*

Correspondence should be addressed to Masaya Iwamuro; iwamuromasaya@yahoo.co.jp

Academic Editor: Hideto Kawaratani

A 68-year-old Japanese woman presented with a solitary pedunculated polyp in the duodenum. Endoscopic ultrasonography showed multiple cystic structures in the polyp. The polyp was successfully resected by endoscopic snare polypectomy and pathologically diagnosed as Brunner's gland hamartoma. Because hamartomatous components were not identified in the stalk of the polyp, we speculate that the stalk developed from traction of the normal duodenal mucosa. When a solitary, pedunculated polyp with cystic structure within the submucosa is found in the duodenum, Brunner's gland hamartoma should be considered in the differential diagnosis, despite the rarity of the disease. This case underscores the usefulness of endoscopic ultrasonography for the diagnosis of duodenal subepithelial tumors.

1. Introduction

Brunner's glands, also called duodenal glands, are found in the submucosa of the duodenum, typically in the duodenal bulb and in the second portion of the duodenum proximal to the sphincter of Oddi. Brunner's glands produce a mucus-rich, bicarbonate-containing, alkaline secretion that aids in neutralizing the acidic content of chyme and gastric acid, providing an alkaline milieu to optimize intestinal absorption and lubricate the intestinal walls [1]. Lesions associated with Brunner's gland vary from hyperplasia, hamartoma, and, in rare instances, adenocarcinoma [1–3].

We recently encountered a patient with a pedunculated polyp in the second portion of the duodenum, which was covered with intact duodenal mucosa. The polyp was successfully resected by endoscopic snare polypectomy. The diagnosis of Brunner's gland hamartoma was based on pathological analysis of the resected specimen. In this report, we speculate the mechanism of morphogenesis of this pedunculated feature, mainly focusing on the pathological characteristics. Moreover, we discuss differential diagnosis of duodenal lesions showing submucosal origin.

2. Case Report

A 68-year-old Japanese woman underwent barium follow-through examination for the upper gastrointestinal tract as part of a routine medical screening. A pedunculated polyp was detected in the duodenum (Figure 1). The patient was referred to our hospital for further investigation and treatment of the polyp. The patient had been taking medication for hyperlipidemia but had no history of gastrointestinal diseases. A physical examination revealed no abnormalities, and there was no evidence of peripheral lymphadenopathy. Laboratory findings revealed an elevated level of total cholesterol to 254 mg/dL, but levels of carcinoembryonic antigen and carbohydrate antigen 19-9 and blood cell counts were within normal ranges. Esophagogastroduodenoscopy

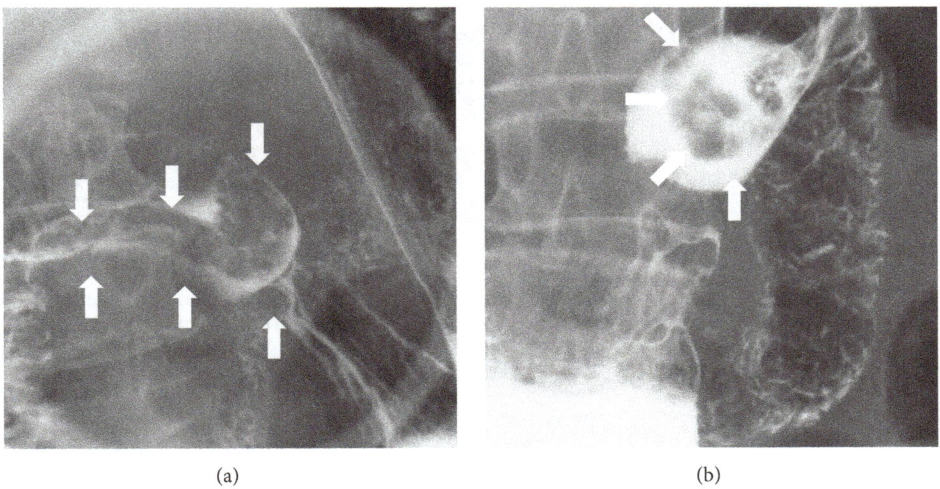

(a) (b)

FIGURE 1: Barium follow-through examination images. A pedunculated polyp can be identified in the duodenum (arrows).

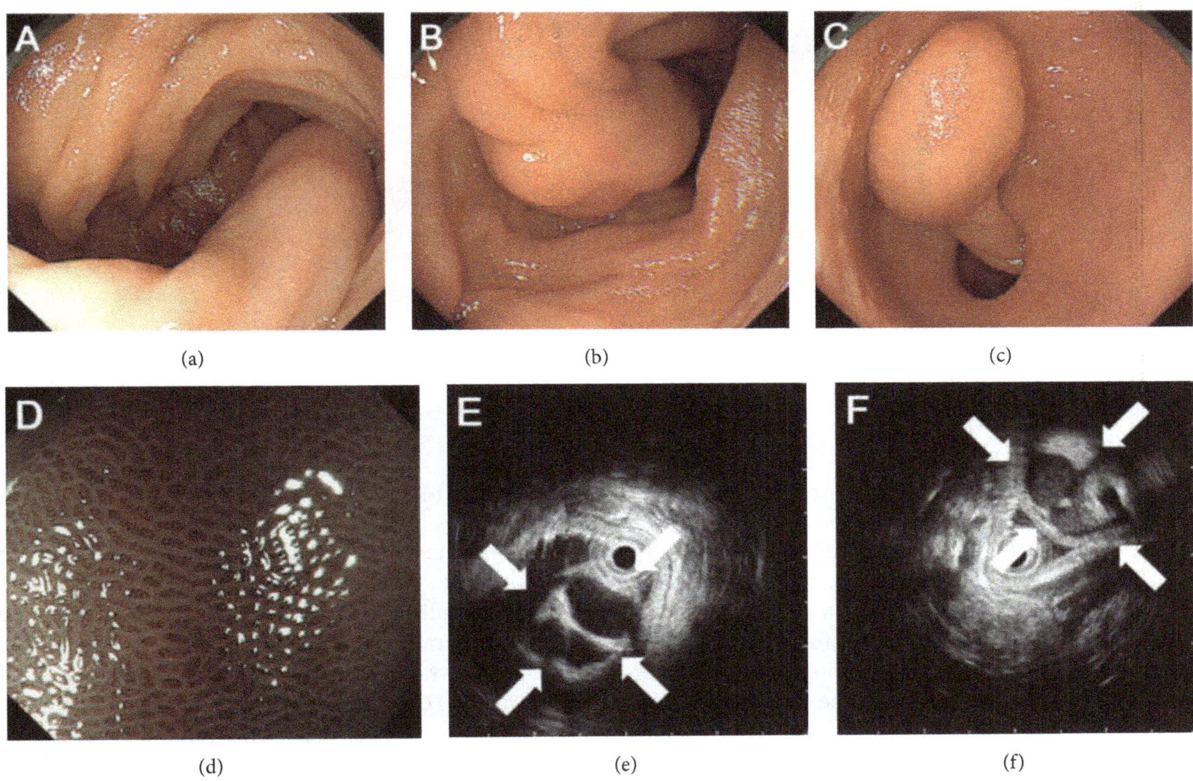

(a) (b) (c)

(d) (e) (f)

FIGURE 2: Endoscopy images. Esophagogastroduodenoscopy results showed a pedunculated polyp measuring approximately 20 mm ((a), (b)). The polyp was easily extended to the stomach by traction with biopsy forceps (c). Magnifying observation with narrowband imaging revealed that the surface of the polyp was entirely covered with intact duodenal mucosa (d). Endoscopic ultrasonography showed multiple cystic structures ((e), (f), arrows).

showed a pedunculated polyp in the duodenal second portion. The head of the polyp was approximately 20 mm in size (Figures 2(a) and 2(b)). There were no erosions or ulcers in the polyp. The tumor had long stalk; therefore it easily migrated to the stomach (Figure 2(c)). Magnifying observation with narrowband imaging confirmed that the surface was entirely covered with intact duodenal mucosa, suggesting a subepithelial origin of the tumor (Figure 2(d)). Endoscopic ultrasonography visualized at least three cystic structures in the polyp head (Figures 2(e) and 2(f)). Based on the macroscopic and ultrasonography features, Brunner's gland hamartoma was highly suspected.

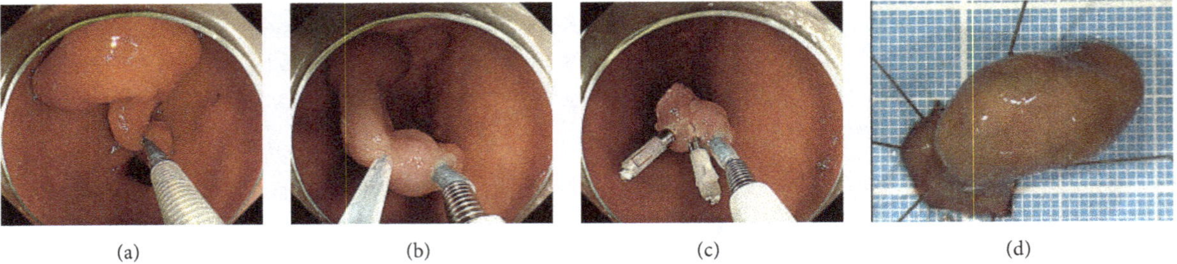

(a) (b) (c) (d)

FIGURE 3: Endoscopic resection of the polyp. During the procedure, the stalk was strangulated with a detachable snare (a). The polyp was then resected by snare polypectomy (b). The cut surface was closed with two metal clips (c). The size of the resected specimen was 26 × 19 mm (d).

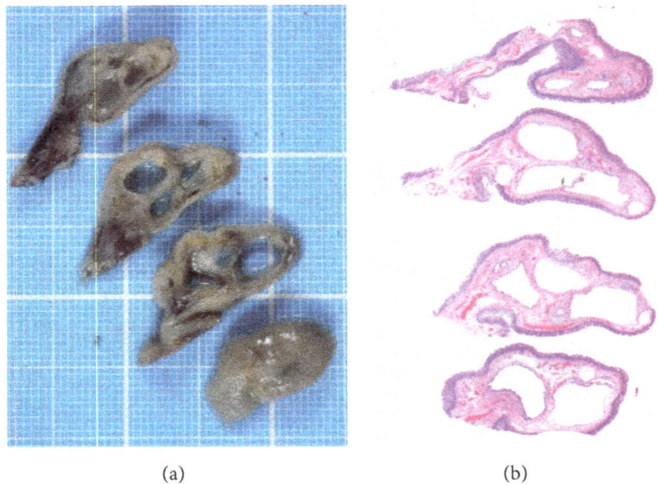

(a) (b)

FIGURE 4: Images of the resected specimen. Macroscopically, multiple cystic structures can be observed in the head of the polyp, whereas no cyst is visible in the stalk.

The patient agreed to undergo endoscopic resection of the polyp to prevent duodenal obstruction due to impaction of the tumor. First, we repositioned the polyp from the duodenum to the stomach by traction with biopsy forceps. The stalk was then strangulated with a detachable snare (Figure 3(a)). Next, the polyp was successfully resected using snare polypectomy (Figure 3(b)). Although there was no bleeding from the resected section, the cut surface was closed with two metal clips (Figure 3(c)). The size of the resected specimen was 26 × 19 mm (Figure 3(d)). Macroscopically, multiple cystic structures were observed in the head of the polyp, whereas no cyst was detected in the stalk (Figure 4). Pathological evaluation revealed a lobular arrangement of proliferated Brunner's glands separated by fibromuscular septa at the head of the polyp (Figures 5(a) and 5(b)). Stromal cell proliferation was also noted. In contrast, Brunner's glands were only partly identified in the stalk (Figures 5(c) and 5(d)). Multiple blood vessels and abundant adipose tissue were observed in the stalk. The cystic structure present in the head of the polyp was lined with columnar cells without atypia, indicating that the cysts consisted of dilated ducts of Brunner's glands (Figures 5(e) and 5(f)).

3. Discussion

Brunner's gland hyperplasia and hamartoma are two representative lesions that arise from Brunner's gland. Although distinct definitions do not exist that discriminate the two lesions, generally hyperplasia indicates multiple lesions less than 1 cm, whereas hamartoma refers to a solitary lesion larger than 1 cm [2, 3]. Macroscopically, Brunner's gland hyperplasia appears as multiple, sessile, submucosal nodules mostly identified in the duodenal bulb and/or in the second portion of the duodenum. Brunner's gland hamartoma typically appears as a polypoid, pedunculated lesion ranging in size from 0.7 to 12 cm, with a mean of 4 cm [1]. Pathologically, Brunner's gland hyperplasia is characterized by an excessive number of Brunner's glands separated by fibrous septa. Brunner's gland hamartoma consists of Brunner's glands, ducts, smooth muscle, adipose tissue, and lymphoid cells [4–6]. In the present patient, Brunner's gland hamartoma appeared with the typical morphology, presenting as a solitary pedunculated polypoid mass with a stalk consisting of normal duodenal mucosa [3, 6, 7]. Dislocation of the polyp head from the duodenum to the gastric lumen has also been described previously [8].

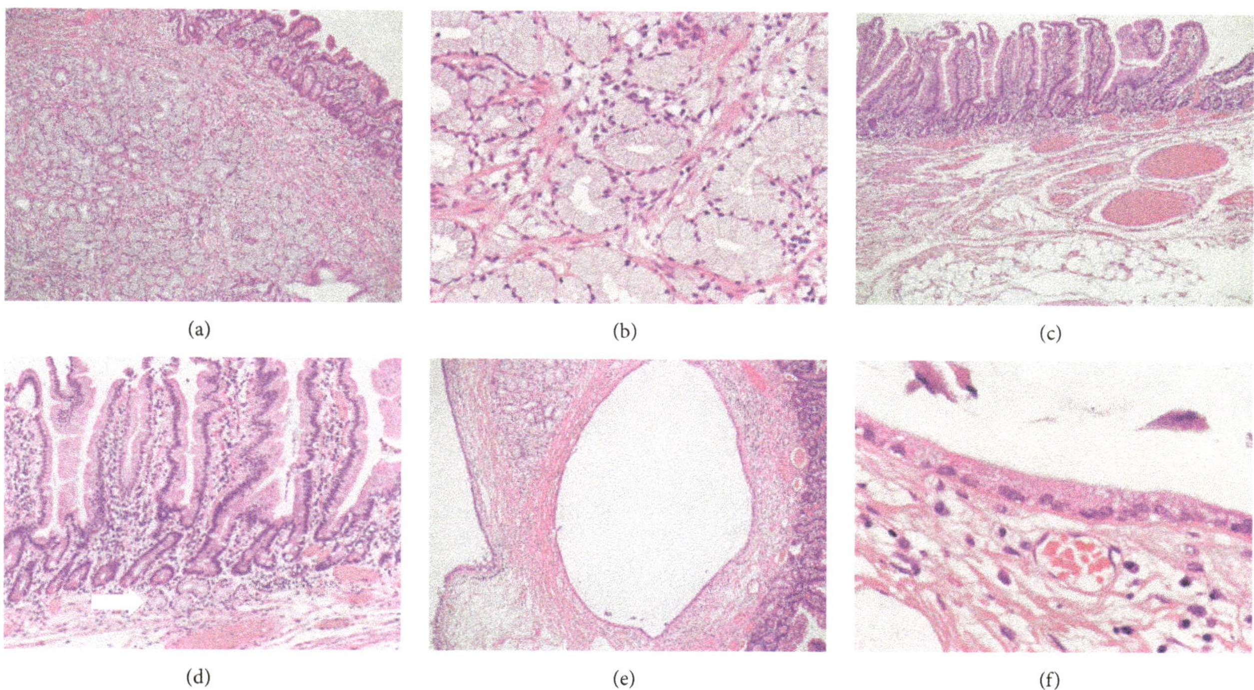

FIGURE 5: Pathological images. Stromal cell proliferation and lobular arrangement of proliferated Brunner's glands separated by fibromuscular septa are visible in the head of the polyp ((a), ×4; (b), ×20). In the stalk, multiple blood vessels and adipose tissues can be seen ((c), ×4; (d), ×10). Brunner's glands are only partly visible in the stalk ((d), arrow). The cystic structure visible in the head of the polyp is lined with columnar cells ((e), ×4; (f), ×40). Based on the pathological features, a diagnosis of Brunner's gland hamartoma was reached.

Patients with Brunner's gland hamartoma may be asymptomatic and the lesion is usually discovered incidentally [9]. Possible symptoms caused by Brunner's gland hamartoma include duodenal obstruction, intussusception, obstructive jaundice, pancreatitis, and bleeding [1, 3, 4]. Thus, resection is indicated for symptomatic or large lesions to relieve or prevent complications [10]. Successful treatment has been reported using endoscopic resection techniques such as snare polypectomy and endoscopic mucosal resection [11–15].

Pathological evaluation of Brunner's gland hamartoma in the present patient revealed that the polyp head consisted of proliferated Brunner's glands in lobules, stromal cells, and marked cystic dilatation lined by columnar cells (Figures 5(a), 5(b), 5(e), and 5(f)). In contrast, such hamartomatous components were not present in the stalk (Figures 5(c) and 5(d)). Consequently, we speculate that peristalsis of the duodenum acted as a traction force on the hamartoma. The mucosa and submucosa were then extended, resulting in the final formation of the stalk. Because the hamartoma was localized at the head of the polyp, the complete resection of the lesion could easily be performed by cutting the stalk using an endoscopic snare polypectomy procedure. In our case, we considered that when performing endoscopic resection of Brunner's gland hamartoma, prevention of hemorrhage or hemostasis was important, since multiple blood vessels were identified in the stalk in our patient (Figure 5(c)). We used a detachable snare before resection of the polyp and it was quite useful to prevent bleeding from the cut surface (Figure 3).

Various types of subepithelial tumors occur in the duodenum, varying from Brunner's gland hyperplasia, Brunner's gland hamartoma, neuroendocrine tumors, gastrointestinal stromal tumors, leiomyomas, ectopic pancreas, lipomas, gangliocytic paragangliomas, lymphomas, and varices [3]. Among these, Brunner's gland hamartomas, lipomas, and gangliocytic paragangliomas can be pedunculated. Lipomas appear as a soft, round, yellowish mass covered with a smooth surface. Endoscopic ultrasonography shows a homogenous, hyperechoic mass in the submucosal layer. Gangliocytic paragangliomas are rare tumors characterized by triphasic cellular differentiation composed of epithelioid neuroendocrine cells, spindle cells with Schwann cell differentiation, and ganglion cells [16–18]. The tumor presents as a single lesion in the duodenum exhibiting a polypoid, pedunculated, or sessile tumor [19]. On endoscopic ultrasonography, gangliocytic paragangliomas are typically seen as an isoechoic mass in the submucosal layer [20]. Hizawa et al. reviewed the endoscopic ultrasonography features of six cases of Brunner's gland hamartoma and they noted that single or multiple cystic structures within the submucosa could be detected in four patients and solid echogenicity in the remaining two patients [10, 21]. Although the cystic structure may be found in the duodenum in association with Brunner's gland hyperplasia, duplication cyst, ectopic pancreas, central necrosis of gastrointestinal stromal tumor, pancreatic pseudocyst, and varices, these lesions do not present a pedunculated appearance. Therefore, endoscopic ultrasonography provides endoscopists with an important tool with which to diagnose pedunculated lesions in the duodenum.

In conclusion, we treated a patient with Brunner's gland hamartoma showing pedunculated morphology. Hamartomatous components were observed in the head of the polyp, suggesting that the stalk resulted from the traction of the normal duodenal mucosa. When a solitary, pedunculated polyp with cystic structure is identified at the duodenum, it is important for clinicians to consider Brunner's gland hamartoma in the differential diagnosis, despite the rarity of the disease.

References

[1] T. Nakabori, S. Shinzaki, T. Yamada et al., "Atypical duodenal ulcer and invagination caused by a large pedunculated duodenal Brunner's gland hamartoma," *Gastrointestinal Endoscopy*, vol. 79, no. 4, pp. 679–680, 2014.

[2] B. Muezzinoglu, H. Ustun, B. Demirhan, and F. Hilmioglu, "Brunner's gland adenoma: case report," *New Zealand Medical Journal*, vol. 108, no. 992, p. 14, 1995.

[3] P. Chattopadhyay, A. K. Kundu, S. Bhattacharyya, and A. Bandyopadhyay, "Diffuse nodular hyperplasia of Brunner's gland presenting as upper gastrointestinal haemorrhage," *Singapore Medical Journal*, vol. 49, no. 1, pp. 81–83, 2008.

[4] J. A. Levine, L. J. Burgart, K. P. Batts, and K. K. Wang, "Brunner's gland hamartomas: clinical presentation and pathological features of 27 cases," *American Journal of Gastroenterology*, vol. 90, no. 2, pp. 290–294, 1995.

[5] N. D. Patel, A. D. Levy, A. K. Mehrotra, and L. H. Sobin, "Brunner's gland hyperplasia and hamartoma: imaging features with clinicopathologic correlation," *American Journal of Roentgenology*, vol. 187, no. 3, pp. 715–722, 2006.

[6] K. Kim, S. J. Jang, H. J. Song, and E. Yu, "Clinicopathologic characteristics and mucin expression in Brunner's gland proliferating lesions," *Digestive Diseases and Sciences*, vol. 58, no. 1, pp. 194–201, 2013.

[7] J. Sedano, R. Swamy, K. Jain, and S. Gupta, "Brunner's gland hamartoma of the duodenum," *The Annals of the Royal College of Surgeons of England*, vol. 97, no. 5, pp. e70–e72, 2015.

[8] K.-M. Chen, M.-H. Chang, and C.-C. Lin, "A duodenal tumor with intermittent obstruction," *Gastroenterology*, vol. 146, no. 4, pp. e7–e8, 2014.

[9] M. Powers, G. S. Sayuk, and H. L. Wang, "Brunner gland cyst: report of three cases," *International Journal of Clinical and Experimental Pathology*, vol. 1, no. 6, pp. 536–538, 2008.

[10] L. Lu, R. Li, G. Zhang, Z. Zhao, W. Fu, and W. Li, "Brunner's gland adenoma of duodenum: report of two cases," *International Journal of Clinical and Experimental Pathology*, vol. 8, no. 6, pp. 7565–7569, 2015.

[11] Y.-Y. Chen, W.-W. Su, M.-S. Soon, and H.-H. Yen, "Hemoclip-assisted polypectomy of large duodenal Brunner's gland hamartoma," *Digestive Diseases and Sciences*, vol. 51, no. 9, pp. 1670–1672, 2006.

[12] Y.-P. Gao, J.-S. Zhu, and W.-J. Zheng, "Brunner's gland adenoma of duodenum: a case report and literature review," *World Journal of Gastroenterology*, vol. 10, no. 17, pp. 2616–2617, 2004.

[13] D. T. Walden and N. E. Marcon, "Endoscopic injection and polypectomy for bleeding Brunner's gland hamartoma: case report and expanded literature review," *Gastrointestinal Endoscopy*, vol. 47, no. 5, pp. 403–407, 1998.

[14] O. Kehl, H. Buhler, B. Stamm, and R. W. Amman, "Endoscopic removal of a large, obstructing and bleeding duodenal Brunner's gland adenoma," *Endoscopy*, vol. 17, no. 6, pp. 231–232, 1985.

[15] E. Shemesh, S. Ben Horin, I. Barshack, and S. Bar-Meir, "Brunner's gland hamartoma presenting as a large duodenal polyp," *Gastrointestinal Endoscopy*, vol. 52, no. 3, pp. 435–436, 2000.

[16] H. K. Park and H. S. Han, "Duodenal gangliocytic paraganglioma with lymph node metastasis," *Archives of Pathology and Laboratory Medicine*, vol. 140, no. 1, pp. 94–98, 2016.

[17] A. G. Hernandez, E. D. Lanuza, A. C. Matias et al., "Large gangliocytic paraganglioma of the duodenum: a rare entity," *World Journal of Gastrointestinal Surgery*, vol. 7, no. 8, pp. 170–173, 2015.

[18] Y. Okubo, T. Nemoto, M. Wakayama et al., "Gangliocytic paraganglioma: a multi-institutional retrospective study in Japan," *BMC Cancer*, vol. 15, no. 1, article 269, 2015.

[19] B. W. Scheithauer, F. E. Nora, J. Lechago et al., "Duodenal gangliocytic paraganglioma. Clinicopathologic and immunocytochemical study of 11 cases," *American Journal of Clinical Pathology*, vol. 86, no. 5, pp. 559–565, 1986.

[20] T. J. Loftus, J. L. Kresak, D. H. Gonzalo, G. A. Sarosi Jr., and K. E. Behrns, "Duodenal gangliocytic paraganglioma: a case report and literature review," *International Journal of Surgery Case Reports*, vol. 8, pp. 5–8, 2015.

[21] K. Hizawa, K. Iwai, M. Esaki et al., "Endosonographic features of Brunner's gland hamartomas which were subsequently resected endoscopically," *Endoscopy*, vol. 34, no. 12, pp. 956–958, 2002.

Aberrant Pancreatic Tissue in a Mediastinal Enteric Duplication Cyst: A Rarity with Review of Literature

Meha Mansi,[1] Nidhi Mahajan,[1] Sonam Mahana,[1] C. R. Gupta,[2] and Anup Mohta[2]

[1]*Department of Pathology, Chacha Nehru Bal Chikitsalaya, New Delhi, India*
[2]*Department of Pediatric Surgery, Chacha Nehru Bal Chikitsalaya, New Delhi, India*

Correspondence should be addressed to Nidhi Mahajan; nidhi0615@gmail.com

Academic Editor: Chia-Tung Shun

Mediastinal enteric duplication cysts are a rare congenital malformation encountered mainly in neonates and infants. It is a distinct entity within the family of foregut duplication cysts. It can present with respiratory distress due to mass effect and hence surgical excision is the preferred treatment. Histologically, it is characterised by a double layered smooth muscle wall with intestinal lining epithelium. We report a case of mediastinal enteric duplication cyst with aberrant pancreatic tissue in a neonate due to its rarity and early presentation. A neonate presented with respiratory distress and a cystic mass in the right posterior mediastinum. The lesion was excised and on histopathological analysis the diagnosis of mediastinal enteric duplication cyst was made. Also, aberrant pancreatic tissue which has been reported rarely was noted in this case. We discuss this case and review similar cases reported in literature.

1. Introduction

Mediastinal enteric duplication cysts are rare congenital malformations seen in neonates and infants. They are a type of foregut duplication cysts, with the other subtypes being bronchogenic and esophageal cyst [1]. The clinical presentation of these cysts depends upon the anatomic site of the gut involved, mass effect of the cyst, and symptoms or complications related to the ectopic mucosal lining which may be present in the cyst. This being extremely important in children as functional gastric mucosa may lead to excessive acid secretion and perforation and ectopic pancreatic tissue may lead to hypoglycaemic attacks. Both the presentations are difficult to diagnose especially in paediatric population. We report a case of mediastinal enteric duplication cyst with aberrant pancreatic tissue in the submucosa for its rarity and dubious radiological features and also review in parallel the literature.

2. Case Report

A 29-day-old neonate weighing 4.2 kg was referred with respiratory distress since day four of life. The child was born of a nonconsanguineous marriage, at 37 weeks, with birth weight of 3.5 kg. The pregnancy and delivery were unremarkable. At admission, the child had poor activity with respiratory rate of 30/minute and pulse rate of 140/minute. Heart sounds were normal. There was decreased air entry on the right side. Biochemical investigations were normal. On the X-ray, a homogeneous opacity was seen in the right middle and lower lung fields with shift of mediastinum to the left (Figure 1). No vertebral defect was seen. In view of pneumothorax, a chest tube was put. Ultrasound, however, showed a well-defined cystic lesion in the right lower lung field. Contrast-enhanced computerised tomography confirmed the presence of a well-defined multilocular cystic collection in the posterior aspect of middle and lower zone of right lung (Figure 2). The hematological profile and serum biochemistry were within the normal limits. Based on the clinical and radiological findings, differential diagnosis of a duplication cyst or congenital cystic adenomatoid malformation was suggested. The patient underwent right thoracotomy with excision of the cyst. The chest was approached by right thoracotomy through the 5th intercostal space. Intraoperatively, a large tense cyst measuring 5 × 4 × 3.5 cms was noted

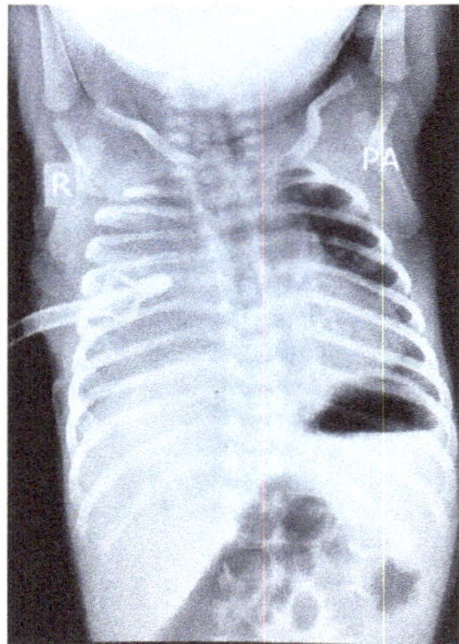

FIGURE 1: Chest radiograph showing a homogeneous opacity in the right middle and lower lung fields with shift of mediastinum to left.

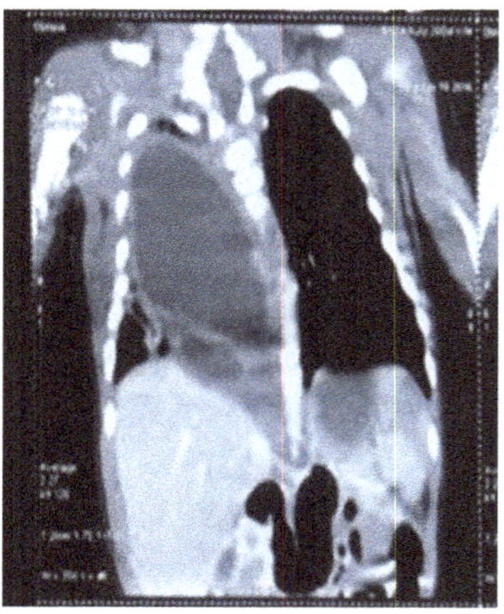

FIGURE 2: Computed tomography scan showed a well-defined fluid attenuation lesion with broad base towards the mediastinum with few loculations.

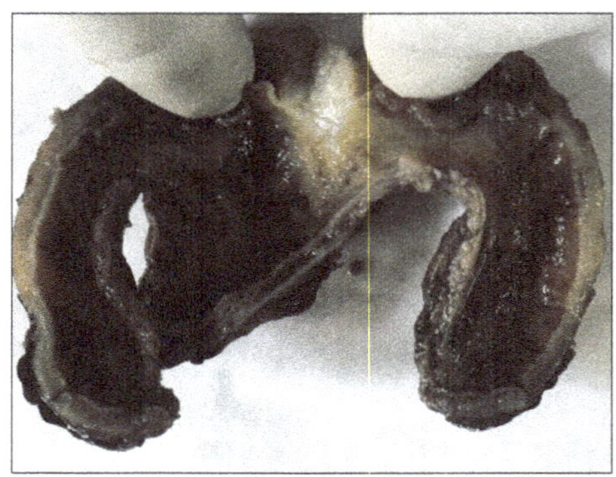

FIGURE 3: Specimen comprising of a unilocular mass with thickened wall and inner surface markedly congested.

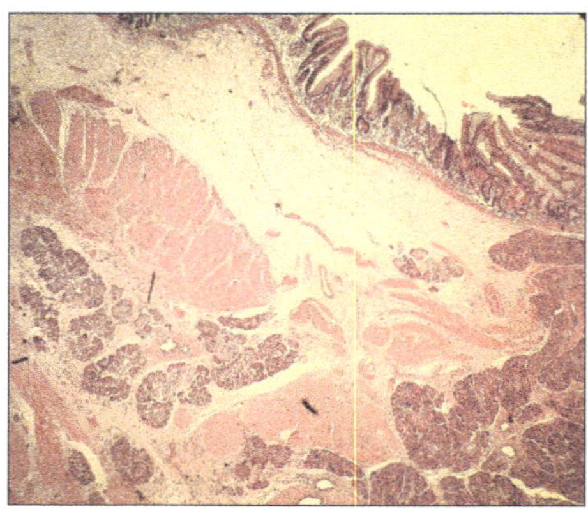

FIGURE 4: Microphotograph showing scanner view of the cyst wall showing double layered intestinal wall with normal intestinal mucosa and pancreatic rests within the muscularis (Hematoxylin & Eosin, 40x).

arising from the posterior mediastinum densely adherent to the lower esophagus and the diaphragm. No communication with the esophageal lumen was present. The cyst was slowly dissected free from both the structures. The cyst could be separated easily from the lung parenchyma. The vertebra was also normal.

On gross pathological examination, the cyst was greyish brown, multiloculated with wall thickness of 0.5 cm (Figure 3). Microscopic sections showed a cyst wall lined by intestinal epithelium with a double layered muscular wall. Aberrant pancreatic tissue was noted in the submucosa and muscularis propria (Figures 4 and 5). Though the Islets of Langerhans were not seen, isolated endocrine cells were seen scattered amidst the exocrine acini. Final histopathological diagnosis of an enteric duplication cyst with ectopic pancreatic rest was suggested. The postoperative course was uneventful. The patient is doing well at follow-up and has not developed any complications.

3. Discussion

The term duplication cyst was first introduced in 1711 by Blassius and Bremer [1]. Gastrointestinal tract duplication cysts are rare congenital malformations seen in infants and children. Midgut duplication cysts are the commonest, followed by foregut and hindgut duplication cysts. Foregut duplication cysts constitute 10% of all mediastinal tumors [1]. They are further classified on the basis of their embryonic origin into bronchogenic, esophageal, and enteric duplication cysts.

Mediastinal enteric cyst is rare and in 60% cases these cysts are diagnosed in neonates and infants with a slight male preponderance [2]. In a case series reported by Cohen et al., out of 15 foregut cysts, none was of enteric type [1]. Enteric cysts associated with vertebral anomalies are called neurenteric cysts. These are usually seen associated with vertebral anomalies like vertebral fusion, scoliosis, anterior and posterior spina bifida, hemivertebrae, diastomyelia, and absence of vertebra [3].

Mediastinal enteric cyst is usually seen in the right posterior mediastinum. It normally presents with pressure symptoms like respiratory distress due to pressure on the

Table 1

Study	Age and sex	Duplication cyst type	Ectopic tissue type
Qazi et al., 1990 [4]	8 years/M	Esophageal gastroenteric duplication cyst	Pancreatic
Prasad et al., 2002 [5]	1 day/M	Mediastinal enteric duplication cyst	Pancreatic
Anagnostou et al., 2009 [2]	2 days/F	Mediastinal enteric duplication cyst	Pancreatic
Present case	4 days/M	Mediastinal enteric duplication cyst	Pancreatic

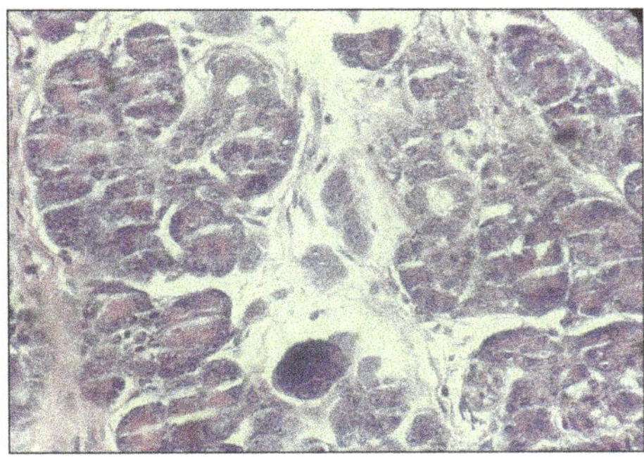

Figure 5: Microphotograph showing acini with cells having abundant eosinophilic granular cytoplasm (Hematoxylin & Eosin, 400x).

bronchi or lung, cough, cyanosis, retrosternal pain, and dysphagia. Children may present with recurrent chest infections. Hematemesis may occur if there is a communication with the esophagus. Ectopic gastric mucosa can be present, leading to peptic ulceration, haemorrhage, or perforation. The current case also presented with respiratory distress and showed a left mediastinal shift.

X-ray of a duplication cyst is an extremely important first-line investigation. Lateral and posterior-anterior views detect maximum lesions and show a homogeneous mass in the posterior mediastinum, usually on the right side. Ultrasonography has limited value; however, on endoscopic ultrasound, a duplication cyst appears as an anechoic or hypoechoic homogeneous cystic lesion with regular margins. Contrast-enhanced computerised tomography confirmed the presence of a well-defined homogeneously enhancing multilocular cystic lesion located in or adjacent to the wall of the part of alimentary canal.

Histopathologically, the cyst shows smooth muscle wall lined by enteric type epithelium. Ectopic gastric lining may be present. Pancreatic tissue in the mediastinum appears as a part of germ cell tumors or as pseudocysts; its presence in the wall of enteric cysts is extremely rare and to the best of our knowledge has been reported only thrice in literature [5] (Table 1). The etiology behind an ectopic rest in the present case is unclear but it has been postulated as pancreatic cell migration and heteroplasia [6]. It is of importance as functional pancreatic tissue may produce insulin and lead to erratic unexplained hypoglycemic episodes in such patients. In the current case, the cyst wall showed unremarkable intestinal lining mucosa with a good volume of ectopic pancreatic rest which was nonfunctional in our case as child had no history suggestive of hypoglycemia and normal biochemistry.

Differentiation from other cystic lesions of the mediastinum like neurenteric cyst, pericardial cyst, thymic cyst, bronchogenic cysts, meningocele, lymphangioma, mature cystic teratoma, cystic schwannomas, cystic thymomas, and cystic tubercular lymphadenitis is important as it has important implications in further management of the patient.

Neurenteric cyst shows variable lining epithelium from respiratory, transitional to squamous. The wall shows variably thickened muscularis layer along with few nerve twigs and dystrophic neurons. There may be evidence of calcification. Pericardial cysts are usually thin walled, benign, filled with clear fluid, and lined by mesothelium. Thymic cysts may be unilocular or multilocular and are thin walled tense cysts filled with brown fluid showing pericystic fibrosis with inflammation, haemorrhage, and cholesterol clefts in the wall [7]. Lymphangiomas are extremely rare, usually present later in life till they obtain significant sizes, and histologically characterised by flattened endothelial lining of the wall filled with lymphatic fluid. Cystic teratomas are rare and usually seen in young adults and comprise of elements from all germ cell lines, especially hair follicles and sebaceous glands.

Thoracoscopic surgical excision of the cyst is the mainstay of treatment with comprehensive supportive care. This resolves the majority of the cases and is associated with minimal morbidity. Few cases which have esophageal or vertebral connections need thoracotomy. In our case, the cyst was quite large in size and expertise in thoracoscopy was not available; hence, the patient was taken up for thoracotomy. To conclude, early intervention is needed in these cases before the patient becomes symptomatic as these lesions, once symptomatic, tend to be associated with higher intraoperative complications and, if left untreated, may be complicated by perforation, obstruction, or haemorrhage. It is important for the pathologists to be aware of the vast differential diagnosis of mediastinal cysts on histopathology which would require thorough sampling to arrive at a correct diagnosis. An active search for ectopic gastric/pancreatic rests is recommended, for both its academic importance and clinical correlation in symptomatic patients.

References

[1] B. J. Birmole, B. K. Kulkarni, A. S. Vaidya, and S. S. Borwankar, "Intrathoracic enteric foregut duplication cyst.," *Journal of Postgraduate Medicine*, vol. 40, no. 4, pp. 228–230, 1994.

[2] E. Anagnostou, V. Soubasi, E. Agakidou, C. Papakonstantinou, N. Antonitsis, and M. Leontsini, "Mediastinal gastroenteric cyst in a neonate containing respiratory-type epithelium and pancreatic tissue," *Pediatric Pulmonology*, vol. 44, no. 12, pp. 1240–1243, 2009.

[3] R. Carachi and A. Azmy, "Foregut duplications," *Pediatric Surgery International*, vol. 18, no. 5-6, pp. 371–374, 2002.

[4] F. M. Qazi, K. R. Geisinger, J. B. Nelson, J. R. Moran, and M. B. Hopkins III, "Symptomatic congenital gastroenteric duplication cyst of the esophagus containing exocrine and endocrine pancreatic tissues," *American Journal of Gastroenterology*, vol. 85, no. 1, pp. 65–67, 1990.

[5] A. Prasad, Y. K. Sarin, S. Ramji, V. S. Suri, A. Sinha, and V. Malhotra, "Mediastinal enteric duplication cyst containing aberrant pancreas," *Indian Journal of Pediatrics*, vol. 69, no. 11, pp. 961–962, 2002.

[6] M. Iglesias Sentís, J. Belda Sanchís, J. M. Gimferrer Garolera, M. Catalán Biela, M. Rubio Garay, and J. Ramírez Ruz, "Mediastinal enteric cyst: unusual clinical presentation and histopathology," *Archivos de Bronconeumologia*, vol. 40, no. 4, pp. 185–187, 2004.

[7] G. M. Graeber, L. D. Thompson, D. J. Cohen, L. D. Ronnigen, J. Jaffin, and R. Zajtchuk, "Cystic lesion of the thymus. An occasionally malignant cervical and/or anterior mediastinal mass," *Journal of Thoracic and Cardiovascular Surgery*, vol. 87, no. 2, pp. 295–300, 1984.

37

Hematochezia: An Uncommon Presentation of Colonic Tuberculosis

Fares Ayoub,[1] Vikas Khullar,[2] Harry Powers,[1] Angela Pham,[2] Shehla Islam,[3] and Amitabh Suman[2]

[1]*Department of Medicine, University of Florida, Gainesville, FL 32608, USA*
[2]*Department of Medicine, Division of Gastroenterology, University of Florida, Gainesville, FL 32608, USA*
[3]*Department of Medicine, Division of Infectious Disease, University of Florida, Gainesville, FL 32608, USA*

Correspondence should be addressed to Fares Ayoub; fares.ayoub@medicine.ufl.edu

Academic Editor: Tetsuo Hirata

Abdominal tuberculosis (TB) is an uncommon entity in the United States. Colonic TB is reported in 2-3% of patients with abdominal TB. It is frequently misdiagnosed as Crohn's disease or carcinoma of the colon due to their shared clinical, radiographic, and endoscopic presentations. We present a case of a 72-year-old male with colonic tuberculosis presenting as hematochezia. Our patient presented with shortness of breath and weight loss. Chest X-ray demonstrated ill-defined bilateral parenchymal opacities in the perihilar, mid, and lower lung zones. The patient was diagnosed and treated for community acquired pneumonia, with no improvement. Hematochezia complicated by symptomatic hypotension developed later in the course of admission. Colonoscopy revealed multiple ulcers at the anus and transverse and ascending colon as well as the cecum with stigmata of bleeding. Biopsy of a sigmoid ulcer was consistent with colonic tuberculosis. Antitubercular therapy was initiated, but the patient passed away secondary to multiorgan failure 29 days into admission.

1. Introduction

After a resurgence in the incidence of tuberculosis (TB) infections in the United States between 1985 and 1992 due to the human immunodeficiency virus (HIV) epidemic, the incidence of TB had annually declined. However, as of 2015, TB incidence has leveled in the US and TB elimination (defined as <1 TB case per 1 million persons annually) remains elusive [1]. Gastrointestinal tuberculosis is a manifestation of extrapulmonary tuberculosis. In 2014, extrapulmonary TB constituted 20.57% of TB cases reported to the CDC and continues to be a missed diagnosis for providers not considering TB in their differential diagnoses [2].

Tuberculosis affecting the gastrointestinal tract was recognized as early as the fourth century BC in texts by Hippocrates [3]. While TB of the gastrointestinal tract is not as common as pulmonary TB, it is an important cause for TB related morbidity and mortality. The pathophysiology of this form of tuberculosis involves spread of mycobacteria to the gastrointestinal tract by number of means: hematogenous spread, swallowing of sputum contaminated with live *M. tuberculosis* bacilli, ingestion of contaminated food, or direct spread from adjacent organs [4]. The terminal ileum and the ileocecal valve are the most commonly affected parts, followed by the ascending colon which is usually affected through continuous involvement extending from the cecum. This predilection for the terminal ileum has been attributed to the presence of large amounts of lymphoid tissue and the longer contact duration of gastrointestinal contents with the lumen [5].

Classically, gastrointestinal TB may present with fever, weight loss, anorexia, abdominal pain, nausea, vomiting, or diarrhea. Hematochezia is a less common presentation [5]. Physical exam findings are nonspecific but may include abdominal tenderness, ascites, and hepatomegaly [4, 5]. Diagnosis is often delayed, as this form of tuberculosis is commonly misdiagnosed as Crohn's disease or carcinoma of the colon due to their similar clinical, radiographic, and endoscopic presentations [5, 6]. Laboratory testing is also nonspecific but may reveal anemia, leukocytosis, increased alkaline phosphatase, and hypoalbuminemia. A chest X-ray may demonstrate evidence of pulmonary TB; however, a normal reading does not exclude disease, as only 15–20% of intestinal TB is associated with active pulmonary TB [7]. CT scanning of the abdomen can exhibit mural thickening, extramural inflammation, and strictures [8]. Colonoscopy can demonstrate ulceration, nodularity, polyps, and luminal narrowing. Mukewar et al. found ulceration to be the most common lesion, found in 88% of patients. Ulcers were largely linear, transverse, or circumferential, covered with yellowish or whitish exudates and surrounding mucosa was inflamed with edema and nodularity. Other lesions found on colonoscopy include polyps which mimicked carcinoma of the colon, as well as unnegotiable luminal narrowing in a smaller subset of patients [5]. Biopsy of colonic ulcers typically demonstrates either caseating or noncaseating granulomas with predominantly lymphocytic chronic inflammation. Acid-fast bacilli (AFB) staining can demonstrate the presence of mycobacteria; however, in one series, this was reported to be positive in only 36% of cases. Other diagnostic tests include tissue culture, PCR, and immunostaining [9].

Treatment of gastrointestinal tuberculosis is analogous to the treatment of pulmonary TB, with 2 months of conventional antituberculous therapy (rifampicin, isoniazid, pyrazinamide, and ethambutol), followed by rifampicin and isoniazid for an additional 4 months [10]. Surgical resection may be required in cases of severe stricture causing high-grade intestinal obstruction.

2. Case

A 72-year-old African American male with no past medical history was hospitalized for shortness of breath and unintentional weight loss for a month prior to presentation. On further questioning, he reported that his shortness of breath had developed over the past year and was associated with an intermittent dry cough. A few days prior to presentation, he had developed fatigue, subjective fever, and chills. He was otherwise asymptomatic. At the time of presentation, he had a blood pressure of 134/85 mmHg, a heart rate of 128 bpm, a respiratory rate of 18 bpm, and an oral temperature of 37.1°C. On physical examination, he appeared to be cachectic. His chest and abdominal exams were within normal limits. The remainder of the examination was unremarkable.

Laboratory testing revealed a myriad of abnormalities. A complete blood count was significant for normocytic anemia with a hemoglobin of 12 g/dL and an MCV of 81.0 fL as well as thrombocytosis with a platelet count of 552 × 10^3/microliter. A metabolic panel revealed hyponatremia with a sodium level of 123 mmol/L, hyperkalemia with a potassium of 6.2 mmol/L, acute renal failure with a creatinine of 8.0 mg/dL and a BUN of 98 mg/dL, and an elevated anion gap metabolic acidosis with a pH of 7.3, a serum CO2 of 11 mmol/L, and an anion gap of 28 mmol/L. Testing for human immunodeficiency virus (HIV) was negative. Urinalysis was remarkable for pyuria with >180 WBC/high

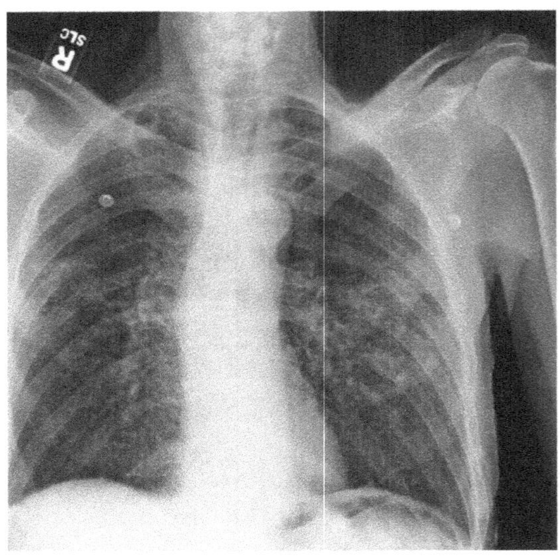

Figure 1: Posteroanterior chest X-ray demonstrating extensive ill-defined bilateral parenchymal opacities in the perihilar, mid, and lower lung zones.

powered field and a negative urine nitrite. This was thought to indicate sterile pyuria, as conventional urine culture techniques were initially negative. A chest X-ray revealed extensive ill-defined bilateral parenchymal opacities in the perihilar, mid, and lower lung zones (Figure 1). The patient was admitted to the hospital for further management of acute renal failure and respiratory abnormalities. Blood and urine cultures were obtained. The patient was hydrated with intravenous normal saline and intravenous ceftriaxone therapy was initiated for a tentative diagnosis of community acquired pneumonia. Over the course of the following three days, the patient's hemoglobin decreased from 12 g/dL to 8 g/dL. A fecal immunohistochemical test for blood in stool was positive and the gastroenterology consult service recommended both an upper endoscopy and lower endoscopy.

Esophagogastroduodenoscopy was unremarkable. Colonoscopy was marred by inadequate bowel preparation but was significant for diverticulosis in the sigmoid and descending and transverse colon with purulent discharge associated with one diverticular opening. It also demonstrated an ulcer in the sigmoid colon which was biopsied (Figure 2). The presence of other ulcers was unclear due to the poor bowel preparation. These findings raised suspicion for acute diverticulitis and the patient's antimicrobial coverage was broadened to include ciprofloxacin and metronidazole. The following day the patient passed a large amount of blood per rectum, developed hypotension with a blood pressure of 79/49 mmHg, and was transferred to the medical intensive care unit. A repeat urgent colonoscopy revealed multiple ulcers at the anus and transverse and ascending colon as well as the cecum; the terminal ileum appeared normal (Figure 3).

A CT scan of the chest obtained for acute hypoxic respiratory failure showed extensive patchy consolidation and reticulonodular opacities throughout the lungs with a 1.3 cm cavitary lesion in the right apex as well as mediastinal and

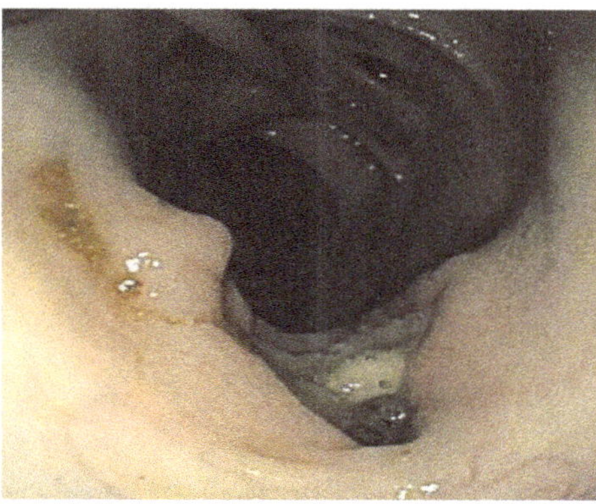

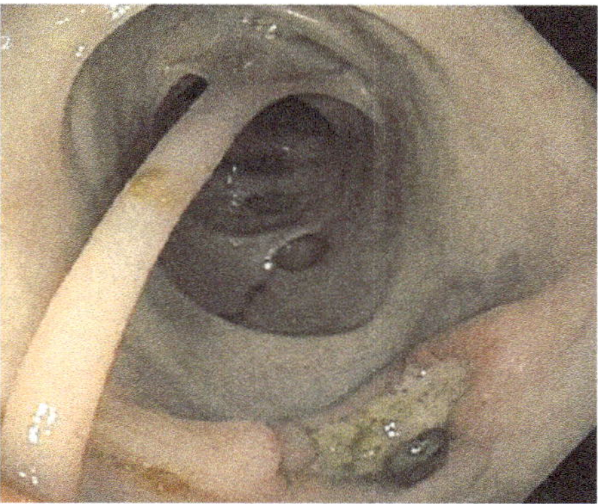

FIGURE 2: First colonoscopy: extensive diverticulosis and solitary ulcer in the sigmoid colon.

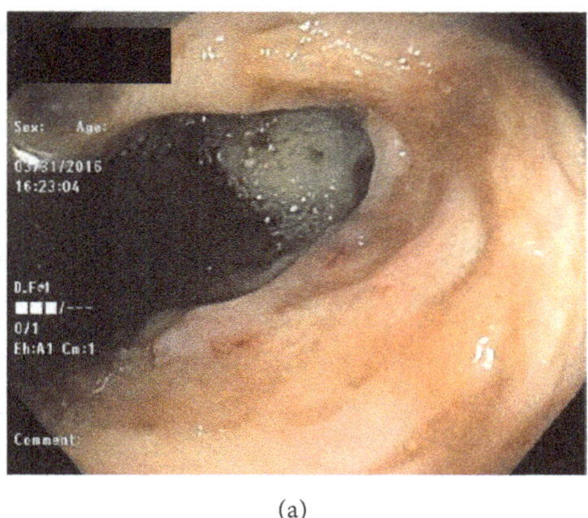

(a)

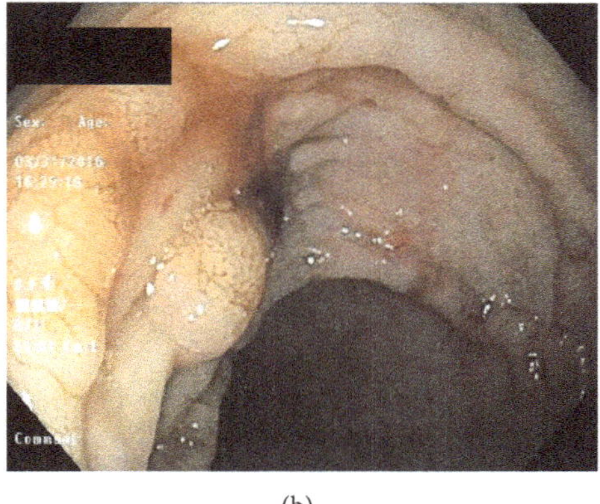

(b)

FIGURE 3: Second colonoscopy: (a) cecal ulcer and (b) transverse colon ulcer.

hilar lymphadenopathy. These findings were suspicious for atypical infection (Figure 4). The patient underwent bronchoscopy with bronchoalveolar lavage and a lavage sample was AFB stain positive. Pathology of the sigmoid ulcer biopsy revealed focal active colitis with cryptitis, crypt abscesses, and mild stromal lymphoplasmacytic inflammation. AFB stain of the sigmoid ulcer biopsy was positive with findings consistent with mycobacterium (Figure 5). AFB stain of a urine sample obtained to explain sterile pyuria was also positive. The patient was placed under respiratory isolation and was started on appropriate antitubercular therapy.

Over the course of our patient's hospitalization, his clinical condition continued to decline. Multiorgan failure requiring vasopressor support later ensued and the patient ultimately passed away 29 days into admission.

3. Discussion

We present a case of diffuse systemic tuberculosis (TB) infection involving the colon, urinary tract, and lungs complicated by multiorgan failure and death. Unique to our patient was the lack of typical risk factors for TB infection. The patient had no history of travel to TB endemic areas and denied incarceration, homelessness, or exposure to infected individuals. It remains unclear where the patient may have contracted the infection; however, earlier exposure to infected individuals or family members that the patient does not recall is possible. Also unique in our patient's case is the presentation of colonic tuberculosis with hematochezia causing hemodynamic instability. Rectal bleeding is a rare presentation of colonic TB; only a handful of case reports have documented this manifestation [11].

Our patient's initial colonoscopy findings of a rectal ulcer, as well as diverticulosis showing signs of active infection, were highly suspicious for acute diverticulitis (Figure 2). However, initial colonoscopy was marred by poor bowel preparation and did not demonstrate the extent of colonic involvement with ulceration and there was low suspicion of active tuberculosis as a potential cause for the patient's drop in hemoglobin. Given our patient's advanced age as well as the presence of multiple diverticulae, angiodysplastic changes in colonic vessels were also part of our differential for lower gastrointestinal bleeding. However, massive hematochezia the following day prompted repeat colonoscopy which showed multiple new ulcers involving all segments of the colon, raising concern for an infectious process (Figure 3). No biopsies were obtained during the second colonoscopy due to active bleeding. Acid-fast stain of the sigmoid ulcer biopsy obtained during the first colonoscopy showed acid-fast organisms consistent with mycobacteria (Figure 5).

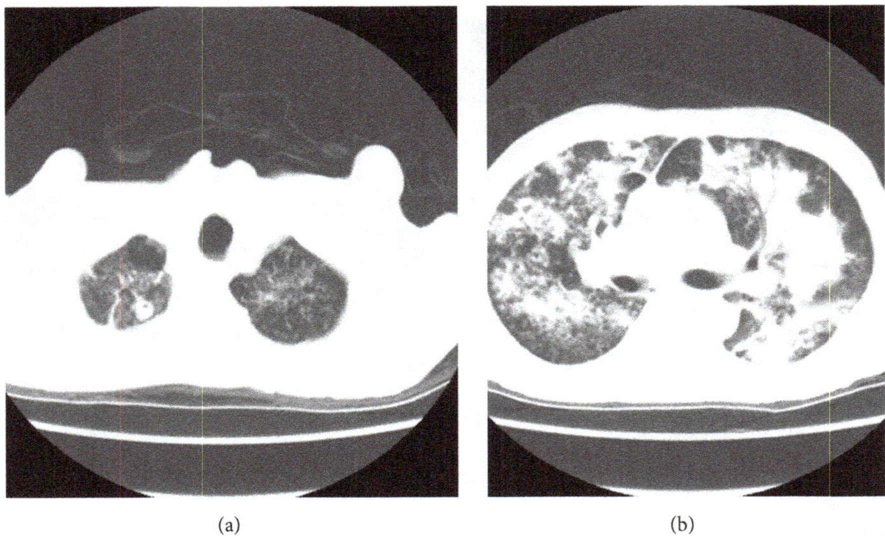

FIGURE 4: CT chest with IV contrast taken on day 13. (a) shows right upper lobe cavitary lesion. (b) shows multilobar consolidation.

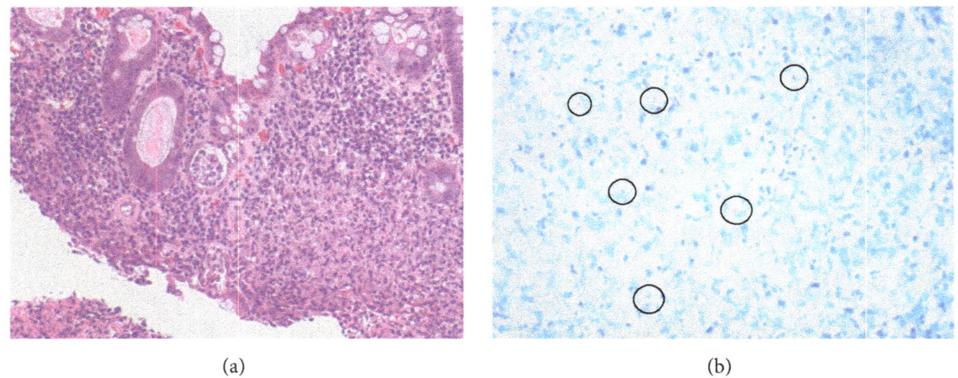

FIGURE 5: (a) 20x hematoxylin and eosin (H&E) stain demonstrating active colitis with crypt abscess and an ill-defined defined granulomatous area. (b) 40x AFB stain of the splenic flexure with necrotizing granuloma and acid-fast bacilli (circled).

Tuberculosis remains a "great mimicker" and must continue to be part of the differential diagnosis in cases of colitis especially in individuals who have additional findings suspicious for infection on chest imaging. While staining for acid-fast bacilli is not routine practice in pathology laboratories, this should be considered in select patients who present with concerns for infection, especially both in the lungs and in the gastrointestinal tract. As described above however, only 15–20% of intestinal TB is associated with active pulmonary TB, thus providers must maintain a high index of suspicion to allow early diagnosis and management.

Our case also serves as a reminder for the importance of postexposure testing and prophylaxis in healthcare workers. Nosocomial transmission of TB in the healthcare setting is well described; cases of multidrug resistant TB transmitted to providers and patients in hospitals have also been reported [12, 13]. In hospitals that receive more than 200 TB admissions a year, incidence of hospital worker infection has been reported to be as high as 10% a year [14].

Hospital-based infection control programs are essential in the control of such transmission. Airborne infection isolation rooms (previously termed negative pressure isolation rooms) should be utilized for patients with suspected or confirmed tuberculosis. N95 masks that filter particles ≥1 micrometer in diameter with at least 95 percent efficiency should be utilized by healthcare staff and offered to visitors of patients with suspected or confirmed tuberculosis. Nonessential invasive diagnostic procedures ought to be postponed unless absolutely necessary [15].

Providers exposed to patients with active pulmonary tuberculosis should be assessed for symptoms suggestive of active TB infection (hemoptysis, weight loss, and fever) and, if present, should undergo chest X-ray with sputum acid-fast stain and culture. Providers without symptoms of active infection are to undergo tuberculin skin testing or an interferon-gamma release assay at baseline and again 8 to 12 weeks postexposure [12].

In our case, all providers who may have been exposed to the patient underwent interferon-γ release assay testing (QuantiFERON, Cellestis Ltd., Australia) at baseline and 8 weeks postexposure. The patient's family members were also contacted and offered screening and appropriate treatment for TB.

References

[1] J. L. Salinas, G. Mindra, M. B. Haddad, R. Pratt, S. F. Price, and A. J. Langer, "Leveling of tuberculosis incidence—United States, 2013–2015," *Morbidity and Mortality Weekly Report*, vol. 65, no. 11, pp. 273–278, 2016.

[2] Department of Health and Human Services (US DHHS), Centers for Disease Control and Prevention (CDC), and Division of TB Elimination, "Online Tuberculosis Information System (OTIS), National Tuberculosis Surveillance System, United States, 1993–2014," CDC WONDER Online Database, January 2016. Data for all years updated by June 5, 2015, http://wonder.cdc.gov/tb-v2014.html.

[3] T. A. Sheer and W. J. Coyle, "Gastrointestinal tuberculosis," *Current Gastroenterology Reports*, vol. 5, no. 4, pp. 273–278, 2003.

[4] K. D. Horvath and R. L. Whelan, "Intestinal tuberculosis: return of an old disease," *The American Journal of Gastroenterology*, vol. 93, no. 5, pp. 692–696, 1998.

[5] S. Mukewar, S. Mukewar, R. Ravi, A. Prasad, and K. S. Dua, "Colon tuberculosis: endoscopic features and prospective endoscopic follow-up after anti-tuberculosis treatment," *Clinical and Translational Gastroenterology*, vol. 3, article e24, 2012.

[6] Y. Lee, S. Yang, J. Byeon et al., "Analysis of colonoscopic findings in the differential diagnosis between intestinal tuberculosis and crohn's disease," *Endoscopy*, vol. 38, no. 6, pp. 592–597, 2006.

[7] B. Nagi, R. Kochhar, D. K. Bhasin, and K. Singh, "Colorectal tuberculosis," *European Radiology*, vol. 13, no. 8, pp. 1907–1912, 2003.

[8] W.-K. Lee, F. Van Tonder, C. J. Tartaglia et al., "CT appearances of abdominal tuberculosis," *Clinical Radiology*, vol. 67, no. 6, pp. 596–604, 2012.

[9] K. M. Kim, A. Lee, K. Y. Choi, K. Y. Lee, and J. J. Kwak, "Intestinal tuberculosis: clinicopathologic analysis and diagnosis by endoscopic biopsy," *The American Journal of Gastroenterology*, vol. 93, no. 4, pp. 606–609, 1998.

[10] V. K. Kapoor, "Abdominal tuberculosis," *Postgraduate Medical Journal*, vol. 74, no. 874, pp. 459–467, 1998.

[11] M. Kela, V. B. Agrawal, R. Sharma, R. Agarwal, and A. Agarwal, "Ileal tuberculosis presenting as a case of massive rectal bleeding," *Clinical and Experimental Gastroenterology*, vol. 2, article 129, 2009.

[12] M. S. Bader and D. S. McKinsey, "Postexposure prophylaxis for common infectious diseases," *American Family Physician*, vol. 88, no. 1, pp. 25–32, 2013.

[13] Centers for Disease Control (CDC), "Nosocomial transmission of multidrug-resistant tuberculosis to health-care workers and HIV-infected patients in an urban hospital—Florida," *Morbidity and Mortality Weekly Report*, vol. 39, no. 40, pp. 718–722, 1990.

[14] D. Menzies, A. Fanning, L. Yuan, and M. Fitzgerald, "Tuberculosis among health care workers," *New England Journal of Medicine*, vol. 332, no. 2, pp. 92–98, 1995.

[15] Centers for Disease Control and Prevention, "Guidelines for preventing the transmission of Mycobacterium tuberculosis in health-care settings, 2005," MMWr 54.RR-17, 2–107, 2005.

38

Gastric Metastasis from Renal Cell Carcinoma, Clear Cell Type, Presenting with Gastrointestinal Bleeding

Mouhanna Abu Ghanimeh,[1] Ayman Qasrawi,[2] Omar Abughanimeh,[2] Sakher Albadarin,[3] and John H. Helzberg[4]

[1] *Internal Medicine Department, Division of Gastroenterology, Henry Ford Hospital, Detroit, MI, USA*
[2] *Internal Medicine Department, University of Missouri-Kansas City School of Medicine, Kansas City, MO, USA*
[3] *Division of Gastroenterology, University of Missouri-Kansas City School of Medicine, Kansas City, MO, USA*
[4] *Saint Luke's Hospital of Kansas City, University of Missouri-Kansas City School of Medicine, Kansas City, MO, USA*

Correspondence should be addressed to Mouhanna Abu Ghanimeh; mouhannaka87@yahoo.com

Academic Editor: Naohiko Koide

Renal cell carcinoma (RCC) accounts for 80–85% of all primary renal neoplasms. Although RCC can metastasize to any organ, gastric metastases from RCC are exceedingly rare. A 67-year-old male presented with melena and acute blood loss anemia. The patient had a history of RCC that had been treated with a radical nephrectomy. He had a recent myocardial infarction and was receiving double antiplatelet therapy. After hemodynamic stabilization, esophagogastroduodenoscopy showed a polypoid mass in the gastric fundus. The mass was excised. Histological and immunohistochemical evaluation were consistent with clear cell RCC. The polypoid lesion is consistent with a late solitary metastasis.

1. Introduction

Renal cell carcinoma (RCC) is the most common cancer originating from the kidney [1]. Lungs, bones, liver, and brain are the most common sites of RCC metastasis [2, 3]. Uncommon metastatic sites, including the gastrointestinal tract [2–4], have also been reported. Gastric metastasis from RCC is rare [5, 6]. Gastric metastases are typically asymptomatic, single, and located in the gastric body or fundus [5, 6]. If they are symptomatic, then gastrointestinal bleeding and anemia are the most common presentations [5, 6]. RCC has the potential for late solitary metastasis. Isolated gastric metastasis from RCC can occur up to 20 years after radical nephrectomy [7]. Immunohistochemistry is useful and increasingly utilized in the diagnosis of RCC [8, 9]. The prognosis in patients with metastatic RCC is generally poor, with a five-year survival rate of 5–30% [10]. Treatment options include embolization and epinephrine injection for bleeding and endoscopic resection or surgery [11–16]. Surgical resection remains the best therapeutic option for a solitary gastric metastasis, resulting in significant survival prolongation in eligible patients [8].

2. Case Summary

A 67-year-old man presented with multiple episodes of melena. His past medical history involved polycystic kidney disease, live donor renal transplantation in 2002 with chronic immunosuppression, and metastatic left-sided RCC that had been treated with radical nephrectomy and the resection of a pulmonary metastasis in 2014. The patient had chronic kidney disease, stage 3, and a recent ST segment elevation myocardial infarction with percutaneous coronary intervention and drug eluting stent insertion. The patient was on 81 mg of aspirin daily and 90 mg of ticagrelor twice daily.

His vital signs on presentation were blood pressure of 121/82 mmHg, pulse of 105 bpm, and oral temperature of 97.7°F (36.5 C). On physical examination, the patient was pale and in mild distress. Abdominal and cardiopulmonary exams

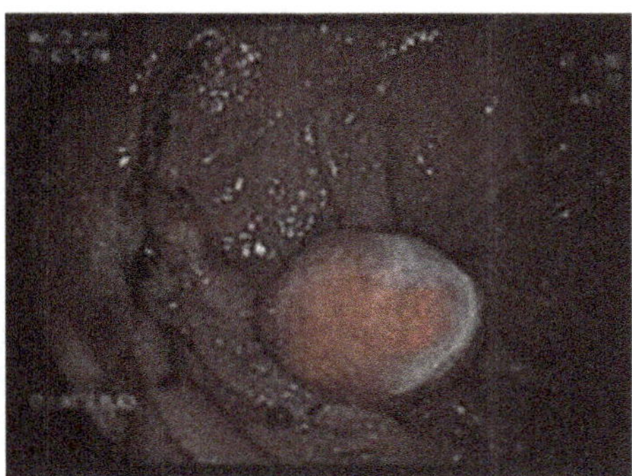

FIGURE 1: EGD showing a 2.5 to 3.0 cm polypoid mass in the gastric fundus.

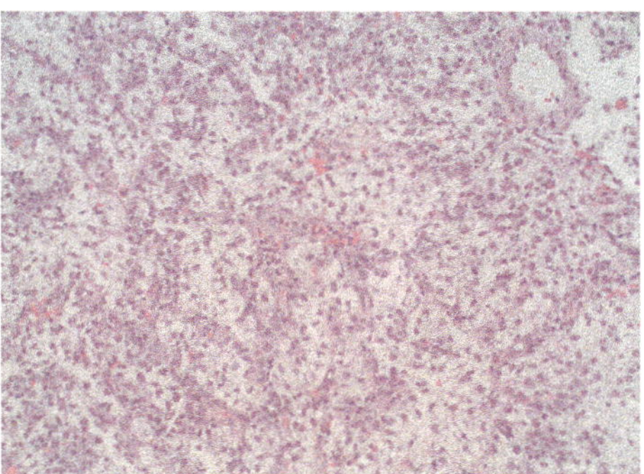

FIGURE 2: Histological evaluation including H&E staining, showing a tumor comprising nests and fascicles of cells with abundant clear cytoplasm and moderately pleomorphic nuclei with prominent eosinophilic nucleoli.

were unremarkable. Initial laboratory evaluation included a hemoglobin (Hb) level of 8.8 g/dl (normal: 13.5–17.5 g/dl), white blood cell (WBC) count of 11,300/cmm (normal: 4,000–11,000/cmm), platelet count of 344,000 cmm (normal: 150,000–450,000/cmm), serum creatinine level of 2.3 mg/dl (normal: 0.9–1.2 mg/dl), aspartate aminotransferase level of 27 units/L (normal: 15–46 units/L), alanine aminotransferase level of 14 units/L (normal: 13–69 units/L), alkaline phosphatase level of 117 units/L (normal: 42–140 units/L), and international normalized ratio of 1.2. The patient was admitted for stabilization and further evaluation of gastrointestinal bleeding.

The patient was intravenously given 80 mg pantoprazole, followed by 8 mg/hour continuous infusion. A total of 2 units of packed red blood cells were transfused. Aspirin and ticagrelor were initially held. On hospitalization day 1, the patient was hemodynamically stable and his Hb level increased to 9.9 g/dl after transfusion. The gastroenterology service proceeded with esophagogastroduodenoscopy (EGD). The EGD (Figure 1) showed a 2.5 to 3.0 cm polypoid mass in the gastric fundus. The polyp was completely removed with a polypectomy snare and cautery. Bleeding occurred after polyp removal, and hemostasis was achieved via local epinephrine injection and the application of two Cook hemostasis clips.

The histological examination (Figure 2) demonstrated a submucosal tumor comprising nests and fascicles of cells with abundant clear cytoplasm and moderately pleomorphic nuclei with prominent eosinophilic nucleoli. A background vascular network and acute and chronic inflammation were observed. Immunohistochemical staining (Figure 3) was positive for pan-keratin PAX2 and PAX8. Both the morphology and immune phenotypes were most consistent with metastatic clear cell RCC, comparable with the right lung lesion resected in 2014.

The patient was observed overnight in the intensive care unit. His Hb levels were unchanged, and he remained hemodynamically stable. Aspirin and ticagrelor treatments were resumed. The oncology service decided to follow him as an outpatient. Chemotherapy was not initiated with his recent gastrointestinal blood loss and myocardial infarction. He is following up now with the oncology and cardiology clinics and has been doing well about 1 year after his presentation.

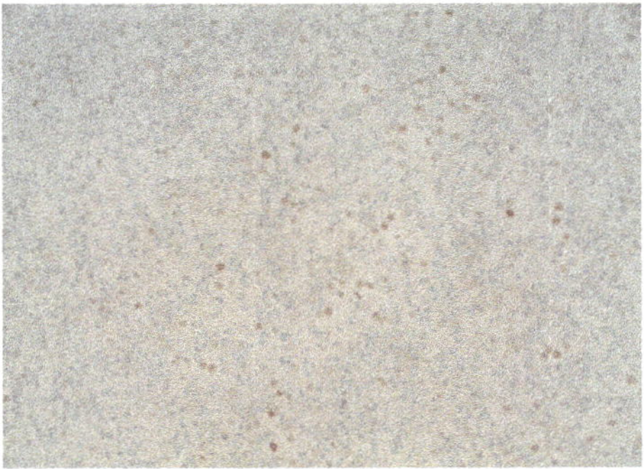

FIGURE 3: Positive immunohistochemical staining for PAX-2, consistent with clear cell RCC.

3. Discussion

RCC is the most common cancer originating from the kidney. This cancer is responsible for 80 to 85% of all primary renal neoplasms and accounts for 3% of all adult malignancies [1]. RCC has an abundant blood supply and can metastasize to any organ [2, 3]. The most common sites of metastasis include the lungs, bones, liver, and brain [2, 3]. However, RCCs can also metastasize to unusual sites, including the pancreas, thyroid gland, adrenal gland, skeletal muscle, and skin [4]. Studies have reported that a metastasis is detected in approximately 30% of RCC patients on initial presentation [3].

Gastric metastases from RCC are exceedingly rare [5, 6]. Pollheimer et al. [5] reported 5 patients who developed gastric metastases from an Austrian database of 2,082 RCC patients. In one instance, an isolated gastric metastasis from RCC was reported 20 years after radical nephrectomy [7]. Table 1 summarizes the reported cases of gastric metastases from RCC in English literature.

Most RCC gastric metastases are located in the gastric body and fundus. Single tumors predominate over multiple tumors [6]. Histologically, these metastases are situated in the submucosa [3, 12]. Clear cell histology is the predominant form of RCC. The presence of clear cell morphology in any unknown lesion should prompt the pathologist to consider

TABLE 1: Reported cases of gastric metastases from RCC in English literature.

Case and reference	Age (years), sex	Gastrointestinal symptoms	Location	Gross appearance	Histology	Treatment
Sullivan et al. 1980 [17]	69, male	Bleeding	Antrum	Mass, single	Not specified	Antrectomy
Boruchowicz et al. 1995 [18]	48, male	Dysphagia	Fundus	Polypoid, single	Clear cell	Chemotherapy
Blake et al. 1995 [11]	63, male	Bleeding	Not specified	Not specified	Not specified	Embolization
Odori et al. 1998 [19]	58, male	Not specified	Not specified	Ulcerated, single	Clear cell	Total gastrectomy with regional lymph node dissection
Picchio et al. 2000 [12]	64, female	Bleeding	Body	Polyp, single	Clear cell	Subtotal gastrectomy
Mascarenhas et al. 2001 [20]	66, male	Bleeding	Body	Ulcerated, single	Clear cell	Partial gastrectomy
Kobayashi et al. 2004 [21]	78, male	Anemia	Lower one-third of stomach	Mass, single	Not specified	Gastrectomy
Kok Wee et al. 2004 [7]	60, male	Bleeding	Body	2 lesions, protruding and ulcerated	Clear cell	Endoscopic therapy
Lamb et al. 2005 [13]	69, male	Bleeding	Body	Mass, single	Clear cell	Embolization, octreotide
Riviello et al. 2006 [22]	68, male	Bleeding	Fundus	Mass, single	Clear cell	Total gastrectomy, chemotherapy
Pezzoli et al. 2007 [15]	78, male	Anemia	Body	Polyps, multiple	Clear cell	Endoscopic mucosal resection
Saidi and Remine 2007 [23]	Not specified	Bleeding	Body	Polyp, single	Clear cell	Wedge resection
Pollheimer et al. 2008 [5]	69, male	Epigastric pain, Nausea, vomiting	Body	Mass, single	Clear cell	Tamoxifen
Pollheimer et al. 2008 [5]	77, male	No symptoms	Antrum	Ulcerated, single	Clear cell	Interferon
Pollheimer et al. 2008 [5]	83, female	Bleeding	Antrum	Mass, multiple	Clear cell	Endoscopic therapy, interferon
Pollheimer et al. 2008 [5]	65, female	Bleeding	Not specified	Multiple	Clear cell	Endoscopic therapy
Pollheimer et al. 2008 [5]	69, male	Anemia, epigastric pain	Body	Multiple	Clear cell	Endoscopic therapy, sunitinib
Kibria et al. 2009 [24]	53, male	Bleeding	Fundus	Polypoid, single	Clear cell	None
Yamamoto et al. 2009 [8]	74, male	Bleeding	Body	Polypoid, single	Not specified	Wedge resection
Tiwari et al. 2010 [25]	58, female	Bleeding	Antrum	Polypoid, single	Clear cell	Subtotal gastrectomy
García-Campelo et al. 2010 [26]	75, male	No symptoms	Fundus and body	Polypoid, multiple	Not specified	Sunitinib
Sugasawa et al. 2010 [27]	69, male	Anemia	Fundus	Ulcerated, single	Clear cell	Wedge resection
Eslick and Kalantar 2011 [28]	65, male	Bleeding	Lower stomach	Polypoid, single	Clear cell	Polypectomy
Kim et al. 2012 [29]	79, male	Abdominal pain	Body	Erosive, single	Clear cell	Partial gastrectomy
Xu et al. 2012 [30]	60, male	Anemia	Body	Polyp, multiple	Clear cell	Polypectomy, sunitinib, sorafenib
Siriwardana et al. 2012 [31]	71, male	Anemia	Not specified	Polypoid, single	Clear cell	Endoscopic mucosal resection

Table 1: Continued.

Case and reference	Age (years), sex	Gastrointestinal symptoms	Location	Gross appearance	Histology	Treatment
Namikawa et al. 2012 [32]	65, male	Not specified	Body	Polypoid, single	Clear cell	Wedge resection
Rodrigues et al. 2012 [33]	45, female	Bleeding	Body	Ulcerated, single	Not specified	Sunitinib
Chibbar et al. 2013 [34]	69, female	Anemia	Body	Polypoid, single	Clear cell	Endoscopic mucosal resection
Rita et al. 2014 [6]	77, male	Bleeding, abdominal pain	Body	Polypoid, single	Clear cell	Endoscopic resection
Greenwald et al. 2014 [35]	62, male	No symptoms	Fundus	Mass, single	Clear cell	Partial gastrectomy
Costa et al. 2014 [36]	66, female	Anemia	Body	Ulcerated, single	Not specified	Laparoscopic wedge resection
Kumcu et al. 2014 [37]	59, male	Bleeding, weight loss	Body	Polypoid, single	Clear cell	Partial gastrectomy
Sakurai et al. 2014 [38]	62, male	Bleeding, anemia	Body	Mass, single	Clear cell	Partial gastrectomy
Forman et al. 2015 [39]	76, female	Bleeding, anemia	Cardia	Mass, single	Clear cell	Not specified
Kongnyuy et al. 2016 [40]	68, male	Anemia, bleeding	Fundus	Mass, single	Clear cell	Not specified
Our case 2016	67, male	Bleeding	Fundus	Polypoid, single	Clear cell	Polypectomy, plan for chemotherapy

the possibility of metastatic RCC, even in the absence of a prior diagnosis [30]. Endoscopically, the metastasis typically appears as a polypoid submucosal-like tumor with a central depression.

In general, the outcome with metastatic RCC is poor with 5-year survival rates of 5–30% [10]. Patients with a single metastasis fare better than those with multiple metastases.

Immunohistochemistry, particularly for vimentin and PAX-2, is a useful adjunct in the diagnosis of RCC [8, 9]. Vimentin is an intermediate filament protein expressed in normal renal tissues [8], and PAX-2 is a transcription factor required for the development and proliferation of renal tubules [9]. Both proteins are expressed in 85% of metastatic clear cell RCCs [8, 9].

Consent

Informed consent was obtained from the patient to publish the details of this case report.

Disclosure

This manuscript is a detailed description of a previous abstract which was presented at the annual meeting of the American College of Gastroenterology (ACG) 2016 in Las Vegas and it was published as an abstract in a special supplement of the American Journal of Gastroenterology.

Authors' Contributions

Mouhanna Abu Ghanimeh, Ayman Qasrawi, and Omar Abughanimeh wrote and revised the manuscript. Sakher Albadarin edited the manuscript. John H. Helzberg performed the EGD, provided images, and reviewed and edited the final manuscript.

References

[1] R. L. Siegel, K. D. Miller, and A. Jemal, "Cancer statistics, 2016," *CA: A Cancer Journal for Clinicians*, vol. 66, no. 1, pp. 7–30, 2016.

[2] J. D. Maldazys and J. B. deKernion, "Prognostic factors in metastatic renal carcinoma," *Journal of Urology*, vol. 136, no. 2, pp. 376–379, 1986.

[3] Y. Satomi, Y. Senga, M. Nakahashi et al., "A clinical and statistical study of 333 cases of renal cell carcinoma. III. Operations, operative findings and results," *Nihon Hinyokika Gakkai Zasshi*, vol. 78, no. 8, pp. 1394–1402, 1987.

[4] V. T. DeVita, T. S. Lawrence, and S. A. Rosenberg, *Cancer: Principles and Practice of Oncology*, Wolters Kluwer Health/Lippincott Williams & Wilkins, Philadelphia, Pa, USA, 8th edition, 2008.

[5] M. J. Pollheimer, T. A. Hinterleitner, V. S. Pollheimer, A. Schlemmer, and C. Langner, "Renal cell carcinoma metastatic to the stomach: Single-centre experience and literature review," *BJU International*, vol. 102, no. 3, pp. 315–319, 2008.

[6] H. Rita, A. Isabel, C. Iolanda et al., "Treatment of gastric metastases from renal cell carcinoma with endoscopic therapy," *Clinical Journal of Gastroenterology*, vol. 7, no. 2, pp. 148–154, 2014.

[7] L. Kok Wee, R.-Y. Shyu, L.-F. Sheu, T.-Y. Hsieh, J.-C. Yan, and P.-J. Chen, "Metastatic renal cell cancer," *Gastrointestinal Endoscopy*, vol. 60, no. 2, p. 265, 2004.

[8] D. Yamamoto, Y. Hamada, S. Okazaki et al., "Metastatic gastric tumor from renal cell carcinoma," *Gastric Cancer*, vol. 12, no. 3, pp. 170–173, 2009.

[9] N. Gokden, M. Gokden, D. C. Phan, and J. K. McKenney, "The utility of PAX-2 in distinguishing metastatic clear cell renal cell carcinoma from its morphologic mimics: An immunohistochemical study with comparison to renal cell carcinoma marker," *American Journal of Surgical Pathology*, vol. 32, no. 10, pp. 1462–1467, 2008.

[10] S. C. Campbell and C. N. Andrew, "Renal tumours," in *Campbell-Walsh Urology*, pp. 1582–1605, Sounders Elsevier Pub, 9th edition, 2007.

[11] M. A. Blake, A. Owens, D. P. O'Donoghue, and D. P. MacErlean, "Embolotherapy for massive upper gastrointestinal haemorrhage secondary to metastatic renal cell carcinoma: Report of three cases," *Gut*, vol. 37, no. 6, pp. 835–837, 1995.

[12] M. Picchio, A. Paioletti, E. Santini et al., "Gastric metastasis from renal cell carcinoma fourteen years after radical nephrectomy," *Acta Chirurgica Belgica*, vol. 100, no. 5, pp. 228–230, 2000.

[13] G. W. A. Lamb, J. Moss, R. Edwards, and M. Aitchison, "Case Report: Octreotide as an adjunct to embolisation in the management of recurrent bleeding upper gastrointestinal metastases from primary renal cell cancer," *International Urology and Nephrology*, vol. 37, no. 4, pp. 691–693, 2005.

[14] P. H. Patel, R. S. K. Chaganti, and R. J. Motzer, "Targeted therapy for metastatic renal cell carcinoma," *British Journal of Cancer*, vol. 94, no. 5, pp. 614–619, 2006.

[15] A. Pezzoli, V. Matarese, S. Boccia, L. Simone, and S. Gullini, "Gastrointestinal bleeding from gastric metastasis of renal cell carcinoma, treated by endoscopic polypectomy.," *Endoscopy*, vol. 39, p. E52, 2007.

[16] T. Klatte, N. Kroeger, U. Zimmermann, M. Burchardt, A. S. Belldegrun, and A. J. Pantuck, "The contemporary role of ablative treatment approaches in the management of renal cell carcinoma (RCC): Focus on radiofrequency ablation (RFA), high-intensity focused ultrasound (HIFU), and cryoablation," *World Journal of Urology*, vol. 32, no. 3, pp. 597–605, 2014.

[17] W. G. Sullivan, E. B. Cabot, and R. E. Donohue, "Metastatic renal cell carcinoma to stomach," *Urology*, vol. 15, no. 4, pp. 375–378, 1980.

[18] A. Boruchowicz, P. Desreumaux, V. Maunoury et al., "Dysphagia revealing esophageal and gastric metastases of renal carcinoma," *The American Journal of Gastroenterology*, vol. 90, no. 12, pp. 2263-2264, 1995.

[19] T. Odori, Y. Tsuboi, K. Katoh et al., "A solitary hematogenous metastasis to the gastric wall from renal cell carcinoma four years after radical nephrectomy," *Journal of Clinical Gastroenterology*, vol. 26, no. 2, pp. 153-154, 1998.

[20] B. Mascarenhas, B. Konety, and J. T. Rubin, "Recurrent metastatic renal cell carcinoma presenting as a bleeding gastric ulcer after a complete response to high-dose interleukin-2 treatment," *Urology*, vol. 57, article 168, no. 1, 2001.

[21] O. Kobayashi, H. Murakami, T. Yoshida et al., "Clinical diagnosis of metastatic gastric tumors: clinicopathologic findings and prognosis of nine patients in a single cancer center," *World Journal of Surgery*, vol. 28, no. 6, pp. 548–551, 2004.

[22] C. Riviello, I. Tanini, G. Cipriani et al., "Unusual gastric and pancreatic metastatic renal cell carcinoma presentation 10 years after surgery and immunotherapy: a case report and a review of literature," *World Journal of Gastroenterology*, vol. 12, no. 32, pp. 5234–5236, 2006.

[23] R. F. Saidi and S. G. Remine, "Isolated gastric metastasis from renal cell carcinoma 10 years after radical nephrectomy [4]," *Journal of Gastroenterology and Hepatology (Australia)*, vol. 22, no. 1, pp. 143-144, 2007.

[24] R. Kibria, K. Sharma, S. A. Ali, and P. Rao, "Upper gastrointestinal bleeding revealing the stomach metastases of renal cell carcinoma," *Journal of Gastrointestinal Cancer*, vol. 40, no. 1-2, pp. 51–54, 2009.

[25] P. Tiwari, A. Tiwari, M. Vijay et al., "Upper gastro-intestinal bleeding - rare presentation of renal cell carcinoma," *Urology Annals*, vol. 2, no. 3, pp. 127–129, 2010.

[26] R. García-Campelo, M. Quindós, D. Dopico Vázquez et al., "Renal cell carcinoma: Complete pathological response in a patient with gastric metastasis of renal cell carcinoma," *Anti-Cancer Drugs*, vol. 21, no. 1, pp. S13–S15, 2010.

[27] H. Sugasawa, T. Ichikura, S. Ono et al., "Isolated gastric metastasis from renal cell carcinoma 19 years after radical nephrectomy," *International Journal of Clinical Oncology*, vol. 15, no. 2, pp. 196–200, 2010.

[28] G. D. Eslick and J. S. Kalantar, "Gastric metastasis in renal cell carcinoma: A case report and systematic review," *Journal of Gastrointestinal Cancer*, vol. 42, no. 4, pp. 296–301, 2011.

[29] M.-Y. Kim, H.-Y. Jung, K. D. Choi et al., "Solitary synchronous metastatic gastric cancer arising from T1b renal cell carcinoma: A case report and systematic review," *Gut and Liver*, vol. 6, no. 3, pp. 388–394, 2012.

[30] J. Xu, S. Latif, and S. Weia, "Metastatic renal cell carcinoma presenting as gastric polyps: A case report and review of the literature," *International Journal of Surgery Case Reports*, vol. 3, no. 12, pp. 601–604, 2012.

[31] H. P. P. Siriwardana, M. H. Harvey, S. S. Kadirkamanathan, B. Tang, D. Kamel, and R. Radzioch, "Endoscopic mucosal resection of a solitary metastatic tumor in the stomach: A case report," *Surgical Laparoscopy, Endoscopy and Percutaneous Techniques*, vol. 22, no. 3, pp. e132–e134, 2012.

[32] T. Namikawa, J. Iwabu, H. Kitagawa, T. Okabayashi, M. Kobayashi, and K. Hanazaki, "Solitary gastric metastasis from a renal cell carcinoma, presenting 23 years after radical nephrectomy," *Endoscopy*, vol. 44, no. 2, pp. E177–E178, 2012.

[33] S. Rodrigues, P. Bastos, and G. MacEdo, "A rare cause of hematemesis: Gastric metastases from renal cell carcinoma," *Gastrointestinal Endoscopy*, vol. 75, no. 4, pp. 894-895, 2012.

[34] R. Chibbar, J. Bacani, and S. Zepeda-Gómez, "Endoscopic mucosal resection of a large gastric metastasis from renal cell carcinoma," *ACG Case Reports Journal*, vol. 1, no. 1, pp. 10–12, 2013.

[35] D. Greenwald, E. Aljahdli, D. Nepomnayshy et al., "Synchronous gastric metastasis of renal cell carcinoma with absence of gastrointestinal symptoms," *ACG Case Reports Journal*, vol. 1, no. 4, pp. 196–198, 2014.

[36] T. N. Costa, F. R. Takeda, U. Ribeiro, and I. Cecconello, "Palliative laparoscopic resection of renal cell carcinoma metastatic to the stomach: Report of a case," *World Journal of Surgical Oncology*, vol. 12, no. 1, article no. 394, 2014.

[37] E. Kumcu, M. Gönültas, and H. Ünverdi, "Gastric metastasis of a renal cell carcinoma presenting as a polypoid mass," *Endoscopy*, vol. 46, supplement 1, no. UCTN:E464, 2014.

[38] K. Sakurai, K. Muguruma, S. Yamazoe et al., "Gastric metastasis from renal cell carcinoma with gastrointestinal bleeding: a case report and review of the literature," *International Surgery*, vol. 99, no. 1, pp. 86–90, 2014.

[39] J. Forman, J. Marshak, Y. A. Tseng et al., "Image of the month: gastric metastasis of renal clear cell carcinoma," *The American Journal of Gastroenterology*, vol. 110, article 15, no. 1, 2015.

[40] M. Kongnyuy, S. Lawindy, D. Martinez et al., "A rare case of the simultaneous, multifocal, metastatic renal cell carcinoma to the ipsilateral left testes, bladder, and stomach," *Case Reports in Urology*, vol. 2016, Article ID 1829025, 3 pages, 2016.

Identification of Abnormal Biliary Anatomy Utilizing Real-Time Near-Infrared Cholangiography: A Report of Two Cases

Joseph Bozzay, Diego Vicente, Elliot M. Jessie, and Carlos J. Rodriguez

Walter Reed National Military Medical Center, 8901 Rockville Pike, Bethesda, MD 20889, USA

Correspondence should be addressed to Joseph Bozzay; joseph.d.bozzay.mil@mail.mil

Academic Editor: Gregory Kouraklis

Biliary duct anomalies are commonly encountered during laparoscopic cholecystectomy. Advancements in the field of surgery allow for enhanced intraoperative detection of these abnormalities. Fluorophore injection and near-infrared (NIR) imaging can provide real-time intraoperative anatomic feedback without intraoperative delays and ionizing radiation. This report details two cases where the PINPOINT Endoscopic Fluorescence Imaging System (NOVADAQ, Ontario, Canada) was used to identify anomalies of the biliary tree and guide operative decision-making.

1. Introduction

The laparoscopic cholecystectomy is one of the most common procedures performed by general surgeons today [1]. Anomalous biliary and arterial anatomy can be encountered in up to 50% of cases and can lead to intraoperative challenges, particularly in patients with significant inflammatory changes [2]. Traditionally, intraoperative cholangiography (IOC) has been very useful for the detection of such biliary tree anomalies [1, 3]. However, IOC requires additional participants in the operative procedure, exposes the patient and operative team to ionizing radiation, and can prolong the case [1, 3].

Fluorescent cholangiography (FC) is a technique that can be easily performed with intravenous fluorophore injection and intraoperative near-infrared (NIR) imaging to view its dissemination throughout the biliary system [1, 4, 5]. This allows for real-time feedback during the operation, thereby eliminating logistics associated with performing IOC. There are multiple systems available, including PINPOINT Endoscopic Fluorescence Imaging System (NOVADAQ, Ontario, Canada), the NIR/ICG system (KARL STORZ, Tuttlingen, Germany), and the STRYKER Infrared Fluorescence (IRF) Imaging System (STRYKER Endoscopy, San Jose, CA). Our institution owns a PINPOINT system which was used for our NIR FC. We present two cases where this technology was utilized to identify anomalous biliary and arterial anatomy in patients undergoing laparoscopic cholecystectomy. In addition to summarizing the basics of NIR FC, this report will also discuss NIR FC clinical trials and the various surgical applications of NIR.

2. Case Report 1

Our first patient was a 29-year-old female with a recent episode of gallstone pancreatitis without ultrasound evidence of cholecystitis. An indeterminate preoperative MRCP failed to rule out retained stones in the biliary tree; therefore, IOC was planned. Her past medical history was notable for familial adenomatous polyposis (FAP) and primary hyperparathyroidism. Her past surgical history included a parathyroidectomy, appendectomy, total proctocolectomy with ileal pouch-anal anastomosis and protective ileostomy, reversal of ileostomy, and laparoscopic ventral hernia repair with intra-abdominal mesh placement. Given her multiple intra-abdominal surgeries, ventral mesh, and recent medical history, she was considered a potential challenging laparoscopic case and it was felt that PINPOINT NIR could offer intraoperative assistance and guidance for the expected dissection.

The patient was injected with 1 mL (2.5 mg) of indocyanine green (ICG) at anesthesia induction. In order to avoid trocar placement through the mesh, a 12 mm trocar was placed via direct visualization in the left upper quadrant, just

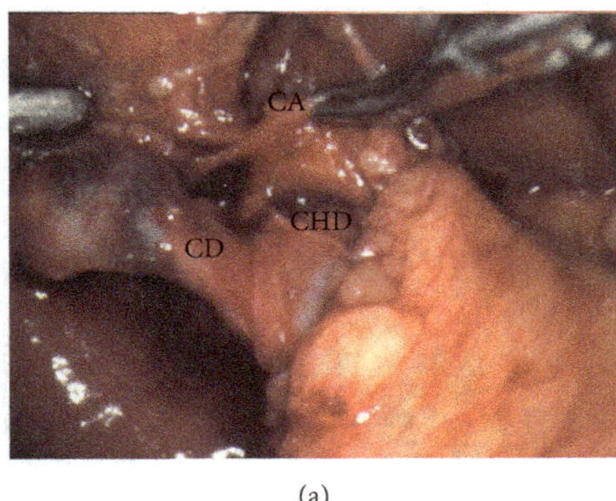

(a)

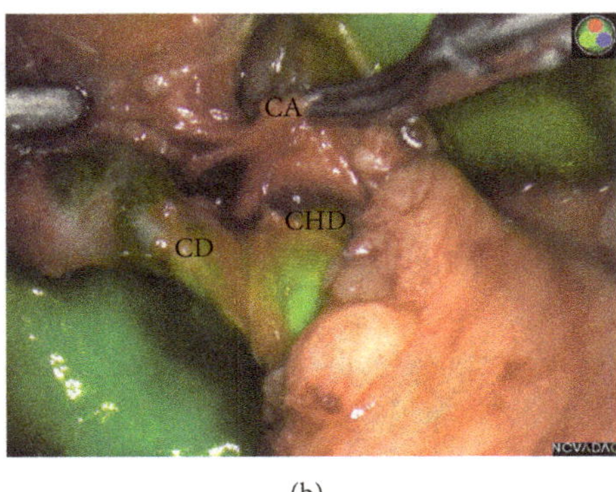

(b)

Figure 1: White light view (panel a) and PINPOINT view (panel b) of the laparoscopic cholecystectomy in the patient with a short cystic duct. CA: cystic artery, CHD: common hepatic duct, and CD: cystic duct.

off the tip of the 11th rib; two 5 mm trocars were placed in the usual subcostal position of the right upper quadrant; and one 5 mm trocar was placed midline, in the subxiphoid position. Eventually, a 10 mm trocar was placed lateral to the mesh, in the left lower quadrant for improved visualization of the gallbladder.

A 10 mm 30° PINPOINT NIR equipped laparoscope was placed through the 12 mm port to provide visualization of the biliary tree. Dense adhesions between small bowel, liver edge, and gallbladder were encountered during dissection to expose the gallbladder. As dissection proceeded towards the infundibulum, FC was periodically performed by selecting the PINPOINT NIR mode on the camera. This allowed us to quickly switch between white light mode and NIR mode (Figures 1(a) and 1(b)). FC easily visualized the gallbladder, a shortened cystic duct, and the common hepatic/cystic duct confluence.

FC allowed for early detection of the confluence of the cystic and common hepatic duct, thus enabling safe, blunt dissection of Calot's Triangle in the setting of a shortened cystic duct. This confluence was not easily seen with the regular white light mode (Figure 1(a)).

After performing a preoperatively planned IOC which was unremarkable, we proceeded to divide the cystic duct. However, we did not feel that the duct was of adequate length for three clips as we were concerned that the distal clip might entrain the biliary tree confluence leading to stricture. Two clips were placed on the cystic duct and two were placed on the infundibulum in order to prevent bile spillage during removal of the gallbladder from the fossa. The gallbladder was removed without difficulty.

On pathologic evaluation, the gallbladder did have evidence of chronic cholecystitis and contained multiple gallstones. The patient recovered without incident from the surgery and was discharged from the hospital the next day. She was seen in clinic and had no complaints. In this case, FC allowed for early identification and safe dissection of a short cystic duct in a challenging patient requiring extensive dissection associated with prior surgery and inflammatory changes from acute pancreatitis and chronic cholecystitis.

3. Case Report 2

Our second patient was a 71-year-old female who had just undergone an endoscopic retrograde cholangiopancreatogram (ERCP) extraction of a common bile duct stone following an episode of gallstone pancreatitis. Her past medical history was notable for paroxysmal atrial fibrillation, but she was otherwise healthy.

As with the first patient, this patient received 1 mL (2.5 mg) of IV ICG at the time general anesthesia was induced. Standard Hasan infraumbilical, subxiphoid (1–5 mm), and RUQ (2–5 mm) ports were placed. Significant adhesions between the liver and abdominal wall were present which suggested Fitz-Hugh-Curtis disease. Once these adhesions were released, the fundus was identified, grasped, and retracted in a cephalad manner.

Dissection of the critical structures revealed the cystic artery to be anterior to the cystic duct with origination from either the proper or right hepatic artery. PINPOINT NIR confirmed that the cystic duct coursed posterior to the cystic artery (Figure 2) and aided in direct visualization of abnormal anatomy. The cystic artery and cystic duct were ligated with clips, divided in standard fashion, and the gallbladder was removed.

The patient was discharged from the hospital without incident on the first postoperative day.

4. Discussion

PINPOINT is the laparoscopic version of the open SPY system. There are other fluorescent cholangiography systems including the NIR/ICG system from KARL STORZ and the STRYKER Infrared Fluorescence (IRF) Imaging System. It utilizes a white light camera and an NIR fluorescence excitation and acquisition system with ICG as the fluorophore [4, 6]. Through pressing a camera-mounted button, PINPOINT can display simultaneous video modes to include conventional white light high definition, fluorescence only, and composite NIR-ICG overlay modes [4–6]. ICG binds to plasma proteins after IV injection, thus enabling it to remain within the intravascular system; however, it only remains

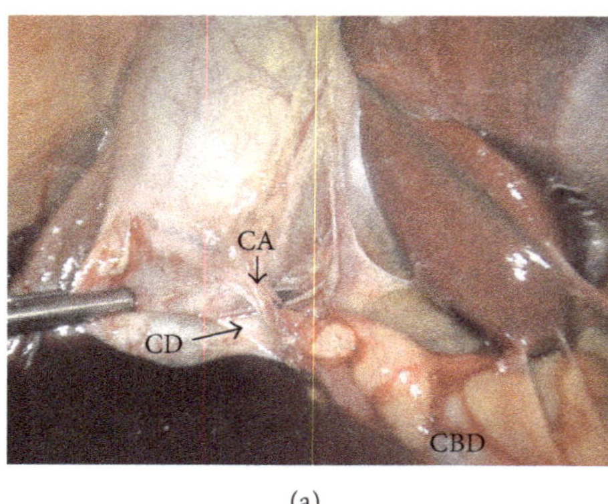

(a)

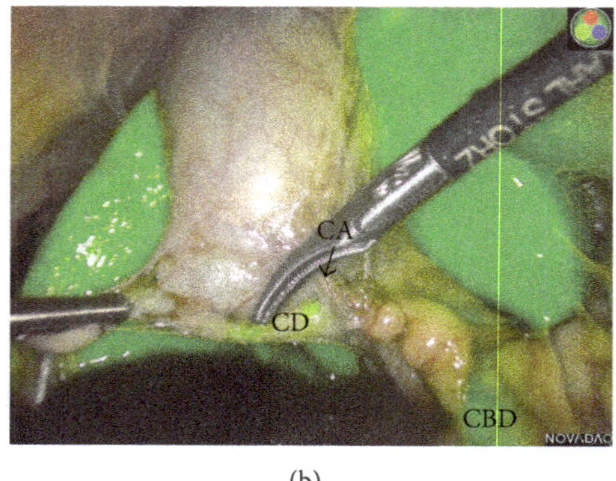

(b)

FIGURE 2: White light view (panel a) and PINPOINT view (panel b) of the laparoscopic cholecystectomy in the patient with a long cystic duct and an anterior cystic artery. CA: cystic artery, CBD: common bile duct, and CD: cystic duct.

in the intravascular space for about three minutes [4–6]. Bound ICG is readily taken up by the liver and is then excreted, unchanged, through the biliary system [1, 5, 7]. ICG is excreted into the bile within minutes after injection and reaches peak concentration at about two hours; however, preoperative injection allows for 30–45 minutes to reach the biliary tree in sufficient concentration to fluoresce when exposed to NIR [1]. Our institution's experience has shown with these and other cases that NIR will continue to show hepatobiliary system enhancement well over two hours after injection.

ICG injection is generally well tolerated with anaphylactic reaction being an exceedingly rare but serious risk [4, 5]. It contains no more than 5% of sodium iodide and so it should be used cautiously in patients who have an allergy to iodides or iodinated imaging agents [4, 5].

Real-time NIR imaging has proven applications to biliary surgery. Matsui and colleagues found that NIR florescence allowed for good identification of biliary anatomy during open or laparoscopic surgery, and they were able to immediately identify damaged or constricted ducts. They concluded that NIR FC provides sensitive and prolonged identification of biliary anatomy and assessment of functional status [7]. A case report with video shows active PINPOINT use to identify an anomalous duct which was thought to be an aberrant right hepatic duct [8]. This helped direct appropriate management of the cystic duct and the patient had no complications [8].

Hutteman and colleagues found ICG-NIR useful for visualizing the common bile duct and biliary anastomoses during pancreaticoduodenectomy and suggested that it could be beneficial in biliary cases with difficult surgical anatomy, as was apparent in our cases [9]. To further evaluate this hypothesis, NIR FC is currently the subject of a randomized study evaluating operative time and safety of operative technique (including bile duct injury and resident autonomy and identification of structures) compared to normal laparoscopic cholecystectomy methods [10]. Another clinic trial by Cleveland Clinic, Florida, has been designed to evaluate the effectiveness of NIR FC compared to standard white light for identifying extrahepatobiliary structures [11]. The multicenter FALCON trial in Netherlands is randomizing patients to either NIR FC or conventional laparoscopic imaging and comparing the time to identification of the "critical view of safety" in addition to other endpoints [12]. These ongoing clinical studies may help determine which patients will benefit the most from the use of NIR FC and if surgical outcomes are affected by its use.

In addition to biliary imaging, NIR-ICG fluorescence has widespread application in surgery to include intraoperative vascular perfusion assessment of myocutaneous flap perforators and hollow viscus anastomoses, as well as oncologic procedures [5, 13, 14]. It is extensively used in the field of plastic surgery to determine the predicted viability of myocutaneous pedicled and free flaps and for assessing skin viability in complex abdominal wall reconstruction cases [5, 13]. Additionally, a recent systemic review concluded that microperfusion techniques utilizing florescent dyes may help guide the management of colorectal anastomosis and impact postoperative complications [15]. In the recent PILLAR II study, NIR was used to intraoperatively assess anastomotic perfusion during colorectal surgery and guide the management of the anastomosis [4]. The cases that had anastomotic adjustments based on NIR perfusion assessment did not develop anastomotic leaks. Shimada et al. reported that ICG fluorescent imaging was useful for evaluating the blood supply to esophagectomy anastomoses but did not find that it reduced the rate of anastomotic leaks in their population of 40 patients [16]. Real-time fluorescence imaging is also being used in the field of surgical oncology to detect disease and improve debulking and wide local excisions and anatomically delineate surrounding structures during organ removal [14]. The ability of NIR to differentiate various tissues offers an advantage over preclinical imaging and the limitations of the human eyesight [14]. Future clinical trials will help further characterize the advantages and limitations of these approaches and determine the impact of NIR on surgical outcomes.

Advances in the field of surgery have allowed surgeons to develop new techniques and to improve operative outcomes. Obvious advantages of NIR FC include real-time anatomic biliary mapping, ease of use, and no need for additional equipment. NIR FC may prove to be a valuable asset in the operating room. Future well-designed studies, such as the one described above, will be useful in this area. Certain patient populations such as those with inflammation or tissue distortion around the gallbladder may benefit from more routine use of NIR FC systems when undergoing laparoscopic cholecystectomy.

Authors' Contributions

Joseph Bozzay, Elliot M. Jessie, and Carlos J. Rodriguez contributed to conception of the study. Joseph Bozzay and Carlos J. Rodriguez contributed to drafting of manuscript. Joseph Bozzay, Diego Vicente, Elliot M. Jessie, and Carlos J. Rodriguez contributed to critical revision.

References

[1] T. Ishizawa, Y. Bandai, M. Ijichi, J. Kaneko, K. Hasegawa, and N. Kokudo, "Fluorescent cholangiography illuminating the biliary tree during laparoscopic cholecystectomy," *British Journal of Surgery*, vol. 97, no. 9, pp. 1369–1377, 2010.

[2] D. V. Kostov and G. L. Kobakov, "Six rare biliary tract anatomic variations: implications for liver surgery," *The Eurasian Journal of Medicine*, vol. 43, no. 2, pp. 67–72, 2011.

[3] K. R. Sirinek and W. H. Schwesinger, "Has intraoperative cholangiography during laparoscopic cholecystectomy become obsolete in the era of preoperative endoscopic retrograde and magnetic resonance cholangiopancreatography?" *Journal of the American College of Surgeons*, vol. 220, no. 4, pp. 522–528, 2015.

[4] M. D. Jafari, S. D. Wexner, J. E. Martz et al., "Perfusion assessment in laparoscopic left-sided/anterior resection (PILLAR II): a multi-institutional study," *Journal of the American College of Surgeons*, vol. 220, no. 1, pp. 82.e1–92.e1, 2015.

[5] J. T. Alander, I. Kaartinen, A. Laakso et al., "A Review of indocyanine green fluorescent imaging in surgery," *International Journal of Biomedical Imaging*, vol. 2012, Article ID 940585, 2012.

[6] D. A. Sherwinter, J. Gallagher, and T. Donkar, "Intra-operative transanal near infrared imaging of colorectal anastomotic perfusion: a feasibility study," *Colorectal Disease*, vol. 15, no. 1, pp. 91–96, 2013.

[7] A. Matsui, E. Tanaka, H. S. Choi et al., "Real-time intra-operative near-infrared fluorescence identification of the extrahepatic bile ducts using clinically available contrast agents," *Surgery*, vol. 148, no. 1, pp. 87–95, 2010.

[8] D. A. Sherwinter, "Identification of anomolous biliary anatomy using near-infrared cholangiography," *Journal of Gastrointestinal Surgery*, vol. 16, no. 9, pp. 1814–1815, 2012.

[9] M. Hutteman, J. R. van der Vorst, J. S. D. Mieog et al., "Near-infrared fluorescence imaging in patients undergoing pancreaticoduodenectomy," *European Surgical Research*, vol. 47, no. 2, pp. 90–97, 2011.

[10] Maimonides Medical Center, "The use of fluorescent imaging for intraoperative cholangiogram during laparoscopic cholecystectomy," in *ClinicalTrials.gov*, National Library of Medicine (US), Bethesda, Md, USA, 2011, https://clinicaltrials.gov/ct2/show/NCT01424215.

[11] Cleveland Clinic, "Fluorescent cholangiography vs white light for bile ducts identification," in *ClinicalTrials.gov*, National Library of Medicine (US), Bethesda, Md, USA, 2016, https://clinicaltrials.gov/ct2/show/NCT02702843.

[12] Maastricht University Medical Center, "FALCON: a multicenter randomized controlled trial," in *ClinicalTrials.gov*, NLM Identifier: NCT02558556, National Library of Medicine (US), Bethesda, Md, USA, 2016, https://clinicaltrials.gov/ct2/show/NCT02558556.

[13] C. Holm, M. Mayr, E. Höfter, U. Dornseifer, and M. Ninkovic, "Assessment of the patency of microvascular anastomoses using microscope-integrated near-infrared angiography: a preliminary study," *Microsurgery*, vol. 29, no. 7, pp. 509–514, 2009.

[14] K. E. Tipirneni, J. M. Warram, L. S. Moore et al., "Oncologic procedures amenable to fluorescence-guided surgery," *Annals of Surgery*, 2016.

[15] S. Nachiappan, A. Askari, A. Currie, R. H. Kennedy, and O. Faiz, "Intraoperative assessment of colorectal anastomotic integrity: a systematic review," *Surgical Endoscopy*, vol. 28, no. 9, pp. 2513–2530, 2014.

[16] Y. Shimada, T. Okumura, T. Nagata et al., "Usefulness of blood supply visualization by indocyanine green fluorescence for reconstruction during esophagectomy," *Esophagus*, vol. 8, no. 4, pp. 259–266, 2011.

Case Report and Literature Review Illustrating the Clinical, Endoscopic, Radiologic, and Histopathologic Findings with Prepouch Ileitis after IPAA and Restorative Proctocolectomy for Refractory Ulcerative Colitis

Christienne Shams,[1] Seifeldin Hakim,[1] Mitual Amin,[2] and Mitchell S. Cappell[3]

[1]*Division of Gastroenterology & Hepatology, Department of Medicine, William Beaumont Hospital, 3535 W. Thirteen Mile Rd, Royal Oak, MI 48073, USA*
[2]*Department of Pathology, William Beaumont Hospital and Oakland University William Beaumont School of Medicine, 3601 W Thirteen Mile Rd, Royal Oak, MI 48073, USA*
[3]*Division of Gastroenterology & Hepatology, Department of Medicine, William Beaumont Hospital and Oakland University William Beaumont School of Medicine, 3535 W. Thirteen Mile Rd, Royal Oak, MI 48073, USA*

Correspondence should be addressed to Mitchell S. Cappell; mitchell.cappell@beaumont.edu

Academic Editor: Daniel C. Damin

Prepouch ileitis (PI) is an uncommon complication of ileal pouch anal anastomosis (IPAA) and restorative proctocolectomy (RPC) for treatment of refractory ulcerative colitis (UC). A case is reported of PI in a 16-year-old girl who presented with severe UC that was initially stabilized with infliximab therapy but re-presented 1 year later with severe UC, refractory to infliximab and corticosteroid therapy, which required IPAA and RPC. Her symptoms resolved postoperatively, but she re-presented 1 year later with 10 loose, bloody, bowel movements/day and involuntary 6-Kg weight-loss. Computerized tomographic enterography showed focal narrowing and mucosal enhancement of the pouch and focal narrowing, abnormal mucosal enhancement, and mural thickening of the prepouch ileum. Pouchoscopy revealed exudates and ulcerations in both the pouch and prepouch ileum up to 50 cm proximal to pouch, as confirmed by histopathology of pouch and ileal biopsies. Capsule endoscopy revealed no small intestinal lesions beyond 50 cm from the pouch. She required antibiotics, hydrocortisone enemas, and eventually azathioprine to control her symptoms. She remains asymptomatic 4 years later while chronically administered azathioprine therapy. Comprehensive literature review demonstrates that this case illustrates the classical clinical, radiologic, endoscopic, and histopathologic findings in PI, a relatively rare syndrome.

1. Introduction

Restorative proctocolectomy (RPC) and ileal pouch anal anastomosis (IPAA) are the treatment of choice for ulcerative colitis (UC) refractory to medical therapy, for UC with severe dysplasia or colon cancer, and sometimes for familial adenomatous polyposis [1–4]. This surgery becomes necessary in 10-30% of patients within one decade after diagnosis of UC [1]. Outcomes are generally favorable, lasting up to 20 years [4]. Prepouch ileitis (PI) affects about 4% of patients undergoing RPC and IPAA [2, 5]. A case is reported of PI after RPC and IPAA, illustrating the classical clinical, radiologic, endoscopic, and histopathologic findings of this rare syndrome.

2. Case

A 16-year-old girl with no significant past medical history presented with bloody diarrhea, abdominal cramps, tenesmus, failure to thrive, and 6-Kg weight-loss during the prior 3 months. Physical examination was unremarkable

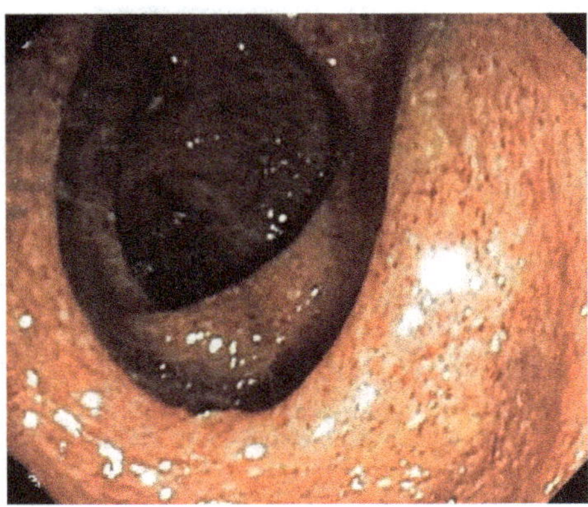

FIGURE 1: Colonoscopy with intubation of terminal ileum shows diffusely erythematous and granular mucosa with focal exudation affecting the rectum through ascending colon, with sparing of the cecum and terminal ileum. The endoscopic findings are consistent with UC.

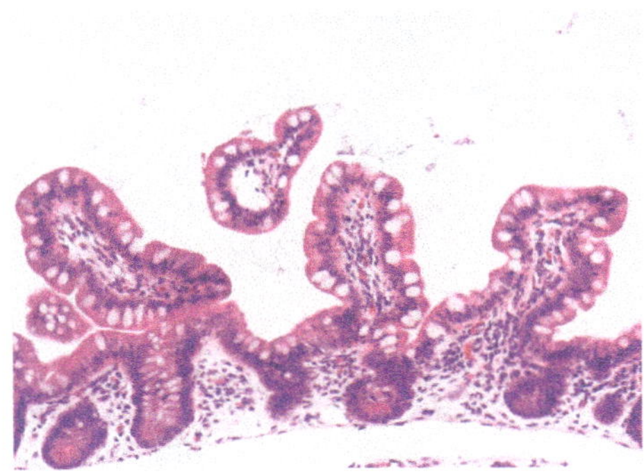

FIGURE 2: Photomicrograph of histopathology with H&E stain of biopsy specimen shows normal ileal mucosa prior to postoperative occurrence of prepouch ileitis, with relatively normal villous height and preserved villous-to-crypt ratio.

except for age-adjusted BMI at the eleventh percentile. Abdominal examination revealed a soft, nontender abdomen and normoactive bowel sounds. Laboratory analysis revealed leukocyte count=8.1 bil/L, hemoglobin=11.4 g/dL, and platelets=207 bil/L. The alkaline phosphatase is 125 U/L, with other parameters of liver function and parameters of renal function within normal limits. Colonoscopy with terminal ileal intubation revealed severely erythematous and granular mucosa with focal exudation from rectum to ascending colon, findings consistent with UC (**Figure 1**), and revealed endoscopically normal appearing cecum and terminal ileum. Histopathologic analysis of colonic biopsies revealed chronic colitis, with a moderate neutrophilic and lymphocytic mucosal infiltrate, crypt distortion, and scattered crypt abscesses. The cecum and terminal ileum appeared histologically normal (**Figure 2**). She was treated with infliximab 5 mg/Kg, with initial symptomatic relief, but re-presented 1 year later with recurrent bloody diarrhea and failure to thrive, despite compliance with infliximab therapy. She developed infliximab antibodies necessitating escalating the infliximab dose, and adding extended-release budesonide 9 mg/day and azathioprine 2 mg/kg/day (after determining that her TPMT (thiopurine methyltransferase) activity was within normal limits). Her symptoms, however, progressed despite therapeutic infliximab levels. She underwent RPC and IPAA for refractory UC, which successfully controlled her symptoms but re-presented one year postoperatively with abdominal pain, 10 loose and bloody bowel movements/day, and involuntary 5-Kg-weight-loss. Fecal lactoferrin and calprotectin levels were elevated. Stool for ova and parasites, bacterial cultures, and *Clostridium difficile* toxin A and B by polymerase chain reaction (PCR) were unremarkable. C-reactive protein (CRP) level was elevated. Computerized tomographic enterography (CTE) showed focal narrowing and enhancement of mucosa within the J-pouch and abnormal mucosal enhancement, mural thickening, and narrowing of afferent ileal limb (**Figures 3(a) and 3(b)**). Pouchoscopy showed moderate exudation and ulcerations in J-pouch (**Figure 4(a)**) and in afferent ileal limb up to 50 cm (**Figure 4(b)**). Histopathologic analysis of J-pouch and afferent ileal limb biopsies revealed chronic active inflammation, highly consistent with pouchitis and PI (**Figure 5**). Immunohistochemistry of ileal biopsies for cytomegalovirus was negative. Capsule endoscopy revealed no small intestinal lesions more proximal than 50 cm in the afferent limb. Ciprofloxacin 500 mg twice daily and metronidazole 500 mg thrice daily were administered for the pouchitis and PI, but this treatment was subsequently escalated to include extended-release budesonide 9 mg/day and daily hydrocortisone enemas. As symptoms persisted, azathioprine 2 mg/kg/day was added, which successfully controlled her symptoms 3 months after initiating the azathioprine therapy. Six months after initiating the azathioprine therapy her fecal lactoferrin and calprotectin levels were within the normal range. At four years of follow-up, the patient has continued to be asymptomatic while chronically taking azathioprine, with normal CRP and erythrocyte sedimentation rate (ESR) levels.

3. Discussion

Despite lack of standard definition, PI is described as histologically evident mucosal inflammation extending beyond the reconstructed pouch up to 50 cm proximally in the afferent limb, and it is usually associated with endoscopically apparent erosions, ulcerations, erythema, and friability in the ileum that had appeared normal at endoscopy before undergoing the surgery [1, 4, 6, 7].

The incidence of PI after RPC and IPAA ranged in two large studies from 4.4% to 6% [1, 8]. PI occurs more frequently in patients who are young, who underwent early colectomy for UC, and who developed intestinal symptoms soon after undergoing RPC and IPAA, possibly because these factors are markers of biologically aggressive UC [1, 7]. Smoking cigarettes does not significantly affect the rate or severity of PI, despite smoking ameliorates UC and pouchitis [1, 2, 9]. Sex does not significantly affect the rate of PI, but males are more likely to develop pouchitis and *Clostridium difficile* infections than females [10]. Pouch anatomy may affect the

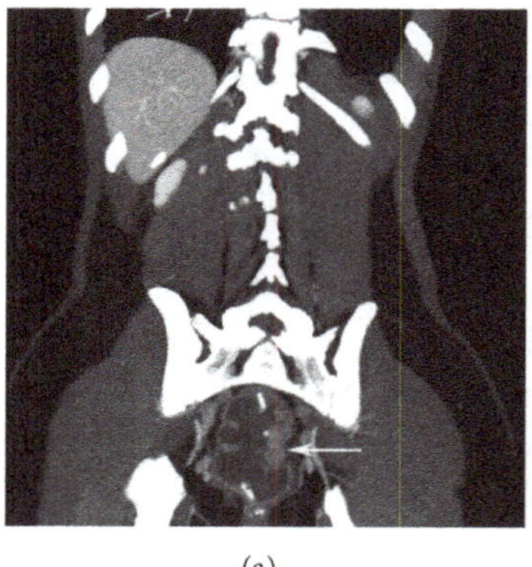
(a)

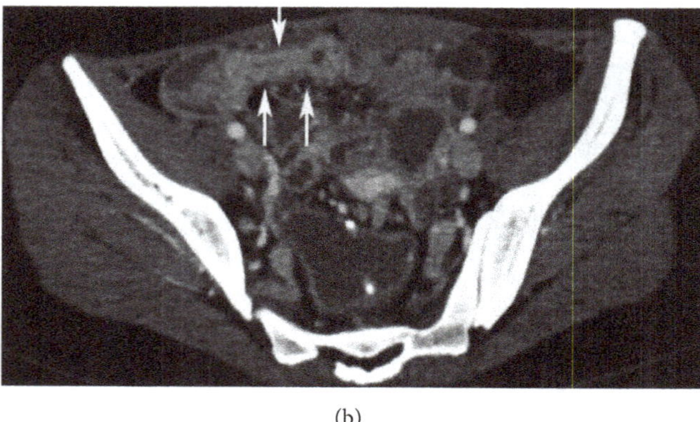
(b)

FIGURE 3: (a) Coronal section of computerized tomographic enterography shows focal mural thickening and enhancement of afferent limb of the J-pouch 1 year after undergoing IPAA and RPC for ulcerative colitis refractory to medical therapy. (b) Transverse section of computerized tomographic enterography shows mucosal hyperenhancement, mural thickening, and luminal narrowing of a 9.4 cm long segment of terminal ileum 1 year after undergoing IPAA and RPC for ulcerative colitis refractory to medical therapy.

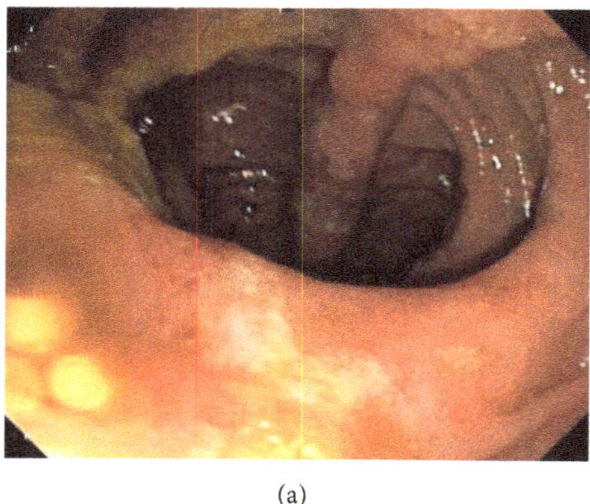
(a)

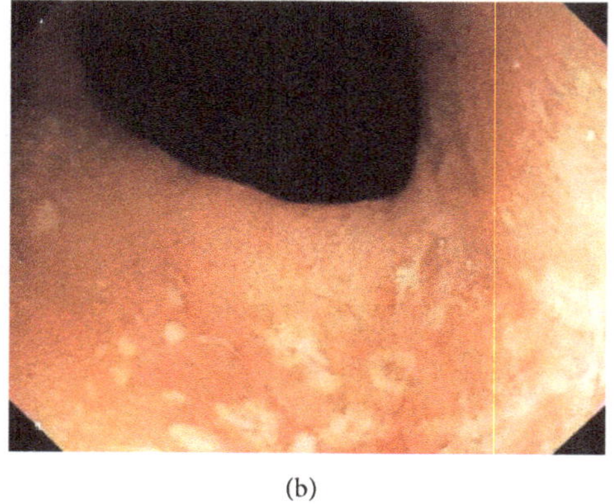
(b)

FIGURE 4: (a) Pouchoscopy shows ulceration and mild inflammation in the J-pouch. (b) Pouchoscopy shows ulceration and mild inflammation in the terminal ileum proximal to the J-pouch.

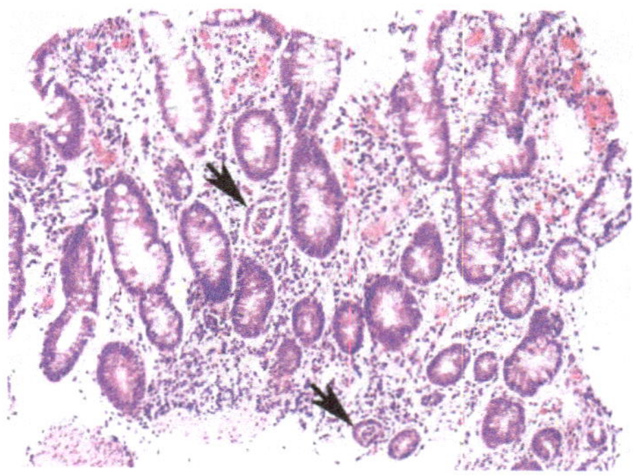

FIGURE 5: Histopathology with H&E shows near total loss of villi, crypt architectural distortion, and crypt abscesses (arrows) in endoscopic biopsies obtained 20 cm from anal verge, findings highly consistent with prepouch ileitis after creation of a J-pouch.

risk of PI, with PI more frequently reported in W-pouches (3.4%) than in S-pouches (2.1%) or J-pouches (1.9%), even though these differences were not statistically significant [11].

PI is strongly associated with PSC in patients with UC as demonstrated by Shen et al. [1, 2, 10]. Moreover, patients with PI and PSC more likely have a concurrent autoimmune disorder, which might contribute to development of PI and pouchitis [2]. The association between PI and PSC might arise from ileal inflammation from abnormal bile acid metabolism in PSC, even though differences in ileal bile acid composition have not yet been described in PI with PSC versus without PSC [2, 9]. PI can sometimes occur in Crohn's disease (CD), but without concomitant PSC [2].

Symptoms of PI include frequent defecation, defecation difficulties, loose stools, flatus, colicky abdominal pain, GI obstruction, and involuntary weight loss [8, 11]. Pouchitis produces similar symptoms [7]. Endoscopic abnormalities with PI include erosions, ulcerations, exudates, erythema, and friability in the ileum beyond the reconstructed pouch up to 50 cm proximally in the afferent limb. Histologic analysis of endoscopic biopsies demonstrates acute or chronic inflammation. Endoscopic and histologic abnormalities in PI are similar to those in pouchitis, except that the endoscopic and histologic abnormalities extend proximally from the pouch and tend to become progressively milder proximally in PI [7, 11]. The diagnosis of PI must be initially confirmed by pouchoscopy and histology, but subsequent flares can be managed clinically, without repeating pouchoscopy [12]. PI can be diagnosed only after excluding infectious ileitis, especially from cytomegalovirus. Iwata et al. [7] reported that serum levels of interleukins (ILs), including IL-1β, IL-6, and IL-8, and of tumor necrosis factor-α are significantly elevated in both pouchitis and PI.

PI and pouchitis respond to the same therapies [1, 7]. Antibiotics and corticosteroids are the mainstays of therapy, with about 75% of patients responding to combined ciprofloxacin and metronidazole antibiotic therapy and about 25% becoming refractory to this therapy [1, 4, 7, 10]. Symptomatic response to antibiotic therapy does not necessarily guarantee mucosal healing [5]. Immunomodulators or biologic therapy is used for refractory patients [1]. PI more frequently requires escalation with immunomodulator or biologic therapy than pouchitis, possibly because PI is associated with autoimmune disorders [1, 2, 7, 10]. Infliximab has some efficacy in refractory patients, while adalimumab is used as salvage therapy in patients with adverse effects or poor response to infliximab [4, 13, 14].

This reported patient presented with many characteristics associated with PI: young age at diagnosis (18 years old), early colectomy (1 year after UC diagnosis), concurrent pouchitis, initial favorable response to RPC and IPAA surgery, and satisfactory symptomatic control of PI achieved after introducing immunomodulators. Specialized tests showed characteristic findings of PI extending to 50 cm beyond the J-pouch including exudation and ulceration on pouchoscopy; mural thickening, mucosal enhancement, and luminal narrowing of the afferent limb on CTE; and absence of lesions in the afferent limb beyond 50 cm proximally on capsule endoscopy [4]. The reported histopathology of ileal biopsies was highly consistent with PI.

PI occurs postoperatively almost exclusively in patients with UC, uncommonly in patients with CD, and extremely rarely in patients with FAP [1]. PI has been postulated to arise after RPC and IPAA for colon cancer with UC or FAP secondary to an altered and pathological ileal milieu (microflora) after surgery [4]. The pathophysiology of PI remains uncertain because of scarce data about this relatively rare condition. Moreover, PI is underreported because patients are routinely treated empirically with antibiotics for symptoms of pouch dysfunction without performing pouchoscopy, and even if pouchoscopy is performed the afferent limb is infrequently intubated [1, 7].

While some authorities believe PI represents CD misdiagnosed as UC before colonic surgery, other authorities believe PI is an extension of existing pouchitis, and still other authorities believe PI is an entirely different disease [1, 15, 16]. Given that PI can sometimes resemble CD in endoscopic appearance and clinical behavior, PI was historically misdiagnosed as CD. However, PI has recently been reported to have histologic and endoscopic characteristics distinct from those of CD [1, 13, 15]; for example, PI is limited to the terminal ileum 50 cm beyond the pouch without proximal small intestinal inflammation [4, 6, 13]. Lorenzo et al. [16] reported that 43% of cases of PI were associated with delayed diagnosis of CD in a study with prolonged postoperative follow-up averaging 20 years in patients who had been diagnosed with UC before surgery; in study patients with UC, PI was uniformly associated with pouchitis, implying a possibly shared pathophysiology of PI and pouchitis from preexistent UC, as previously reported [1, 4–6]. Bell et al. [11] reported only 50% of PI in UC patients is associated with pouchitis, and in these cases PI and pouchitis share histological and morphological similarities. These contradictory findings between Bell et al. [11] and Lorenzo et al. [16] may arise from lack of endoscopic evaluation of the neoterminal ileum during pouchoscopy for presumed pouch failure; ileoscopic evaluation for PI typically occurs much later after symptom onset than evaluation for pouchitis, and the endoscopic and histologic findings may have irreversibly changed after this long delay because of altered ileal microflora [11].

PI may result from mucosal inflammation from reflux into the afferent limb of altered pouch microflora secondary to pouch stasis [1, 3, 5, 10, 11]. Despite a frequent association with UC, Haboubi et al. [6] suggest PI is not necessarily related to UC. While ileal inflammation can occur in patients with unoperated UC from reflux (backwash ileitis), backwash ileitis generally resolves following RPC, while PI initially presents following RPC [11, 17].

Despite its relative rarity, PI should be considered in any patient status-post IPAA and RPC who presents with IPAA complications consistent with pouchitis. Such patients should undergo pouchoscopy with afferent limb intubation. Treatment should be initiated promptly after diagnosis of PI, with addition of immunomodulator or biologic therapy as necessary. This well-documented case report illustrates the clinical, radiologic, endoscopic, and histologic findings of PI, a relatively rare and inadequately understood disease. Further investigations are needed to better understand the pathophysiology of PI.

Conflicts of Interest

All authors report no conflicts of interest. In particular, Dr. Cappell, as a consultant of the United States Food and Drug Administration (FDA) Advisory Committee for Gastrointestinal Drugs, affirms that this paper does not discuss any proprietary confidential pharmaceutical data submitted to the FDA. Dr. Cappell is also a member of the speaker's bureau for AstraZeneca and Daiichi Sankyo, comarketers of Movantik. Dr. Cappell received a onetime honorarium from Mallinckrodt. This work does not discuss any drug manufactured or marketed by AstraZeneca, Daiichi Sankyo, or Mallinckrodt.

Authors' Contributions

Initial draft of manuscript was written by Dr. Shams and Dr. Hakim. Manuscript was thoroughly revised by Dr. Cappell, who functioned as the mentor for Dr. Shams and Dr. Hakim. Dr. Amin performed all the histopathology and wrote the pathologic sections of the manuscript.

References

[1] M. A. Samaan, D. de Jong, S. Sahami et al., "Incidence and Severity of Prepouch Ileitis," *Inflammatory Bowel Diseases*, vol. 22, no. 3, pp. 662–668, 2016.

[2] B. Shen, A. E. Bennett, U. Navaneethan et al., "Primary sclerosing cholangitis is associated with endoscopic and histologic inflammation of the distal afferent limb in patients with ileal pouch-anal anastomosis," *Inflammatory Bowel Diseases*, vol. 17, no. 9, pp. 1890–1900, 2011.

[3] G. Ugolini, G. Rosati, I. Montroni et al., "Prepouch ileitis, myth or reality? The first case with acute abdomen," *Inflammatory Bowel Diseases*, vol. 16, no. 1, pp. 12–14, 2010.

[4] S. D. McLaughlin, S. K. Clark, A. J. Bell, P. P. Tekkis, P. J. Ciclitira, and R. J. Nicholls, "Incidence and short-term implications of prepouch ileitis following restorative proctocolectomy with ileal pouch-anal anastomosis for ulcerative colitis," *Diseases of the Colon & Rectum*, vol. 52, no. 5, pp. 879–883, 2009.

[5] S. D. Mclaughlin, S. K. Clark, A. J. Bell, P. P. Tekkis, P. J. Ciclitira, and R. J. Nicholls, "An open study of antibiotics for the treatment of pre-pouch ileitis following restorative proctocolectomy with ileal pouch-anal anastomosis," *Alimentary Pharmacology & Therapeutics*, vol. 29, no. 1, pp. 69–74, 2009.

[6] N. Haboubi, "Small bowel inflammation in ulcerative colitis," *Colorectal Disease*, vol. 8, no. 5, pp. 373-374, 2006.

[7] T. Iwata, T. Yamamoto, S. Umegae, and K. Matsumoto, "Pouchitis and pre-pouch ileitis developed after restorative proctocolectomy for ulceratrive colitis: A case report," *World Journal of Gastroenterology*, vol. 13, no. 4, pp. 643–646, 2007.

[8] M. Rottoli, C. Vallicelli, E. Bigonzi et al., "Prepouch Ileitis After Ileal Pouch-anal Anastomosis: Patterns of Presentation and Risk Factors for Failure of Treatment," *Journal of Crohn's and Colitis*, vol. 12, no. 3, pp. 273–279, 2018.

[9] E. V. Loftus Jr., G. C. Harewood, C. G. Loftus et al., "PSC-IBD: a unique form of inflammatory bowel disease associated with primary sclerosing cholangitis," *Gut*, vol. 54, no. 1, pp. 91–96, 2005.

[10] B. Shen, F. H. Remzi, B. Nutter et al., "Association between immune-associated disorders and adverse outcomes of ileal pouch-anal anastomosis," *American Journal of Gastroenterology*, vol. 104, no. 3, pp. 655–664, 2009.

[11] A. J. Bell, A. B. Price, A. Forbes, P. J. Ciclitira, C. Groves, and R. J. Nicholls, "Pre-pouch ileitis: A disease of the ileum in ulcerative colitis after restorative proctocolectomy," *Colorectal Disease*, vol. 8, no. 5, pp. 402–410, 2006.

[12] D. S. Pardi, G. D'Haens, B. Shen, S. Campbell, and P. Gionchetti, "Clinical guidelines for the management of pouchitis," *Inflammatory Bowel Diseases*, vol. 15, no. 9, pp. 1424–1431, 2009.

[13] M. Barreiro-de Acosta, O. García-Bosch, R. Souto et al., "Efficacy of infliximab rescue therapy in patients with chronic refractory pouchitis: A multicenter study," *Inflammatory Bowel Diseases*, vol. 18, no. 5, pp. 812–817, 2012.

[14] M. Barreiro-De Acosta, O. García-Bosch, J. Gordillo et al., "Efficacy of adalimumab rescue therapy in patients with chronic refractory pouchitis previously treated with infliximab: a case series," *European Journal of Gastroenterology & Hepatology*, vol. 24, no. 7, pp. 756–758, 2012.

[15] C. Calabrese, A. Fabbri, P. Gionchetti et al., "Controlled study using wireless capsule endoscopy for the evaluation of the small intestine in chronic refractory pouchitis," *Alimentary Pharmacology & Therapeutics*, vol. 25, no. 11, pp. 1311–1316, 2007.

[16] G. Lorenzo, C. Maurizio, L. P. Maria et al., "Ileal pouch-anal anastomosis 20 years later: is it still a good surgical option for patients with ulcerative colitis?" *International Journal of Colorectal Disease*, vol. 31, no. 12, pp. 1835–1843, 2016.

[17] C. Slatter, S. Girgis, H. Huynh, and W. El-Matary, "Pre-pouch ileitis after colectomy in paediatric ulcerative colitis," *Acta Paediatrica*, vol. 97, no. 3, pp. 381–383, 2008.

41

Foreign Body Moves Retrograde through Ileocecal Valve during Colonoscopy

Maria Paparoupa and Markus Bruns-Toepler

Department of Pulmonary Diseases, Infectious Diseases, Gastroenterology, Nephrology and Intensive Care Unit, University Hospital of Giessen, Klinikstr. 33, 35392 Giessen, Germany

Correspondence should be addressed to Maria Paparoupa; maria.paparoupa@yahoo.com

Academic Editor: Yoshihiro Moriwaki

Ingestion of foreign bodies and particularly of button or/and cylindrical batteries is frequent in children and adults with underlying psychiatric diseases. We present a case of a 30-year-old woman with unstable borderline disorder, where overall 4 button and 2 cylindrical batteries were endoscopically removed from her digestive system. During the last session of colonoscopy a peculiar incident was observed, as a cylindrical battery of 15 mm diameter and 43 mm length moved retrograde through ileocecal valve into the small bowel. The foreign body removal from terminal ileum was effective and safe using an endoscopic loop. This report suggests that endoscopic insertion in terminal ileum should be attempted in every colonoscopy session conducted under the indication of foreign body removal, as the possibility of retrograde movement of even large foreign bodies in the colon and through ileocecal valve is given.

1. Introduction

Ingestion of foreign bodies and particularly of button or/and cylindrical batteries is frequent in children and scientific literature is mainly based on pediatric case series [1]. Nevertheless, the phenomenon is also observed in adults, more often in psychiatric patients suffering of unstable borderline disorder. Several reports describe the ingestion of multiple batteries as suicidal attempt or an act aiming to relieve sudden emotional discomfort on this population [2]. The clinical features can be harmless until foreign bodies are disposed through the natural way or take the form of major complications such as esophageal perforation [3], aortic-esophageal fistula [3], tracheoesophageal fistula [4], bowel obstruction or perforation [2] and even spondylodiscitis [5], and airway impaction [6]. Endoscopic treatment is preferred as high rates of removal success, low incidence of complications, and reduced hospitalization make it favorable towards surgical approach [7]. We present a case of endoscopic removal of overall 4 button and 2 cylindrical batteries from the digestive system of a young woman, where a peculiar incident of a foreign body moving retrograde through ileocecal valve was observed.

2. Case Presentation

The 30-year-old woman was admitted to our intensive care unit after being endotracheal intubated in emergency setting due to possible battery ingestion. The patient was suffering from a severe borderline personality disorder with a long medical history of recurrent suicide attempts and numerous incidents of nonsuicidal self-injury (NSSI) causing deep scarves on her arms and breasts. She was living in a residence specialized on giving care that ensures the surveillance of members with refractory psychiatric disorders who were unable to get integrated into community. Approximately one hour before her admission the patient called social servers for help and confessed having swallowed an uncertain number of different types of batteries while being unattended. Although relief of sudden emotional stress with no suicidal attention was her given motive, the patient refused to follow emergency physician to the hospital and became violent, which led to application of sedative-hypnotic drugs and subsequently to prehospital endotracheal intubation.

The general physical examination on the board revealed signs of acute abdomen and laboratory tests were unremarkable. An immediate upper intestinoscopy was undertaken

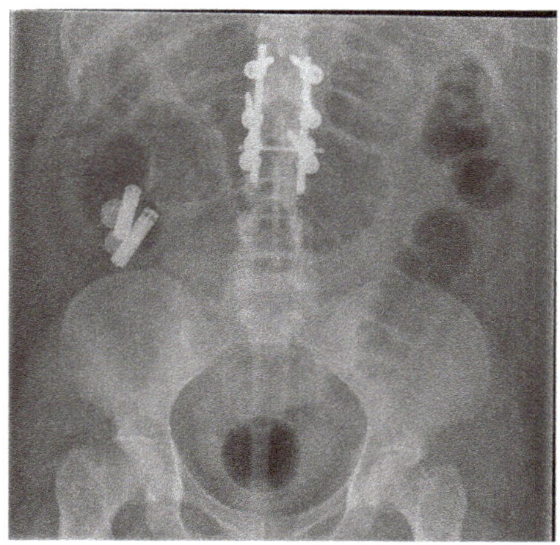

FIGURE 1: X-ray presenting a cluster of four batteries, two button batteries, and two cylindrical ones in Right Lower Quadrant (RLQ) of abdomen.

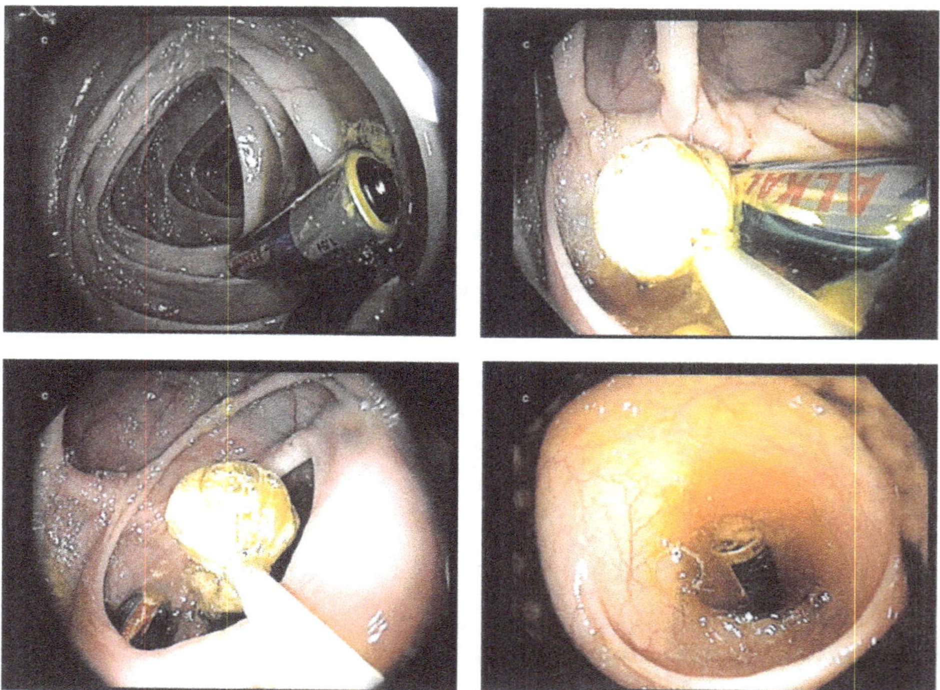

FIGURE 2: Having captured the third battery in a Dormia basket, we could see the last cylindrical one, in the background of endoscopic field deep in cecum.

in order to exclude esophageal impaction and two button batteries were removed from the stomach of the patient. Preparation for colonoscopy was initiated. As the total number of digested foreign bodies remained uncertain an X-ray of abdomen was performed 12 hours after starting colon prep. As shown in Figure 1 two more button batteries and two cylindrical ones were found to form a cluster in Right Lower Quadrant (RLQ) of abdomen. Having concerns that the batteries were already oxidated or even stuck in terminal ileum, we proceeded immediately with lower intestinal endoscopy.

Under the implementation of endoscopic loops and Dormia basket, three of overall four batteries were removed from cecum as they have already passed into colon. Having captured the third one, we could see the last cylindrical battery in the background of endoscopic field deep in cecum (Figure 2). Surprisingly after inserting colon again in order to remove it, the foreign body was not detectable anymore. The examination was unsuccessfully repeated over three sessions with careful inspection of the colonic loops from cecum to rectum. We supposed subsequently that the battery could

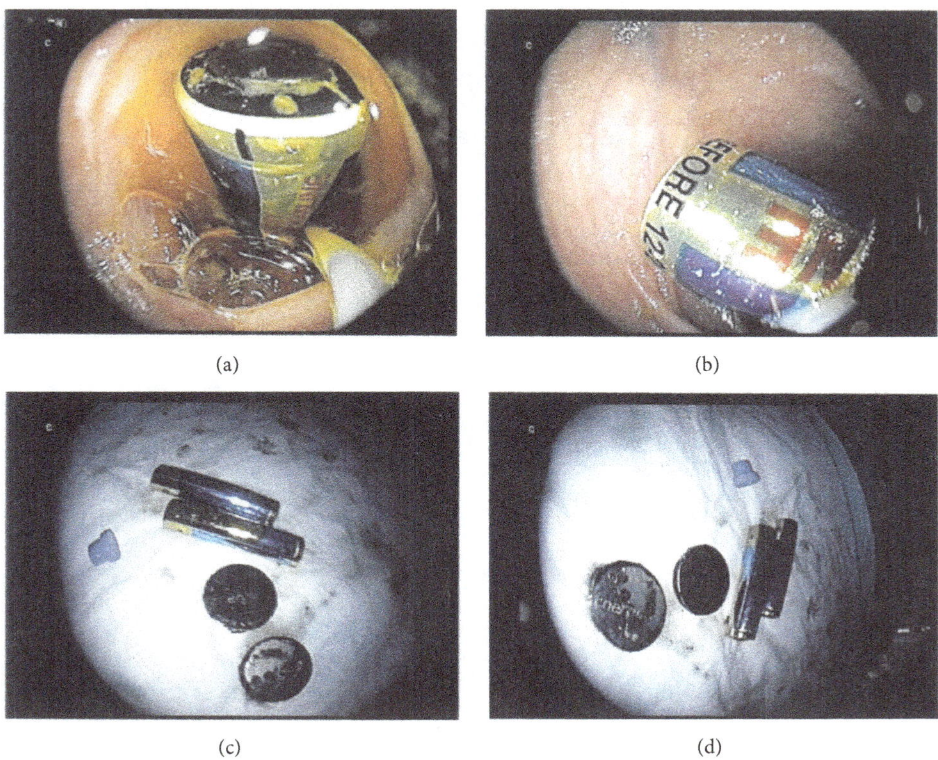

FIGURE 3: The cylindrical battery was detected in terminal ileum, grasped with an endoscopic loop and pulled through the valve ((a) and (b)). All four batteries are presented after their removal per anus ((c) and (d)).

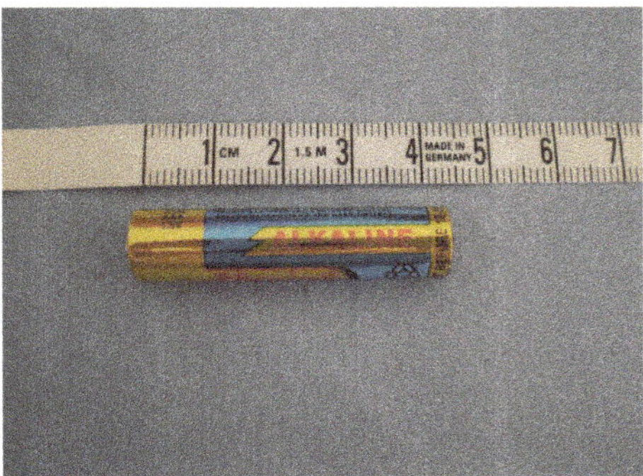

FIGURE 4: The length of the cylindrical battery was more than 4 cm.

have moved retrograde into small bowel. We negotiated colonoscope through the ileocecal valve, detected the foreign body in terminal ileum, grasped it with an endoscopic loop, pulled it through the valve, and removed it per anus (Figure 3). The length of the battery was more than 4 cm (Figure 4) with a diameter of 15 mm.

3. Discussion

There have been reports of small bowel obstruction secondary to battery ingestion, which have been managed surgically [2]. In our case two button and two cylindrical batteries passed through ileocecal valve, although radiological assessment of their exact position in the bowel was difficult and we had to proceed with endoscopic evaluation. Our main concern was the oxidation of the button batteries as several hours ago two of such foreign bodies were removed from the stomach of the patient and we could already macroscopically detect multiple oxidative erosions on their surface. Unfortunately no picture documentation of the upper intestinoscopy of this case has been preserved. Release of toxic metals in the gastrointestinal system can lead to intoxication through heavy metals like Cadmium (Cd), Hydrargyrum (Hg), and others, as elsewhere described in the literature [8]. Another factor which accelerated our decision to perform endoscopic removal of the batteries, though missing signs of small bowel obstruction, was the reported possibility of bowel perforation, as batteries interact with each other and electrical discharge, leading to severe tissue damage, can be produced. According to a retrospective review of case series, the anatomic direction of the battery's negative pole was a predictive risk factor of long term complications due to button battery impaction [9]. The experimental work of Yasui in rats showed that, prior to leakage of the cell alkali, ulceration or perforation of the digestive mucosa occurred due to electric discharge of the battery and this effect was independent of fasted state or acidic environment [10].

In our case, after uncomplicated colonoscopic removal of two button and one cylindrical batteries, the retrograde movement of the last cylindrical one through ileocecal valve was observed. We suppose that a foreign body of such diameter (43 mm) and length (15 mm) was able to move backwards through a tight pathway being forced by intestinal peristaltic waves and elevated liquid and air pressure in colon during colonoscopy session. The retrograde movement of a battery in gastrointestinal system has been described before in a case where battery has moved from the stomach to esophagus after administration of ipecac [1]. To our knowledge, this is the first report of a retrograde movement through ileocecal valve. Colonoscopic removal of the foreign body from terminal ileum was effective and safe. Tissue damage, perforation, and small bowel obstruction could be prevented. The postinterventional course of the patient was uneventful and normal bowel activity was present within few hours. This report suggests that endoscopic insertion in terminal ileum should be attempted in every colonoscopy session conducted under the indication of foreign body removal, as the possibility of retrograde movement of even large foreign bodies in the colon and through ileocecal valve is given.

References

[1] T. Litovitz and B. F. Schmitz, "Ingestion of cylindrical and button batteries: an analysis of 2382 cases," *Pediatrics*, vol. 89, no. 4, part 2, pp. 747–757, 1992.

[2] L. Dunphy, M. Maatouk, M. Raja, and R. O'Hara, "Ingested cylindrical batteries in an incarcerated male: a caustic tale!," *BMJ Case Reports*, vol. 2015, article 1503, 2015.

[3] A. V. Barabino, P. Gandullia, S. Vignola, S. Arrigo, L. Zannini, and P. Di Pietro, "Lithium battery lodged in the oesophagus: a report of three paediatric cases," *Digestive and Liver Disease*, vol. 47, no. 11, pp. 984–986, 2015.

[4] S. Fuentes, I. Cano, M. I. Benavent, and A. Gómez, "Severe esophageal injuries caused by accidental button battery ingestion in children," *Journal of Emergencies, Trauma and Shock*, vol. 7, no. 4, pp. 316–321, 2014.

[5] H. Eshaghi, S. Norouzi, G. Heidari-Bateni, and S. Mamishi, "Spondylodiscitis: a rare complication of button battery ingestion in a 10-month-old boy," *Pediatric Emergency Care*, vol. 29, no. 3, pp. 368–370, 2013.

[6] C. I. Cruz and D. Patel, "Impacted button-battery masquerading as croup," *Journal of Emergency Medicine*, vol. 45, no. 1, pp. 30–33, 2013.

[7] G. Geraci, C. Sciume', G. Di Carlo, A. Picciurro, and G. Modica, "Retrospective analysis of management of ingested foreign bodies and food impactions in emergency endoscopic setting in adults," *BMC Emergency Medicine*, vol. 16, no. 1, article 42, 2016.

[8] W. Rebhandl, I. Steffan, P. Schramel et al., "Release of toxic metals from button batteries retained in the stomach: an in vitro study," *Journal of Pediatric Surgery*, vol. 37, no. 1, pp. 87–92, 2002.

[9] M. J. Eliason, J. M. Melzer, J. R. Winters, and T. Q. Gallagher, "Identifying predictive factors for long-term complications following button battery impactions: a case series and literature review," *International Journal of Pediatric Otorhinolaryngology*, vol. 87, pp. 189–202, 2016.

[10] T. Yasui, "Hazardous effects due to alkaline button battery ingestion: an experimental study," *Annals of Emergency Medicine*, vol. 15, no. 8, pp. 901–906, 1986.

Successful Endoscopic Treatment of Bouveret Syndrome in a Patient with Choledochoduodenal Fistula Complicating Duodenal Ulcer

Syed Hasan,[1] Zubair Khan,[1] Umar Darr,[1] Toseef Javaid,[1] Nauman Siddiqui,[1] Jamal Saleh,[1] Abdallah Kobeissy,[1,2] and Ali Nawras[1,2]

[1]*Department of Internal Medicine, University of Toledo Medical Center, Toledo, OH, USA*
[2]*Division of Gastroenterology, University of Toledo, Toledo, OH, USA*

Correspondence should be addressed to Zubair Khan; zubair.khan@utoledo.edu

Academic Editor: Engin Altintas

Introduction. Cholecystoduodenal fistulas represent the most common type of bilioenteric fistulas while choledochoduodenal fistulas account for only 1–25% of cases. Bilioenteric fistula cases are associated with cholelithiasis and are rarely associated with duodenal peptic ulcers. Here we present the first case of Bouveret syndrome secondary to choledochoduodenal fistula complicating peptic duodenal ulcer managed successfully via endoscopic mechanical lithotripsy. *Case*. 86-year-old male with a medical history significant for coronary artery disease and stage 3 colorectal cancer status after resection and chemoradiation presented with intractable sharp abdominal pain worse postprandially for one week in duration, associated with early satiety, anorexia, and 5 lbs weight loss in one week. CT abdomen showed possible choledochoduodenal fistula and a distended stomach. An esophagogastroduodenoscopy (EGD) was performed revealing a large 2.5–3 cm stone lodged in the duodenal bulb at the base of duodenal ulcer with a fistula opening beneath it. The stone was extracted in 2 pieces via mechanical lithotripsy. Endoscopic ultrasound of the CBD revealed Rigler's triad. *Conclusion*. Bouveret syndrome is mostly associated with cholecystoduodenal fistula and has high mortality and morbidity due to underlying comorbid conditions and elderly age. Patients are not always fit for surgical management, and endoscopic management is not always successful.

1. Introduction

Cholecystoduodenal fistulas represent the most common type of bilioenteric fistulas while choledochoduodenal fistulas account for only 1–25% of bilioenteric fistulas cases [1]. Although 75–90% of bilioenteric fistula cases are associated with cholelithiasis [1, 2] only 5-6% of them are associated with duodenal peptic ulcers [2–4].

The passage of a large gallstone through a cholecystoduodenal fistula and the subsequent impaction in the duodenum causing gastric outlet obstruction are a rare occurrence and this is known as Bouveret syndrome. This type of gallstone ileus was first described by the Beaussier in 1770 and again by Leon Bouveret in 1896 [5]. It is more prevalent in the elderly and in females, with a reported median age of 74 years and a female-to-male ratio of 1.9 [6–9]. It is mostly caused by cholecystoduodenal fistula or rarely cholecystogastric fistula.

Because of the older age and significant comorbid conditions in patients presenting with Bouveret syndrome, the mortality (60%) and morbidity (12–33%) are relatively high and necessitate early and quick removal of the stone by the least invasive procedure [5, 10].

2. Case Study

This is an 86-year-old male patient with a past medical history significant for coronary artery disease and stage 3 colorectal cancer status after resection and chemoradiation that presented from an outlying facility for intractable sharp abdominal pain that was worse postprandially, one week in

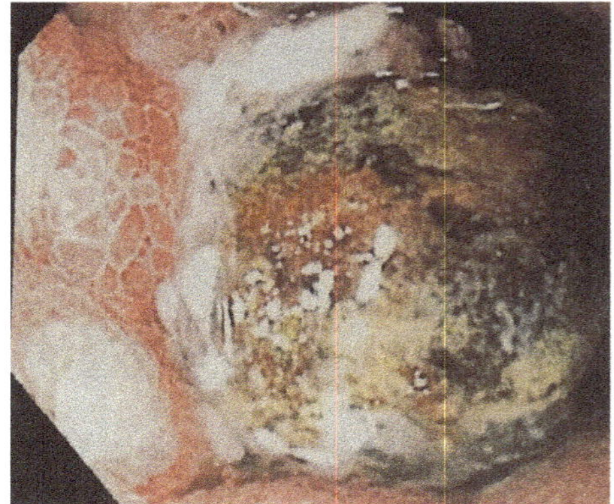

FIGURE 1: Impacted gallstone in duodenum.

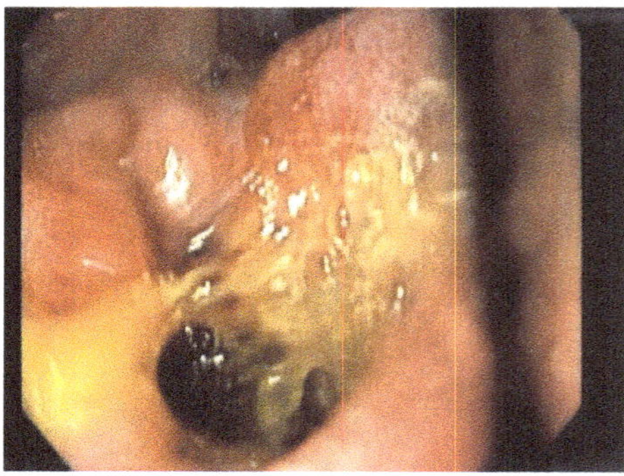

FIGURE 2: Choledochoduodenal fistula at the base of ulcer.

duration, associated with early satiety, anorexia, and 5 lbs weight loss in the last week. Physical exam revealed mild-to-moderate epigastric tenderness and right hypochondrial tenderness. The differential diagnosis before any further work-up was peptic ulcer disease, cholecystitis, or metastasis from colorectal cancer to gastroduodenal region. A CT scan of the abdomen at the outlying facility showed possible choledochoduodenal fistula, distended stomach, and a cyst in the tail of the pancreas. An esophagogastroduodenoscopy (EDG) was performed revealing a large duodenal bulb ulcer with a stone lodged in it (Figure 1).

The ulcer was 1.5 × 0.5 cm and the suspected choledochoduodenal fistula was identified (Figure 2). The stone was secured with a Roth net, and extraction was attempted.

The stone was pulled successfully into the stomach but could not be pulled through the esophagus without a significant risk of traumatizing the esophagus because of the size of the stone. Thus, it was mechanically crushed into 2 pieces using a biliary mechanical lithotripter and extracted (Figure 3). The stone measured 2.5 × 3 cm in diameter (Figure 4).

The duodenum was then reexamined and a duodenal bulb fistula tract orifice was found on the posterior wall at the base of the ulcer. Examination of the common bile duct (CBD) with endoscopic ultrasound (EUS) revealed regions of high echogenicity with prominent shadowing consistent with pneumobilia and no gallstones in the gall

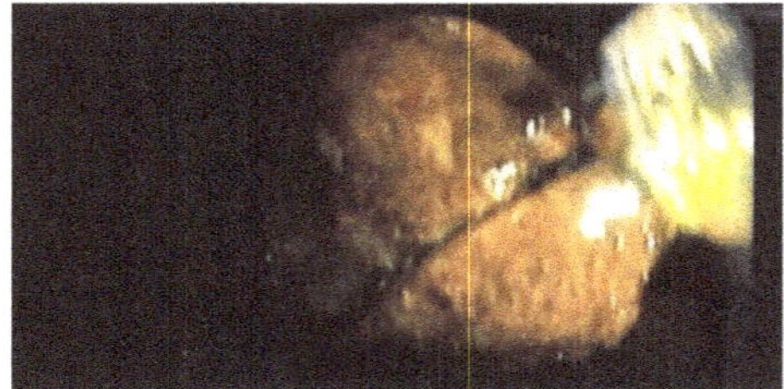

FIGURE 3: Stone in lithotripter.

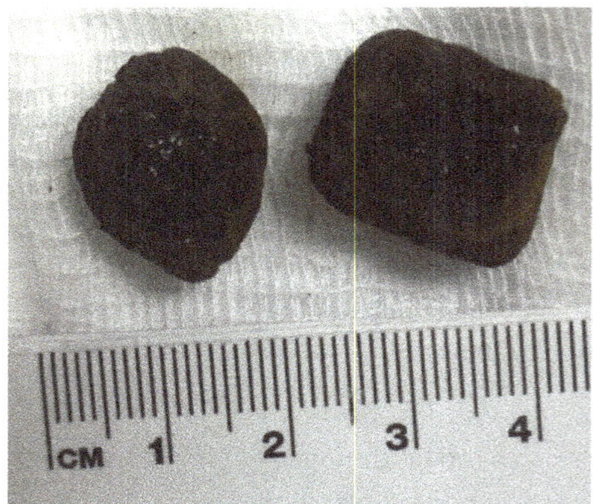

FIGURE 4: Broken gallstone.

bladder. The patient did well after the procedure and his symptoms were completely resolved. He subsequently underwent cholecystectomy and was discharged home on proton pump inhibitors for 8 weeks after one week of hospital stay. He underwent follow-up EGD after 8 weeks at the outside facility that reported resolution of duodenal bulb ulcer and choledochoduodenal fistula. He also underwent HIDA scan and that did not show any biliary-enteric leak.

3. Discussion

The creation of a bilioenteric fistula is a very rare complication of cholelithiasis which affects less than 1% of patients [11]. The fistula can occur anywhere in the GI tract with the most common location being cholecystoduodenal (~ 60%) and cholecystocolic (17%) and cholecystogastric and choledochoduodenal fistulas (5%) [5]. The risk factors for developing bilioenteric fistulas in patients with cholelithiasis include long standing cholelithiasis, repetitive bouts of acute cholecystitis, being a female, age > 60 yrs, and a large calculus (greater than 2 cm) [12].

To the best of our knowledge, this is the first reported case of Bouveret syndrome secondary to choledochoduodenal fistula. All the previous reported cases describe Bouveret syndrome mostly secondary to cholecystoduodenal fistula. Most of the bilioenteric fistulas are associated with cholelithiasis but choledochoduodenal fistulas are unique as they are predominantly attributed to duodenal peptic ulcers (75–80%) and are a rare occurrence [1–3]. The reason for the rarity becomes obvious when one realizes that a duodenal ulcer most typically occurs about 4 cm distal to the pylorus whereas the CBD is about 7 cm distal to the pylorus [13]. Most cases of choledochoduodenal fistulas occur at the posterior wall of the duodenal bulb, and fistulas at the anterior wall of the duodenal bulb are extremely rare [1, 2, 14–16]. Another important fact is that Bouveret syndrome is more prevalent in elderly females but choledochoduodenal fistula is more prevalent in elderly males [15].

For the most part, choledochoduodenal fistulas are incidental findings at upper GI studies and seldom produce any specific symptoms; the symptoms if present are either result of biliary tract obstruction or result of duodenal peptic ulcers [13]. In our case the patient was having impacted gallstone at the duodenal ulcer so he presented with symptoms of Bouveret syndrome. In Bouveret syndrome, findings on presentation are often nonspecific with nausea, distention, and abdominal pain being the most common [17]. And, because of the nonspecific and vague presentation, the diagnosis is often delayed. Radiographic imaging of these patients may reveal a radiolucent gallstone, pyloric, or duodenal obstruction and pneumobilia known as Rigler's triad [10, 17]. Our patient had all three major symptoms and Rigler's triad as identified by Cappell and Davis.

The most frequent sites where stones are found to be impacted are the terminal ilium (50–75%) and proximal ileum and jejunum (20–40%) and rarely the stomach and duodenum [12]. On endoscopy, the gastroduodenal obstruction was noted in nearly all the cases but a review of 128 cases by Cappell and Davis showed the stone itself was only visualized in 69% of cases, while the fistula itself was only visualized in 13% of the cases evaluated [17]. In our patient, the stone was found impacted in the duodenal bulb, obstructing the pyloric outlet. While many options exist for lithotripsy, including electrohydraulic, extracorporeal shockwave, and laser, our patient was treated using mechanical lithotripsy. Despite having various endoscopy techniques, the success rate of these is only 9% [18].

Given the elderly patient population of Bouveret syndrome with significant comorbid conditions, sometimes significant delay in diagnosis requires safe and quick removal of stone to relive the obstruction. The endoscopic removal of the stone is a good option. If the stone is too large for removal through endoscope alone, mechanic, laser, or extracorporeal shockwave lithotripsy may be considered [19]. In the presence of skilled endoscopist and proper facilities, endoscopic retrieval of stone is preferred over invasive procedures like enterolithotomy and cholecystectomy, unless the need arises for it because of other symptoms or in the setting of gallbladder malignancy [19, 20].

In our case beside treating the Bouveret syndrome the other management challenge was duodenal peptic ulcer complicating choledochoduodenal fistulas. Mostly isolated choledochoduodenal fistulas with duodenal peptic ulcers are treated medically with proton pump inhibitors. Surgery must be reserved for patients with poorly controlled or recurrent ulcer symptoms, major ulcer complications, such as perforation, hemorrhage, or obstruction, or exceptional cases with cholangitis or biliary obstruction [16, 21]. As in our case the patient presentation was attributable to Bouveret syndrome that was managed successfully endoscopically, no further intervention was done for choledochoduodenal fistulas beside prescribing proton pump inhibitors for duodenal peptic ulcer.

In conclusion, we report a rare case of choledochoduodenal fistula complicating a duodenal peptic ulcer and the first reported case of Bouveret syndrome secondary to choledochoduodenal fistula which was successfully managed endoscopically. The choledochoduodenal fistulas are rare in this modern era because of the exclusive and universal treatment of peptic ulcer disease with proton pump inhibitors. This case further necessitates the need of early utilization of imaging techniques in the evaluation of elderly patient population presenting with nonspecific gastrointestinal symptoms. Also, based on our experience we would recommend treatment of cases of Bouveret syndrome in an institution with skilled endoscopist and advanced facilities as the majority of patient population is not a candidate for invasive interventions.

Disclosure

The abstract of the case report was presented in the ACG meeting 2015.

Authors' Contributions

Syed Hasan and Zubair Khan contributed equally to writing the case report manuscript and major parts of discussion. Umar darr, Toseef Javaid, Nauman Siddiqui, Jamal Saleh, and Abdallah Kobeissy assisted in the literature review. Ali Nawras supervised and reviewed the entire article.

References

[1] M. C. Misra, H. Grewal, and B. M. L. Kapur, "Spontaneous choledochoduodenal fistula complicating peptic ulcer disease—a case report," *The Japanese Journal of Surgery*, vol. 19, no. 3, pp. 367–369, 1989.

[2] Y. Iso, R. Yoh, R. Okita et al., "Choledochoduodenal fistula: a rare complication of a penetrated duodenal ulcer," *Hepato-Gastroenterol*, vol. 43, pp. 489–491, 1996.

[3] S. F. Marshall and R. C. Polk, "Spontaneous internal biliary fistulas," *Surgical Clinics of North America*, vol. 38, no. 3, pp. 679–691, 1958.

[4] P. Shah and R. Ramakantan, "Choledochoduodenal fistula complicating duodenal ulcer," *Journal of Postgraduate Medicine*, vol. 36, pp. 167-168, 1990.

[5] V. K. Mavroeidis, D. I. Matthioudakis, N. K. Economou, and I. D. Karanikas, "Bouveret syndrome—the rarest variant of gallstone ileus: a case report and literature review," *Case Reports in Surgery*, vol. 2013, Article ID 839370, 6 pages, 2013.

[6] A. Koulaouzidis and J. Moschos, "Bouveret's syndrome. narrative review," *Annals of Hepatology*, vol. 6, no. 2, pp. 89–91, 2007.

[7] S. Sultan, I. Doycheva, A. Limaye, A. Suman, and C. E. Forsmark, "Bouveret's syndrome: Case report and review of the literature," *Gastroenterology Research and Practice*, Article ID 914951, 4 pages, 2009.

[8] R. J. Kurtz, T. M. Heimann, and A. B. Kurtz, "Gallstone lleus: a diagnostic problem," *The American Journal of Surgery*, vol. 146, no. 3, pp. 314–317, 1983.

[9] H. F. Newman and J. D. Northup, "The autopsy incidence of gallstones," *Surgery, Gynecology & Obstetrics*, vol. 109, no. 1, pp. 1–13, 1959.

[10] A. Patel and S. Agarwal, "The yellow brick road of bouveret syndrome," *Clinical Gastroenterology and Hepatology*, vol. 12, no. 8, p. A24, 2014.

[11] Y. A. Masannat, S. Caplin, and T. Brown, "A rare complication of a common disease: Bouveret syndrome, a case report," *World Journal of Gastroenterology*, vol. 12, no. 16, pp. 2620-2621, 2006.

[12] C. Iancu, R. Bodea, N. Al Hajjar, D. Todea-Iancu, O. Bălă, and I. Acalovschi, "Bouveret syndrome associated with acute gangrenous cholecystitis," *Journal of Gastrointestinal and Liver Diseases*, vol. 17, no. 1, pp. 87–90, 2008.

[13] M. Michowitz, C. Farago, I. Lazarovici, and M. Solowiejczyk, "Choledochoduodenal fistula: a rare complication of duodenal ulcer," *The American Journal of Gastroenterology*, vol. 79, no. 5, pp. 416–420, 1984.

[14] M. Naga and M. S. Mogawer, "Choledochoduodenal fistula: a rare sequel of duodenal ulcer," *Endoscopy*, vol. 23, no. 5, pp. 307-308, 1991.

[15] M. G. Sarr, A. J. Shepard, and G. D. Zuidema, "Choledochoduodenal fistula: An unusual complication of duodenal ulcer disease," *The American Journal of Surgery*, vol. 141, no. 6, pp. 736–740, 1981.

[16] C. E. Bickham Jr., "Choledochoduodenal fistula: a rare complication of duodenal ulcer. Report of three cases," *The Medical Annals of the District of Columbia*, vol. 42, no. 5, pp. 217–221, 1973.

[17] M. S. Cappell and M. Davis, "Characterization of Bouveret's syndrome: a comprehensive review of 128 cases," *The American Journal of Gastroenterology*, vol. 101, no. 9, pp. 2139–2146, 2006.

[18] A. S. Lowe, S. Stephenson, C. L. Kay, and J. May, "Duodenal obstruction by gallstone (Bouveret's syndrome): A review of the literature," *Endoscopy*, vol. 37, no. 1, pp. 82–87, 2005.

[19] J. F. B. Chick, N. R. Chauhan, J. C. Mandell, D. A. T. De Souza, R. J. Bair, and B. Khurana, "Traffic jam in the duodenum: Imaging and pathogenesis of Bouveret syndrome," *Journal of Emergency Medicine*, vol. 45, no. 4, pp. e135–e137, 2013.

[20] M. M. Alsolaiman, C. Reitz, A. T. Nawras, J. B. Rodgers, and B. J. Maliakkal, "Bouveret's syndrome complicated by distal gallstone ileus after laser lithotropsy using Holmium: YAG laser," *BMC Gastroenterology*, vol. 2, article 15, 2002.

[21] E. R. Feller, A. L. Warshaw, and R. H. Schapiro, "Observations on management of choledochoduodenal fistula due to penetrating peptic ulcer," *Gastroenterology*, vol. 78, no. 1, pp. 126–131, 1980.

Indocyanine-Green Fluorescence-GUIDED Liver Resection of Metastasis from Squamous Cell Carcinoma Invading the Biliary Tree

Sara Benedicenti, Sarah Molfino, Marie Sophie Alfano, Beatrice Molteni, Paola Porsio, Nazario Portolani, and Gian Luca Baiocchi

Department of Clinical and Experimental Sciences, Surgical Clinic, University of Brescia, Brescia, Italy

Correspondence should be addressed to Sarah Molfino; sarahmolfino@gmail.com

Academic Editor: Hideto Kawaratani

Background. The concept of fluorescence-guided navigation surgery based on indocyanine green (ICG) is a developing interest in many fields of surgical oncology. The technique seems to be promising also during hepatic resection. *Case Presentation.* We reported our experience of ICG-fluorescence-guided liver resection of metastasis located at VIII Couinaud's segment from colon squamous cell carcinoma of a 74-year-old male patient. *Results.* After laparotomy, the fluorescing tumour has been clearly identified on the liver surface. We have also identified that a large area of fluorescent parenchyma that gets from the peripheral of the lesion up to the portal pedicle such as the neoplasia would interest the right biliary tree in the form of neoplastic lymphangitis. This datum was not preoperatively known. *Conclusion.* Fluorescent imaging navigation liver resection could be a feasible and safe technique helpful in identifying additional characteristics of lesion. It could be a powerful tool but further studies are required.

1. Introduction

Indocyanine green (ICG) is a water-soluble, anionic, amphiphilic tricarbocyanine molecule that emits fluorescence upon illumination with near infrared light [1, 2].

For several years, it has been used in ophthalmic angiography and for determining cardiac output and hepatic function [3]. However, it has only recently showed practicability and feasibility in the field of surgical oncology [4–9].

Focusing on liver metastases, many studies showed how near infrared fluorescence imaging using indocyanine green is a promising technique to intraoperatively visualize the contrast between hepatic lesions and normal liver tissue in real time and how it could be considered a powerful tool to help surgery in the "fluorescent-guided surgery" [10–12].

Referring to the surgical treatment of colon cancer metastatic disease, liver resection is allowed in about 20% of patients [13]. The problem of getting a complete removal of tumour is the presence of residual foci of tumour cells, associated with tumour recurrence and lower survival rates.

In this case the "ICG-fluorescence-based navigation" can be a useful tool in order to locate supplementary lesions that could have been missed with current imaging techniques, such as computer tomography (CT), magnetic resonance imaging, and ultrasonography (US) [12].

Based on recent studies that suggest the effective utility of Photodynamic-Eye (PDE) assessment of ICG fluorescence (PDE + ICG) combined with Intraoperative Ultrasound (IOUS) for ensuring the complete surgical removal of liver metastases from colorectal cancer [14–16], we report our experience with the use of this technique during resection of liver metastasis from colon squamous cell carcinoma, invading the biliary tree.

2. Case Report

A 74-year-old male patient was admitted to our hospital in March 2017 to undergo liver resection to treat a malignant hepatic lesion diagnosed with CT and PET and a fine-needle biopsy positive for squamous carcinoma. The hepatic tumour discovered during follow-up for a previous bladder cancer submitted to endoscopic surgery three years before measured 22 mm in diameter and was located in the VIII Couinaud's segment [17] of the liver in association with three smaller

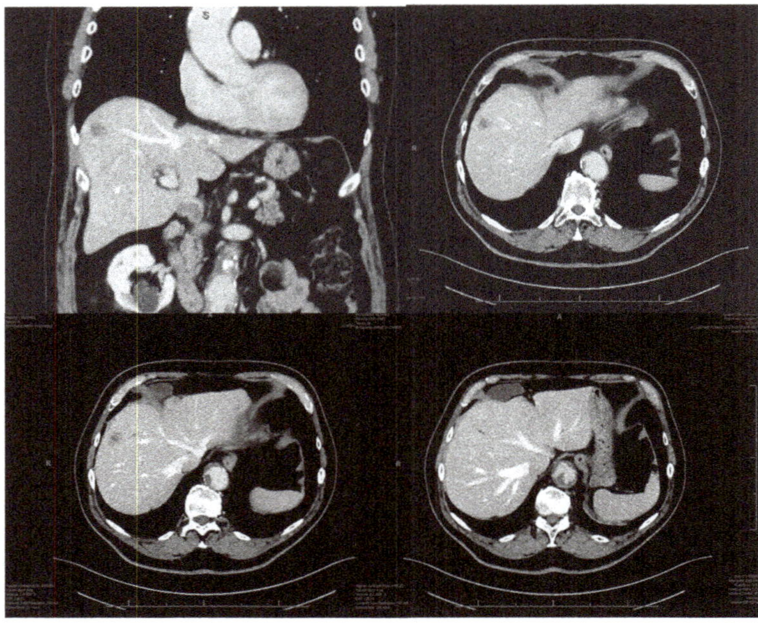

FIGURE 1: Preoperative CT imaging of hepatic lesion.

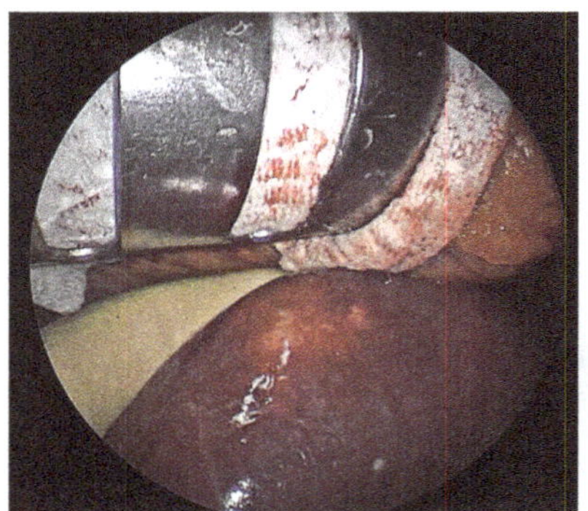
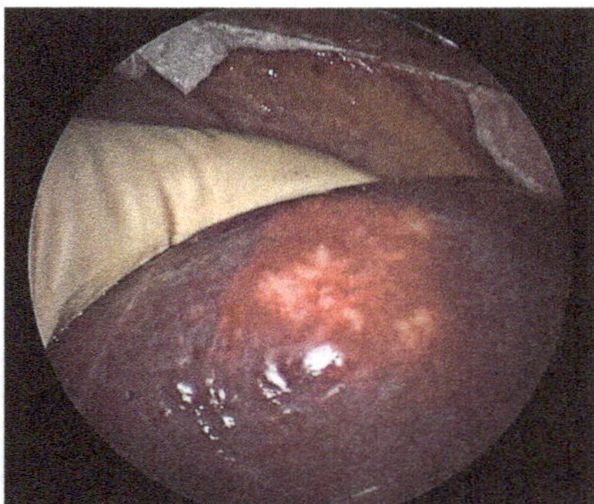
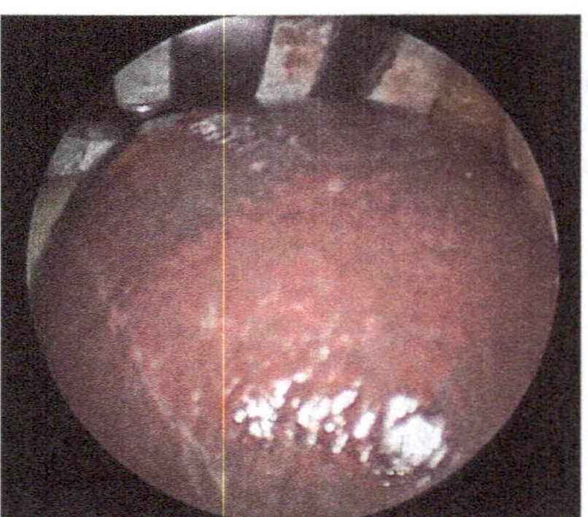

FIGURE 2: Intraoperative visualization of metastatic lesion at the liver surface.

hypodense liver lesions with a focal dilatation of peripheral biliary tree (Figure 1).

The case is discussed with radiologists, oncologists, and pathologists of our hospital. Even if the lesion had been the single site of disease; due to the proximity/doubtful infiltration of the lesion to the biliary tree, we decided to submit the patient to an explorative staging laparotomy and possible palliative surgery.

Our internal protocol states that during the preadmission every patient who is a candidate for a liver resection is subjected to a routine liver function test with ICG to determinate the most appropriate surgical procedures [18]: 0,5 mg/Kg ICG are routinely injected intravenously up to seven days before surgery to evaluate the ICG retention rate at 15 min (R15). In our case 45 mg of ICG was intravenously administrated to test hepatic function, ten days before the surgery (patient R15 = 8.9).

Thanks to the ICG property of being fluorescent with the light emitted from the photodynamic eye of the laparoscopic system in our possession, it is possible to visualize the lesion during the surgical procedure. To this target, timing of administration and dose of ICG are key points.

Several studies have demonstrated that the effective dose of ICG depends on the timing of injection; in particular, if the function liver test had been performed more than 7 days before surgery it would have been necessary to administer an adjunctive dose (0,1 mg/Kg) the day before [10]. In this case, it was necessary to administrate an adjunctive dose of ICG the day before the surgery (9 mg of ICG injected intravenously). After laparotomy, exploration of the abdominal cavity, and exposure of the liver, we easily confirmed the superficial lesion in the VIII Couinaud's segment. The liver surface has been analysed with the fluorescent imaging system. The fluorescing tumour has been clearly identified and defined on the liver surface, as shown in Figure 2. We have also identified that a large area of fluorescent parenchyma that gets from the peripheral of the lesion up to the portal pedicle such as the neoplasia would interest the right biliary tree in the form

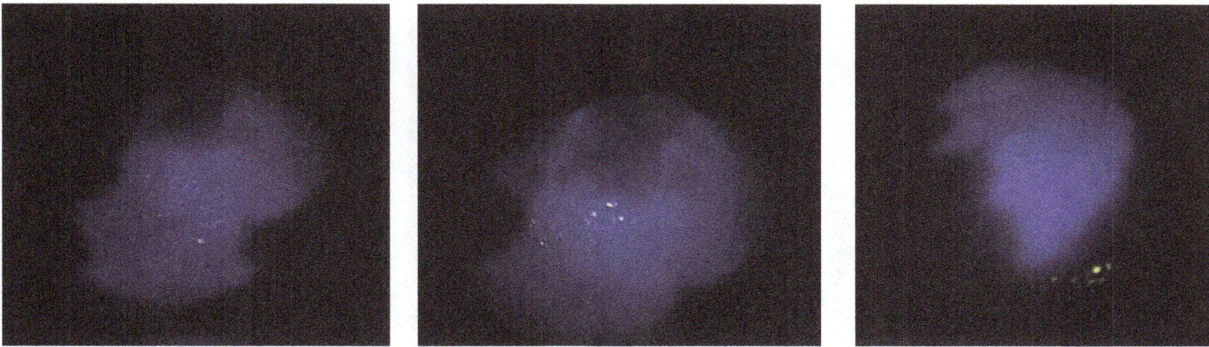

FIGURE 3: Intraoperative visualization with ICG-PDE system: the small lesion with rim staining around the tumour and the fluorescence emitted region from the cholestatic area.

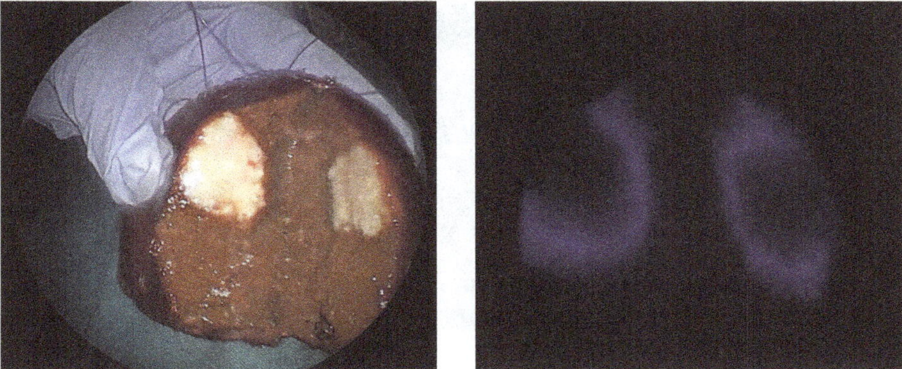

FIGURE 4: Normal and fluorescent pattern of the tumour in the resected specimen (rim fluorescence type).

of neoplastic lymphangitis (Figure 3). This datum was not preoperatively known.

A right hepatectomy would have been the oncologically correct surgical procedure due to the infiltration of right biliary duct. Considering the probable metastatic nature of the lesion, the absence of a clearly primary lesion, the age, the comorbidities, and the small size of residual liver, we have decided to perform an atypical segmental resection of S8 associated with cholecystectomy and lymphadenectomy of the hepatic pedicle nodes, including the area of impaired biliary excretion.

At the histological examination, the lesion, the lymph nodes of the hepatic pedicle region, and the right biliary branch, respectively, resulted in hepatic metastases from squamous cell carcinoma and sites of metastatic location. As expected the resection margin was interested by neoplasia.

In particular, the histological examination showed the following:

(i) Macroscopical exam: the neoplasia, in a site, appears to be in contact with the resection margin

(ii) Microscopical exam: parenchymal hepatic section that showed metastatic localization of squamous carcinoma moderately differentiated. The neoplasia interest the surgery resection margin.

In this case, fluorescent imaging has revealed a fluorescing ring around the hepatic metastasis (Figure 4). The fluorescence of the cholestatic area was shown on the cut surface (Figure 5).

3. Discussion

ICG-fluorescent imaging techniques have begun to be used in hepatobiliary procedures in the last few years. These techniques are expected to complement conventional imaging techniques without having the purpose to replace all of the roles of conventional techniques. It provides simultaneous, real time, and high resolution identification of many type of different structures and, particularly during the navigation surgery application, could be a helpful tool to discover adjunctive lesions and identify segmental staining and biliary tree visualization [9, 11, 15, 19, 20].

The major advantage of this system is that it overlays fluorescent images on the background colour images. This property can make it easier for a surgeon to understand the exact location of the fluorescing lesions (liver cancer/or bile ducts) on the surrounding structures as compared with that in the conventional fluorescent imaging system [16, 21].

The fluorescent imaging of segmental cholestasis region, caused by the duct tumour invasion or thrombi and demonstrated at the intraoperative PDE-visualization, could be explained by the fact that ICG has been retained in the noncancerous liver parenchyma due to bile ducts obstruction and the consecutive altered biliary excretion in this tissue [22].

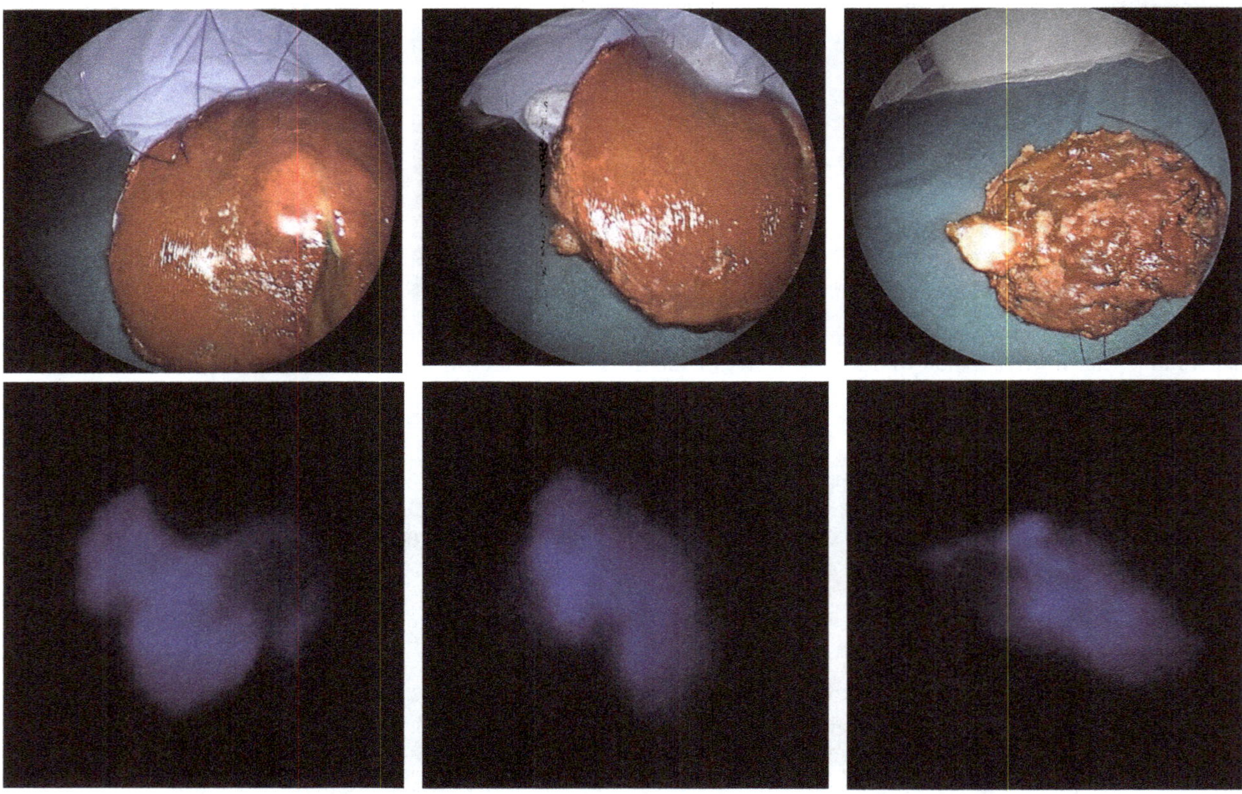

FIGURE 5: Visualization of cholestatic area by fluorescence on the cut surface.

Our case report shows how feasibility and safety of this procedure could help to identify additional characteristics of the lesion, such as the cholestasis area around the lesion itself and infiltration of the biliary tree too with minimal adjunctive costs [23–25]. So it could be simple and helpful to guide a surgical procedure.

4. Conclusion

The major advantages of fluorescent imaging are its feasibility and safety. Once ICG is preoperatively administered for liver function testing, we can obtain fluorescent images of tumour and cholestasis regions in real time by simply placing the camera imaging on the liver surface before the resection, during the liver resection, and over surgical specimens.

Further and ongoing studies are required to better define the feasibility and usefulness of this technique.

References

[1] E. Engel, R. Schraml, T. Maisch et al., "Light-induced decomposition of indocyanine green," *Investigative Ophthalmology & Visual Science*, vol. 49, no. 5, pp. 1777–1783, 2008.

[2] Indocyanine Green kit, "PULSION," http://dailymed.nlm.nih.gov/dailymed/drugInfo.cfm?id=15096, 2010.

[3] L. A. Yannuzzi, "Indocyanine green angiography: a perspective on use in the clinical setting," *American Journal of Ophthalmology*, vol. 151, no. 5, pp. 745–751, 2011.

[4] C. A. Morton, S. B. Brown, S. Collins et al., "Guidelines for topical photodynamic therapy: Report of a workshop of the British Photodermatology Group," *British Journal of Dermatology*, vol. 146, no. 4, pp. 552–567, 2002.

[5] B. Lam, M. P. Wong, S. L. Fung et al., "The clinical value of autofluorescence bronchoscopy for the diagnosis of lung cancer," *European Respiratory Journal*, vol. 28, no. 5, pp. 915–919, 2006.

[6] S. Tobis, J. K. Knopf, C. R. Silvers et al., "Near infrared fluorescence imaging after intravenous indocyanine green: Initial clinical experience with open partial nephrectomy for renal cortical tumors," *Urology*, vol. 79, no. 4, pp. 958–964, 2012.

[7] W. Stummer, S. Stocker, S. Wagner et al., "Intraoperative detection of malignant gliomas by 5-aminolevulinic acid- induced porphyrin fluorescence," *Neurosurgery*, vol. 42, no. 3, pp. 518–526, 1998.

[8] M. Kusano, Y. Tajima, K. Yamazaki, M. Kato, M. Watanabe, and M. Miwa, "Sentinel node mapping guided by indocyanine green fluorescence imaging: A new method for sentinel node navigation surgery in gastrointestinal cancer," *Digestive Surgery*, vol. 25, no. 2, pp. 103–108, 2008.

[9] F. Ogata, M. Narushima, M. Mihara, R. Azuma, Y. Morimoto, and I. Koshima, "Intraoperative lymphography using indocyanine green dye for near-infrared fluorescence labeling in lymphedema," *Annals of Plastic Surgery*, vol. 59, no. 2, pp. 180–184, 2007.

[10] T. Abo, A. Nanashima, S. Tobinaga et al., "Usefulness of intraoperative diagnosis of hepatic tumors located at the liver surface and hepatic segmental visualization using indocyanine green-photodynamic eye imaging," *European Journal of Surgical Oncology (EJSO)*, vol. 41, no. 2, pp. 257–264, 2015.

[11] K. Norihiro and I. Takeaki, "Clinical application of fluorescence imaging of liver cancer using indocyanine green," *Liver Cancer*, no. 1, pp. 15–21, 2012.

[12] A. Peloso, E. Franchi, M. C. Canepa et al., "Combined use of intraoperative ultrasound and indocyanine green fluorescence imaging to detect liver metastases from colorectal cancer," *HPB*, vol. 15, no. 12, pp. 928–934, 2013.

[13] G. Folprecht, A. Grothey, S. Alberts, H.-R. Raab, and C.-H. Köhne, "Neoadjuvant treatment of unresectable colorectal liver metastases: Correlation between tumour response and resection rates," *Annals of Oncology*, vol. 16, no. 8, pp. 1311–1319, 2005.

[14] T. Aoki, D. Yasuda, Y. Shimizu et al., "Image-guided liver mapping using fluorescence navigation system with indocyanine green for anatomical hepatic resection," *World Journal of Surgery*, vol. 32, no. 8, pp. 1763–1767, 2008.

[15] K. Gotoh, T. Yamada, O. Ishikawa et al., "A novel image-guided surgery of hepatocellular carcinoma by indocyanine green fluorescence imaging navigation," *Journal of Surgical Oncology*, vol. 100, no. 1, pp. 75–79, 2009.

[16] T. Ishizawa, N. Fukushima, and J. Shibahara, "Real-time identification of liver cancer by using indocyanine green fluorescent imaging," *American cancersociety*, 2009.

[17] Y. Sakamoto, N. Kokudo, Y. Kawaguchi, and K. Akita, "Clinical Anatomy of the Liver: Review of the 19th Meeting of the Japanese Research Society of Clinical Anatomy," *Liver Cancer*, vol. 6, no. 2, pp. 146–160, 2017.

[18] G. Torzilli, M. Makuuchi, K. Inoue et al., "No-mortality liver resection for hepatocellular carcinoma in cirrhotic and noncirrhotic patients: Is there a way? A prospective analysis of our approach," *JAMA Surgery*, vol. 134, no. 9, pp. 984–992, 1999.

[19] T. Ishizawa, Y. Bandai, M. Ijichi, J. Kaneko, K. Hasegawa, and N. Kokudo, "Fluorescent cholangiography illuminating the biliary tree during laparoscopic cholecystectomy," *British Journal of Surgery*, vol. 97, no. 9, pp. 1369–1377, 2010.

[20] H. Takahashi, N. Zaidi, and E. Berber, "An initial report on the intraoperative use of indocyanine green fluorescence imaging in the surgical management of liver tumorss," *Journal of Surgical Oncology*, vol. 114, no. 5, pp. 625–629, 2016.

[21] T. Ishizawa, S. Tamura, K. Masuda et al., "Intraoperative fluorescent cholangiography using indocyanine green: a biliary road map for safe surgery," *Journal of the American College of Surgeons*, vol. 208, no. 1, pp. e1–e4, 2009.

[22] N. Harada, T. Ishizawa, A. Muraoka et al., "Fluorescence Navigation Hepatectomy by Visualization of Localized Cholestasis from Bile Duct Tumor Infiltration," *Journal of the American College of Surgeons*, vol. 210, no. 6, pp. e2–e6, 2010.

[23] Y. Fujisawa, Y. Nakamura, Y. Kawachi, and F. Otsuka, "A custom-made, low-cost intraoperative fluorescence navigation system with indocyanine green for sentinel lymph node biopsy in skin cancer," *Dermatology*, vol. 222, no. 3, pp. 261–268, 2011.

[24] L. Sorrentino, A. Sartani, G. Pietropaolo et al., "A Novel Indocyanine Green Fluorescence-Guided Video-Assisted Technique for Sentinel Node Biopsy in Breast Cancer," *World Journal of Surgery*, pp. 1–10, 2018.

[25] A. McGregor, S. N. Pavri, C. Tsay, S. Kim, and D. Narayan, "Use of Indocyanine Green for Sentinel Lymph Node Biopsy: Case Series and Methods Comparison," *Plastic and Reconstructive Surgery - Global Open*, vol. 5, no. 11, Article ID e1566, 2017.

Pseudoephedrine Induced Ischemic Colitis: A Case Report and Review of Literature

Muhammad Aziz,[1] Asad Pervez,[2] Rawish Fatima,[3] and Ajay Bansal[2]

[1] *Department of Internal Medicine, University of Kansas Medical Center, Kansas City, KS, USA*
[2] *Department of Gastroenterology and Hepatology, University of Kansas Medical Center, Kansas City, KS, USA*
[3] *Department of Internal Medicine, Dow University of Health Sciences, Karachi, Pakistan*

Correspondence should be addressed to Muhammad Aziz; maziz2@kumc.edu

Academic Editor: Hideto Kawaratani

Ischemic colitis due to medications is common, and a number of cases have been described with pseudoephedrine as the culprit agent. We present here an interesting case of a healthy female with no risk factors who developed pseudoephedrine induced ischemic colitis. This case serves to remind the healthcare providers about the utmost importance of obtaining a comprehensive history to aid with the diagnosis.

1. Introduction

Ischemic colitis is caused due to the sudden interruption of blood supply of the bowel, which results in ischemic injury particularly to the watershed areas. Risk factors associated with ischemic colitis include age, female gender, cardiovascular conditions, autoimmune diseases, hypercoagulable state, and medications [1].

Various case reports have been published linking ischemic colitis to numerous medications [1]. We present an interesting case of a patient with no medical comorbidities who presented with ischemic colitis likely associated with pseudoephedrine.

2. Case Report

A 54-year-old previously healthy Caucasian female with otherwise unremarkable past medical history presented to emergency department with one-day history of hematochezia and abdominal pain. The patient described crampy left lower quadrant pain with no aggravating or relieving factors. She had a total of five bowel movements since symptom onset with the first bowel movement containing stool mixed with bright red blood followed by predominantly bloody stools. She took no medications on a regular basis and denied having a screening colonoscopy for colorectal cancer at age 50. She reported symptoms of upper respiratory tract infection (cold, sneeze, and cough) for which she took three doses of 120 mg pseudoephedrine purchased from a local grocery store for 1 day prior to symptom onset. Her maternal grandfather had prostate cancer but there was no significant gastrointestinal tumor history in the family. She was a nonsmoker and reported drinking socially (roughly one standard drink) once a week.

Her admission vitals were within normal limits. Physical examination was consistent with mild tenderness on the left side of abdomen and hypoactive bowel sounds. Rectal examination showed bright red blood without any stool in the rectal canal. Her laboratory values were significant for mild anemia with hemoglobin of 11.5 mg/dl, hematocrit of 34.5%, erythrocyte sedimentation rate 31 mm/hr, and C-reactive protein 2.15 mg/dl. A computed tomography scan revealed mild to moderate mural thickening of the descending/sigmoid colon consistent with colitis without pericolonic abscess, ascites, or free air (Figure 1). An infectious workup was obtained including blood cultures, stool cultures, gastrointestinal panel for *Clostridium difficile*, and gastrointestinal viruses but was negative. She was resuscitated with intravenous fluids.

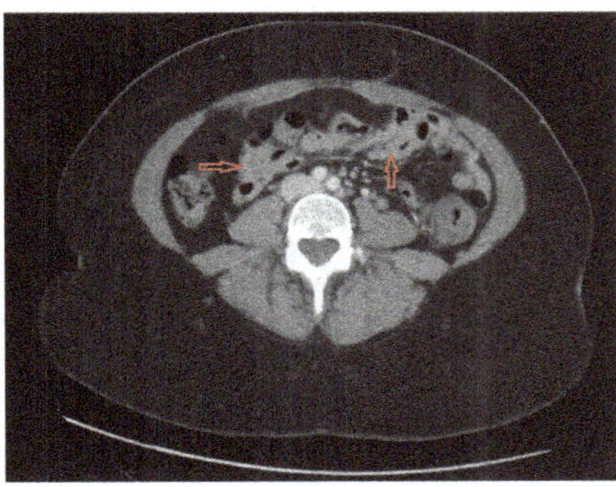

FIGURE 1: Transverse section of computed tomography scan demonstrating mild to moderate mural thickening of the descending/sigmoid colon (arrows) consistent with colitis without pericolonic abscess, ascites, or free air.

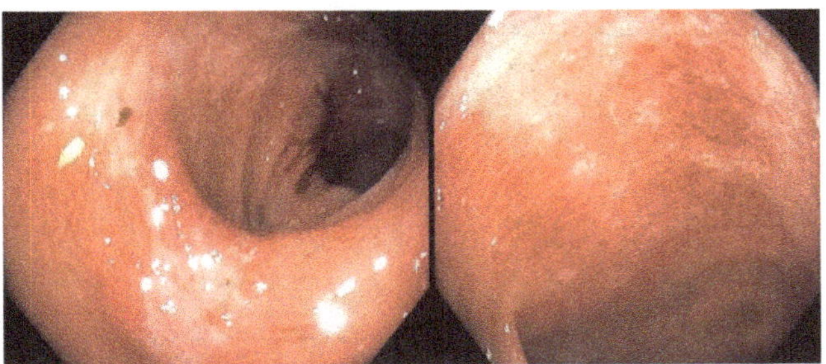

FIGURE 2: Colonoscopy demonstrating segmental moderate inflammation in the sigmoid colon, descending colon, and splenic flexure.

The patient underwent colonoscopy which demonstrated segmental moderate inflammation in the sigmoid colon, descending colon and splenic flexure along with internal and external hemorrhoids. There was evidence of submucosal hemorrhages with mild edema in the aforementioned segments of the colon (Figure 2). Endoscopic findings were highly suspicious of ischemic colitis. Several biopsies were obtained from the inflamed areas which exhibited focal lamina propria eosinophilic change with mild crypt attenuation and loss of goblet cells consistent with mild ischemic changes. There was no evidence of chronic inflammation.

She was observed in the hospital for 3 days and her diet was progressed slowly. Her bloody bowel movements ceased after 1 day in the hospital and patient was counseled and educated regarding avoidance of pseudoephedrine and over the counter medications for symptomatic management.

3. Discussion

This case demonstrates the occurrence of ischemic colitis in an otherwise healthy female who did not have any major risk factors that would predispose her to ischemic colitis. Medications are an increasingly common cause of ischemic colitis [1], which led us to do an extensive inquiry into over the counter drugs, herbal medications, complementary, and alternative management. The fact that the patient improved with conservative measures and has remained disease free since recovering from her initial injury favors medication as the culprit for causing ischemic colitis as opposed to a thrombotic or autoimmune disease. The patient scored an 8 on the Naranjo scoring system which classifies this event as a probable drug reaction [2] (Table 1). A thorough workup for autoimmune conditions was not carried out as the patient did not have any other symptoms and has also been disease-free since her discharge. Similarly, anticoagulation workup was not performed as the patient did not have evidence of clots or thrombus on the CT scan obtained nor did she have a previous history of thromboembolism.

Data are available in the literature on various medications causing ischemic colitis with different mechanisms of action [1]. Drugs such as norepinephrine, ephedrine, phenylephrine, phentermine, methamphetamine, vasopressin, epinephrine, cocaine, ergotamine, triptans, and ephedra cause vasoconstriction in the bowel predisposing the gut to ischemia particularly at the watershed area. Antihypertensive medications such as angiotensin converting enzyme inhibitors, diuretics, calcium channel blockers, and nitrates can cause ischemia by decreasing preload and reducing the blood supply to the affected organ. Thromboembolism is implicated with the use of oral contraceptive use and hormones. Other novel mechanisms have been proposed for other medications such as vasculitis with gold salts and increase colonic luminal pressure and subsequently decreased blood supply by alosetron [3]. Several other medications are implicated with causing ischemic colitis but the mechanism of action is unclear [4].

Pseudoephedrine is a commonly used over the counter medication for cold and allergy symptoms. It is a sympathomimetic drug with a direct agonistic effect on α- and $\beta 2$-adrenergic receptors causing vasoconstriction of blood vessels and relaxation of smooth muscles in the bronchi, respectively. This sympathomimetic action is likely responsible for causing ischemia in the gut as mentioned with other drugs related to same category above. After an extensive literature search, we found ten cases that suggested pseudoephedrine as the culprit agent for causing ischemic colitis [5–11] (Table 2). The dose of pseudoephedrine ingested varied across these cases with a range of 60 mg/day to 900 mg/day. Similarly, the duration of pseudoephedrine use ranged from as minimal as 5 days to 2 years. All the cases recovered uneventfully except one that required immediate surgical intervention with right-sided ischemic colitis. Our case is unique as our patient took only 3 doses of 120 mg of the drug for just one day and developed symptoms. This is the lowest possible exposure reported in the literature.

In conclusion, medications are an important factor that predisposes an individual to develop ischemic colitis. Our case report exemplifies that pseudoephedrine may cause ischemic colitis. Moreover, we would like to stress to healthcare providers (clinicians, nurse practitioners, assistant physicians, and medical students) the importance of detailed history and review of medications including prescription drugs, over the counter medications, herbal supplements, and alternative treatments to aid in the diagnosis of this condition.

TABLE 1: Naranjo scoring algorithm for determining possibility of drug reaction, scoring: ≥ 9 = definite ADR, 5-8 = probable ADR, 1-4 = possible ADR, and 0 = doubtful ADR.

	Question	Yes	No	NA	Points
1.	Are there previous conclusive reports on this reaction? Yes (+1) No (0) NA (0)	X			1
2.	Did the adverse events appear after the suspected drug was given? Yes (+2) No (-1) NA (0)	X			2
3.	Did the adverse reaction improve when the drug was discontinued or a specific antagonist was given? Yes (+2) No (-1) NA (0)	X			2
4.	Did the adverse reaction appear when the drug was readministered? Yes (+2) No (-1) NA (0)			X	0
5.	Are there alternative causes that could have caused the reaction? Yes (-1) No (+2) NA (0)		X		2
6.	Did the reaction reappear when a placebo was given? Yes (-1) No (+1) NA (0)			X	0
7.	Was the drug detected in any body fluid in toxic concentrations? Yes (+1) No (0) NA (0)			X	0
8.	Was the reaction more severe when the dose was increased, or less severe when the dose was decreased? Yes (+1) No (0) NA (0)			X	0
9.	Did the patient have a similar reaction to the same or similar drugs in any previous exposure? Yes (+1) No (0) NA (0)			X	0
10.	Was the adverse event confirmed by any objective evidence? Yes (+1) No (0) NA (0)	X			1

TABLE 2: Previously reported dosing for pseudoephedrine in patients presenting with ischemic colitis.

S. No	Author	Year	Dose and Frequency	Sequela
1.	Schneider	1995	Pseudoephedrine 240 mg daily for 5 days	Resolved
2.	Dowd	1999	Three patients used pseudoephedrine 120 mg twice daily for 7 days and one patient used 120 mg daily for 6 months	Resolved
3.	Lichtenstein et al.	2000	Sudafed (Pseudoephedrine) 120 mg twice daily for 5 days	Resolved
4.	Klestov et al.	2001	Nucosef daily (14.9 mg codeine + 60 mg pseudoephedrine) for 2 years and 900 mg daily pseudoephedrine before each hospitalizations.	First hospitalization: Right hemicolectomy Second hospitalization: ileocolic resection
5.	Traino et al.	2004	Pseudoephedrine 240 mg per day for 7 days + tramadol 150 mg per day for chronic back pain	Resolved
6.	Sherid et al.	2014	Sudafed (Pseudoephedrine) 120 mg twice daily for 5 days	Resolved
7.	Ambesh et al.	2017	Pseudoephedrine hydrochloride, 10 mg four times daily for 1 month	Resolved
8.	Aziz et al.	2018	Pseudoephedrine 120 mg × 3 in one day	Resolved

Consent

Informed consent was obtained from the patient via telephone after confirming patient's name, MRN, and DOB.

Authors' Contributions

Author guarantor is Muhammad Aziz. Muhammad Aziz was involved in manuscript writing and literature search. Other authors critically reviewed the manuscript and performed literature search on their own.

References

[1] P. D. R. Higgins, K. J. Davis, and L. Laine, "Systematic review: the epidemiology of ischaemic colitis," *Alimentary Pharmacology & Therapeutics*, vol. 19, no. 7, pp. 729–738, 2004.

[2] C. A. Naranjo, U. Busto, and E. M. Sellers, "A method for estimating the probability of adverse drug reactions," *Clinical Pharmacology & Therapeutics*, vol. 30, no. 2, pp. 239–245, 1981.

[3] M. Sherid and E. D. Ehrenpreis, "Types of colitis based on histology," *Disease-a-Month*, vol. 57, no. 9, pp. 457–489, 2011.

[4] K. Bielefeldt, "Ischemic Colitis as a Complication of Medication Use: An Analysis of the Federal Adverse Event Reporting System," *Digestive Diseases and Sciences*, vol. 61, no. 9, pp. 2655–2665, 2016.

[5] R. P. Schneider, "Ischemic colitis caused by decongestant?" *Journal of Clinical Gastroenterology*, vol. 21, no. 4, pp. 335-336, 1995.

[6] J. Dowd, D. Bailey, K. Moussa, S. Nair, R. Doyle, and J. A. Culpepper-Morgan, "Ischemic colitis associated with pseudoephedrine: Four cases," *American Journal of Gastroenterology*, vol. 94, no. 9, pp. 2430–2434, 1999.

[7] G. R. Lichtenstein and N. S. Yee, "Ischemic coliris associated with decongestant use," *Annals of Internal Medicine*, vol. 132, no. 8, article 682, 2000.

[8] A. Klestov, P. Kubler, and J. Meulet, "Recurrent ischaemic colitis associated with pseudoephedrine use," *Internal Medicine Journal*, vol. 31, no. 3, pp. 195-196, 2001.

[9] A. A. Traino, N. A. Buckley, and M. L. Bassett, "Probable ishemic colitis caused by pseudoephedrine with tramadol as a possible contributing factor," *Annals of Pharmacotherapy*, vol. 38, no. 12, pp. 2068–2070, 2004.

[10] M. Sherid, S. Samo, H. Husein, S. Sulaiman, and J. A. Vainder, "Pseudoephedrine-induced ischemic colitis: Case report and literature review," *Journal of Digestive Diseases*, vol. 15, no. 5, pp. 276–280, 2014.

[11] P. Ambesh, S. Siddiqui, C. Obiagwu et al., "Pseudoephedrine Associated Ischemic Colitis," *American Journal of Therapeutics*, p. 1, 2018.

Pneumatosis Coli Formation via Counterperfusion Supersaturation in a Patient with Severe Diarrhea

Eric Vecchio, Sehrish Jamot, and Jason Ferreira

Rhode Island Hospital and Brown University, USA

Correspondence should be addressed to Eric Vecchio; eric.vecchio@gmail.com

Academic Editor: Naohiko Koide

We present the case of an elderly male patient with known multiple myeloma who was hospitalized with profuse watery diarrhea and abdominal pain after a course of induction chemotherapy. Intestinal intramural gas was found on imaging and the diagnosis of pneumatosis intestinalis was confirmed by colonoscopy. We propose counterperfusion supersaturation as the etiology for this patient's pneumatosis coli via disruption of homeostasis between nitrogen and hydrogen normally present in the bowel. His condition was successfully treated with antidiarrheal medications and inhaled oxygen as well as intravenous hydration, and he eventually completed multiple myeloma directed chemotherapy with an excellent response. In this report, we discuss how clinicians can improve management of pneumatosis intestinalis by understanding the proposed pathophysiology.

1. Introduction

Pneumatosis intestinalis (PI) is a radiographic finding, which describes intestinal intramural air. It is frequently benign and does not typically require intervention [1, 2]. It is a rare condition affecting men and women equally and usually presents between the fourth and seventh decades of life [3]. Etiologies vary widely and range from idiopathic and benign to life threatening. The pathogenesis of this finding relies on the suspected origin of the intramural gas and the path it took to arrive in the bowel wall. Treatment is mainly supportive; however, additional therapy directed at the disease process responsible for producing pneumatosis intestinalis is typically required. In this report we present a case of pneumatosis intestinalis believed to be caused by counterperfusion supersaturation.

2. Case Report

An 86-year-old male with a past medical history significant for IgG lambda light chain multiple myeloma, congestive heart failure, and atrial fibrillation on anticoagulation presented for evaluation of abdominal pain, increasing abdominal distention, and inability to pass flatus or bowel movements for two days. Prior to his ileus-like symptoms, he experienced anorexia, rigors, and severe watery diarrhea for several days in correlation with the completion of his second cycle of Revlimid (lenalidomide), Velcade (bortezomib), and dexamethasone induction chemotherapy for multiple myeloma.

On presentation, he was afebrile and hypotensive to 72/42. Physical exam demonstrated a pale man with dry oral mucosa and a mildly tender, tympanitic abdomen without peritoneal signs. On laboratory examination he was found to have a white blood cell count of 4.6 x10^9/L, hemoglobin of 8.1 g/dl, platelets of 15 x10^9/L, creatinine of 2.35 mg/dL (baseline of 0.9 mg/dL), and lactic acid of 2.3 meq/L. A non-contrast abdominal computerized tomography (CT) scan was performed, which demonstrated diffuse colonic distention with submucosal and intraluminal gas, distended fluid-filled distal small bowel loops, and innumerable small submucosal lesions covering the surface of the colon (Figures 1 and 2). The clinical picture and data were interpreted as concern for an infectious colitis, but extensive stool testing including clostridium difficile toxin polymerase chain reaction, giardia antigen, cryptosporidium antigen, and stool cultures were all negative.

Initially, the diagnosis of bortezomib-induced ileus was entertained; however, the patient's diarrhea quickly resumed once he had been fluid resuscitated. He continued to

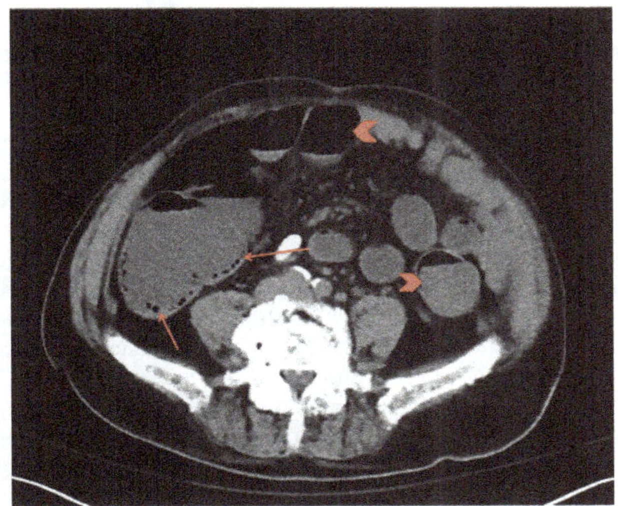

FIGURE 1: CT scan notable for colonic distention with submucosal and intraluminal gas (arrow), distended fluid-filled distal small bowel loops (arrowhead).

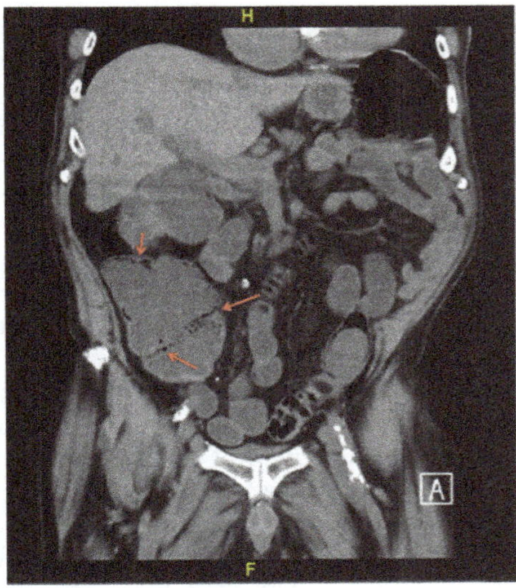

FIGURE 2: Coronal view with colonic wall thickening and submucosal and intraluminal air (arrow).

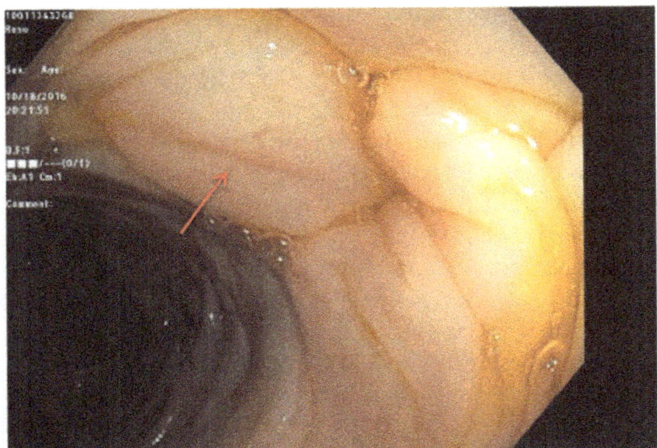

FIGURE 3: Pneumatosis coli of the transverse colon (arrow).

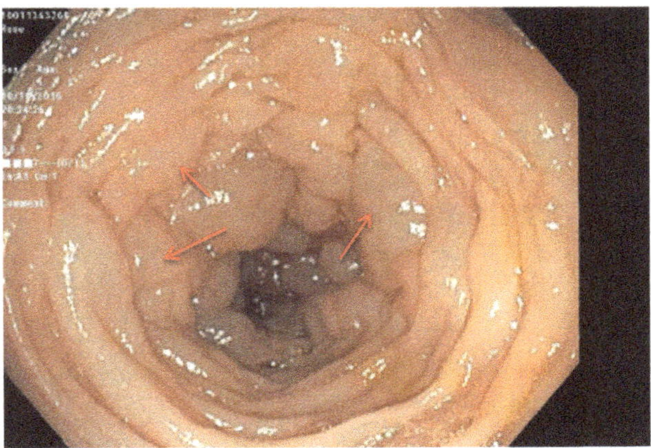

FIGURE 4: Pneumatosis coli of the descending colon (arrows).

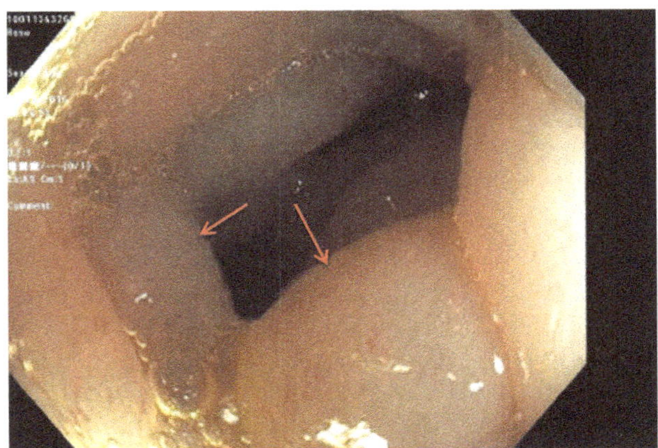

FIGURE 5: Pneumatosis coli of the sigmoid colon (arrows).

have watery stools requiring rectal tube placement without improvement on piperacillin-tazobactam and metronidazole. The gastroenterology service was consulted to determine the etiology of his diarrhea and abdominal pain, at which point the diagnosis of pneumatosis coli was considered. Repeat CT scan with IV contrast was requested and revealed bowel wall thickening of the transverse and proximal descending colon as well as multiple mildly thickened mid and distal small bowel loops. Based on the updated CT findings, concern for underlying typhlitis arose and the patient was maintained on empiric antibiotic therapy. Due to continued voluminous watery diarrhea, hypotension requiring constant fluid administration, severe hypokalemia, and little to no improvement on antibiotics, the patient was prepped for colonoscopy for direct visualization of the abnormal appearing bowel on imaging.

On colonoscopy, the colonic mucosa was normal appearing except for the presence of diffuse intramural gas consistent with pneumatosis coli (Figures 3–5). Biopsies of the colonic lesions were obtained and sent for pathological evaluation. After confirming the diagnosis of pneumatosis coli on colonoscopy, the objective for patient care shifted to controlling stool output with antidiarrheal agents. Treatment was successful using a combination of diphenoxylate/atropine,

MS16-9681, B1 (Procedure Date: 10/18/2016) - (PP201619402 A1) *Target population: Amyloid*

Antibodies To [Clone/Reagent]	*Result*
Kappa light chains [polyclonal ab]	NEGATIVE
Lambda light chains [polyclonal ab]	FOCALLY POSITIVE
Amyloid A [mc1]	STRONG SIGNAL
Amyloid P protein [polyclonal ab]	STRONG SIGNAL
Transthyretin [EPR3219]	STRONG SIGNAL

SPECIAL STAIN SUMMARY

MS16-9681, B1 (Procedure Date: 10/18/2016) - Colon, descending (PP201619402 A1)
Target population: Amyloid

Special Stain	*Result*
Amyloid / Congo Red, Alkaline	Positive for apple-green birefringence

Figure 6: Pathology result of colonic biopsy confirming diagnosis of gastrointestinal amyloidosis.

cholestyramine, and loperamide. The surgical pathology of the colonic biopsies returned positive for apple green birefringence on Congo red stain consistent with gastrointestinal amyloidosis (Figure 6). The patient received continued treatment directed towards his multiple myeloma, which was thought to have caused the amyloidosis. The patient had a dramatic response to chemotherapy with resolution of his gastrointestinal symptoms.

3. Discussion

3.1. Pathophysiology. Pneumatosis intestinalis is the term used to describe pockets of gas found within the wall of the intestine. Determination of the origin of the deposited gas can help us understand the mechanisms by which pneumatosis intestinalis can occur. Gas can be found in the intestinal lumen due to ingestion of air, production by flora, production by invasive pathogenic gas-producing bacteria; can diffuse from nearby mesenteric blood vessels; or can be of pulmonary origin. One theorized mechanism for gas deposition within the luminal wall involves intraluminal air dissecting into the wall of the intestine via mucosal defects. Bacterial invasion of the intestinal wall by gas-producing organisms can also lead to deposition of gas in the submucosa of the intestine. Gas from ruptured lung parenchyma can dissect into the mediastinum to the retroperitoneum, from where it can eventually track along perivascular tissue planes to deposit in the wall of the bowel [2]. Finally, counterperfusion supersaturation is a mechanism by which gas diffusion gradients (particularly nitrogen and hydrogen) between the bowel and mesenteric blood vessels are disrupted. Specifically, gas cysts tend to occur in close proximity to blood vessels on the mesenteric border of the colon. Normally the colon lumen serves as a hydrogen source and a nitrogen sink, whereas the circulation is a hydrogen sink and a nitrogen source. This establishes a homeostatic exchange of the two gases. In scenarios where this steady state is perturbed, gas can deposit within the luminal wall and can be perpetuated until the ongoing pathology is properly addressed [4].

3.2. Presentation. Symptomatology of PI is largely nonspecific and is attributed to the underlying condition causing pneumatosis intestinalis. Frequently, patients present with diarrhea, abdominal pain, abdominal distention, nausea, vomiting, and weight loss if the diarrhea is protracted and mucous in the stool. Interestingly, PI is one of the differential diagnoses associated with sterile pneumoperitoneum [3].

3.3. Diagnosis. Diagnosis of pneumatosis intestinalis is largely imaging based. It can be diagnosed on X-ray, ultrasound, CT, and endoscopy among other modalities. Abdominal radiographs can demonstrate pneumatosis intestinalis in two-thirds of cases [5]. Ultrasonography can also be used to demonstrate pneumatosis intestinalis, which manifests itself as bright echoes found in the intestinal wall. The majority of studies investigating the presence of intraluminal gas relate to diagnosis of intestinal ischemia. Multidetector-row CT (MDCT) is the most commonly used method of imaging when it comes to sensitivity of detecting intramural gas [6]. In one small study, CT had a specificity of more than 95% for detecting the presence of intramural gas relating to intestinal ischemia. Even more important is the ability of MDCT to quickly image the entire abdomen, increasing the chances that the clinician will be able to identify the cause of the PI and rule out life threatening conditions.

3.4. Complications. Complications occur in about 3% of patients with pneumatosis intestinalis and include volvulus, bowel obstruction, gastrointestinal hemorrhage, and intestinal perforation manifested as pneumoperitoneum [3].

3.5. Management. In general, inhaled oxygen therapy has been cited as early as the 1970s as a treatment for PI [7, 8]. Studies are conclusive in demonstrating that oxygen is beneficial both at various concentrations and delivery routes from nasal cannula to hyperbaric oxygen therapy; however, the optimal dose has not been determined [9]. Oxygen therapy may directly improve symptoms by displacing gases found within the cysts with oxygen, which is subsequently metabolized causing resolution of the cysts [10]. Treatment should also be directed towards the underlying disease resulting in pneumatosis intestinalis as well as management of potential complications of pneumatosis including bowel necrosis, intestinal perforation, and peritonitis.

We believe the pneumatosis intestinalis in this patient formed via counterperfusion supersaturation for a number of reasons. First, his initial presentation with significant hypotension likely resulted in a disruption of the normal nitrogen and hydrogen homeostasis of the intestine by impairing diffusion of nitrogen from the blood to the gut due to low blood pressure. Additionally, chronic disruption of mesenteric vascular permeability as a result of amyloid vasculopathy may have contributed to the formation of pneumatosis intestinalis in this patient. Finally, there was likely an increase in hydrogen in the lumen of the intestine due to reduction in gut hydrogen absorption by intestinal bacteria as a result of antibiotic administration. Since the mucosa was not disrupted on colonoscopy, we do not believe the PI was formed as a result of amyloid deposition throughout the GI tract, despite the presence of amyloid on biopsy.

3.6. Conclusion. The differential for pneumatosis intestinalis is broad and includes both benign and life threatening conditions. Any disease state causing damage to the intestinal blood supply or disruption of the gut microbiome can potentially cause PI. Lack of knowledge of this condition and its proposed pathophysiology may limit timely diagnosis and as a result could cause patient harm. Specifically, patients are at risk for unnecessary surgery, extreme volume depletion, and electrolyte abnormalities due to uncontrolled diarrhea, side effects from antibiotic therapy, and increased hospital length of stay, all of which ultimately can result in poor outcomes and increased healthcare costs.

Pneumatosis intestinalis is a condition caused by the deposition of gas into the bowel wall. Air can make its way into the bowel by a number of pathologic mechanisms, all of which take into account either mucosal injury or pressure/diffusion gradients between body compartments. The diagnosis is imaging based and is best performed with MDCT scan due to its ability not only to identify the finding, but also to potentially reveal the underlying disease process. Treatment of pneumatosis intestinalis itself is supportive consisting of intravenous hydration and inhaled oxygen therapy. Clinical and laboratory evaluation to diagnose the underlying cause of the pneumatosis intestinalis is paramount and careful consideration is necessary prior to initiating aggressive interventions.

References

[1] P. N. Khalil, S. Huber-Wagner, R. Ladurner et al., "Natural history, clinical pattern, and surgical considerations of pneumatosis intestinalis," *European Journal of Medical Research*, vol. 14, no. 6, pp. 231–239, 2009.

[2] S. D. St Peter, M. A. Abbas, and K. A. Kelly, "The spectrum of pneumatosis intestinalis," *JAMA Surgery*, vol. 138, no. 1, pp. 68–75, 2003.

[3] D. C. Sabiston and C. M. Townsend, *Sabiston Textbook of Surgery : The Biological Basis of Modern Surgical Practice*, Elsevier Saunders, Philadelphia, PA, USA, 19th edition, 2012.

[4] T. Florin and B. Hills, "Does counterperfusion supersaturation cause gas cysts in pneumatosis cystoides coli, and can breathing heliox reduce them?" *The Lancet*, vol. 345, no. 8959, pp. 1220–1222, 1995.

[5] J. Jamart, "Pneumatosis cystoides intestinalis. A statistical study of 919 cases," *Acta Hepatogastroenterol (Stuttg)*, vol. 26, pp. 419–422, 1979.

[6] M. Moschetta, A. A. Stabile Ianora, P. Pedote, A. Scardapane, and G. Angelelli, "Prognostic value of multidetector computed tomography in bowel infarction," *La Radiologia Medica*, vol. 114, no. 5, pp. 780–791, 2009.

[7] J. C. Gruenberg, S. K. Batra, and R. J. Priest, "Treatment of Pneumatosis Cystoides Intestinalis With Oxygen," *JAMA Surgery*, vol. 112, no. 1, pp. 62–64, 1977.

[8] M. Miralbés, J. Hinojosa, J. Alonso, and J. Berenguer, "Oxygen therapy in pneumatosis coli - What is the minimum oxygen requirement?" *Diseases of the Colon & Rectum*, vol. 26, no. 7, pp. 458–460, 1983.

[9] G. Gagliardi, I. W. Thompson, M. J. Hershman, A. Forbes, P. R. Hawley, and I. C. Talbot, "Pneumatosis coli: a proposed pathogenesis based on study of 25 cases and review of the literature," *International Journal of Colorectal Disease*, vol. 11, no. 3, pp. 111–118, 1996.

[10] F. Azzaroli, L. Turco, L. Ceroni et al., "Pneumatosis cystoides intestinalis," *World Journal of Gastroenterology*, vol. 17, no. 44, pp. 4932–4936, 2011.

46

Two Cases of Rectal Xanthoma Presenting as Yellowish to Whitish Lesions during Colonoscopy

Masaya Iwamuro,[1,2] Takehiro Tanaka,[3] Daisuke Takei,[1] Yuusaku Sugihara,[1] Keita Harada,[1] Sakiko Hiraoka,[1] Yoshiro Kawahara,[4] and Hiroyuki Okada[1]

[1] *Department of Gastroenterology and Hepatology, Okayama University Graduate School of Medicine, Dentistry and Pharmaceutical Sciences, Okayama 700-8558, Japan*
[2] *Department of General Medicine, Okayama University Graduate School of Medicine, Dentistry and Pharmaceutical Sciences, Okayama 700-8558, Japan*
[3] *Department of Pathology, Okayama University Hospital, Okayama 700-8558, Japan*
[4] *Department of Endoscopy, Okayama University Hospital, Okayama 700-8558, Japan*

Correspondence should be addressed to Masaya Iwamuro; iwamuromasaya@yahoo.co.jp

Academic Editor: Tetsuo Hirata

Two cases of rectal xanthomas are described. One case is that of a 56-year-old Japanese man in whom multiple yellowish spots measuring approximately 3 to 5 mm were observed in the rectum during colonoscopy. The other case is that of a 78-year-old Japanese man in whom colonoscopy showed a whitish plaque of 4 mm in diameter in the rectum. Biopsy examinations performed on both patients revealed the deposition of xanthoma cells within the rectal mucosa. Within the gastrointestinal tract, xanthomas most frequently arise in the stomach, whereas the colorectum is rarely affected. Despite this infrequency, the two cases indicate that xanthomas should be recalled when yellowish to whitish lesions are observed in the colorectum.

1. Introduction

Xanthomas in the alimentary tract are benign mucosal lesions resulting from the aggregation of foamy histiocytes within the gastrointestinal mucosa [1]. Within the gastrointestinal tract, the stomach is the most frequently affected by xanthoma, whereas other parts such as the esophagus, duodenum [2], small intestine, and colorectum usually remain unaffected. Macroscopic features of gastric xanthoma are well known as yellow to white well-demarcated plaques or nodules [3]. Endoscopic images of colorectal xanthoma have rarely been reported in the literature due to their infrequency.

We recently encountered two patients with rectal xanthomas that were observed as yellowish to whitish lesions during colonoscopy. In this report, we focus mainly on the macroscopic characteristics of the colorectal xanthoma and review previously reported cases of this disease.

2. Case Report

2.1. Case 1. A 56-year-old Japanese man was referred to our hospital for investigation of tarry stool. The patient had been consuming lansoprazole, irsogladine, metoprolol, flutoprazepam, and ethyl loflazepate for gastritis, hypertension, and anxiety disorder but had no history of dyslipidemia or diabetes mellitus. A physical examination revealed no abnormalities in his abdomen or xanthomas on his skin, and laboratory findings showed no abnormalities. The levels of cholesterol, triglyceride, and plasma glucose were within normal range. Esophagogastroduodenoscopy showed erosive and atrophic gastritis.

During colonoscopy, multiple yellowish spots measuring approximately 3 to 5 mm were observed in the rectum, in addition to hemorrhoids (Figure 1(a)). Magnifying observation with narrow-band imaging revealed that the pits of the rectal mucosa were intact (Figure 1(b)). Indigo-carmine

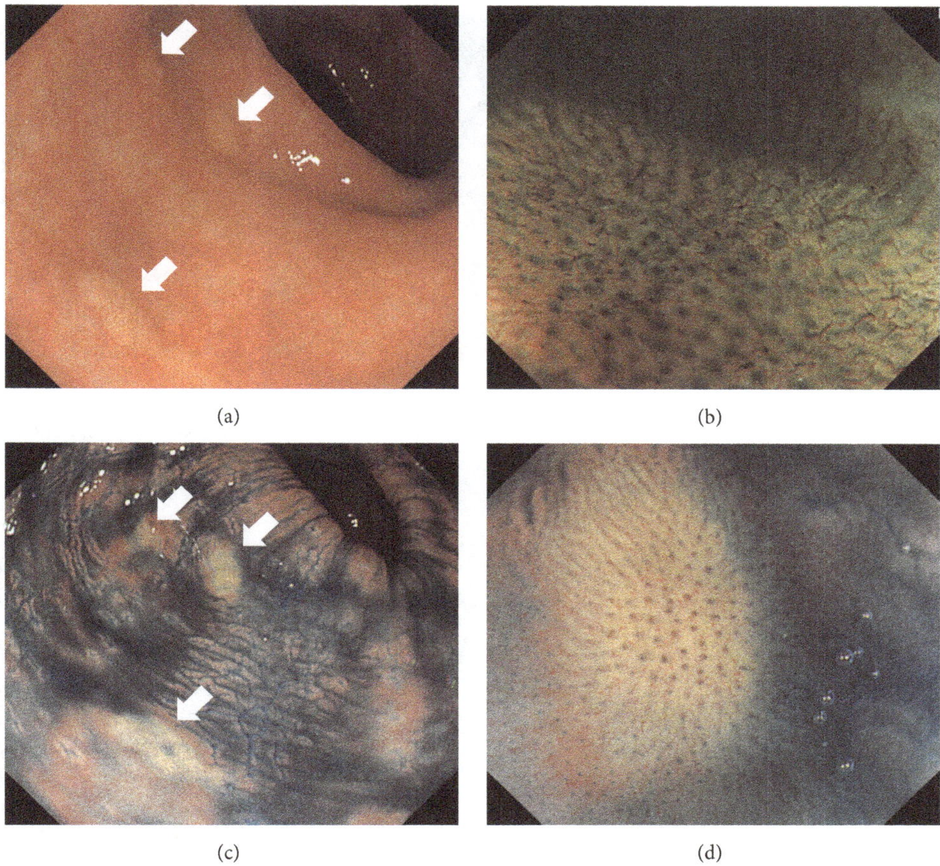

FIGURE 1: Colonoscopy images of case 1. Multiple yellowish spots measuring approximately 3 to 5 mm are seen in the rectum (a). Magnifying observation with narrow-band imaging reveals intact pits of the rectal mucosa (b). Indigo-carmine spraying emphasizes the whitish to yellowish color of the lesions (c, d).

spraying emphasized the whitish to yellowish color of the lesions (Figures 1(c) and 1(d)). Histological analysis of the biopsied samples revealed accumulation of xanthoma cells within the mucosal layer. Consequently, a diagnosis of rectal xanthoma was made.

2.2. Case 2. A 78-year-old Japanese man had been treated for remitting seronegative symmetrical synovitis with pitting edema. The patient underwent colonoscopy for screening purposes. He had been taking 2 mg/day of prednisone but had no history of dyslipidemia or diabetes mellitus. A physical examination revealed no xanthomas on his eyelid or extremities and a blood test revealed that his levels of cholesterol, triglyceride, and plasma glucose were within normal range.

Colonoscopy showed a whitish plaque of 4 mm in diameter in the rectum (Figure 2). Biopsy examination revealed massive deposition of xanthoma cells within the rectal mucosa (Figure 3), leading to the diagnosis of rectal xanthoma.

3. Discussion

In the two cases presented, rectal xanthomas were observed as yellowish to whitish lesions during colonoscopy. As described above, typical gastric xanthomas are well-demarcated whitish plaques or nodules. Similarly, cases with xanthomas in the sigmoid colon and rectum, showing multiple, well-defined, and whitish-yellow lesions, have been previously reported [4, 5]. Weinstock et al. reported a case consistent with xanthoma presenting as flat, yellow, and irregularly shaped lesions in the sigmoid colon [6]. Endoscopic images presented in their report show a hexagonal-shaped appearance, which is not similar to the macroscopy of gastric xanthomas. The case report by Moran and Fogt, which did not present endoscopic images, described a xanthoma in the rectosigmoid colon as polypoid in appearance [7]. Miliauskas et al. reported that, by reviewing their four cases and nine previously reported cases, papules were observed in eight cases and polyps were noted in three cases [8, 9]. Nakasono et al. summarized 28 colorectal xanthomas biopsied from 25 patients. Xanthomas were located in the sigmoid colon (17/28 lesions) and rectum (11/28 lesions) [9]. Macroscopically, 23 lesions presented sessile appearance and the remaining five lesions were pedunculated. Twelve of the xanthoma lesions were reddish, five were whitish, two were yellow-whitish, and one was normal color. Consequently, the morphology of colorectal xanthomas varies from flat, sessile to pedunculated lesions, with yellowish, yellow-whitish, whitish, and even reddish colors.

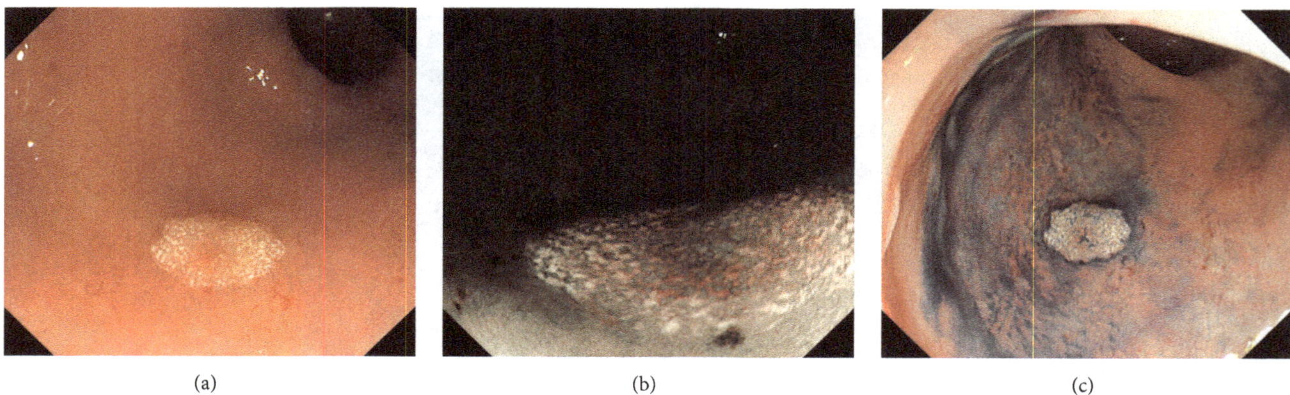

(a) (b) (c)

FIGURE 2: Colonoscopy images of case 2. A whitish plaque of 4 mm in diameter in the rectum is seen (a). Narrow-band imaging (b) and indigo-carmine spraying (c) show whitish lesions more clearly.

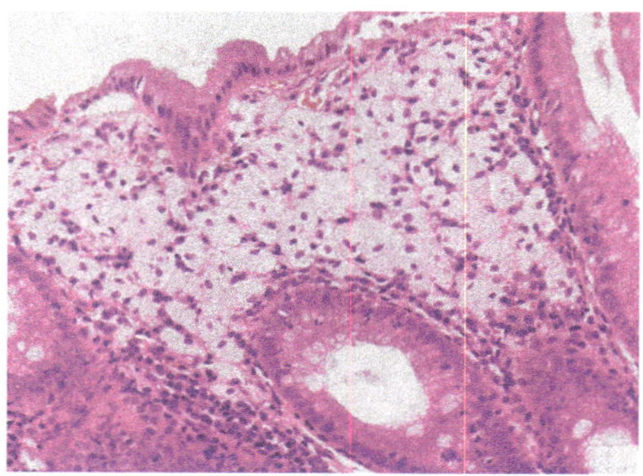

FIGURE 3: Pathological image of case 2. Biopsy examination reveals massive deposition of xanthoma cells within the rectal mucosa.

Endoscopists must recall this entity as a differential diagnosis when they observe whitish lesions in the colorectum regardless. In the two cases we presented, narrow-band imaging highlighted lesions that were yellowish to whitish in color. Moreover, observation under magnification revealed intact pits in the rectal mucosa. We propose that the intact pits reflect undamaged epithelial cells observed by histopathological examination of biopsy specimens. However, since this observation is based on only two cases, usefulness of observation under magnification and optical chromoendoscopy techniques such as narrow-band imaging, flexible spectral imaging color enhancement, and i-SCAN for the diagnosis of colorectal xanthomas should be further investigated.

Diseases other than xanthomas that present with yellowish to whitish lesions in the colon include pseudomembranous colitis, lipomas, and lymphomas. Pseudomembranous colitis is a common cause of antibiotic-associated diarrhea. This disease is characterized by elevated yellow-white plaques that coalesce to form pseudomembranes along the colorectal mucosa and can be easily diagnosed based on their endoscopic appearance [10]. Colonic lipomas are generally observed as solitary, soft, spherical, smooth yellowish lesions [11]. Pedunculated and semipedunculated lipomas can be easily diagnosed, but those with a slightly elevated appearance may be misinterpreted as xanthomas. Lymphomas, particularly the indolent subtypes, sometimes present as whitish, slightly elevated lesions in the colorectum. For instance, follicular lymphomas in the colorectum are identified as papular, polypoid, or flat elevated lesions [12]. While the color of the lymphoma lesions is not grossly different than that of the surrounding intact mucosa, colorectal xanthomas, as observed in this report, do show a definite color contrast between the lesions and surrounding mucosa.

Microscopically, foamy macrophages are generally confined to the lamina propria mucosae of the colorectum; the muscularis mucosae or submucosa is rarely affected. Nakasono et al. reported that hyperplastic change was identified in the surface epithelium in 22/28 lesions [9]. In addition, thickening of the basement membrane of the surface epithelium, cell debris, and proliferation of the capillaries were frequently observed. In contrast, the two presented cases lack hyperplastic change in the epithelium. In case 2, we speculate that the accumulation of foamy cells itself accounts for the slightly elevated morphology since prominent deposition of foamy cells exists in the lamina propria mucosae (Figure 3).

Although cutaneous and tendinous xanthomas occur in relation to hyperlipidemia, gastrointestinal xanthomas are not associated with dyslipidemia [3, 7, 13]. Miliauskas et al. reported that, among four cases with colorectal xanthomas, none had hyperlipidemia and only one had diabetes mellitus [7, 8]. The two cases presented did not have metabolic disorders, including increased lipid levels and diabetes mellitus. Gastrointestinal xanthomas are asymptomatic and believed to be harmless [8, 9]. Therefore, no specific treatment is considered necessary for colorectal xanthomas.

The etiology of colorectal xanthomas remains unknown. Xanthomas in the stomach are assumed to arise as an inflammatory response to focal mucosal damage and chronic injury such as chronic gastritis [3, 7, 14–16]. The resident macrophages commonly exist in the subepithelial lamina propria of the gastrointestinal tract. Although macrophages are not pathologically noticeable in normal gut mucosa, they can be identified when they phagocytize and accumulate exogenous or endogenous substances [17]. Content of the foamy macrophages in xanthomas is assumed to come from lipids derived from damaged cell membranes [3, 7, 14]. Mucosal damage and chronic injury are believed to be associated with the pathogenesis of colorectal xanthomas [7, 15]. Toxic factors, focal infection, or mechanical damage by peristalsis or contact with feces may cause such injury to the colorectal mucosa [5, 9].

In conclusion, we encountered two patients with rectal xanthomas. Both cases showed yellow to whitish lesions in the rectum. Although colorectal xanthoma can present varied morphology, endoscopists should consider this entity when yellowish to whitish lesions are observed in the colorectum.

References

[1] B. M. Andrejic, S. V. Bozanic, N. S. Solajic, M. A. Djolai, and A. M. Levakov, "Xanthomas of the stomach: a report of two cases," *Bosnian Journal of Basic Medical Sciences*, vol. 12, no. 2, pp. 127–129, 2012.

[2] M. Iwamuro, T. Tanaka, F. Otsuka, and H. Okada, "Xanthoma of the Duodenum," *Internal Medicine*, vol. 55, no. 19, pp. 2899-2900, 2016.

[3] S. Basyigit, A. Kefeli, Z. Asilturk, F. Sapmaz, and B. Aktas, "Gastric Xanthoma: A review of the literature," *Shiraz E Medical Journal*, vol. 16, no. 7, Article ID e29569, pp. 1–5, 2015.

[4] Y. Hisanaga, Y. Akaike, and K. Kuroda, "Xanthoma disseminatum with large plaques confined to the back, pulmonary involvement and multiple intestinal xanthomas," *Dermatology*, vol. 208, no. 2, pp. 164–166, 2004.

[5] W. Remmele, K. Beck, and E. Kaiserling, "Multiple lipid islands of the colonic mucosa. A light and electron microscopic study," *Pathology Research and Practice*, vol. 183, no. 3, pp. 336–346, 1988.

[6] L. B. Weinstock, B. A. Shatz, R. J. Saltman, and K. Deschryver, "Xanthoma of the colon," *Gastrointestinal Endoscopy*, vol. 55, no. 3, p. 410, 2002.

[7] A. M. Moran and F. Fogt, "70-year-old female presenting with rectosigmoid (Colonic) xanthoma and multiple benign polyps - case report," *Polish Journal of Pathology*, vol. 61, no. 1, pp. 42–45, 2010.

[8] J. R. Miliauskas, "Rectosigmoid (colonic) xanthoma: a report of four cases and review of the literature," *Pathology*, vol. 34, no. 2, pp. 144–147, 2002.

[9] M. Nakasono, M. Hirokawa, N. Muguruma et al., "Colorectal xanthomas with polypoid lesion: report of 25 cases," *APMIS*, vol. 112, no. 1, pp. 3–10, 2004.

[10] D. M. Tang, N. H. Urrunaga, H. De Groot, E. C. von Rosenvinge, G. Xie, and L. J. Ghazi, "Pseudomembranous colitis: not always caused by clostridium difficile," *Case Reports in Medicine*, vol. 2014, Article ID 812704, 4 pages, 2014.

[11] G. Martinez-Mier, A. B. Ortiz-Bayliss, R. Alvarado-Arenas, and M. A. Carrasco-Arroniz, "Caecum lipoma: A rare cause of lower gastrointestinal bleeding," *BMJ Case Reports*, vol. 2014, 2014.

[12] M. Iwamuro, H. Okada, K. Takata et al., "Colorectal manifestation of follicular lymphoma," *Internal Medicine*, vol. 55, no. 1, pp. 1–8, 2016.

[13] A. G. Coates, T. T. Nostrant, J. A. P. Wilson, W. O. Dobbins III, and F. P. Agha, "Gastric xanthomatosis and cholestasis - A causal relationship," *Digestive Diseases and Sciences*, vol. 31, no. 9, pp. 925–928, 1986.

[14] J. Lechago, "Lipid islands of the stomach: An insular issue?" *Gastroenterology*, vol. 110, no. 2, pp. 630–632, 1996.

[15] P. A. Bejarano, J. Aranda-Michel, and C. Fenoglio-Preiser, "Histochemical and immunohistochemical characterization of foamy histiocytes (muciphages and xanthelasma) of the rectum," *American Journal of Surgical Pathology*, vol. 24, no. 7, pp. 1009–1015, 2000.

[16] N. Bassullu, I. Turkmen, S. Uraz et al., "Xanthomatous hyperplastic polyps of the stomach: Clinicopathologic study of 5 patients with polypoid gastric lesions showing combined features of gastric xanthelasma and hyperplastic polyp," *Annals of Diagnostic Pathology*, vol. 17, no. 1, pp. 72–74, 2013.

[17] X. Sagaert, T. Tousseyn, G. De Hertogh, and K. Geboes, "Macrophage-related diseases of the gut: a pathologist's perspective," *Virchows Archiv*, vol. 460, no. 6, pp. 555–567, 2012.

Gastric MALT Lymphoma with Increased Plasma Cell Differentiation Showing Unique Endoscopic Features

Masaya Iwamuro,[1] Takehiro Tanaka,[2] Kenji Nishida,[3] Seiji Kawano,[1] Yoshiro Kawahara,[4] Shogen Ohya,[5] Tadashi Yoshino,[3] and Hiroyuki Okada[1]

[1] *Department of Gastroenterology and Hepatology, Okayama University Graduate School of Medicine, Dentistry, and Pharmaceutical Sciences, Okayama 700-8558, Japan*
[2] *Department of Pathology, Okayama University Hospital, Okayama 700-8558, Japan*
[3] *Department of Pathology, Okayama University Graduate School of Medicine, Dentistry, and Pharmaceutical Sciences, Okayama 700-8558, Japan*
[4] *Department of Endoscopy, Okayama University Hospital, Okayama 700-8558, Japan*
[5] *Kawaguchi Medical Clinic, Okayama 700-0913, Japan*

Correspondence should be addressed to Masaya Iwamuro; iwamuromasaya@yahoo.co.jp

Academic Editor: Yucel Ustundag

A 62-year-old woman was diagnosed with extranodal marginal zone lymphoma of mucosa-associated lymphoid tissue (MALT lymphoma) with increased plasma cell differentiation of the stomach. Esophagogastroduodenoscopy showed slightly elevated, whitish lesions in the gastric body. Magnifying endoscopic observation revealed that the gastric surface epithelium was swollen, but the structure was not destroyed or diminished. Elongated, tortuous vasculature was observed on the surface of the whitish lesions. The patient underwent eradication treatment for *Helicobacter pylori*, which resulted in complete remission. Although the appearance of abnormal vessels and the destruction of gastric epithelial structure are the typical features of gastric MALT lymphoma during magnifying endoscopy, the present case showed different features, which were rather similar to those observed in a previously reported case of gastric plasmacytoma. The current case indicates that magnifying endoscopic features are not uniform among gastric MALT lymphomas.

1. Introduction

Extranodal marginal zone lymphoma or mucosa-associated lymphoid tissue (MALT lymphoma) is one of the most common non-Hodgkin lymphomas arising in the gastrointestinal tract, particularly in the stomach [1]. Gastric MALT lymphomas exhibit various types of morphologies, ranging from erosions/ulcers, early gastric cancer-like lesions, whitish mucosa, and cobblestone appearance to submucosal tumor [2]. Magnifying endoscopic observation of gastric MALT lymphomas shows typical features such as the appearance of abnormal vessels and the destruction of gastric epithelial structure [3–5]. Since these features disappear when pathological remission is achieved [5], understanding these features is essential for proper detection and management of gastric MALT lymphomas.

Recently, we encountered a case of gastric MALT lymphoma with increased plasma cell differentiation. The gastric lesions exhibited unique endoscopic features, showing slightly elevated, whitish lesions, with a swollen epithelium but intact epithelial structure. Elongated, tortuous vasculature was observed on the surface of the whitish lesions, suggesting the deposition of whitish substances beneath the gastric epithelium. These features identified in magnifying endoscopic observation were similar to those observed in a previously reported case of gastric plasmacytoma [6]. In this report, we focus mainly on the pathologic and endoscopic features of our patient.

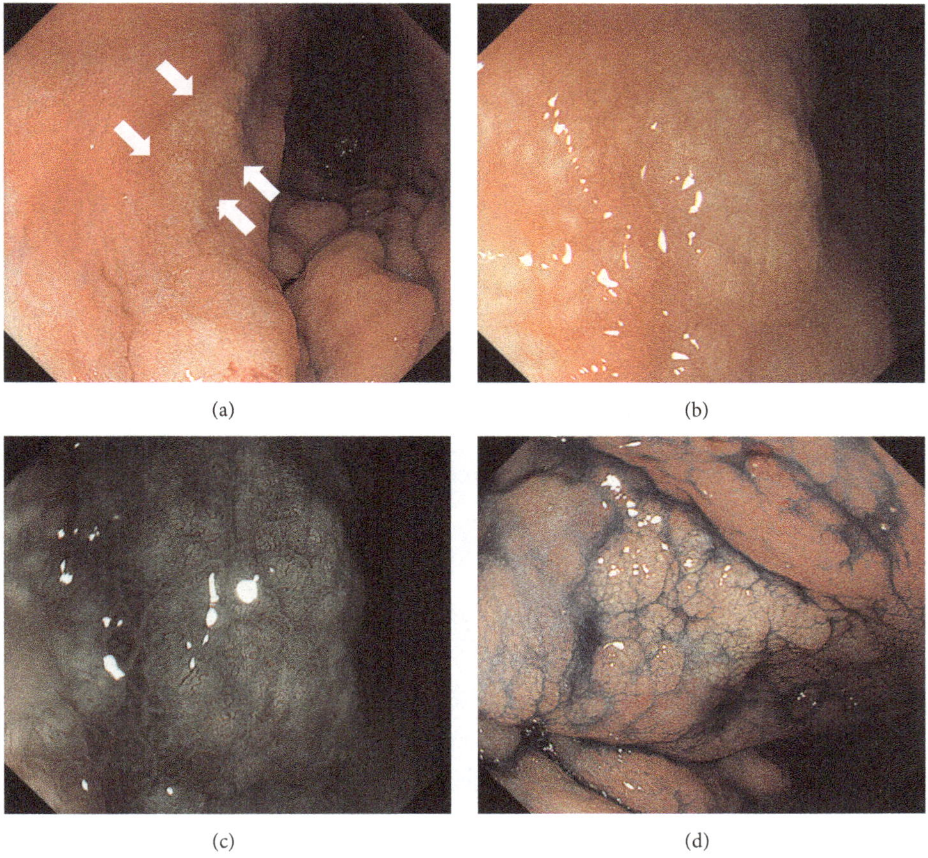

FIGURE 1: Esophagogastroduodenoscopy images. Slightly elevated, whitish lesions are observed in the gastric body ((a) arrows). Magnifying endoscopic observation with white light (b) and with narrow-band imaging (c) reveals that the gastric surface epithelium is swollen, but the structure is not destroyed or diminished. Whitish area is emphasized after indigo carmine spraying (d).

2. Case Report

A 62-year-old woman tested positive for serum anti-*Helicobacter pylori* IgG antibody at her annual medical checkup. Subsequently, she underwent esophagogastroduodenoscopy at her family clinic, which revealed a whitish area in the gastric body. The patient was referred to Okayama University Hospital for further investigation and treatment. She had been taking rosuvastatin for hyperlipidemia and had no history of gastrointestinal diseases. A physical examination revealed no abnormalities, and there were no lymphadenopathies or hepatosplenomegaly. Laboratory findings including hemoglobin, lactate dehydrogenase, soluble interleukin-2 receptor, and immunoglobulin M, G, and A levels were within the normal ranges. There was no M protein in serum or urine protein electrophoresis. Monoclonal protein was not identified in the serum or urine by using immunoelectrophoresis. Esophagogastroduodenoscopy (GIF-H260Z; Olympus, Tokyo, Japan) showed slightly elevated, whitish lesions in the gastric body (Figure 1(a)). Magnifying endoscopic observation with white light (Figure 1(b)) and with narrow-band imaging (Figure 1(c)) revealed that the gastric surface epithelium was swollen, but the structure was not destroyed or diminished. Elongated, tortuous vasculature was observed on the surface of the whitish lesions, suggesting the deposition of whitish substances beneath the gastric epithelium.

Biopsy samples from the gastric lesions showed dense, diffuse infiltration of small-to-medium-sized monocytoid cells and plasma cells and multiple Dutcher bodies (Figure 2). Lymphoepithelial lesions were absent. Immunohistochemistry analysis showed that the infiltrating cells were positive for CD20 and BCL2, while they were negative for CD3, CD10, and cyclin D1 (Figure 3). In situ hybridization for immunoglobulin light chains showed expression of monoclonal immunoglobulin light chain κ in these cells (Figures 3(f) and 3(g)). Few tumor cells were positive for Ki-67 staining, indicating few mitotic cells. The diagnosis of gastric MALT lymphoma with plasma cell differentiation was made based on these pathological features. Fluorescence in situ hybridization (FISH) analysis for t(11;18)(q21;q21) translocation revealed no fusion genes of *BIRC3-MALT1*, although extra copies of *MALT1* were identified in 32.0% of the monocytoid cells (Figure 4), indicating trisomy of chromosome 18 [2, 7]. Chromosome banding of the bone marrow aspirate showed a normal karyotype of 46, XX, indicating no congenital chromosomal abnormalities.

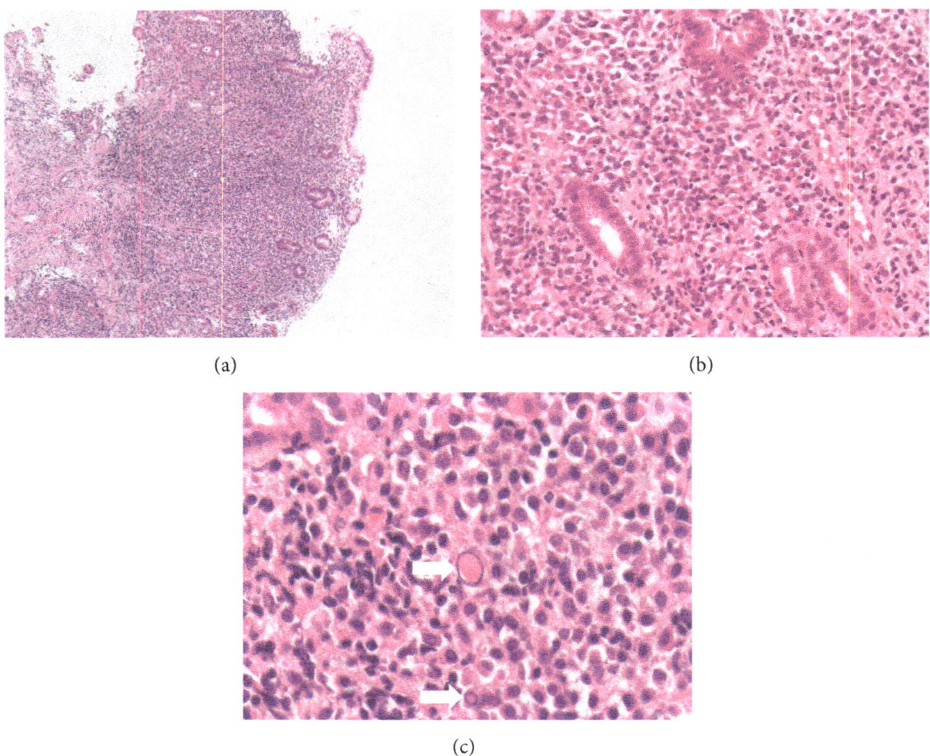

FIGURE 2: Pathological images. Hematoxylin and eosin staining shows dense, diffuse infiltration of small-to-medium-sized monocytoid cells and plasma cells (a, b) and multiple Dutcher bodies ((c) arrows).

Colonoscopy showed no infiltration of monocytoid B-cells. Bone marrow aspiration and a biopsy also showed no monocytoid B-cells. Contrast-enhanced computed tomography imaging of the neck, chest, abdomen, and pelvis demonstrated no lymph node enlargement or organ involvement. Positron emission tomography disclosed tracer uptake in the gastric body, but there was no uptake in other organs. Based on these findings, the patient was diagnosed with primary gastric MALT lymphoma exhibiting prominent plasma cell differentiation.

Since the patient tested positive for *H. pylori* infection serologically and pathologically and as the urea breath test showed positive results, eradication of *H. pylori* was performed as a first-line therapy for gastric MALT lymphoma. Esophagogastroduodenoscopy performed three months after successful eradication of *H. pylori* revealed that the whitish lesions had disappeared (Figure 5). Remission was pathologically confirmed on the biopsied specimen.

3. Discussion

Plasma cell differentiation is not a rare event in MALT lymphoma [8]. This feature is reportedly more frequent in thyroid MALT lymphomas than in MALT lymphomas occurring in other organs [9]. Plasma cell differentiation occurs in approximately one-third of the cases of primary gastric MALT lymphomas [1, 10]. However, prominent plasma cell differentiation, as observed in the present case, is rarely observed in gastric MALT lymphomas.

Recently, Park et al. investigated the clinicopathological features of gastric MALT lymphoma with increased plasma cell differentiation [10]. The authors retrospectively compared 36 cases with increased plasma cell differentiation and 16 cases with minimal plasma cell differentiation. They reported that pathological response, that is, complete histologic response or probable minimal residual disease, was more frequently achieved after *H. pylori* eradication in gastric MALT lymphomas with increased plasma cell differentiation, compared with that in lymphomas with minimal plasma cell differentiation (94.4% versus 66.7%). Moreover, relapse was less frequent in cases with increased plasma cell differentiation (5.6% versus 35.7%). These results indicate that increased plasma cell differentiation is an indicator of favorable treatment response. The present patient also showed complete histologic response after successful *H. pylori* eradication.

As described above, the appearance of abnormal vessels and the destruction of gastric epithelial structure have been known as the key magnifying endoscopic features of gastric MALT lymphomas [3–5]. Figure 6 shows the endoscopic images of typical gastric MALT lymphoma in a 46-year-old Japanese woman. There were two whitish lesions in the gastric body (Figure 6(a)), with branched vessels and faded gastric epithelial structure (Figure 6(b)), as observed in the magnifying observation. Ono et al. reported the disappearance of

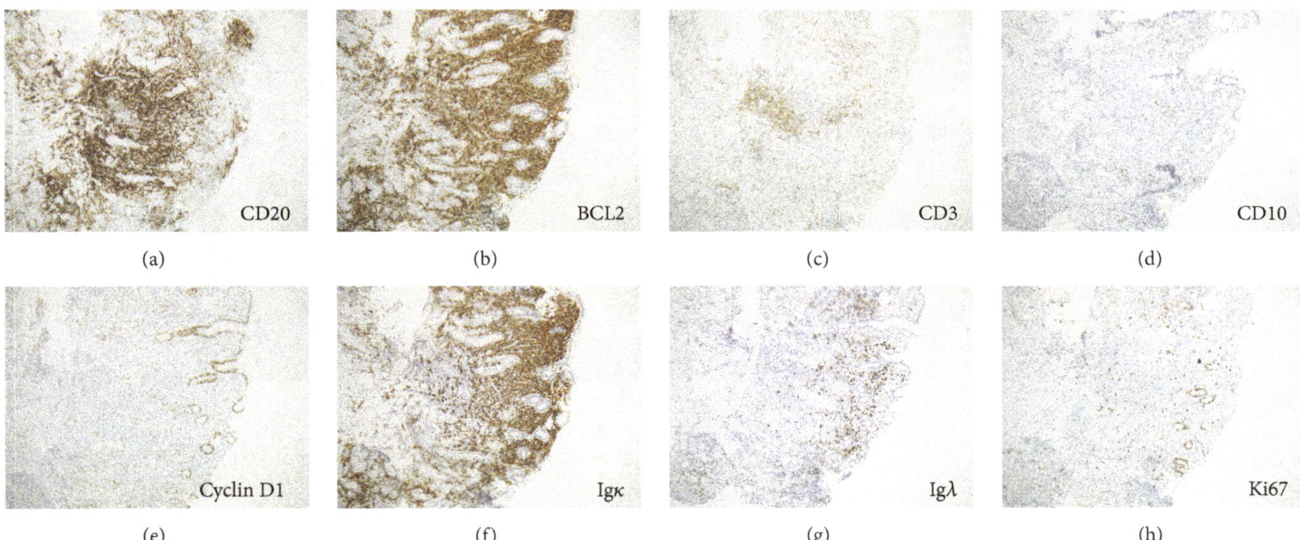

FIGURE 3: Pathological images with immunostaining. The infiltrating cells are positive for CD20 (a) and BCL2 (b), while they are negative for CD3 (c), CD10 (d), and cyclin D1 (e). In situ hybridization for immunoglobulin light chains shows positive results for immunoglobulin light chain κ (f) and negative results for light chain λ (g).

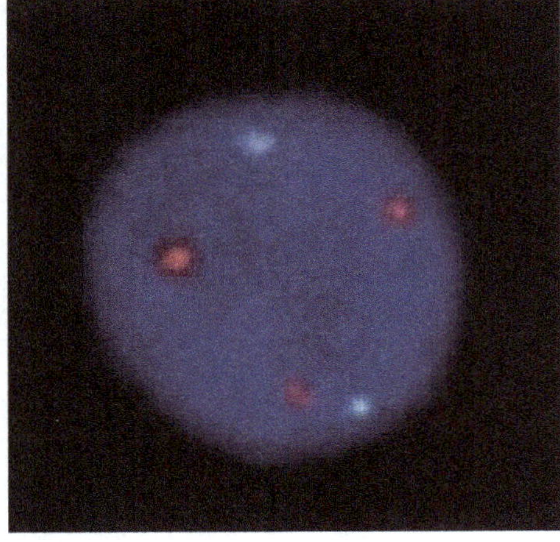

FIGURE 4: Fluorescence in situ hybridization image. Analysis for t(11;18)(q21;q21) translocation reveals no fusion genes of *BIRC3-MALT1*, although extra copies of *MALT1* are identified, indicating trisomy of chromosome 18.

gastric pits and appearance of abnormal vessels in all 11 of their patients with gastric MALT lymphoma [3]. Moreover, after achieving a complete response of MALT lymphoma, abnormal vessels were no longer detected and gastric pits reemerged, although with an irregular size and formation pattern throughout the lesion; moreover, the subepithelial capillary network had unequal diameters. Subsequently, the same group investigated the magnifying endoscopic features of 21 patients with gastric MALT lymphoma and reported that nonstructural areas and abnormal vessels were positive in all lymphoma lesions (100%) before initiating treatment [5]. In addition, swelling of the crypt epithelium, which was termed as "ballooning," was noted in 11 patients (52.4%). Nonaka et al. used the term "tree-like appearance," which was defined as abnormal blood vessels resembling branches from the trunk of a tree, in which the gastric glandular structure was lost. The authors reported that they identified the tree-like appearance in 12 out of 16 patients with gastric MALT lymphoma (75.0%) during magnifying esophagogastroduodenoscopy observation with narrow-band imaging [4, 11, 12]. Consequently, unusually shaped vasculature and destruction of gastric pits with a nonstructural pattern appear to be representative features of untreated gastric MALT lymphomas.

In the present patient, although swelling of the gastric surface epithelium was observed, the structure of gastric pits was intact. Vasculature on the lesion showed an elongated, tortuous appearance, but it was not "tree-like." Therefore, the magnifying endoscopic features of the present case were different from those of typical gastric MALT lymphomas. Nevertheless, we noticed several similarities between the magnifying endoscopic features of the present case and a case of gastric plasmacytoma reported by Harada et al. [6], in which the gastric lesion was described as a discolored, slightly elevated area with tortuous superficial vessels.

Extramedullary plasmacytoma is defined as an accumulation of neoplastic monoclonal plasma cells occurring in the extraosseous site without evidence of a systemic plasma cell proliferative disorder [13, 14]. Several authors have noted that the distinction between plasmacytoma and MALT lymphoma with plasma cell differentiation is sometimes ambiguous [8, 15]. Meanwhile, Meyerson et al. investigated both diseases and related disorders by using flow cytometric analysis and described that plasma cells observed in marginal zone lymphoma resembled normal precursor plasma cells, whereas those observed in plasma cell myeloma were similar to more mature marrow plasma cells [16]. Regardless of the pathogeneses of the two diseases, the similarities in the endoscopic images observed in the present case and the

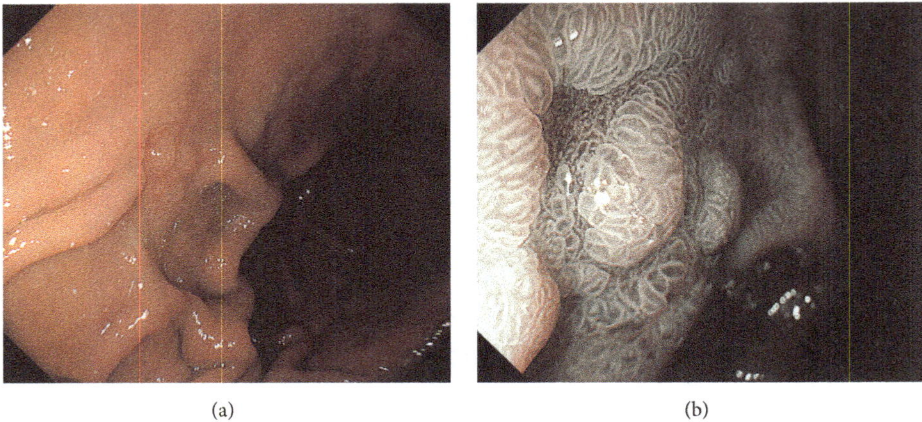

FIGURE 5: Esophagogastroduodenoscopy images after treatment. Three months after successful eradication of *H. pylori*, the whitish lesions disappeared.

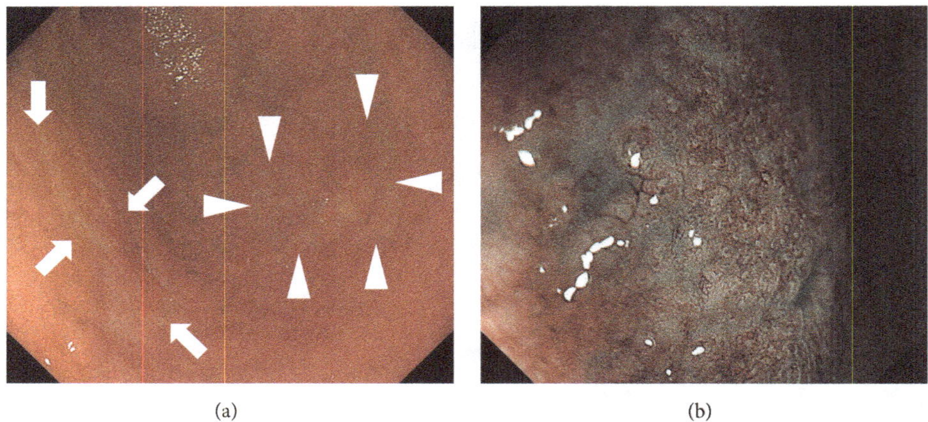

FIGURE 6: Endoscopic images of typical gastric MALT lymphoma. Two whitish lesions are observed in the gastric body ((a) arrows and arrowheads). Magnifying observation reveals branched vessels and fading of the gastric epithelial structure (b).

case of plasmacytoma reported by Harada et al. [6] may reflect common pathological features shared between the two cases, for example, proliferation of plasma cells. However, further studies are required to determine the macroscopic morphologies of gastric MALT lymphoma with increased plasma cell differentiation, as we had previously encountered another case of this disease, which showed a lack of gastric pits and the presence of abnormal vessels [7].

Another feature that may concern the outcome of the present case is extra copies of *MALT1*, which was observed in FISH analysis (Figure 4). Recently, we investigated 146 patients with gastric MALT lymphoma and found extra copies of *MALT1* in 31 patients (21.2%) and t(11;18) translocation in 27 patients (18.5%) [2]. Analysis of the patient outcome revealed that *H. pylori* eradication alone resulted in complete remission in 13 (61.9%) patients with extra copies of *MALT1*. The response rate to *H. pylori* eradication in this patient group was similar to that of patients without chromosomal aberrations (72.1%). However, although the difference was not statistically significant, event-free survival of the patients with extra copies of *MALT1* tended to be inferior to that of the patients without chromosomal aberration ($p = 0.10$). Therefore, we speculate that patients with additional copies of *MALT1*, including the present patient, may require more frequent clinical follow-ups to monitor disease progression and relapse.

In conclusion, this patient with gastric MALT lymphoma with increased plasma cell differentiation was treated. Although the gastric epithelium was swollen and elongated, tortuous vasculature was observed, branched microvessels were absent, and the gastric pits were preserved, under magnifying observation. These images were different from the typical features of gastric MALT lymphoma, but were similar to those of a previously reported case of gastric plasmacytoma. This case indicates that magnifying endoscopic features are not uniform among gastric MALT lymphomas and that increased plasma cells may be responsible for such atypical features.

References

[1] P. G. Isaacson, A. Chott, S. Nakamura, H. K. Muller-Hermelink, N. L. Harris, and S. H. Swerdlow, "Extranodal marginal zone lymphoma of mucosa-associated lymphoid tissue (MALT lymphoma)," in *WHO Classification of Tumours of Haematopoietic and Lymphoid Tissues*, S. H. Swerdlow, E. Campo, N. L. Harris, E. S. Jaffe, S. A. Pileri, and H. Stein, Eds., pp. 214–217, IARC, Lyon, France, 4th edition, 2008.

[2] M. Iwamuro, R. Takenaka, M. Nakagawa et al., "Management of gastric mucosa-associated lymphoid tissue lymphoma in patients with extra copies of the MALT1 gene," *World Journal of Gastroenterology*, vol. 23, no. 33, pp. 6155–6163, 2017.

[3] S. Ono, M. Kato, Y. Ono et al., "Characteristics of magnified endoscopic images of gastric extranodal marginal zone B-cell lymphoma of the mucosa-associated lymphoid tissue, including changes after treatment," *Gastrointestinal Endoscopy*, vol. 68, no. 4, pp. 624–631, 2008.

[4] K. Nonaka, K. Ohata, N. Matsuhashi et al., "Is narrow-band imaging useful for histological evaluation of gastric mucosa-associated lymphoid tissue lymphoma after treatment?" *Digestive Endoscopy*, vol. 26, no. 3, pp. 358–364, 2014.

[5] S. Ono, M. Kato, Y. Ono et al., "Target biopsy using magnifying endoscopy in clinical management of gastric mucosa-associated lymphoid tissue lymphoma," *Journal of Gastroenterology and Hepatology*, vol. 26, no. 7, pp. 1133–1138, 2011.

[6] S. Harada, S. Fukunishi, T. Takeuchi et al., "Magnifying narrow-band imaging endoscopy for the diagnosis of gastric primary extramedullary plasmacytoma: A first case report," *Endoscopy*, vol. 46, pp. E435–E436, 2014.

[7] H. Ishikawa, M. Iwamuro, H. Okada et al., "Recurrence after radiotherapy for gastric mucosa-associated lymphoid tissue (MALT) lymphoma with trisomy 18," *Internal Medicine*, vol. 54, no. 8, pp. 911–916, 2015.

[8] Y. Chong, C. S. Kang, W. J. Oh, T.-J. Kim, and E. J. Lee, "Nodal involvement of extranodal marginal zone lymphoma with extreme plasmacytic differentiation (Mott cell formation) simulating plasma cell neoplasm and lymphoplasmacytic lymphoma," *Blood Research*, vol. 49, no. 4, pp. 275–278, 2014.

[9] S. Kaba, M. Hirokawa, S. Kuma et al., "Cytologic findings of primary thyroid MALT lymphoma with extreme plasma cell differentiation: FNA cytology of two cases," *Diagnostic Cytopathology*, vol. 37, no. 11, pp. 815–819, 2009.

[10] S. Park, S. Ahn, M. Hong, and Y. H. Ko, "Increased plasmacytic differentiation in gastric mucosa–associated lymphoid tissue lymphomas: Helicobacter pylori eradication response and IgG4+ plasma cell association," *Human Pathology*, vol. 59, pp. 113–119, 2017.

[11] K. Nonaka, K. Ishikawa, M. Shimizu et al., "Gastrointestinal: Gastric mucosa-associated lymphoma presented with unique vascular features on magnified endoscopy combined with narrow-band imaging," *Journal of Gastroenterology and Hepatology*, vol. 24, no. 10, p. 1697, 2009.

[12] K. Nonaka, "A case of gastric mucosa-associated lymphoid tissue lymphoma in which magnified endoscopy with narrow band imaging was useful in the diagnosis," *World Journal of Gastrointestinal Endoscopy*, vol. 4, no. 4, pp. 151–156, 2012.

[13] Y. J. Han, S. J. Park, M. I. Park et al., "Solitary Extramedullary Plasmacytoma in the Gastrointestinal Tract: Report of Two Cases and Review of Literature," *The Korean Journal of Gastroenterology*, vol. 63, no. 5, pp. 316–320, 2014.

[14] G. Wen, W. Wang, Y. Zhang, S. Niu, Q. Li, and Y. Li, "Management of extramedullary plasmacytoma: Role of radiotherapy and prognostic factor analysis in 55 patients," *Chinese Journal of Cancer Research*, vol. 29, no. 5, pp. 438–446, 2017.

[15] T. J. Molina, P. Lin, S. H. Swerdlow, and J. R. Cook, "Marginal zone lymphomas with plasmacytic differentiation and related disorders," *American Journal of Clinical Pathology*, vol. 136, no. 2, pp. 211–225, 2011.

[16] H. J. Meyerson, J. Bailey, J. Miedler, and F. Olobatuyi, "Marginal zone B cell lymphomas with extensive plasmacytic differentiation are neoplasms of precursor plasma cells," *Cytometry Part B - Clinical Cytometry*, vol. 80, no. 2, pp. 71–82, 2011.

Microwave Thermal Ablation in an Unusual Case of Malignant and Locally Advanced Rare Tumor of Pancreas in ASA IV Old Male Patient

Francesco D'Amico,[1,2] Michele Finotti,[1,2] Chiara Di Renzo,[1] Alessio Pasquale,[1] Alessandra Bertacco,[1] Giorgio Caturegli,[2] Gabriel E. Gondolesi,[3] and Umberto Cillo[1]

[1]*Department of Surgery, Oncology and Gastroenterology, Hepatobiliary Surgery and Liver Transplantation, Padova University, Padova, Italy*
[2]*Department of Surgery, Division of Transplantation and Immunology, Yale University, New Haven, CT, USA*
[3]*Department of Surgery, Favaloro Foundation, Buenos Aires University, Buenos Aires, Argentina*

Correspondence should be addressed to Francesco D'Amico; drdamico@hotmail.com

Academic Editor: Gregory Kouraklis

Pancreatic intraductal papillary-mucinous neoplasm is a rare primary neoplasm of unknown pathogenesis. This kind of tumor represents 0.2–2.7% of all pancreatic cancers and they may proceed to malignant lesions. In this study, we describe a case of pancreatic intraductal papillary-mucinous tumor (4.3 cm) with normal tumoral markers and nuclear atypia. We perform also a systematic review of the literature on MEDLINE and find only one relevant study that used microwave ablation for the palliative treatment of pancreatic tumor. We describe the case of a 70-year-old Caucasian male who was diagnosed with a pancreatic tumor with biliary tree dilatation. The patient underwent computed tomography (CT), percutaneous biopsy, and an endoscopic positioning of prosthesis in the biliary tree. Due to the worsening of jaundice and cholestasis, and considering the severe systemic disease status, palliative surgery with microwave thermoablation in the head of pancreas was performed. No complications were observed. The hospitalization lasted for 11 days after surgery, with normal liver and pancreatic lab tests at discharge. The patient followed a line of chemotherapy for 6 months with a complete response for 8 months. One month after the treatment, a staging CT scan was performed showing the size of the cephalopancreatic lesion had decreased from 43 to 35 mm with signs of complete ablation. The patient had a total response at the imaging of 10 months. One year later, a CT scan follow-up showed progression of the pancreatic disease. The disease remained stable for 18 months. The patient died due to cardiovascular complications with an overall survival of 30 months. Microwave ablation in our case report has been demonstrated to be feasible and safe without complications. It can be used as a phase of multimodality treatment in patients with severe systemic disease status and advanced intraductal papillary-mucinous neoplasm.

1. Introduction

Pancreatic intraductal papillary-mucinous neoplasm (IPMN) is caused by proliferation of mucin-producing neoplastic epithelia and characterized by cystic or saccular dilation of the branch duct (BD-IPMN) and/or main duct (MD-IPMN) [1]. The natural behavior of these neoplasms could proceed to malignant lesions. Cells of different oncogenetic potential can be found in the same tumor, representing the natural progression of the disease (adenomas, low- and high-grade dysplasia to in situ carcinoma, to invasive and metastatic carcinoma). Correct distinction between MD-IPMN and BD-IPMN is essential, as the potential malignant evolution of BD is about 25% (ranging from 6% to 46%) while that of MD is 70% [2], and the prevalence of carcinoma in MD can be high (60% to 92%) [1, 3–6].

The international consensus guidelines of 2012 allow an evidence-based management of IPMN [1]. Pancreatic resections are indicated for MD-IPMN because of the high rate

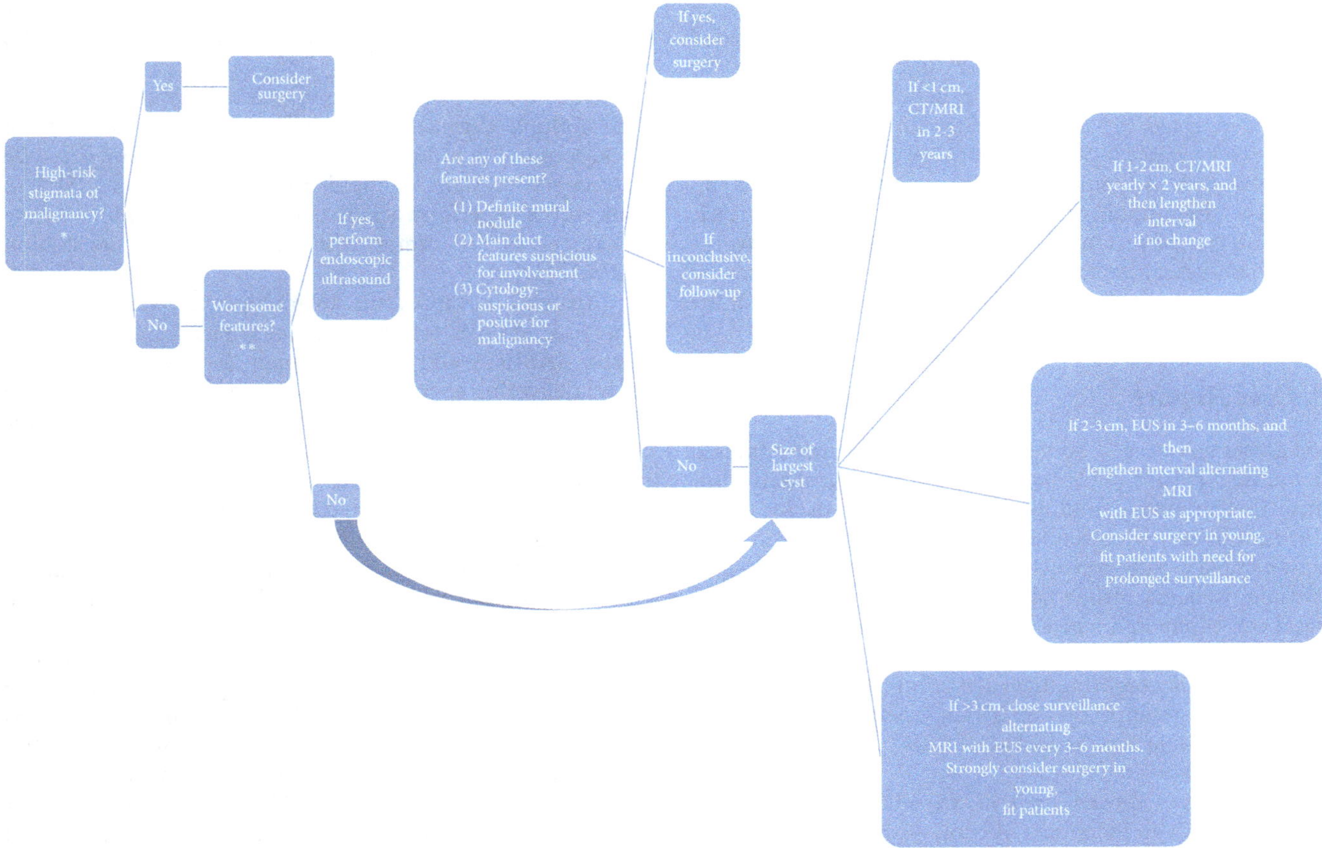

FIGURE 1: Decisional algorithm for management of IPMN and MCN (international consensus guidelines 2012) [1]. *(A) Obstructive jaundice in a patient with cystic lesion of the head of the pancreas; (B) enhancing solid component within cyst; (C) main pancreatic duct > 10. **(A) Cyst > 3 cm; (B) thickened/enhancing cyst walls; (C) main duct size 5–9 mm; (D) nonenhancing mural nodule; (E) abrupt change in caliber of pancreatic duct with distal pancreatic atrophy.

of malignancy, while the correct management and follow-up of BD-IPMN are debated. These guidelines divide BD-IPMN into two categories: BD-IPMN with "high-risk stigmata" and "worrisome features." High-risk stigmata include obstructive jaundice, an enhanced solid component, and dilation of the main pancreatic duct (MPD) to a diameter equal to or more than 10 mm. Worrisome features include history of pancreatitis, maximal cyst diameter equal to or greater than 30 mm, a thickened and enhanced cyst wall, MPD diameter of 5–9 mm, nonenhanced mural nodules, abrupt change in the caliber of MPD with distal pancreatic atrophy, and lymphadenopathy. Pancreatectomy is not automatically recommended for patients with worrisome features and follow-up should be considered [7] (Figure 1).

IPMNs are mostly asymptomatic, but can present with long-standing hyperlipasemia, but the most common symptom is acute pancreatitis, due to duct obstruction from mucus or from papillary proliferation. In a recent study at the University of Brescia, Baiocchi et al. [8] followed 40 patients with IPMN during the period from 1992 to 2007 and found less than 50% were symptomatic (principally showing acute pancreatitis at the clinical visit). Since the majority of the patients with IPMN are asymptomatic, the diagnosis is often incidental. Diagnosis of IPMNs, according to the most recent international consensus guidelines of 2012, should be based on imaging studies and typical anatomical and pathological features [1]. The current gold-standard method for the diagnosis of IPMN is Cholangio-Wirsung Magnetic Resonance Imaging (MRI), which appears superior to CT because of better contrast resolution, facilitating recognition of septae, nodules, and duct communications [7]. The specificity of Cholangio-Wirsung MRI in differentiating benign from malignant lesions is increased by using 18-Fludeoxyglucose Positron Emission Tomography (18-FDG-PET, specificity raised from 43% to 100%) [9].

Endoscopic retrograde cholangiopancreatography (ERCP) offers the possibility of performing brushing or biopsy. On the other hand, ERCP may increase the risk of some complications, such as acute pancreatitis. The Surgical Clinic of Brescia [8] evaluated the effects of ERCP and its complications: 50% of the IPMN patients submitted to ERCP developed an iatrogenic pancreatitis. These risk factors explain why the international consensus guidelines for the management of IPMN recommend not to use routine ERCP for sampling of fluid or brushings.

Generally, IPMN can be approached surgically in 90–100% of cases. Pancreatectomy is highly recommended for patients with high-risk stigmata in consideration of the low 5-year survival rates (ranging between 31% and 54%). Patients resected for in situ carcinoma have a median of 5-year survival of 80–90%, 50–70% for invasive carcinoma, and 40%–50% if lymph nodal metastases are present [3]. However, these findings considered cases where pancreatic resection is feasible. On the contrary, we present a case where pancreatic resection for a MD-IPMN evolving to cancer could not be performed due to the performance status of the patient.

2. Case Report

We present a case of a 70-year-old Caucasian male admitted to our department in October 2010 due to generalized jaundice. The patient had multiple chronic conditions: hypertensive cardiopathy with double ischemic heart attack, being an active smoker, with previous history of pleurisy with pleural effusion, ischemic stroke five years priorly, and a history of basal cell carcinoma and a treated malignant melanoma in the head.

Due to his comorbidities, according to physical status classification system of the American Society of Anaesthesiologists, the patient was defined as ASA IV (patient with severe systemic disease).

Blood tests showed high direct bilirubin (8.4 mg/dL) associated with an increment of cholestasis indices. Tumoral markers were negative (CEA and Ca 19-9).

The patient underwent an abdominal ultrasound followed by a CT scan that showed a hypodense and non-homogeneous expansive formation (43 mm) in the head of the pancreas with concomitant dilatation of the intra- and extrahepatic biliary tree, without dilatation of Wirsung duct. The lesion was in direct contact of the gastroduodenal artery (GDA) without infiltration. The patient referred to our center completed the staging with an abdominal magnetic resonance plus angiography (MRA) (Figure 2(a)).

Endoscopic retrograde cholangiopancreatography (ERCP) demonstrated a complete obstruction of the intrapancreatic common bile duct. A plastic stent was placed to reduce the bilirubin level and resolve the biliary-tree dilatation.

Percutaneous fine-needle aspiration cytology (FNAC) suggested single or small papillary clusters of epithelial cells with some crowded and hyperchromatic nuclei. These findings were considered compatible with IPMN with high-grade dysplasia.

Due to worsening jaundice and cholestasis, in December 2010 the patient underwent exploratory laparotomy in order to evaluate whether to perform a palliative surgery. The laparoscopic approach due to the severe cardiopathy of the patient was contraindicated.

An exploration of the abdomen was performed, in order to rule out previously undetected metastases. The gastrocolic ligament was divided to access the *bursa omentalis* and a partial Kocher manoeuvre was performed to expose the pancreatic head with the identification of the lesion.

Intraoperative ultrasound studies demonstrated a new evidence of infiltration of the superior mesenteric vein (SMV) and GDA.

Due to the patient's age, his severe systemic disease, and multiple chronic conditions (ASA IV), we decided not to keep on with a duodenocephalopancreatectomy (despite intraoperative signs of rapid progression of the IPMN to cancer) but to perform a palliative surgery and a mini invasive treatment of the tumor with microwave thermoablation (MWA) [19].

An AMICA (apparatus for microwave ablation) system was used. MWA was performed using a 2.45 MHz generator (AMICA-GEN, HS Hospital Service SpA, Aprilia, Italy) delivering energy through a 14- or 16-gauge internally cooled coaxial antenna (AMICA PROBE, HS Hospital Service SpA, Aprilia, Italy), featuring a miniaturized quarter wave impedance transformer (referred to as minichoke) for reflected wave confinement. All procedures were performed under ultrasonographic (US) guidance (Hitachi Hi Vision 6500 convex). The probe was placed directly in the center of the lesion under US guidance, keeping safe margins from the Wirsung and bile ducts.

In order to avoid iatrogenic damage due to the heat produced by the microwave needle, we also placed cold wet gauze over the inferior vena cava and the duodenum was perfused continuously with cold saline solution through a nasogastric tube placed in the second portion of the duodenum.

We performed two cycles of MWA, 60 seconds each, at 20 Watts of power. The effect of the treatment was monitored during the procedure by US. We used a single 3-0 Vicryl stitch to close the microwave needle track in order to prevent possible pancreatic fistula.

In this particular case, the open procedure, compared to a percutaneous approach, allowed us to achieve a complete ablation of the tumor (two cycles with a better volume of necrosis) with high grade of safety.

We completed the procedure with a Roux-Y anastomosis and gastroenteroanastomosis.

The patient had an uneventful recovery without complications and was discharged on the 11th postoperative day with normal liver and pancreatic laboratory tests.

One month after the treatment, a staging CT was performed showing no dilatation of intra- and extrahepatic biliary tree. The size of the cephalopancreatic lesion decreased from 43 to 35 mm with signs of complete ablation (no contrast medium uptake). No lymphadenopathy or metastatic disease was detected (Figure 2(b)).

The patient began a line of chemotherapy from January to July 2011 (12 cycles with Oxaliplatin) and he did not show progression at CT scan for 10 months.

In October 2011, CT scan follow-up (Figure 2(c)) showed progression of the pancreatic disease (40 mm from 35 mm with suspected initial infiltration of duodenum) with single liver metastases (5 mm at the left hepatic lobe).

The disease remained stable for 18 months with normal level of bilirubin but increasing levels of tumor marker (CA 19-9 from 2763, February 2011, up to 7000, November 2011).

The patient died in June 2013 from cardiovascular complications with an overall survival (OS) of 30 months (Table 1).

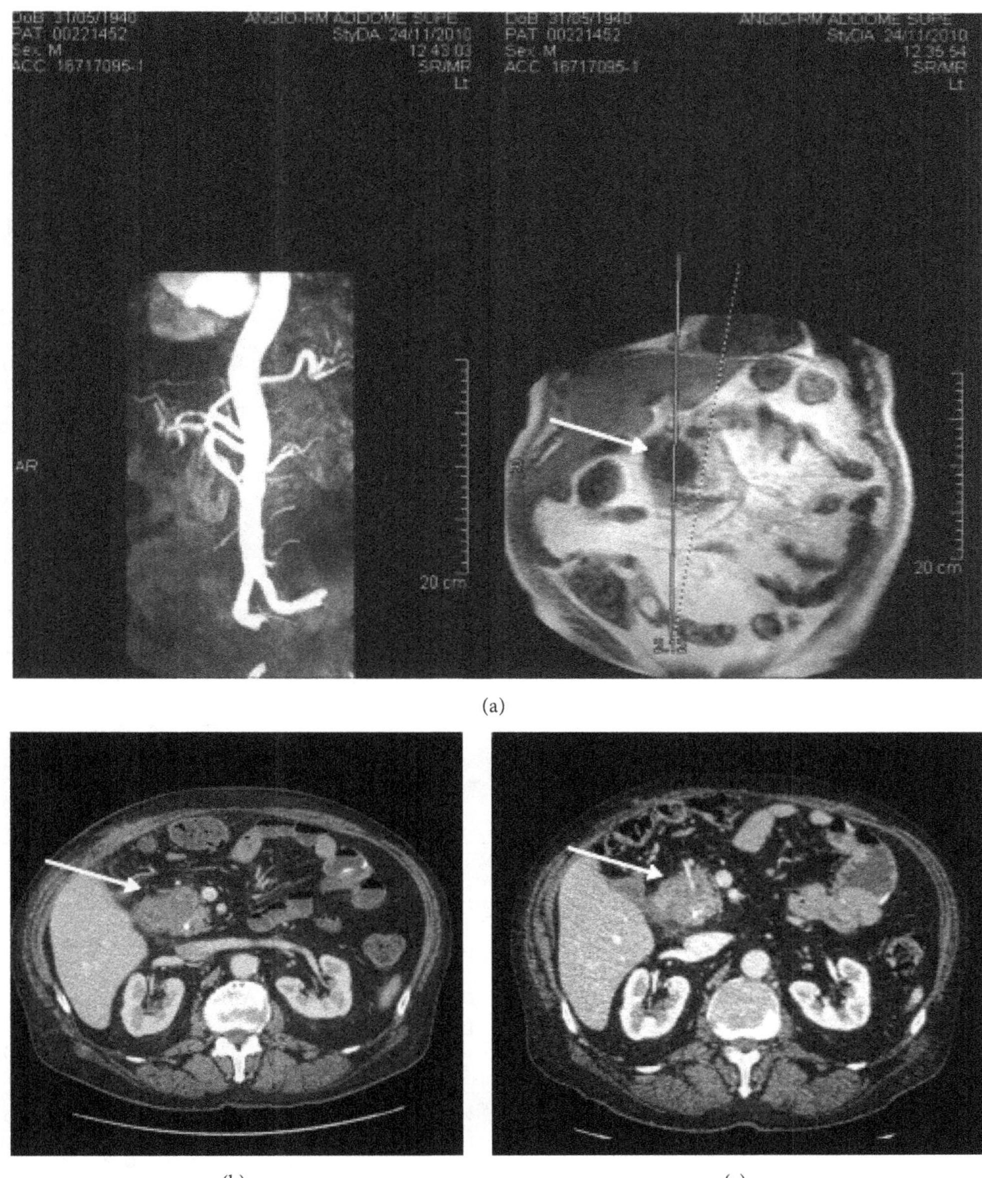

Figure 2: (a) Preoperative staging with an abdominal magnetic resonance plus angiography (MRA) with normal superior and inferior mesenteric and splenic artery. (b) CT scan one month after the treatment. The size of the cephalopancreatic lesion decreased from 43 to 35 mm with sign of complete ablation (no contrast medium uptake). (c) CT scan 10-month follow-up. Progression of the pancreatic disease (40 mm from 35 mm) with suspected initial infiltration of duodenum. The arrows in (a), (b), and (c) refer to the cephalopancreatic lesion.

3. Discussion

Our case report described a MD-IPMN, which evolved to a locally advanced pancreatic cancer (LAPC), considered unresectable, due to the performance status of the patient and the stage of the disease (infiltration of the superior mesenteric vein and infiltration of the gastroduodenal artery).

Furthermore, we have to consider that the diagnosis of IPMN is essentially histological after pancreatic resection. In our case report, the preoperative diagnostic tools suggested MD-IPMN, but imaging studies and intraoperative findings suggested a malignant evolution (pancreatic cancer) in a patient considered unresectable for cardiovascular disease.

Recent studies showed an increase of OS in patients affected by pancreatic cancer treated with adjuvant therapy compared to patients treated with surgery alone. The patients who can receive more benefit from the treatment are the ones with higher stage disease [20]. In particular, treatment with gemcitabine seems to be the adjuvant treatment of choice for patients with resected invasive pancreatic cancer [21].

Despite the advances in chemotherapy and chemoradiotherapy regimen, unresectable locally advanced pancreas carcinoma remains a disease with poor prognosis with reported

TABLE 1: Outcomes, type of ablation, and complications in premalignant pancreatic lesions: review of the literature. CTP: cystic tumors of the pancreas; PNET: primitive neuroectodermal tumor; EUS: endoscopic ultrasonography; CR: complete resolution; NA: not available.

Author	Lesion type	Number	Treatment	Median area of ablation, mm (range)	Outcome	Major complications
Gan et al. 2005 [10]	CTP	25	EUS guided ethanol Lavage	19.4 (6–30)	CR 35%	None
Oh et al. 2008 [11]	CTP	14	EUS guided ethanol Lavage + paclitaxel	25.5 (17–52)	CR 79%	Acute pancreatitis ($n = 1$) Abdominal pain ($n = 1$)
Oh et al. 2009 [12]	CTP	10	EUS guided ethanol Lavage + paclitaxel	29.5 (20–68)	CR 60%	Mild pancreatitis ($n = 1$)
DeWitt et al. 2009 [13]	CTP	42	Randomised double blind: saline versus ethanol	22.4 (10–58)	CR 33%	Abdominal pain ($n = 5$) Pancreatitis ($n = 1$) Cystic bleeding ($n = 1$)
Oh et al. 2011 [14]	CTP	52	EUS guided ethanol Lavage + paclitaxel	31.8 (17–68)	CR 62%	Mild pancreatitis ($n = 1$)
Levy et al. 2012 [15]	PNET	8	EUS guided ethanol Lavage and intraoperative ethanol Lavage	16.6 (8–21)	NA	Peritumoral bleeding ($n = 3$)
Pai et al. 2013 [16]	CTP + PNET	8	EUS guided RFA	38	CR 25%	None
Park et al. 2016 [17]	CTP	91	Ethanol	30 (20–50)	CR 45%	Acute pancreatitis ($n = 3$)
Moyer et al. 2016 [18]	CTP	10	Ethanol or saline plus paclitaxel and gemcitabine	30	CR 75%	Acute pancreatitis ($n = 1$)

median survival of 9–13 months [22]. Locoregional ablative therapies can be considered possible alternative treatments. Liver tumors are an example where ablative approach has been safely used for a long time. The pancreas, however, entails the risk of complications of associating injuries, especially in relation to duodenum and major vessels.

We performed a systematic literature review using the PubMed and EMBASE databases and the Cochrane Library for studies published in the English language up to December 1, 2016. Only articles that described microwave ablation in unresectable IPMN were initially included. There is no case of MWA used to specifically treat IPMN that could be retrieved; therefore, we increased our search to LAPC.

Table 1 summarizes outcomes, type of ablation, and complications using ablative therapies in premalignant pancreatic disease, as reported in the literature.

Radiofrequency ablation (RFA) is the most common thermal ablation therapy used for LAPC. One study showed a survival rate of 22% with a median follow-up of 12 months [23]. A more recent study showed safety and feasibility of RFA under ultrasonography guidance in 22 patients. The median postablation survival time was 6 months [24]. Experience with MW ablation for unresectable LAPC is limited. The largest case series [25] considered 15 patients in a period between 2004 and 2006 in which all partial necrosis was achieved with no major procedure-related morbidity or mortality using MWA. The longest patient follow-up was 22 months, but the median survival was only 13 months [25].

Our case reports an overall survival after MWA of 30 months. Despite encouraging results, MWA for LAPC as well as its efficacy together with chemoradiotherapy is under investigation, without any conclusive data currently available regarding indication and best ablation protocol for LAPC.

4. Conclusions

Most clinical ablative experience for LAPC exists with RFA. There is actually no previous case of microwave thermal ablation use to treat specifically IPMN in rapid progression to cancer. Our case report showed that MWA can be considered a safe and efficacious alternative treatment as a palliative surgery when resection of IPMN is not feasible. However long-term data or randomized controlled trials are required to further characterize this treatment.

Abbreviations

IPMN: Intraductal papillary-mucinous neoplasm
BD-IPMN: Intraductal papillary-mucinous neoplasm branch duct
MD-IPMN: Intraductal papillary-mucinous neoplasm main duct

ERCP: Endoscopic retrograde cholangiopancreatography
MRI: Magnetic Resonance Imaging
CT: Computed tomography
ASA: American Society of Anaesthesiologists
MRA: Magnetic resonance angiography
FNAC: Fine-needle aspiration cytology
MCN: Mucinous cystic neoplasm
MPD: Main pancreatic duct
MWA: Microwave ablation
LAPC: Locally advanced pancreatic cancer
RFA: Radio frequency ablation
GDA: Gastroduodenal artery
SMV: Superior mesenteric vein
OS: Overall survival.

Consent

Written informed consent was obtained from the patient for publication of this case report and any accompanying images. No name or initials appear in the paper and in the pictures attached.

Disclosure

This paper was presented at X World Congress of IHPBA 2012 Poster and SIC (Italian Society of Surgery) 2013 Poster.

Authors' Contributions

Francesco D'Amico and Alessandra Bertacco contributed to study conception and design. Francesco D'Amico, Michele Finotti, Chiara Di Renzo, and Alessio Pasquale contributed to acquisition of data. Francesco D'Amico, Gabriel E. Gondolesi, and Alessandra Bertacco contributed to analysis and interpretation of data. Michele Finotti, Chiara Di Renzo, Alessio Pasquale, and Giorgio Caturegli contributed to drafting of manuscript. Francesco D'Amico, Gabriel E. Gondolesi, and Umberto Cillo contributed to critical revision. Francesco D'Amico and Umberto Cillo performed the surgery.

References

[1] M. Tanaka, C. Fernández-del Castillo, V. Adsay et al., "International consensus guidelines 2012 for the management of IPMN and MCN of the pancreas," *Pancreatology*, vol. 12, no. 3, pp. 183–197, 2012.

[2] M. Tanaka, S. Chari, V. Adsay et al., "International consensus guidelines for management of intraductal papillary mucinous neoplasms and mucinous cystic neoplasms of the pancreas," *Pancreatology*, vol. 6, no. 1-2, pp. 17–32, 2006.

[3] R. Salvia, C. Fernández-Del Castillo, C. Bassi et al., "Main-duct intraductal papillary mucinous neoplasms of the pancreas: clinical predictors of malignancy and longterm survival following resection," *Annals of Surgery*, vol. 239, no. 5, pp. 678–687, 2004.

[4] S. Fritz, M. Klauss, F. Bergmann et al., "Small (Sendai negative) branch-duct IPMNs: Not harmless," *Annals of Surgery*, vol. 256, no. 2, pp. 313–320, 2012.

[5] R. S. Tang, B. Weinberg, D. W. Dawson et al., "Evaluation of the Guidelines for Operative Management of Pancreatic Branch-Duct Intraductal Papillary Mucinous Neoplasm," *Clinical Gastroenterology and Hepatology*, vol. 6, no. 7, pp. 815–819, 2008.

[6] Y. Watanabe, K. Nishihara, Y. Niina et al., "Validity of the management strategy for intraductal papillary mucinous neoplasm advocated by the international consensus guidelines 2012: a retrospective review," *Surgery Today*, vol. 46, no. 9, pp. 1045–1052, 2016.

[7] L. L. Berland, S. G. Silverman, R. M. Gore et al., "Managing incidental findings on abdominal CT: white paper of the ACR incidental findings committee," *Journal of the American College of Radiology*, vol. 7, no. 10, pp. 754–773, 2010.

[8] G. L. Baiocchi, N. Portolani, G. Missale et al., "Intraductal papillary mucinous neoplasm of the pancreas (IPMN): Clinicopathological correlations and surgical indications," *World Journal of Surgical Oncology*, vol. 8, article no. 25, 2010.

[9] C. Sperti, S. Bissoli, C. Pasquali et al., "18-Fluorodeoxyglucose positron emission tomography enhances computed tomography diagnosis of malignant intraductal papillary mucinous neoplasms of the pancreas," *Annals of Surgery*, vol. 246, no. 6, pp. 932–937, 2007.

[10] S. I. Gan, C. C. Thompson, G. Y. Lauwers, B. C. Bounds, and W. R. Brugge, "Ethanol lavage of pancreatic cystic lesions: initial pilot study," *Gastrointestinal Endoscopy*, vol. 61, no. 6, pp. 746–752, 2005.

[11] H.-C. Oh, D. W. Seo, T. Y. Lee et al., "New treatment for cystic tumors of the pancreas: EUS-guided ethanol lavage with paclitaxel injection," *Gastrointestinal Endoscopy*, vol. 67, no. 4, pp. 636–642, 2008.

[12] H.-C. Oh, D. W. Seo, S. C. Kim et al., "Septated cystic tumors of the pancreas: Is it possible to treat them by endoscopic ultrasonography-guided intervention?" *Scandinavian Journal of Gastroenterology*, vol. 44, no. 2, pp. 242–247, 2009.

[13] J. DeWitt, K. McGreevy, C. M. Schmidt, and W. R. Brugge, "EUS-guided ethanol versus saline solution lavage for pancreatic cysts: a randomized, double-blind study," *Gastrointestinal Endoscopy*, vol. 70, no. 4, pp. 710–723, 2009.

[14] H. Oh, D. W. Seo, T. J. Song et al., "Endoscopic ultrasonography-guided ethanol lavage with paclitaxel injection treats patients with pancreatic cysts," *Gastroenterology*, vol. 140, no. 1, pp. 172–179, 2011.

[15] M. J. Levy, G. B. Thompson, M. D. Topazian, M. R. Callstrom, C. S. Grant, and A. Vella, "US-guided ethanol ablation of insulinomas: a new treatment option," *Gastrointestinal Endoscopy*, vol. 75, no. 1, pp. 200–206, 2012.

[16] M. Pai, H. Senturk, S. Lakhtakia et al., "351 Endoscopic Ultrasound Guided Radiofrequency Ablation (EUS-RFA) for Cystic

Neoplasms and Neuroendocrine Tumors of the Pancreas," *Gastrointestinal Endoscopy*, vol. 77, no. 5, pp. AB143–AB144, 2013.

[17] J. K. Park, B. J. Song, J. K. Ryu et al., "Clinical Outcomes of Endoscopic Ultrasonography-Guided Pancreatic Cyst Ablation," *Pancreas*, vol. 45, no. 6, pp. 889–894, 2016.

[18] M. Moyer, C. Dye, S. Sharzehi et al., "Is alcohol required for effective pancreatic cyst ablation? The prospective randomized CHARM trial pilot study," *Endoscopy International Open*, vol. 04, no. 05, pp. E603–E607, 2016.

[19] M. G. Keane, K. Bramis, S. P. Pereira, and G. K. Fusai, "Systematic review of novel ablative methods in locally advanced pancreatic cancer," *World Journal of Gastroenterology*, vol. 20, no. 9, pp. 2267–2278, 2014.

[20] M. T. McMillan, R. S. Lewis, J. A. Drebin et al., "The efficacy of adjuvant therapy for pancreatic invasive intraductal papillary mucinous neoplasm (IPMN)," *Cancer*, vol. 122, no. 4, pp. 521–533, 2016.

[21] J. P. Neoptolemos, D. D. Stocken, H. Friess et al., "A Randomized Trial of Chemoradiotherapy and Chemotherapy after Resection of Pancreatic Cancer," *The New England Journal of Medicine*, vol. 350, no. 12, pp. 1200–1210, 2004.

[22] V. Heinemann, M. Haas, and S. Boeck, "Neoadjuvant treatment of borderline resectable and non-resectable pancreatic cancer," *Annals of Oncology*, vol. 24, no. 10, pp. 2484–2492, 2013.

[23] R. Girelli, I. Frigerio, A. Giardino et al., "Results of 100 pancreatic radiofrequency ablations in the context of a multimodal strategy for stage III ductal adenocarcinoma," *Langenbeck's Archives of Surgery*, vol. 398, no. 1, pp. 63–69, 2013.

[24] P. G. Arcidiacono, S. Carrara, M. Reni et al., "Feasibility and safety of EUS-guided cryothermal ablation in patients with locally advanced pancreatic cancer," *Gastrointestinal Endoscopy*, vol. 76, no. 6, pp. 1142–1151, 2012.

[25] N. J. Lygidakis, S. K. Sharma, P. Papastratis et al., "Microwave ablation in locally advanced pancreatic carcinoma-a new look," *Hepato-gastroenterology*, vol. 54, no. 77, pp. 1305–1310, 2006.

A Rare Case of Esophageal Adenocarcinoma with Urinary Bladder Metastasis

Heather Katz,[1] Rahoma E. Saad,[2] Krista Denning,[3] and Toni O. Pacioles[1]

[1]*Department of Hematology/Oncology, Joan C. Edwards School of Medicine, Marshall University, 1600 Medical Center Dr, Huntington, WV 25701, USA*
[2]*Department of Internal Medicine, Joan C. Edwards School of Medicine, Marshall University, 1600 Medical Center Dr, Huntington, WV 25701, USA*
[3]*Department of Pathology, Joan C. Edwards School of Medicine, Marshall University, 1600 Medical Center Dr, Huntington, WV 25701, USA*

Correspondence should be addressed to Heather Katz; katzh@marshall.edu

Academic Editor: Daniel C. Damin

Metastatic esophageal adenocarcinoma to the urinary bladder is extremely rare. We describe a previously healthy 49-year-old female with recent diagnosis of adenocarcinoma of the gastroesophageal junction with metastatic disease to the liver. Biopsy was positive for human epidermal growth factor receptor 2 (HER2) by Fluorescence In Situ Hybridization (FISH). She received six cycles of Cisplatin, 5-Fluorouracil, and Herceptin and subsequently developed symptomatic anemia and hematuria. Cystoscopy with retroflexion was performed and she received a transurethral resection of bladder tumor with fulguration. Pathology of the bladder tumor revealed similar morphology to her liver metastasis and immunohistochemical stains were consistent with metastatic esophageal cancer. Three weeks after being diagnosed with metachronous urinary bladder metastasis from esophageal adenocarcinoma primary, she expired. She only received her first cycle of palliative chemotherapy with Ramucirumab and Paclitaxel.

1. Introduction

Esophageal cancer is the eighth most common cancers and the sixth cause of all cancer death worldwide [1]. The two main histological subtypes of esophageal cancer are squamous cell carcinoma (SCC) and adenocarcinoma [1–4]. Esophageal cancer is a highly fatal malignancy [1–4]. In United States, the overall 5-year survival rate for esophageal adenocarcinoma is less than 20% [1–5]. The high mortality from esophageal cancer is attributed to local invasion and distant spread of this malignancy [1–5]. Metastasis of esophageal cancer usually occurs to regional lymph nodes, lungs, liver, brain, bone, and peritoneum [6, 7]. Distant metastasis of esophageal cancer to urinary bladder is extremely rare and has only been reported twice worldwide [7, 8].

We report the third case of metastasis to the urinary bladder from the esophagus; however this is the first case of metachronous metastasis despite being treated previously with six cycles of chemotherapy with Cisplatin, 5-Fluorouracil, and Trastuzumab.

2. Case Report

A 49-year-old female with a past medical history of gastroesophageal reflux disease, anemia, and anxiety presented initially with symptoms of early satiety, feeling bloated, fullness, vomiting, dysphagia to solids, and a 36-pound weight loss over the past 6 months. She has a 35-pack year history of smoking. There is no family history of cancer. On physical exam, her vitals were stable and her exam was pertinent for cachexia and paleness of the skin and conjunctiva. Labs revealed iron deficiency anemia with hemoglobin of 10 g/dL and elevated alkaline phosphatase 171 units/L.

Due to her complaints and findings of iron deficiency, esophagogastroduodenoscopy (EGD) was done and showed a mass at the distal esophagus causing a tight stricture

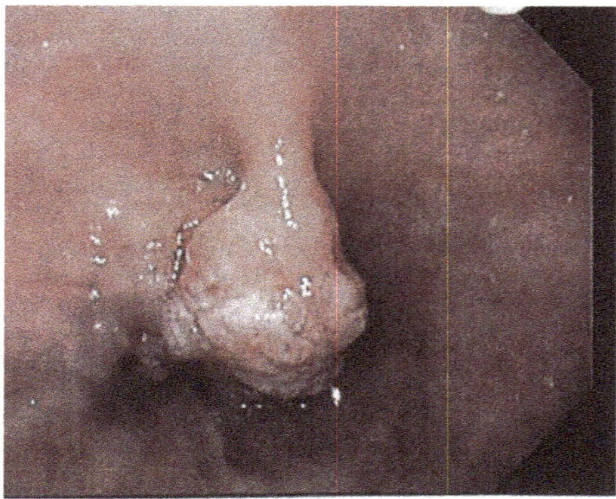

Figure 1: Esophageal tumor seen during EGD.

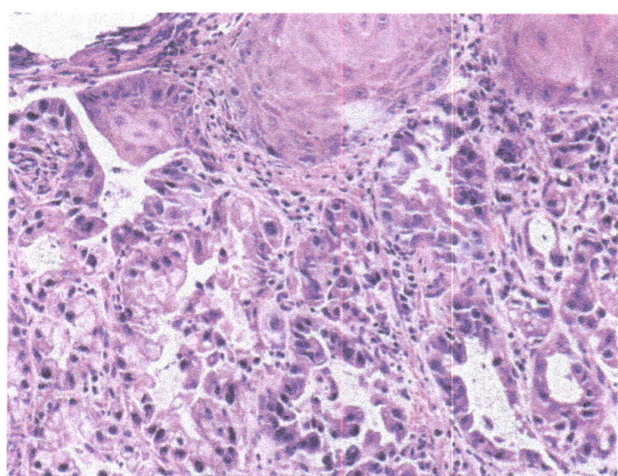

Figure 2: H&E stain of the esophageal tumor showing adenocarcinoma.

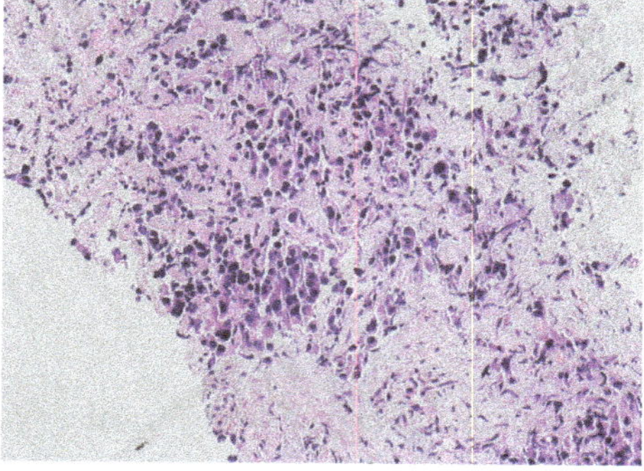

Figure 3: H&E stain from liver biopsy with morphologically similar cells to the esophagus biopsy.

(Figure 1). The biopsy showed adenocarcinoma of the esophagus (Figure 2). Endoscopic ultrasound revealed a hypoechoic mass that was seen at the junction invading all the layers of the esophageal wall up to the capsule of the liver. Two 6.5 mm lymph nodes were seen around the mass due to the stricture. Further staging was performed with computed tomography (CT) chest, abdomen, and pelvis. CT scan of the chest with contrast showed mild thickening of the distal esophagus without other findings. CT scan of the abdomen and pelvis revealed retroperitoneal adenopathy most prominent in the para-aortic location measuring up to 1.9 × 1.7 cm and extending along the internal and external iliac chain as

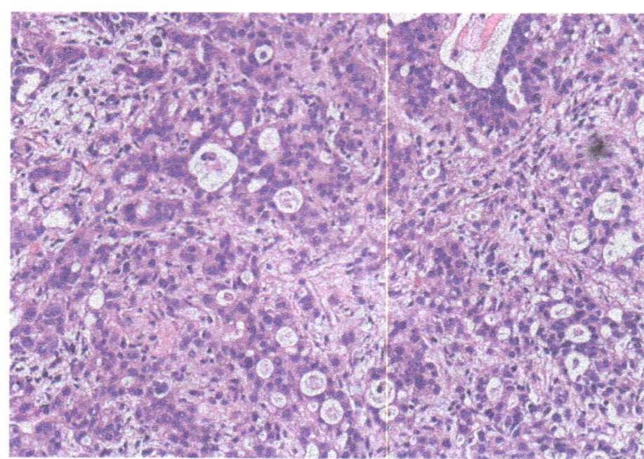

Figure 4: H&E stain of the bladder tumor with morphologically similar cells to the esophagus biopsy.

well as hypodense lesions within the liver. The liver lesions were biopsied and the cells were morphologically similar to the cells from the esophageal tumor (Figure 3). Final pathology revealed poorly differentiated adenocarcinoma, consistent with patient known diagnosis of adenocarcinoma of the esophagus.

HER2 immunohistochemical staining was negative with weak (1+) discontinuous membranous staining; however Fluorescence In Situ Hybridization (FISH) for HER2 was performed and was positive, with HER2 amplified HER2/CN17 ratio: 3.8.

Positron emission tomography scan was performed 6 months after diagnosis showed a hypermetabolic subcarinal lymph node showing a peak standardized uptake value (SUV) of 5 and diffuse hypermetabolic activity involving the distal esophagus into the proximal stomach, peak SUV 13.0. There was also a hypermetabolic mass in the right lobe of the liver measuring approximately 3 cm in size showing a peak SUV of 11.0. There were no other areas of abnormal radiotracer accumulation.

She completed six cycles of Cisplatin, 5-Fluorouracil, and Herceptin; however prior to the last cycle the patient was found to have symptomatic anemia and upon further questioning hematuria.

A cystoscopy with retroflexion and transurethral resection of bladder tumor with fulguration was performed. Pathology was compared to the previous biopsy of the liver and was thought to be morphologically similar (Figure 4). Immunohistochemical (IHC) stains showed cytokeratin 7 positive, cytokeratin 20 positive (Figure 5), Caudal Type Homeobox 2 (CDX2) positive (Figure 6), GATA3 negative in neoplastic cells (Figure 7), and Uroplakin negative in neoplastic cells (Figure 8). The morphologic and immunohistochemical findings were consistent with metastatic esophageal carcinoma. The patient was then started on palliative immunotherapy and chemotherapy with Ramucirumab and Paclitaxel and completed one cycle before receiving hospice care and ultimately expiring one week later.

3. Discussion

Esophageal cancer is the eighth most common cancer and the sixth cause of all cancer deaths worldwide [1]. While

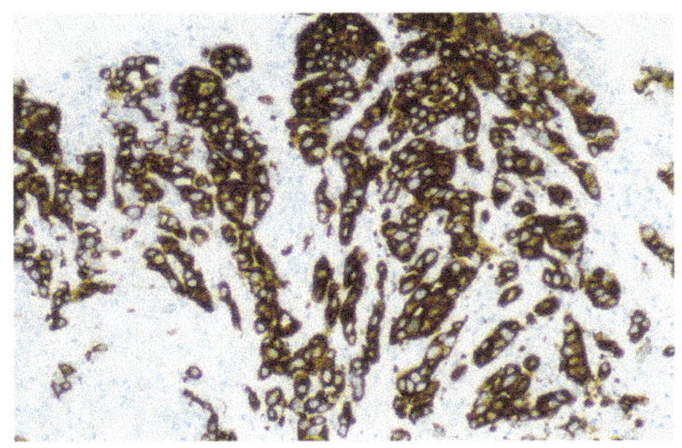

FIGURE 5: Bladder tumor with CK20 positive stain.

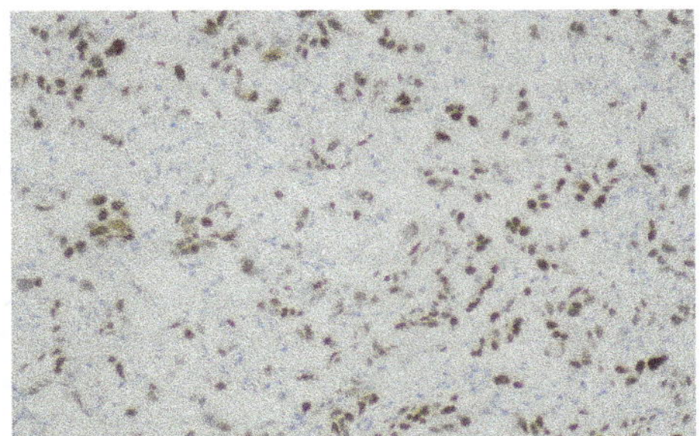

FIGURE 6: Bladder tumor with positive stain for CDX2.

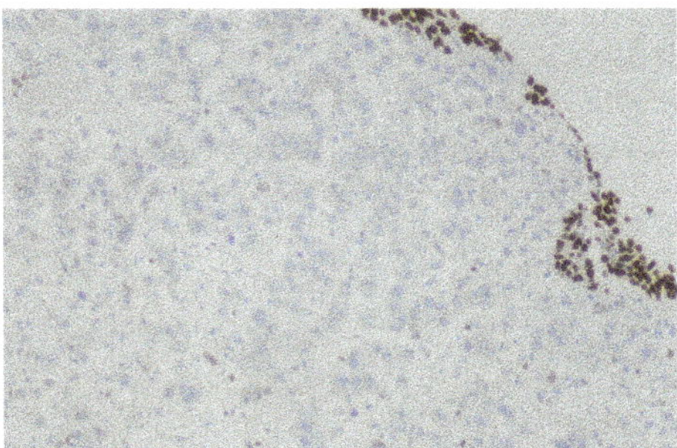

FIGURE 7: Bladder tumor with negative stain for GATA 3 in neoplastic cells.

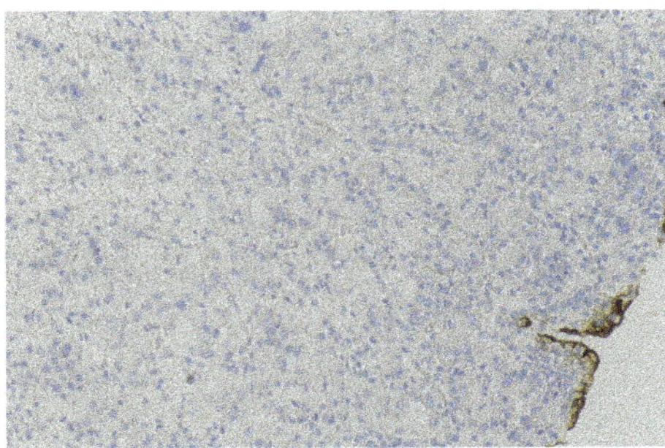

FIGURE 8: Bladder tumor with negative stain for Uroplakin in neoplastic cells.

squamous cell carcinoma of the esophagus is the most common histological subtype of esophageal cancer globally, in western countries, adenocarcinoma has become the predominant subtype [1–5]. Risk factors for adenocarcinoma of the esophagus include gastroesophageal reflux disease (GERD), obesity, and smoking [1–5].

There are 5 main routes of metastasis of esophageal and gastric cancer: (1) direct invasion; (2) lymphatic spread; and (3) hematogenous, (4) transperitoneal, and (5) intraluminal implantation [6]. The most common areas of esophageal cancer metastasis are to the liver and peritoneum [6–8], regional lymph nodes, lung, pleura, stomach, kidney, adrenals, and bone [8]. The urinary bladder is an extremely rare site of metastasis. Velcheti and Govindan [7] reviewed 264 cases of metastatic disease to the bladder and found the most common primary site to be genitourinary, colorectal, melanoma, breast, stomach, unknown primary, choriocarcinoma, lung, and pancreas. After an extensive literature search, there have only been two cases of metastatic disease to the bladder originating from the esophagus described in the literature.

Schuurman et al. [8] described a case of a 53-year-old male who presented with abdominal pain and difficulty in swallowing. He received an EGD with biopsy and was diagnosed with adenocarcinoma of the esophagus. Metastatic workup showed no obvious distant metastasis; however a thickened dorsal bladder wall was noted and biopsy revealed malignant tumor consistent with adenocarcinoma of the esophagus. Matsumoto et al. [9] described a case of a 74-year-old man presenting with gross hematuria and workup revealed an intrapelvic tumor invading the bladder, rectum, sigmoid colon, and left ilium. Pathologic diagnosis of the intrapelvic tumor was moderately differentiated squamous cell carcinoma. Preoperatively, gastrointestinal fiberscopy with biopsy revealed moderately differentiated squamous cell carcinoma. The intrapelvic tumor that invaded the bladder was diagnosed as metastatic tumor from esophageal cancer. While the cases described by Schuurman et al. and Matsumoto et al. discussed synchronous bladder metastasis at time of diagnosis, our patient had metachronous bladder metastasis despite completing a course of chemotherapy for esophageal cancer with liver metastasis.

Immunohistochemical staining is essential to capture the correct diagnosis and establish metastatic versus primary disease. In the present case, immunohistochemistry (IHC) stained positive for CK7, CK20, and CDX2 and negative for Uroplakin and GATA3 (Table 1). This confirmed the diagnosis of esophageal adenocarcinoma with metastasis to urinary bladder and excluded primary adenocarcinoma in the bladder which was crucial to ensure appropriate treatment. Gastrointestinal tumors stain for cytokeratins 7 and 20, or CDX-2, a homeobox gene protein expressed in nuclei of the intestinal epithelium that functions as a tumor suppressor gene [10]. CDX-2 has been shown to be sensitive and specific for gastrointestinal tumors, including esophageal adenocarcinoma [11]. This marker is absent in bladder carcinoma. High-molecular weight cytokeratins, cytokeratin 7, cytokeratin 20, and GATA-3 have previously been used to diagnose bladder cancer [12]. A specific antigen such as Uroplakin III appears specific to urothelial origin and has been used more recently [13].

TABLE 1: Immunohistochemistry stains used to diagnose primary esophageal cancer, metastasis from an esophageal primary cancer, and primary bladder cancer.

Immunohistochemistry stains	Esophageal tumor	Liver biopsy (neoplastic cells)	Bladder biopsy (neoplastic cells)	*Primary* bladder cancer
CK7	+	+	+	+
CK20	+	+	+	+
CDX-2	+	+	+	−
GATA-3	−	−	−	+
Uroplakin	−	−	−	+

This is the first case of metachronous metastatic esophageal cancer to the urinary bladder and will be a useful adjunct to the current literature. This case highlights the importance of comprehensive evaluations and further workups in patients being treated for metastatic esophageal cancer who present with hematuria and symptomatic anemia. Although rare, in patients with esophageal cancer who present with these symptoms, metastatic disease from an esophageal primary tumor should be in the differential diagnosis.

References

[1] K. J. Napier, M. Scheerer, and S. Misra, "Esophageal cancer: a review of epidemiology, pathogenesis, staging workup and treatment modalities," *World Journal of Gastrointestinal Oncology*, vol. 6, no. 5, pp. 112–120, 2014.

[2] H. Pohl, B. Sirovich, and H. G. Welch, "Esophageal adenocarcinoma incidence: are we reaching the peak?" *Cancer Epidemiology Biomarkers and Prevention*, vol. 19, no. 6, pp. 1468–1470, 2010.

[3] M. F. Buas and T. L. Vaughan, "Epidemiology and risk factors for gastroesophageal junction tumors: understanding the rising incidence of this disease," *Seminars in Radiation Oncology*, vol. 23, no. 1, pp. 3–9, 2013.

[4] L. S. Engel, W. Chow, T. L. Vaughan et al., "Population attributable risks of esophageal and gastric cancers," *JNCI Journal of the National Cancer Institute*, vol. 95, no. 18, pp. 1404–1413, 2003.

[5] A. Dubecz, I. Gall, N. Solymosi et al., "Temporal trends in long-term survival and cure rates in esophageal cancer: a SEER database analysis," *Journal of Thoracic Oncology*, vol. 7, no. 2, pp. 443–447, 2012.

[6] J. Makker, N. Karki, B. Sapkota, M. Niazi, and P. Remy, "Rare presentation of gastroesophageal carcinoma with rectal metastasis: a case report," *American Journal of Case Reports*, vol. 17, pp. 611–615, 2016.

[7] V. Velcheti and R. Govindan, "Metastatic cancer involving bladder: a review," *The Canadian Journal of Urology*, vol. 14, no. 1, pp. 3443–3448, 2007.

[8] J. P. Schuurman, T. S. De Vries Reilingh, S. M. Roothaan, R. T. Bijleveld, and M. J. Wiezer, "Urinary bladder metastasis from an esophageal adenocarcinoma: a case report," *American Journal of Gastroenterology*, vol. 104, no. 6, pp. 1603-1604, 2009.

[9] Y. Matsumoto, H. Mibu, Y. Kagebayashi, and Y. Miyasaka, "Metastatic intrapelvic tumor from esophageal cancer: a case report," *Hinyokika Kiyo*, vol. 50, no. 10, pp. 725–727, 2004.

[10] E. Suh, L. Chen, J. Taylor, and P. G. Traber, "A homeodomain protein related to caudal regulates intestine-specific gene transcription," *Molecular and Cellular Biology*, vol. 14, no. 11, pp. 7340–7351, 1994.

[11] R. W. Phillips, H. F. Frierson Jr., and C. A. Moskaluk, "Cdx2 as a marker of epithelial intestinal differentiation in the esophagus," *American Journal of Surgical Pathology*, vol. 27, no. 11, pp. 1442–1447, 2003.

[12] M. B. Amin, K. Trpkov, A. Lopez-Beltran, D. Grignon, and Members of the ISUP Immunohistochemistry in Diagnostic Urologic Pathology Group, "Best practices recommendations in the application of immunohistochemistry in the bladder lesions: report from the International Society of Urologic Pathology consensus conference," *The American Journal of Surgical Pathology*, vol. 38, no. 8, pp. e20–e34, 2014.

[13] O. Kaufmann, J. Volmerig, and M. Dietel, "Uroplakin III is a highly specific and moderately sensitive immunohistochemical marker for primary and metastatic urothelial carcinomas," *American Journal of Clinical Pathology*, vol. 113, no. 5, pp. 683–687, 2000.

Acute Hepatitis due to Garcinia Cambogia Extract, an Herbal Weight Loss Supplement

Akshay Sharma,[1] Elisa Akagi,[1] Aji Njie,[1] Sachin Goyal,[2] Camelia Arsene,[3] Geetha Krishnamoorthy,[4] and Murray Ehrinpreis[5]

[1]*Resident, Department of Internal Medicine, Sinai-Grace Hospital, Detroit Medical Center/Wayne State University, USA*
[2]*Fellow, Department of Internal Medicine, Division of Gastroenterology, Detroit Medical Center/Wayne State University, USA*
[3]*Clinical Research Director, Sinai-Grace Hospital; Associate Program Director, Transitional Medicine Residency Program, Sinai-Grace Hospital, Detroit Medical Center/Wayne State School of Medicine, Detroit, MI, USA*
[4]*Associate Program Director, Department of Internal Medicine, Sinai-Grace Hospital, Detroit Medical Center/Wayne State University, USA*
[5]*Program Director, Department of Internal Medicine, Division of Gastroenterology, Detroit Medical Center/Wayne State University, USA*

Correspondence should be addressed to Akshay Sharma; g.akshaysharma@gmail.com

Academic Editor: Yucel Ustundag

The Drug Induced Liver Injury Network reports dietary supplements as one of the most important causes of drug induced hepatotoxicity, yet millions of people use these supplements without being aware of their potential life-threatening side effects. Garcinia cambogia (GC) extract is an herbal weight loss supplement, reported to cause fulminant hepatic failure. We present a case of a 57-year-old female with no previous history of liver disease, who presented with acute hepatitis due to GC extract taken for weight loss, which resolved after stopping it and got reaggravated on retaking it. Obtaining a history of herbal supplement use is critical in the evaluation of acute hepatitis.

1. Introduction

Fighting obesity can be challenging, and dietary supplements advertised as "slimming aids" are being widely used by people to manage weight loss [1]. Some of these supplements have potential life-threatening side effects. Extract of Garcinia cambogia (GC), a tropical fruit, is sold as a weight loss supplement. Hydroxycitric acid (HCA) is the active ingredient in GC that is associated with fat metabolism and weight loss. Hepatotoxicity due to GC extract has been reported, including cases of fulminant hepatic failure [1]. We present a case of acute hepatitis due to GC extract, which resolved after stopping the supplement and got reaggravated on retaking it.

2. Case Presentation

A 57-year-old female with no previous history of liver disease presented with abdominal pain and vomiting for one day. The abdominal pain was described as 7/10 in severity, nonradiating, and diffuse, but most intense in the right upper quadrant. She denied previously experiencing any similar pain. She denied fever or chills but reported 3 episodes of nonbloody, nonbilious emesis after the pain started. There was a history of heart failure with preserved ejection fraction. She had been taking vitamins A and D and an herbal supplement for weight loss but she denied the use of any prescription weight loss medications. She denied using alcohol, acetaminophen, or any illicit drugs. Her vital signs were normal. Physical examination was significant for diffuse abdominal tenderness without any rigidity or guarding. There was no hepatosplenomegaly or scleral icterus. Laboratory evaluation revealed an alanine aminotransferase (ALT) of 738 U/L [normal: 7-55 U/L], aspartate aminotransferase (AST) of 856 U/L [normal: 8-48 U/L], and an alkaline phosphatase of 80 U/L [normal: 45-115 U/L]. Her total bilirubin was 2.4 mg/dL [normal: 0.1-1.2 mg/dL] and direct bilirubin was 1.4 mg/dL [normal: 0-0.4 mg/dL]. International normalized

Table 1: CIOMS/RUCAM scale.

Criteria	Score
1. Time from drug intake until reaction onset	
5-90 days	+2
<5 or >90 days	+1
2. Time from drug withdrawal until reaction onset	
<15 days	+1
>15 days	0
3. Alcohol risk	
Present	+1
Absent	0
4. Age risk factor	
>55 years	+1
<55 years	0
5. Course of reaction	
>50% improvement within 8 days	+3
>50% improvement within 30 days	+2
Worsening or <50% improvement in 30 days	-1
6. Concomitant therapy	
Time to onset incompatible	0
Time to onset compatible but with unknown reaction	-1
Time to onset compatible but known reaction	-2
Role proved in the case	-3
None or information not available	0
7. Exclusion of non-drug-related causes	
Rule out	+2
"Possible" to "not investigated"	0
Probable	-3
8. Previous information on hepatotoxicity	
Reaction unknown	0
Reaction published but unlabeled	+1
Reaction labeled in the product's characteristics	+2
9. Response to re-administration	
Positive	+3
Compatible	+2
Negative	-2
Not available or not interpretable	0
Plasma concentration of drug known as toxic	+3
Validated laboratory test with high specificity, sensitivity, and predictive values	Positive: +3 Negative: -3

ratio (INR) was 1.19 [normal: 0.8-1.1] and prothrombin time (PT) was 12.7 seconds [normal 11-13.5 seconds]. Testing for hepatitis A, hepatitis B, hepatitis C, hepatitis E, Herpes-Simplex virus, Ebstein-Barr virus, Parvovirus, and Cytomegalovirus was negative. She had normal vitamins A and D levels ruling out hypervitaminosis as the cause of hepatitis. She tested negative for alcohol and acetaminophen. Anti-smooth muscle antibody, anti-mitochondrial antibody, antinuclear antibody, and anti-liver kidney microsomal antibody were negative. An iron profile was normal. Abdominal ultrasound showed a normal liver with normal echotexture and no biliary ductal dilatation. When the herbal supplement was scrutinized, it was found to be 100% pure GC fruit rind extract. She had consumed two capsules daily as recommended for about one month. Each capsule had 1400 mg of GC extract. She was asked to stop taking the supplement. Her liver enzymes decreased significantly with an ALT of 396 μ/L and AST of 138 μ/L within three days with resolution of her abdominal symptoms. Her total and direct bilirubin came down to 0.6 mg/dL and 0.4 mg/dL, respectively. Her INR and PT also normalized. She had a normal ALT of 25 and AST of 12 in the one-month follow-up visit. Six months later, patient was found to have an elevated ALT of 301 and AST of 69. On interrogation, it was found that she had

TABLE 2: Calculation of CIOMS score in our patient gave a score of 11.

Time from drug intake until reaction onset	5 to 90 days [+2]
Time from drug withdrawal until reaction onset	≤15 days [+1]
Alcohol risk factor	Absent [0]
Age risk factor	≥55 years [+1]
Course of the reaction	>50% improvement 8 days [+3]
Concomitant therapy	Time to onset compatible and known reaction [-2]
Exclusion of non-drug-related causes	Rule out [+2]
Previous information on hepatotoxicity	Reaction published but unlabeled [+1]
Response to re-administration	Positive [+3]

started taking the same supplement again in the desperate need to lose weight. The CIOMS/RUCAM scale, a scoring system (Table 1) that is used to establish the etiology of liver damage when drug induced liver damage is suspected, gave a score of 11 for our patient (Table 2)[2, 3]. The score classifies the drug as highly probable (score ≥ 9), probable (score 6-8), possible (score 3-5), unlikely (score 1-2), and excluded (score 0) as the cause of liver injury [2, 3]. This lead us to conclude that the etiology of the patient's hepatitis was GC extract.

3. Discussion

The Drug Induced Liver Injury Network reports dietary supplements as one of the most important causes of drug induced hepatotoxicity [4]. Yet millions of people use these supplements without being aware of their potential life-threatening side effects. GC is a tropical fruit grown in South East Asia used as a culinary agent due to its sharp, sour taste [5]. Numerous GC products for weight loss are on the market in spite of the reported possible toxicity associated with the regular use of these supplements [5]. The most important ingredient of GC is HCA which blocks adenosine triphosphatase citrate lyase, a catalyst for the conversion process of citrate to acetyl-coenzyme A, which plays a key role in fatty acid, cholesterol, and triglyceride syntheses [5, 6]. HCA was one of the main components of hydroxycut products, recalled after the Food and Drug Administration received reports of 23 cases of hepatotoxicity [7]. GC extract and HCA are proposed to cause weight loss by increasing satiety through regulation of serotonin levels, reducing lipogenesis, and upregulating fat oxidation [5]. A meta-analysis of 9 randomized controlled trials of GC extract for weight loss found that it leads to only a small short term weight loss and causes mainly mild gastrointestinal side effects (average dose of GC extract used was 1-3 g) [7]. Cases of acute liver failure progressing to fulminant hepatic failure requiring liver transplantation have been reported due to GC extract [1, 8]. In the cases of fulminant hepatic failure, biopsy showed significant necrosis and collapse of liver parenchymal architecture. The exact mechanism by which GC extract causes liver injury is still unclear but a recent study on mice demonstrated that it exacerbates steatohepatitis by increasing hepatic collagen accumulation, lipid peroxidation, and levels of proinflammatory cytokines like tumor necrosis factor-alpha and monocyte chemoattractant protein-1 [9]. It also caused an increase in mRNA level of superoxide dismutase and glutathione peroxidase responsible for oxidative stress [9]. Since the patient had been taking vitamins A and D, we looked up the literature but could not find any reports of their interaction with GC extract. As far as we are aware, there is no reported medical treatment for GC extract-induced hepatitis. Acute hepatitis seems to be a reversible side effect of GC extract, which resolves when it is stopped, as demonstrated by our case. Our case also depicts that once resolved, hepatitis can be reinduced by GC extract. There have been no such reports in the literature to the best of our knowledge. Early recognition and discontinuation of GC extract were associated with resolution of the GC extract-induced acute hepatitis and prevented the progression to fulminant hepatic failure. As physicians, it is our responsibility to be informed and educate our patients about all the possible side effects of any supplements that they may be taking. Whenever we come across acute hepatitis of unexplained etiology, obtaining a detailed history of herbal supplement use is of utmost importance.

Consent

Informed patient consent was obtained for publication of the case details.

Disclosure

There are no current or prior papers or online publications, except the following conference presentation: poster presentation at the World Congress of Gastroenterology at ACG meeting in Orlando in October 2017. The authors report no external funding source for this study.

Authors' Contributions

All authors contributed equally to the writing and editing of the manuscript.

References

[1] K. E. Lunsford, A. S. Bodzin, D. C. Reino, H. L. Wang, and R. W. Busuttil, "Dangerous dietary supplements: Garcinia cambogia-Associated hepatic failure requiring transplantation," *World Journal of Gastroenterology*, vol. 22, no. 45, pp. 10071–10076, 2016.

[2] C. Benichou, "Criteria of drug-induced liver disorders," *Journal of Hepatology*, vol. 11, no. 2, pp. 272–276, 1990.

[3] G. Danan and C. Benichou, "Causality assessment of adverse reactions to drugs—I: a novel method based on the conclusions of international consensus meetings: application to drug-induced liver injuries," *Journal of Clinical Epidemiology*, vol. 46, no. 11, pp. 1323–1330, 1993.

[4] N. Chalasani, H. L. Bonkovsky, R. Fontana et al., "Features and outcomes of 899 patients with drug-induced liver injury: the DILIN prospective study," *Gastroenterology*, vol. 148, no. 7, pp. 1340–1352.e7, 2015.

[5] R. B. Semwal, D. K. Semwal, I. Vermaak, and A. Viljoen, "A comprehensive scientific overview of Garcinia cambogia," *Fitoterapia*, vol. 102, pp. 134–148, 2015.

[6] J. Hu, A. Komakula, and M. E. Fraser, "Binding of hydroxycitrate to human ATP-citrate lyase," *Acta Crystallographica, Section D: Structural Biology*, vol. 73, part 8, pp. 660–671, 2017.

[7] I. Onakpoya, S. K. Hung, R. Perry, B. Wider, and E. Ernst, "The use of Garcinia extract (hydroxycitric acid) as a weight loss supplement: a systematic review and meta-analysis of randomised clinical trials," *Journal of Obesity*, vol. 2011, Article ID 509038, 9 pages, 2011.

[8] R. Corey, K. T. Werner, A. Singer et al., "Acute liver failure associated with Garcinia cambogia use," *Annals of Hepatology*, vol. 15, no. 1, pp. 123–126, 2016.

[9] Y.-J. Kim, M.-S. Choi, Y. B. Park, S. R. Kim, M.-K. Lee, and U. J. Jung, "Garcinia cambogia attenuates diet-induced adiposity but exacerbates hepatic collagen accumulation and inflammation," *World Journal of Gastroenterology*, vol. 19, no. 29, pp. 4689–4701, 2013.

Endoscopy- and Monitored Anesthesia Care-Assisted High-Resolution Impedance Manometry Improves Clinical Management

Kaci E. Christian, John D. Morris, and Guofeng Xie

Division of Gastroenterology and Hepatology, University of Maryland School of Medicine, Veterans Affairs Maryland Health Care System, Baltimore, MD 21201, USA

Correspondence should be addressed to Guofeng Xie; gxie@som.umaryland.edu

Academic Editor: Yoshiro Kawahara

Background. High-resolution impedance manometry (HRiM) is the test of choice to diagnose esophageal motility disorders and is particularly useful for identifying achalasia subtypes, which often guide therapy. HRiM is typically performed without sedation in the office setting. However, a substantial number of patients fail this approach. We report our single-center experience on endoscopy-assisted HRiM under monitored anesthesia care (MAC) in adults to demonstrate the feasibility and effectiveness of this approach. *Methods.* Patients who had failed prior HRiM attempts received propofol under MAC. Patients then underwent an upper endoscopy, followed immediately by passage of a Diversateck HRiM motility catheter through the nares and under direct visualization into the stomach, often using the tip of the endoscope to guide the catheter. We then awakened the patients and asked them to perform 10 saline swallows. *Results.* We successfully completed HRiM studies in 14 consecutive patients. Six patients had achalasia; two had esophagogastric junction outflow obstruction; two had absent contractility; one had distal esophageal spasm; one had ineffective esophageal motility; and one had a normal study. The majority of these patients were treated successfully with targeted interventions, including per oral endoscopic myotomy, gastrostomy, botox injection, medical therapy, and dietary modifications.

1. Introduction

Esophageal manometry has become the gold-standard test to diagnose esophageal motility disorders and is also useful in the evaluation of gastroesophageal reflux disease (GERD), noncardiac chest pain, or systemic conditions that may lead to esophageal dysmotility. High-resolution impedance manometry (HRiM) with topography plotting incorporates impedance and manometry sensors, providing information on esophageal peristaltic patterns and pressures. Identification of specific esophageal motility disorders, especially subtypes of achalasia, is important, since this often guides therapeutic options [1]. The procedure is typically performed without sedation in the outpatient setting. However, some patients fail this approach due to a variety of reasons including poor tolerance or anatomic variants precluding intranasal intubation, coiling in the pharynx or esophagus, or hypersensitive gag reflex. In prior studies, 21% of high-resolution manometry studies were technically imperfect and 29% of those were imperfect due to inability to traverse the lower esophageal sphincter (LES) [2]. Twelve percent of the above-mentioned series of imperfect studies were due to inability to complete the minimum number of swallows for reasons including intolerance of the procedure [2], which include inability to intubate the nares or failure to traverse the LES. No standardized alternative techniques exist.

Previous reports trialed using through-the-scope manometric assessment revealed a good correlation between LES pressures obtained by standard manometry. However, these reports were limited by reduced peristaltic wave amplitudes due to the use of dry swallows [3]. Another group reported accurate diagnoses of achalasia and esophageal scleroderma by directly visualizing swallows during videoendoscopy [4]. However, according to the widely accepted Chicago

Table 1: Indication for manometry testing with failure rate as well as reason for failed study.

Indication	N	Failed or limited study	% failed
Refractory GERD	63	21	33%
Lung transplant evaluation	6	1	17%
Dysphagia	91	25	27%
Chest pain	4	0	0%
TOTAL	164	47	29%
Reason for failure	N	% of total	
Gagging	14	29.8%	
Nostrils	20	42.6%	
LES or esophagus	11	23.4%	
Unclear	2	4.3%	
TOTAL	47	100.0%	

classification, this technique lacks the metrics required for a diagnosis of a major motility disorder [5]. More recently, failure to perform transnasal manometry was circumvented by using an endoscopic-assisted over-the-wire technique, which utilized a water-perfusion motility catheter. Successful completion of the manometric study and diagnosis in this cohort resulted in treatment for achalasia (33.3%), change in medication (33.3%), and completion of preoperative assessment (27.7%) [6].

We report our single-center experience on endoscopy- and monitored anesthesia care- (MAC-) assisted high-resolution esophageal impedance manometry in adult patients to demonstrate the feasibility and effectiveness of this technique.

2. Materials and Methods

We evaluated patients who had failed prior attempts at manometry in the office setting for this study. All MAC- and EGD-assisted HRiM studies were performed within one week of prior failed attempts of unsedated HRiM tests. Subjects arrived at the endoscopy suite after fasting for a minimum of 6 hours. Topical anesthesia was provided with Cetacaine (benzocaine 14%, butamben 2%, and tetracaine hydrochloride 2%) spray to the throat and 5 mL of viscous lidocaine 2% solution to the nares. Patients were then sedated using propofol at the anesthetist's discretion in a monitored anesthesia care (MAC) setting. First, while, in the supine position, patients underwent a standard upper endoscopy using an Olympus GIF H180 or H190 gastroscope; an Olympus GIF XP190 scope was required in some cases. A Diversateck HRiM motility catheter was then passed through the right or left nostril into the esophagus and proximal stomach, under direct visualization and guidance with an endoscope. The tip of the catheter was centered directly above the esophagogastric junction (EGJ) prior to entering the stomach. One patient required insertion of a nasopharyngeal trumpeted airway to allow passage of the manometry catheter through the nares due to a history of prior craniofacial surgery. Once the manometry probe was in the correct position, the endoscope was withdrawn. To avoid damaging the motility catheter, endoscopic tools such as biopsy forceps or snares were not used. In some cases, simple endoscopic maneuvers such as opening the EGJ with the neonatal endoscope or gently nudging the tip of the catheter with an endoscope to redirect the motility probe were required to successfully place the motility catheter into the stomach. There was no visible damage to the motility catheter. After allowing sufficient time to awaken (usually 5 to 10 minutes), patients were given 10 consecutive 5-mL boluses of normal saline, followed by 5 mL of a viscous solution (Diversatek Healthcare Inc) as needed, while being in supine position for a total of 10 to 20 swallows. Esophageal muscle functions were recorded using the Diversatek ZVU software. The motility catheter was removed at the end of the procedure. On average, the EGD-assisted HRiM study took about 30 minutes versus 15 to 20 minutes for conventional HRiM test.

3. Results

As shown in Table 1, from January 1, 2017, to December 31, 2017, our institution performed high-resolution esophageal impedance manometry (HRiM) on 164 unique patients. Of these, 63 received manometry/impedance-pH tests to evaluate refractory GERD (38.4%); six manometry/impedance-pH tests were performed as part of lung transplant preoperative evaluation (3.7%); 91 manometry for evaluation of dysphagia (55.5%); and four manometry to evaluate atypical chest pain (2.4%). Forty-seven patients (29%) had an incomplete or limited study either at our institution or on previous attempts with outside providers. Of these, 14 patients were unable to tolerate the procedure due to excessive gagging or coughing (30%); in 20 patients, we were unable to pass the catheter through either nostril (43%), and, in 11 patients (23%), the catheter was unable to traverse the EGJ/LES or was coiled in the distal esophagus. We reviewed the charts of these patients, who either failed unsedated manometry or had known anatomic abnormalities limiting unsedated manometry, and found 14 consecutive patients who underwent MAC-assisted endoscopic probe placement. A brief clinical vignette is presented on these patients below (summarized

TABLE 2: Description and outcomes of MAC- and endoscopy-assisted manometry cases.

	N	%
Age	14	
Sex		
Women	7	50%
Men	7	50%
Indication		
Dysphagia	8	57.1%
Recurrent dysphagia	2	14.3%
Recurrent aspiration, dysphagia	2	14.3%
Lung transplant evaluation, GERD	1	7.1%
Atypical chest pain	1	7.1%
Reason for requiring endoscopic probe placement		
Inability to traverse LES	5	35.7%
Gagging	3	21.4%
Patient discomfort	2	14.3%
EGD indicated	2	14.3%
History of craniofacial fractures	1	7.1%
Looping posterior oropharynx	1	7.1%
Findings/Diagnosis		
Major motility abnormality	11	78.6%
Type II achalasia	4	28.6%
Previously treated achalasia	2	14.3%
EGJOO	2	14.3%
Absent contractility	2	14.3%
DES	1	7.1%
IEM	2	14.3%
Normal	1	7.1%
Treatment recommendations		
Interventions	5	35.7%
POEM	3	21.4%
Botox injection	1	7.1%
PEG	1	7.1%
Medical therapy	3	21.4%
Dietary modification	4	28.6%
Other	2	14.3%

and described in Tables 2 and 3). In summary, 11 of the 14 patients (78.6%) were diagnosed with a major motility disorder based on the most recent Chicago classification of esophageal disorders [7], eight of whom had either a subtype of achalasia or esophagogastric junction outlet obstruction (EGJOO). Five patients underwent procedural interventions including three peroral endoscopic myotomies (POEM) (21.4%), one botulinum toxin (Botox) injection (7.1%), and one percutaneous endoscopic gastrostomy (PEG) (7.1%). Three patients (21.4%) were treated with medical therapy, and, in the remaining six patients, we recommended dietary modification (28.6%) or continuation of previous therapy (14.3%).

Patient 1 was a 32-year-old woman with a history of achalasia with a Heller myotomy at age of eight years. She developed recurrent dysphagia that had been either refractory or with only temporary response, to multiple pneumatic dilations at other institutions. She was unable to tolerate unsedated manometry. The manometry catheter was successfully placed at the time of sedated endoscopy with findings of patent esophagogastric junction (EGJ)/LES, severe ineffective motility and distal esophageal spasm, and a normal IRP consistent with her history of previously treated type III achalasia.

Patient 2 was a 51-year-old woman with prior laparoscopic hiatal hernia repair and Toupet fundoplication with solid and liquid dysphagia and nausea who was being considered for surgical revision. Due to a history of craniofacial fractures and postsurgical anatomy and refusal to undergo unsedated manometry, she required direct visual guidance with an EGD scope for proper passage and positioning of the catheter; her manometry was normal.

Patient 3 was a 62-year-old woman with a prior Nissen fundoplication for GERD followed by repair of type III paraesophageal hernia with Belsey-Mark IV fundoplication two years later who developed dysphagia and regurgitation. She was unable to tolerate unsedated manometry due to severe gagging. Subsequently, the motility catheter was successfully advanced into the proximal stomach with MAC-assisted endoscopic guidance and showed findings of severe ineffective esophageal motility.

Patient 4 was a 71-year-old woman with reflux symptoms and pulmonary fibrosis undergoing evaluation for lung transplantation. Unsedated manometry was attempted but unsuccessful due to inability to traverse the EGJ with the motility catheter. Under endoscopic guidance, the catheter was visualized abutting the distal esophagus just above the EGJ and was successfully guided into the proximal stomach with the assistance of a neonatal endoscope (Olympus GIF XP190). Her motility findings were consistent with type II achalasia. After discussing risks and benefits with the transplant team, patient deferred Heller myotomy and transplant listing.

Patient 5 was a 52-year-old woman with a six-month history of progressively worsening solid and liquid dysphagia associated with a >50 lbs weight loss. Patient discomfort and inability to traverse the EGJ precluded her from completing unsedated manometry. Via endoscopy-assisted manometry, a diagnosis of type II achalasia was made and the patient proceeded to POEM with improvement in Eckardt score from 10 (preop) to 3 (postop).

Patient 6 was an 18-year-old man with progressive dysphagia and an associated 65-lb weight loss who was unable to tolerate insertion of the manometry probe due to severe gagging and discomfort. He underwent MAC-assisted probe placement; direct visualization was needed due to a dilated esophagus and tight gastroesophageal junction. He was diagnosed with type II achalasia and proceeded to POEM with improvement in Eckardt score from 9 to 0.

Patient 7 was an 85-year-old man with solid and liquid dysphagia and an inability to traverse the gastroesophageal

TABLE 3: Summary of MAC- and endoscopy-assisted manometry cases.

#	Age	Sex	Pertinent history	Indication for EGD-Assistance	Diagnosis	Recommendation	Outcome
1	32	F	Achalasia s/p HM	Patient discomfort	Type III achalasia s/p HM	Diet modification	Not available
2	51	F	HH repair, Toupet fundoplication	Prior craniofacial fractures	Normal	N/A	Stable symptoms
3	62	F	Type III PEH s/p fundoplication	Severe gagging	Severe IEM s/p fundoplication	Diet modification	Improved dysphagia
4	71	F	Pulmonary fibrosis, GERD	Inability to traverse LES	Type II achalasia	Follow up with pulmonary	Deferred HM, transplant listing
5	52	F	Progressive dysphagia w/ weight loss	Inability to traverse LES	Type II achalasia	POEM performed	Improved dysphagia; weight gain
6	18	M	Dysphagia w/ weight loss	Severe gagging	Type II achalasia	POEM performed	Improved dysphagia; weight gain
7	85	M	Corkscrew esophagram	Inability to traverse LES	DES	Botox injection performed	Improvement in dysphagia
8	63	M	S/p lung transplant, abnormal esophagram	EGD for possible GEJ stricture	EGJOO	PEG for enteral nutrition	Tolerated PEG; stable lung symptoms
9	65	M	Prior craniofacial surgery	Oropharyngeal looping	EGJOO	Calcium channel blocker	No follow up available
10	66	M	Dysphagia w/ weight loss	Inability to traverse LES	Type II achalasia	POEM performed	Improved dysphagia; weight gain
11	58	M	S/p lung transplant, abnormal esophagram	No prior EGD	IEM	GERD management	Stable
12	24	F	Type I achalasia s/p HM	Patient discomfort	Type I achalasia s/p treatment	Diet modification	Not available
13	61	M	Bird's beak esophagram	Probe looping	Absent contractility	Dietary modification	Long hospital stay
14	75	F	GERD, prior candida esophagitis	Gagging	Absent contractility	Bethanechol	Not available

HH: hiatal hernia; HM: Heller myotomy; PEH: paraesophageal hernia; LES: lower esophageal sphincter; GEJ: gastroesophageal junction; IEM: ineffective esophageal motility; DES: diffuse esophageal spasm; EGJOO: esophagogastric junction outflow obstruction; POEM: peroral endoscopic myotomy.

junction during prior attempts at manometry. He had undergone prior endoscopies with balloon dilation of the mid esophagus with minimal relief. Barium esophagram revealed a corkscrew appearance. He underwent endoscopy-assisted manometry that showed distal esophageal spasm; he was referred for Botox injection 5 cm above the EGJ with significant symptomatic improvement.

Patient 8 was a 63-year-old man with a history of a bilateral lung transplant due to silicosis with episodes of recurrent aspiration and a barium esophagram concerning for a gastroesophageal junction stricture. Due to this known abnormality, direct visualization following standard upper endoscopy exam was used to help advance the manometry probe past a tight lower esophageal sphincter. A diagnosis of EGJ outflow obstruction was made; due to fragile pulmonary status following frequent aspiration events, a percutaneous endoscopic gastrostomy tube was placed following this diagnosis.

Patient 9 was a 65-year-old man with a history of dysphagia who failed awake manometry due to inability to pass the probe through his nares with looping in the posterior oropharynx. He had a history of prior craniofacial surgery. After MAC sedation, attempt to insert the motility catheter via either nostril failed. A trumpeted nasal airway was used to allow passage of the probe through his nares and into the esophagus. Due to difficulty traversing the EGJ, an Olympus GIF XP190 scope was used to help guide the probe into proximal stomach. Manometry revealed EGJ outflow obstruction and he was treated successfully with a calcium channel blocker.

Patient 10 was a 66-year-old man with two years of worsening dysphagia and 40-lb weight loss referred from another institution after an EGD showed a dilated esophagus and inability to traverse the EGJ with the endoscope, suggestive of achalasia. He underwent repeat EGD at our institution, noting a tight EGJ/LES that was traversed with moderate pressure. Under direct visualization, the manometry catheter was placed into the distal esophagus but was unable to be advanced further due to patient's oxygen desaturation that

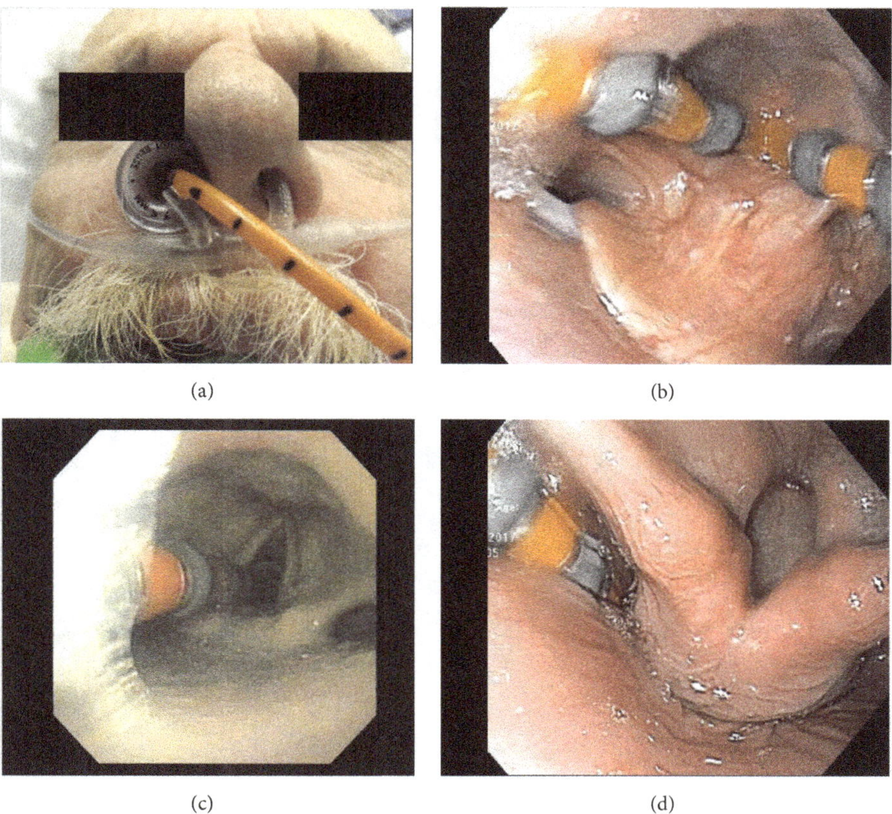

FIGURE 1: Examples of nasopharyngeal and laryngeal issues addressed with MAC-assisted endoscopic placement. (a) Nasal trumpet used for deviated septum and prior sinus surgery. (b) Coiling of the motility catheter in the posterior oropharynx at the vallecula of the epiglottis. (c) Motility catheter visualized in the trachea prior to being endoscopically guided through the upper esophageal sphincter (UES). (d) Successful placement of the motility catheter through the UES.

resolved after propofol infusion was discontinued. Manometry revealed aperistalsis with panesophageal pressurization that, in conjunction with the EGD results and barium esophagram showing tapering of the distal esophagus, was strongly suggestive of type II achalasia. The patient was referred for and underwent successful POEM.

Patient 11 was a 58-year-old man with a history of bilateral lung transplant due to cryptogenic organizing pneumonia referred for recurrent aspiration pneumonia and abnormal esophagram with poor antegrade peristalsis and distal intraesophageal reflux. After failing unsedated probe placement, he underwent EGD with endoscopic placement of the motility catheter into the proximal stomach. Manometry revealed ineffective esophageal motility.

Patient 12 was a 24-year-old woman with a history of Type I achalasia who had undergone Heller myotomy seven years earlier and complained of progressively worsening dysphagia. Unsedated manometry was unsuccessful, as the probe was not able to enter the esophagus. During sedated probe placement with direct visualization, the probe was not able to enter esophagus via the right pyriform sinus. The probe was repositioned to the left pyriform sinus and able to be advanced into proximal stomach. EGD showed evidence of prior myotomy and patent EGJ/LES. Postsurgical type I achalasia was diagnosed based on manometry findings and dietary modifications were recommended.

Patient 13 was a 61-year-old man with a two-year history of solid and liquid dysphagia. An esophagram revealed smooth narrowing of the gastroesophageal junction with incomplete relaxation, a bird's beak appearance, and esophageal dysmotility suggestive of achalasia. Unsedated manometry was attempted and revealed absent peristalsis. However, the probe had looped in the distal esophagus and did not traverse the EGJ. Due to the uncertainty in diagnosis, the patient underwent endoscopy-guided placement of the motility catheter into the proximal stomach under MAC. EGD showed patent EGJ/LES. Manometry confirmed absent contractility and dietary modifications were recommended.

Patient 14 was a 75-year-old woman with a history of atypical chest pain and dysphagia who did not tolerate unsedated manometry due to gagging. She underwent successful placement of the manometry catheter into the proximal stomach with EGD guidance under MAC. EGD showed patent EGJ/LES. Manometry findings were consistent with absent contractility and she was currently treated with Bethanechol.

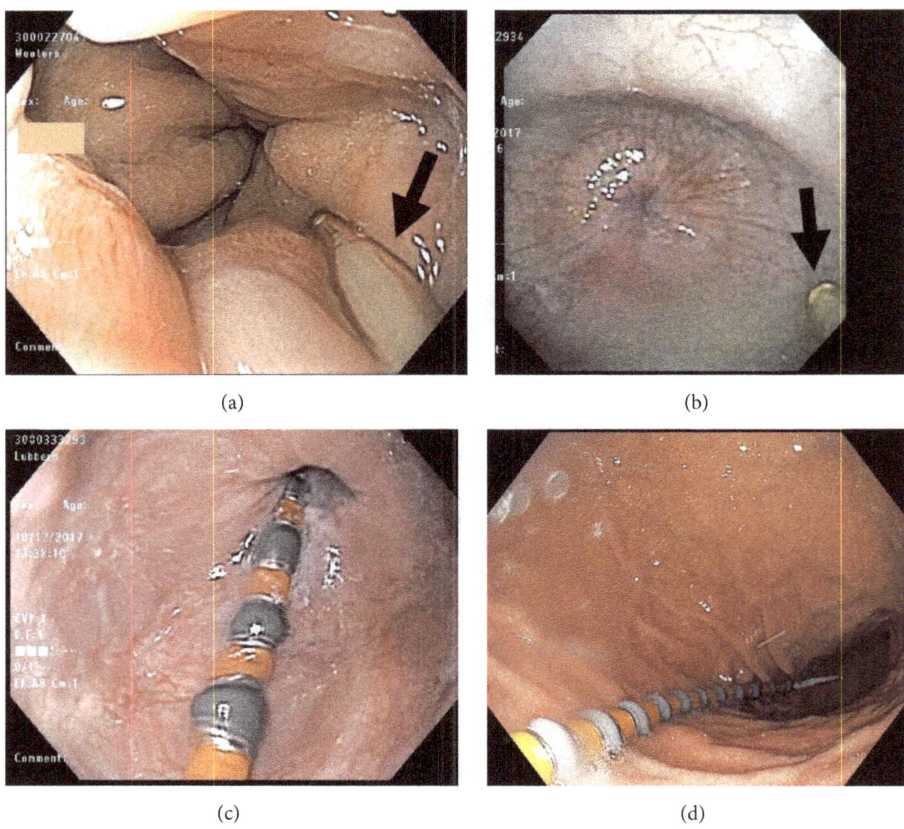

Figure 2: Examples of esophagogastric junction (EGJ) issues addressed with MAC-assisted endoscopic placement. (a) Motility catheter (arrow) hung up at hiatal hernia. (b) Motility catheter (arrow) impeded at tight lower esophageal sphincter (LES) in a patient with achalasia with a tight LES. (c) Motility catheter (arrow) visualized passing through the EGJ under direct visualization. (d) Endoscopic confirmation of successful placement of the motility catheter through the LES into the stomach.

4. Discussion

We report our experience with MAC/endoscopy-assisted HRiM and clinical outcomes in 14 patients in whom unsedated manometry had previously failed or was contraindicated. The approach was used in a subset of our patients in whom manometric data was required prior to referral for possible invasive procedures or in whom there was diagnostic uncertainty. Notably, all procedures were successful without any peri- or postprocedural complications.

This technique effectively overcame anatomical issues related to esophageal tortuosity, distal esophageal dilation, tight LES, deviated septum, or prior craniofacial surgery, respectively. Additionally, patient-related issues such as excessive coughing or gagging and inability to complete the study due to excessive discomfort were managed. Lastly, direct visualization was able to resolve uncertainty in cases with questionable prior manometric findings related to uncertain probe placement. Examples of nasopharyngeal/laryngeal and esophageal/EGJ issues of manometry probe placement are shown in Figures 1 and 2, respectively.

In our experience, the use of endoscopy-assisted HRiM allowed for the successful diagnosis of dysphagia and subsequent treatment with a procedural intervention in a substantial portion of our cohort (35.7% - POEM 21.4%, Botox injection 7.1%, PEG 7.1%), as well as medical therapy in three patients (21.4%), or dietary modifications in four (28.6%). In addition, in four patients (28.6%), the manometry findings supported the decision to defer further interventional procedures, including two patients with previously treated achalasia found to have a normal IRP, and two patients with prior hiatal hernia repair under consideration for surgical revision. Lastly, in one pre-lung transplant patient (Patient #4), a new diagnosis of achalasia assisted the patient in deciding not to pursue lung transplantation after a risk-benefit discussion with the transplant team.

Limitations of this study include the small sample size, retrospective review of the cases, and lack of a controlled comparative group. However, our study does show the potential benefit of pursuing objective HRiM data and a definitive diagnosis in patients who fail initial attempts at unsedated manometry. Due to the additional expense and small increase in risk of complication due to the endoscopic procedure and required sedation, we only selected a subset of our patients in whom there was a particularly high suspicion of a major motility disorder in which a procedural intervention might be beneficial. Also, we selected patients in whom the decision to recommend a surgical procedure was, in large part, dependent on the manometry findings. Furthermore, obtaining a definitive manometric diagnosis for spastic esophageal disorders as the cause of dysphagia becomes increasingly important as POEM emerged as an attractive treatment option [8, 9].

Another potential limitation of this technique is that the effect of anesthesia on esophageal motility is uncertain. Topical anesthetics do not influence the pharyngeal phase of swallowing, once the swallowing reflex is triggered [10]. Propofol does not alter the gastroesophageal pressure gradient but minimally decreases lower esophageal sphincter pressure at higher doses, an effect not seen with moderate doses [11]. Propofol, which is quickly redistributed from the central nervous system to peripheral tissues, has short duration of action [12]. This short duration of action and quick recovery have allowed for the frequent use of propofol in endoscopy to facilitate patient throughput [13]. In our cohort of patients, this feature also allowed a necessary short turnaround time to obtain manometric data with awake supine swallows. Indeed, the large proportion of achalasia and other major motility disorder diagnoses in our patients provides additional evidence that the residual effects of propofol are unlikely to confound acquisition of manometric data when performed after a short wash out period.

In conclusion, endoscopy- and MAC-assisted HRiM can ensure completion of esophageal motility studies in patients otherwise unable to achieve definitive manometric diagnoses. In selected patients with suspected major motility disorders such as achalasia, EGJOO, or spastic esophageal motility disorders, our approach can help guide therapy and result in successful treatment outcomes.

Authors' Contributions

Kaci E. Christian and John D. Morris contributed equally to this paper.

References

[1] J. E. Pandolfino, S. K. Ghosh, J. Rice, J. O. Clarke, M. A. Kwiatek, and P. J. Kahrilas, "Classifying esophageal motility by pressure topography characteristics: A study of 400 patients and 75 controls," *American Journal of Gastroenterology*, vol. 103, no. 1, pp. 27–37, 2008.

[2] S. Roman, P. J. Kahrilas, L. Boris, K. Bidari, D. Luger, and J. E. Pandolfino, "High-resolution manometry studies are frequently imperfect but usually still interpretable," *Clinical Gastroenterology and Hepatology*, vol. 9, no. 12, pp. 1050–1055, 2011.

[3] P. Y. Kwo, A. J. Cameron, and S. F. Phillips, "Endoscopic Esophageal Manometry," *American Journal of Gastroenterology*, vol. 90, no. 11, pp. 1985–1988, 1995.

[4] A. J. Cameron, A. Malcolm, C. M. Prather, and S. F. Phillips, "Videoendoscopic diagnosis of esophageal motility disorders," *Gastrointestinal Endoscopy*, vol. 49, no. 1, pp. 62–69, 1999.

[5] A. J. Bredenoord, M. Fox, P. J. Kahrilas, J. E. Pandolfino, W. Schwizer, and A. J. P. M. Smout, "Chicago classification criteria of esophageal motility disorders defined in high resolution esophageal pressure topography," *Neurogastroenterology & Motility*, vol. 24, supplement 1, pp. 57–65, 2012.

[6] R. Brun, K. Staller, S. Viner, and B. Kuo, "Endoscopically assisted water perfusion esophageal manometry with minimal sedation: Technique, indications, and implication on the clinical management," *Journal of Clinical Gastroenterology*, vol. 45, no. 9, pp. 759–763, 2011.

[7] P. J. Kahrilas, A. J. Bredenoord, M. Fox et al., "The Chicago Classification of esophageal motility disorders, v3.0," *Neurogastroenterology & Motility*, vol. 27, no. 2, pp. 160–174, 2015.

[8] A. M. Sharata, C. M. Dunst, R. Pescarus et al., "Peroral Endoscopic Myotomy (POEM) for Esophageal Primary Motility Disorders: Analysis of 100 Consecutive Patients," *Journal of Gastrointestinal Surgery*, vol. 19, no. 1, pp. 161–170, 2014.

[9] F. Schlottmann, N. J. Shaheen, R. D. Madanick, and M. G. Patti, "The role of Heller myotomy and POEM for nonachalasia motility disorders," *Diseases of the esophagus : official journal of the International Society for Diseases of the Esophagus*, vol. 30, no. 4, pp. 1–5, 2017.

[10] C. Ertekin, N. Kiylioglu, S. Tarlaci, A. Keskin, and I. Aydogdu, "Effect of mucosal anaesthesia on oropharyngeal swallowing," *Neurogastroenterology & Motility*, vol. 12, no. 6, pp. 567–572, 2000.

[11] A. Turan, J. Wo, Y. Kasuya et al., "Effects of dexmedetomidine and propofol on lower esophageal sphincter and gastroesophageal pressure gradient in healthy volunteers," *Anesthesiology*, vol. 112, no. 1, pp. 19–24, 2010.

[12] A. Shafer, V. A. Doze, S. L. Shafer, and P. F. White, "Pharmacokinetics and pharmacodynamics of propofol infusions during general anesthesia," *Anesthesiology*, vol. 69, no. 3, pp. 348–356, 1988.

[13] J. J. Vargo, P. J. Niklewski, J. L. Williams, J. F. Martin, and D. O. Faigel, "Patient safety during sedation by anesthesia professionals during routine upper endoscopy and colonoscopy: an analysis of 1.38 million procedures," *Gastrointestinal Endoscopy*, vol. 85, no. 1, pp. 101–108, 2017.

Portomesenteric Thrombosis Secondary to Acute Cholecystitis: A Case Report

Haseeb Ahmad Chaudhary, Ibrahim Yusuf Abubeker, Kamran Mushtaq, Khaldun Obeidat, and Anand Kartha

Department of Medicine, Hamad Medical Corporation, Doha, Qatar

Correspondence should be addressed to Kamran Mushtaq; bkamrans@hotmail.com

Academic Editor: Olga I. Giouleme

Portomesenteric venous thrombosis (PMVT) is an uncommon clinical problem. Common risk factors include intra-abdominal infections, abdominal surgeries, malignancy, cirrhosis, and inherited thrombophilia. Early recognition and treatment of PMVT are important to avoid serious complications like mesenteric ischemia and infarction. Acute cholecystitis is a clinical condition encountered daily but rarely may be complicated by development of portomesenteric venous thrombosis. Only few cases have been reported of superior mesenteric vein thrombosis secondary to cholecystitis. We report a case of a forty-one-year-old male patient who developed partial portal and superior mesenteric vein thrombosis after mild acute cholecystitis for which surgery had been deferred. Patient had no other identifiable risk factors for thrombosis. Patient was successfully treated with 6 months of anticoagulation with warfarin and complete recanalization of portomesenteric veins was achieved at the end of treatment.

1. Introduction

The prevalence of portal vein thrombosis is about 1% in the general population [1]. Wide variety of causes of portal and superior mesenteric vein thrombosis has been reported before [2]. The three main categorical groups are malignant thrombosis, cirrhotic PVT, and nonmalignant, noncirrhotic PVT [3]. The most common risk factors for PVT are cirrhosis, hepatobiliary malignancies, and pancreatitis [4]. Acquired thrombotic risk factors, such as latent myeloproliferative disorders and prothrombotic genetic defects, have also been identified as major risk factors for PVT [5]. Early recognition of PMVT is important as delayed diagnosis can lead to life threatening complication like mesenteric ischemia and infarction.

2. Case Presentation

We report a case of a forty-one-year-old male patient who presented to our emergency department with chief complaints of abdominal pain and was found to have right upper quadrant tenderness. There was no significant past medical, psychosocial, and family history. Ultrasound of abdomen showed distended gallbladder wall, with wall thickness measuring 7 mm along with pericholecystic fluid suggestive of acute cholecystitis. In addition, a 7 mm calculus was also noted in the cystic duct. Common bile duct diameter was 4 mm and portal vein trunk diameter was 10 mm. A hypodense lesion 11 by 15 mm was also seen in the left lobe of liver suggesting hemangioma. He was diagnosed with mild acute calculous cholecystitis and was discharged on oral antibiotics. He was advised for interval cholecystectomy in 4 weeks.

Sixteen days later, he presented again to the emergency with periumbilical, postprandial abdominal pain. It was associated with nausea and vomiting but no fever, jaundice, or change in bowel habits. On examination, his vital signs were normal, and abdomen was soft with minimal right hypochondrial tenderness, there was no hepatosplenomegaly, and bowel sounds were normal. There was no melena on digital rectal exam.

Laboratory investigation revealed WBC: 6500 x 109/L, Hb:159 gm/l, and PLT:247000 x10^9/L. Coagulation studies

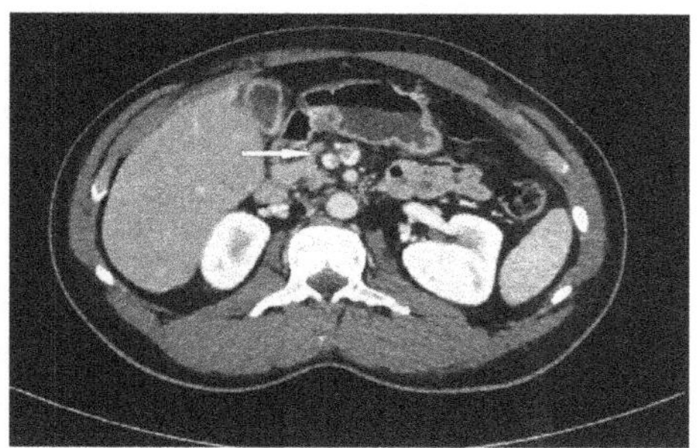

FIGURE 1: Contrast-enhanced CT scan showing pericholecystic fluid and partial filling defect in the superior mesenteric vein (white arrow).

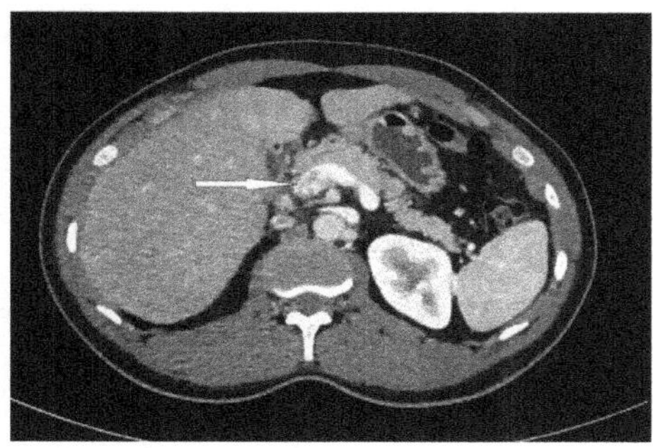

FIGURE 2: Contrast-enhanced CT scan abdomen showing partial filling defect in the portal vein (white arrow).

including prothrombin time, partial thromboplastin time, and INR were normal, and urea, creatinine, and electrolytes were all within normal range. Liver function tests revealed ALT: 29 IU/L, AST: 17 IU/L, ALP:117 IU/L, total bilirubin: 6 umol/l, protein:76 gm/l, and albumin: 41gm/l and CRP was very elevated at 1476 nmol/L (range: 0.76-28.5 nmol/l).

A contrast-enhanced CT scan of the abdomen was performed to rule out any complications as the changing nature of pain was not explained by cholecystitis alone. Apart from confirming the pericholecystic fluid and distended gall bladder, it also showed filling defects in several branches of the superior mesenteric vein and portal vein confluence with partial obliteration of the lumen, suggesting venous thrombosis, and part of the distal small bowel loops demonstrated apparent wall thickening with hyperenhancement and mesenteric congestion (Figures 1 and 2).

Doppler ultrasound study of hepatobiliary system also confirmed the presence of partial thrombosis. Portomesenteric thrombosis is an unusual site for thrombosis so work-up was done to rule out other causes. Antithrombin III activity was 101.2% (normal range 71-116 %), homocysteine: 8 umol/L (range: 5-15 umol/L), and ANA, anticardiolipin IgG, and IgM antibodies were negative. Genetic testing for prothrombin gene mutation 20210 and factor V Leiden mutation was also negative. Flow cytometric analysis of peripheral blood for paroxysmal nocturnal hemoglobinuria was negative. JAK2 mutation was not detected. Alpha-fetoprotein level was normal. MRI abdomen was performed to assess the nature of

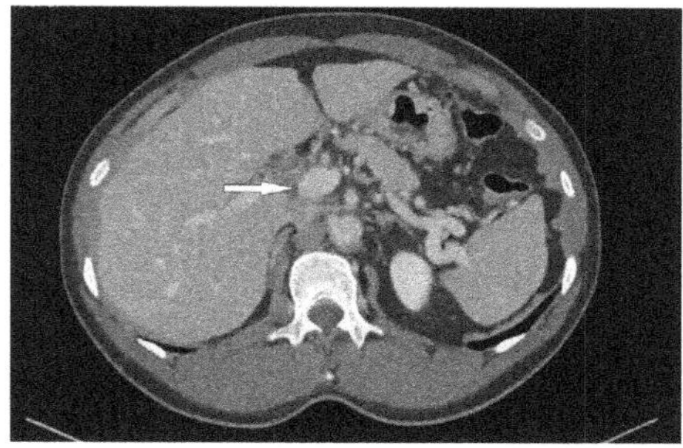

FIGURE 3: Contrast-enhanced CT abdomen after 6 months of anticoagulation showing complete recanalization of previously seen portomesenteric thrombosis.

hypoechoic lesion in the liver seen on the initial ultrasound. MRI abdomen confirmed that the hypoechoic lesion in right lobe of liver was hemangioma and possibility of a primary liver tumour was ruled out.

The patient was started on therapeutic anticoagulation with enoxaparin at 1 mg/kg subcutaneous BID dose and IV Ceftriaxone 2 grams per day along with bowel rest. After 24 hrs the patient was started on warfarin and enoxaparin was continued for 5 days for overlap until his INR was in therapeutic range (2.0-3.0). Patient was discharged after 6 days of hospitalization and appointment with surgical team for cholecystectomy was given. His stay in the hospital was uneventful so a repeat CT scan was not done to look for bowel ischemia. On follow-up at 6 months patient was doing well clinically and completed the warfarin course. Repeat CT abdomen with contrast showed complete recanalization of portal and superior mesenteric veins (Figure 3) and patient is waiting for cholecystectomy.

3. Discussion

Portomesenteric venous thrombosis (PMVT) includes thrombosis involving portal vein and superior mesenteric and/or inferior mesenteric vein. Acute portal or superior mesenteric vein thrombosis often presents with abdominal pain, whereas chronic disease manifests either as an incidental finding on CT or with features of portal hypertension. Contrast-enhanced CT scan of abdomen diagnoses more than 90% of cases and is considered gold standard as it can also diagnose potential complications like mesenteric ischemia and infarction [6]. Our patient's initial presentation with mild acute cholecystitis and later presentation with central abdominal pain led to the decision of contrast-enhanced CT imaging that revealed partial thrombosis of portal and superior mesenteric veins. In contrast to the reported cases before [7], our patient did not have septic cholecystitis with absence of fever, leukocytosis, and near-normal liver function tests on presentation indicating the cholecystitis was of mild nature with raised CRP and US features suggestive of such a diagnosis [8].

Local inflammatory causes of PMVT cholecystitis, cholangitis, hepatitis, appendicitis, diverticulitis, and pancreatitis have all been reported in the past [3]. One-third of these patients have more than one risk factor for thrombosis [9]. Given the vague presentation, high degree of clinical suspicion is required to diagnose patients with PMVT [10]. PMVT remains undiagnosed in several cases and detected incidentally during examination for other reasons [6]. PMVT have also been reported after several intra-abdominal surgeries in which case surgery itself acts as a risk factor for thrombosis [11]. Studies have suggested the incidence of portal vein thrombosis to be higher with laparoscopic surgery than open surgery [12].

PMVT is a rare complication of acute cholecystitis as previously reported; our case is unique in a way that our patient had mild form of cholecystitis and did not undergo surgery and still had portal vein thrombosis which was more extensive and partially involved the superior mesenteric vein as well. The early recognition of this complication of a mild cholecystitis with appropriate medical management can improve outcomes [13] and shorten hospital stay [14]. Prompt recognition is also critically important to avoid life threatening complications like mesenteric ischemia and infarction [15].

Work-up for inherited and acquired thrombophilia conditions was negative, with normal antithrombin III level and homocysteine levels. Advanced imaging with CT and MRI did not reveal any local tumour that could have contributed to the thrombus formation and propagation. The indication to perform MRI Liver was to characterize the hypodense lesion picked up by ultrasonogram in the left lobe of liver, which proved to be a hemangioma. Our patient did not have any evidence of haemolysis but flow cytometry for paroxysmal nocturnal hemoglobinuria was performed to rule out that possibility, JAK2 mutation was also not detected which ruled out polycythaemia vera and essential thrombocytosis [16].

We believe the initial triggering factor for portal vein thrombosis in our case could be the intense inflammatory response caused by the stone in the cystic duct, which sits in close proximity to the draining cystic veins in Calot's triangle [17]. Cystic veins eventually drain into the right portal vein branch through which the thrombosis can propagate if left untreated, although the ultrasound Doppler did not reveal dilatation in the cystic vein in this case.

Nevertheless, with bowel rest, IV hydration, antibiotics, and anticoagulation patient's condition dramatically improved and he was discharged pain-free from the hospital with follow-up. There is newer data emerging on use of direct acting oral anticoagulants and novel oral anticoagulants (NOACs) in PMVT [18, 19]. However, we restricted anticoagulation to warfarin due to the affordability issues of our patient.

4. Conclusion

Portomesenteric vein thrombosis is a rare complication of acute cholecystitis. Early recognition of this complication of cholecystitis with appropriate medical management can improve outcomes and shorten hospital stay and prevent life threatening complications like mesenteric ischemia. PMVT can be successfully treated with oral anticoagulation with warfarin resulting in favourable outcome.

Consent

Informed consent was taken from the patient.

Authors' Contributions

Haseeb A. Chaudhary, Ibrahim Yusuf, and Kamran Mushtaq reviewed the literature, drafted and edited the manuscript, and approved the final manuscript. Khaldun Obeidat and Anand Kartha reviewed the literature and edited and approved the final manuscript. The manuscript was prepared according to ICJME guidelines and CARE guidelines for reporting the case reports.

References

[1] D. Sacerdoti, G. Serianni, S. Gaiani, M. Bolognesi, G. Bombonato, and A. Gatta, "Thrombosis of the portal venous system," *Journal of Ultrasound*, vol. 10, no. 1, pp. 12–21, 2007.

[2] M. El-Wahsh, "A case of portal vein thrombosis associated with acute cholecystitis/pancreatitis or coincidence," *Hepatobiliary & Pancreatic Diseases International*, vol. 5, no. 2, pp. 308–310, May 2006.

[3] J. Trebicka and C. P. Strassburg, "Etiology and complications of portal vein thrombosis," *Viszeralmedizin: Gastrointestinal Medicine and Surgery*, vol. 30, no. 6, pp. 375–380, 2014.

[4] N. V. Jamieson, "Changing perspectives in portal vein thrombosis and liver transplantation," *Transplantation*, vol. 69, no. 9, pp. 1772–1774, 2000.

[5] M. Muneer, H. Abdelrahman, A. El-Menyar, A. Zarour, A. Awad, and H. Al-Thani, "Acute cholecystitis complicated with portal vein thrombosis: A case report and literature review," *American Journal of Case Reports*, vol. 16, pp. 627–630, 2015.

[6] A. K. Singal, P. S. Kamath, and A. Tefferi, "Mesenteric venous thrombosis," *Mayo Clinic Proceedings*, vol. 88, no. 3, pp. 285–294, 2013.

[7] P. Menéndez-Sánchez, D. Gambi-Pisonero, P. Villarejo-Campos, D. Padilla-Valverde, and J. Martín-Fernández, "Septic thrombophlebitis of the portal vein due to acute cholecystitis," *Cirugía y Cirujanos*, vol. 78, no. 5, pp. 439–441, 2010.

[8] T. Juvonen, H. Kiviniemi, O. Niemelä, and M. I. Kairaluoma, "Diagnostic accuracy of ultrasonography and C reactive protein concentration in acute cholecystitis: a prospective clinical study," *European Journal of Surgery*, vol. 158, pp. 365–369, 1992.

[9] H. Toyoda, T. Kumada, T. Tada et al., "Discrepant imaging findings of portal vein thrombosis with dynamic computed tomography and computed tomography during arterial portography in hepatocellular carcinoma: possible cause leading to inappropriate treatment selection," *Clinical Journal of Gastroenterology*, vol. 10, no. 2, pp. 163–167, 2017.

[10] N. Hidajat, H. Stobbe, V. Griesshaber, R. Felix, and R.-J. Schroder, "Imaging and radiological interventions of portal vein thrombosis," *Acta Radiologica*, vol. 46, no. 4, pp. 336–343, 2005.

[11] M. E. Allaix, M. K. Krane, M. Zoccali, K. Umanskiy, R. Hurst, and A. Fichera, "Postoperative portomesenteric venous thrombosis: Lessons learned from 1,069 consecutive laparoscopic colorectal resections," *World Journal of Surgery*, vol. 38, no. 4, pp. 976–984, 2014.

[12] M. Ikeda, M. Sekimoto, S. Takiguchi et al., "High incidence of thrombosis of the portal venous system after laparoscopic splenectomy: a prospective study with contrast-enhanced CT scan," *Annals of Surgery*, vol. 241, no. 2, pp. 208–216, 2005.

[13] T. Sauerbuch, U. T. Hopt, H. Neeff, B. Pötzsch, M. Rössle, and D. Valla, "Management of portal/mesenteric vein occlusion," *Viszeralmedizin: Gastrointestinal Medicine and Surgery*, vol. 30, no. 6, pp. 417–420, 2014.

[14] L. Brunaud, L. Antunes, S. Collinet-Adler et al., "Acute mesenteric venous thrombosis: Case for nonoperative management," *Journal of Vascular Surgery*, vol. 34, no. 4, pp. 673–679, 2001.

[15] S. Occhionorelli, A. La Manna, R. Stano, L. Morganti, and G. Vasquez, "The surgical approach to near-total small bowel infarction in a patient with massive portomesenteric thrombosis. Case report," *Ann Ital Chir*, 2016.

[16] S. K. Austin and J. R. Lambert, "The JAK2V617F mutation and thrombosis," *British Journal of Haematology*, vol. 143, no. 3, pp. 307–320, 2008.

[17] F. Arthur, "The cystic vein: the significance of a forgotten anatomic landmark," *JSLS: Journal of the Society of Laparoendoscopic Surgeons*, vol. 1, no. 3, pp. 263–266, 1997.

[18] A. De Gottardi, J. Trebicka, C. Klinger et al., "Antithrombotic treatment with direct-acting oral anticoagulants in patients with splanchnic vein thrombosis and cirrhosis," *Liver International*, vol. 37, no. 5, pp. 694–699, 2017.

[19] N. M. Intagliata, Z. H. Henry, H. Maitland et al., "Direct Oral Anticoagulants in Cirrhosis Patients Pose Similar Risks of Bleeding When Compared to Traditional Anticoagulation," *Digestive Diseases and Sciences*, vol. 61, no. 6, pp. 1721–1727, 2016.

53

Ischemic Gastropathic Ulcer Mimics Gastric Cancer

Saleh Daher,[1] Ziv Lahav,[2] Ayman Abu Rmeileh,[2] Meir Mizrahi,[3] and Tawfik Khoury[1]

[1] *Division of Gastroenterology and Hepatology, Department of Medicine, Hebrew University-Hadassah Medical Center, P.O. Box 12000, Ein Kerem, 91120 Jerusalem, Israel*
[2] *Department of Internal Medicine, Hebrew University-Hadassah Medical Center, P.O. Box 12000, 91120 Jerusalem, Israel*
[3] *Division of Gastroenterology and Hepatology, Advanced Endoscopy Center, Beth Israel Deaconess Medical Center, Harvard Medical School, 330 Brookline Avenue, Stoneman 458, Boston, MA 02215, USA*

Correspondence should be addressed to Tawfik Khoury; tawfikkhoury1@hotmail.com

Academic Editor: R. J. L. F. Loffeld

Gastric ulcer due to mesenteric ischemia is a rare clinical finding. As a result, few reports of ischemic gastric ulcers have been reported in the literature. The diagnosis of ischemic gastropathy is seldom considered in patients presenting with abdominal pain and gastric ulcers. In this case report, we describe a patient with increasing abdominal pain, weight loss, and gastric ulcers, who underwent extensive medical evaluation and whose symptoms were resistant to medical interventions. Finally he was diagnosed with chronic mesenteric ischemia, and his clinical and endoscopic abnormalities resolved after surgical revascularization of both the superior mesenteric artery and the celiac trunk.

1. Introduction

Chronic mesenteric ischemia classically presents as "abdominal angina," characterized by generalized postprandial abdominal pain lasting up to 3 hours, as well as weight loss and upper-abdominal bruit. Symptoms are not specific and often mistakenly attributed to other gastrointestinal etiologies, such as peptic ulcer or gallstones. Gastric ischemia is not commonly encountered because of the rich collateral blood supply to the stomach, making gastric ulceration from ischemia a rare condition [1–3]. Gastric ischemia manifested as gastric ulcer might result from localized or diffuse vascular insufficiency caused by etiologies such as systemic hypotension, vasculitis, or localized thromboembolism. However, *Helicobacter pylori (HP)* infection is considered to be the major cause of peptic ulcer disease, and the use of nonsteroidal anti-inflammatory drugs (NSAIDs) accounts for the majority of the remainder [4]. Herein we report a long-standing case of chronic mesenteric ischemia where an *HP*-negative gastric ulcer and not associated with the use of NSAIDs was detected in the initial evaluation. The patient's complaints ultimately responded to revascularization surgery, with resolution of his non-NSAID, non-*HP* gastric ulcers.

2. Case Report

A 46-year-old male presented with progressive, mostly postprandial abdominal pain, and significant weight loss of almost 44 lb. in a six-month period.

His medical history was notable for heavy smoking for the past 30 years and cholelithiasis. His medications included 40 mg esomeprazole once a day.

Four months prior to presentation, he underwent an esophagogastroduodenoscopy (EGD) to evaluate similar complaints and was diagnosed with peptic ulcer disease (PUD) with positive *HP*. No improvement followed a course of a high dosage of esomeprazole and *Helicobacter* eradication therapy.

On admission the patient was stable, with a heart rate of 65 beats/min., blood pressure of 110/60 mmHg, and oxygen saturation of 98%. His physical examination was unremarkable except for epigastric tenderness and bilateral temporal and extremities wasting. Laboratory tests revealed normal CBC, kidney, and liver function. His C-reactive protein and erythrocyte sedimentation rate were also unremarkable.

Upon admission, a review of a computed tomography (CT) scan was done in an outpatient setting and revealed fatty liver, thickened gastric wall (Figure 1), and a hypodense

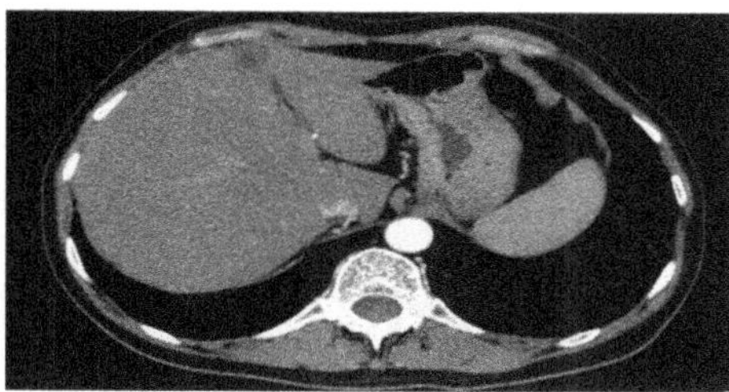

FIGURE 1: Computed tomography (CT) revealed a thickened gastric wall mainly involving the pyloric region.

area in the stomach; however no revision of the gastrointestinal arterial vasculature was done at that time. The patient underwent second EGD that revealed mildly erythematous antral mucosa. An immunohistochemical stain for HP was negative. Random gastric biopsies showed mild chronic active gastritis. The patient was discharged with the impression that he is suffering from active nonspecific gastritis. The dosage of esomeprazole was escalated to 40 mg twice a day. Due to the continuity of his symptoms, a third EGD was performed that showed hyperemic erythematous gastric mucosa with few longitudinal ulcerations that were located on the greater curvature on a preantral location. The pathology examination from gastric biopsies revealed a single focus of markedly atypical glands with necrotic material in the lumen, suspicious of a malignancy. A week later, a fourth EGD showed large ulcerations on the preantral greater and lesser curvatures (Figure 2) with hyperemic intervening mucosa. A pathological examination showed acute gastritis and duodenitis, reactive atypia, negative stain for *HP*, and no signs of intestinal metaplasia or malignancy.

Six weeks later, he was admitted again due to worsening of epigastric pain and further weight loss, overall losing 66 lbs. over 9 months. During the third hospitalization, a diagnosis of ischemia was considered. A CT angiogram showed significant gastric pyloric wall thickening and surrounding small lymphadenopathy, several new splenic infarcts, and significant narrowing and obstruction in the origin of the superior mesenteric artery (SMA) and the origin of the celiac trunk with mild stenosis of the inferior mesenteric artery (IMA) origin (Figure 3). A vascular surgery consult was obtained and open surgical revascularization was recommended given our patient's young age and lack of comorbidities. The patient underwent a surgical bypass with expanded polytetrafluoroethylene (ePTFE) graft between the right common iliac artery and the SMA with extension graft to the hepatic artery that resulted in significant clinical improvement and weight gain. Repeat EGD following the surgical bypass revealed mild gastritis and duodenitis with resolution of the gastric ulcers.

3. Discussion

Gastric ulceration as a direct result of chronic mesenteric ischemia is a rare condition. The normal mesenteric arterial blood supply relies on three major branches of the abdominal aorta: the celiac trunk, the SMA, and the IMA. Most of the gastric blood supply is through the celiac artery. However, the stomach receives additional blood from a rich collateral mesenteric circulation that makes the stomach less vulnerable to ischemic insult. While an isolated stenosis of the celiac trunk is usually well tolerated, a concomitant compromised SMA blood supply can be enough to cause ischemic gastric ulcer [5–7]. The clinical presentation of ischemic gastropathy is often misinterpreted. Classic symptoms include sitophobia, postprandial abdominal pain, and weight loss [8]. However, the concomitant occurrence of more nonspecific symptoms, such as vomiting, diarrhea, and nausea, can complicate the clinical presentation [9], and the abdominal pain that is typical of mesenteric ischemia is incorrectly attributed to the presence of a gastric ulcer.

Gastric ulcers are usually attributed to more common etiologies, such as *HP* infection or NSAIDs. The irregular, ill-defined endoscopic characteristics of these gastric ulcers may also raise a suspicion of gastric malignancy, especially when weight loss is reported. Histology from a gastric ulcer usually reveals nonspecific findings of inflammation and reactive changes that usually lead to a diagnosis of gastritis [8].

Revascularization is the appropriate treatment in cases of ischemic gastropathy. This may be either by surgery or by angioplasty, with or without the use of stents [7].

The choice of the revascularization method (open versus endovascular) is generally based on patient's age and comorbidities, as well as the anatomy of vascular lesions [10–12]. For young patients without contraindications for open surgery, open surgical revascularization may be the preferred initial approach [13].

In most cases, after successful revascularization, the endoscopic findings disappear within months, while the clinical symptoms resolve within few days [14].

We have described herein a patient with recurrent postprandial abdominal pain, significant weight loss, and an HP-negative gastric ulcer without history of NSAID use. The similarity of symptoms between chronic mesenteric ischemia and gastric cancer, and the presence of gastric ulcers, led us to ruling out a malignancy, despite the fact that the clinical presentation was classic for chronic mesenteric ischemia. Finally, our patient was diagnosed with severe SMA and celiac stenosis, which most probably caused the gastric ulceration due to the concomitant compromised collateral mesenteric circulation, with complete clinical and endoscopic resolution after successful revascularization.

This case highlights the need to be aware of this occurrence. We believe that increased awareness and knowledge of this disease can result in a much faster diagnosis, specifically with the increasing availability of noninvasive imaging by CT or MRI angiography that can rapidly exclude gastrointestinal vascular incompetence [15].

In conclusion, it is extremely important to fully investigate nonhealing, ill-defined gastric ulcers for the possibility of malignancy; however, gastric ulcers that mimic gastric cancer, that are resistant to treatment, or that are *HP*-negative with no history of NSAID use should be investigated for a possible ischemic etiology, especially in patients with concomitant atherosclerotic vascular disease.

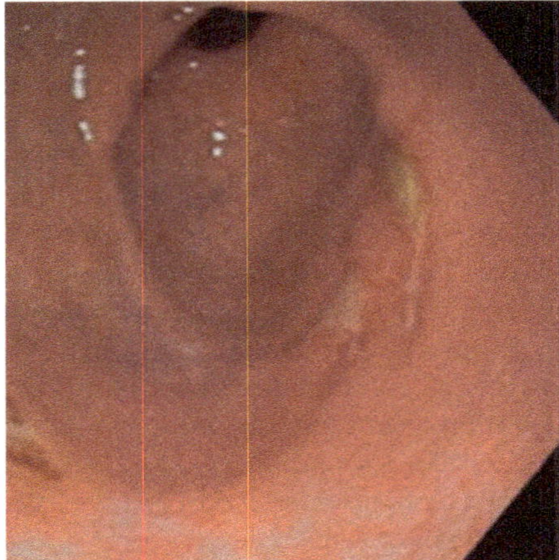
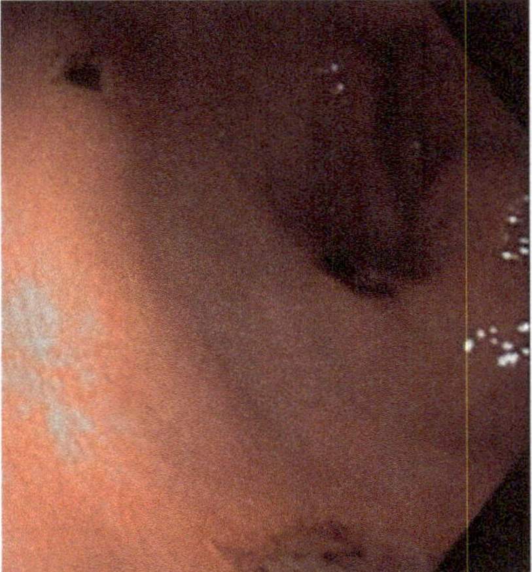

FIGURE 2: EGD showed multiple gastric ulcers in the body of the stomach, fundus, and pylorus.

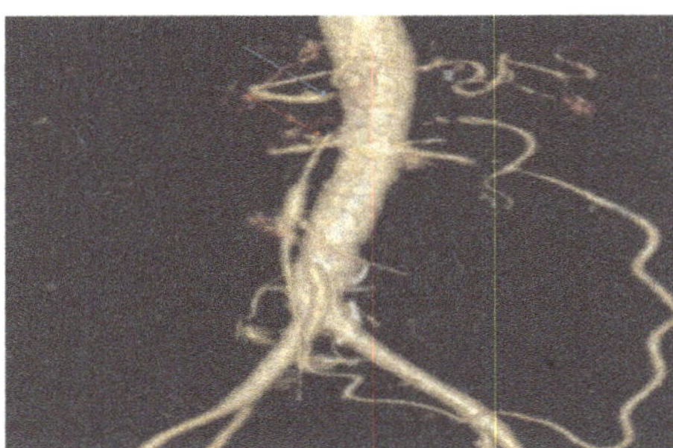

FIGURE 3: Computed tomography (CT) angiogram shows stenosis of the SMA and celiac trunk origins.

Authors' Contributions

Tawfik Khoury, Saleh Daher, and Meir Mizrahi treated the patient and followed him up. Tawfik Khoury, Ziv Lahav, Meir Mizrahi, and Saleh Daher contributed to the acquisition and interpretation of data. All authors contributed to the drafting of the paper, critical revision, and final approval of the version submitted to the journal.

References

[1] G. Lanciault and E. D. Jacobson, "The gastrointestinal circulation," *Gastroenterology*, vol. 71, no. 5, pp. 851–873, 1976.

[2] K. M. Casey, T. M. Quigley, R. A. Kozarek, and E. J. Raker, "Lethal nature of ischemic gastropathy," *The American Journal of Surgery*, vol. 165, no. 5, pp. 646–649, 1993.

[3] M. Turan, M. Şen, E. Canbay, K. Karadayi, and E. Yildiz, "Gastric necrosis and perforation caused by acute gastric dilatation: report of a case," *Surgery Today*, vol. 33, no. 4, pp. 302–304, 2003.

[4] F. K. L. Chan and W. K. Leung, "Peptic-ulcer disease," *The Lancet*, vol. 360, no. 9337, pp. 933–941, 2002.

[5] G. Mercogliano, O. Tully, and D. Schmidt, "Gastric ischemia treated with superior mesenteric artery revascularization," *Clinical Gastroenterology and Hepatology*, vol. 5, no. 4, p. A26, 2007.

[6] J.-P. Richieri, B. Pol, and M.-J. Payan, "Acute necrotizing ischemic gastritis: clinical, endoscopic and histopathologic aspects," *Gastrointestinal Endoscopy*, vol. 48, no. 2, pp. 210–212, 1998.

[7] L. J. Brandt and S. J. Boley, "AGA technical review on intestinal ischemia. American Gastrointestinal Association," *Gastroenterology*, vol. 118, no. 5, pp. 954–968, 2000.

[8] J. Haberer, N. N. Trivedi, J. Kohlwes, and L. Tierney Jr., "Clinical problem-solving. A gut feeling," *The New England Journal of Medicine*, vol. 349, no. 1, pp. 73–78, 2003.

[9] R. C. Bakker, D. P. M. Brandjes, P. Snel, J. A. Lawson, J. Lindeman, and D. Batchelor, "Malabsorption syndrome associated with ulceration of the stomach and small bowel caused by chronic intestinal ischemia in a patient with hyperhomocysteinemia," *Mayo Clinic Proceedings*, vol. 72, no. 6, pp. 546–550, 1997.

[10] R. S. M. Davies, M. L. Wall, S. H. Silverman et al., "Surgical versus endovascular reconstruction for chronic mesenteric ischemia: a contemporary UK series," *Vascular and Endovascular Surgery*, vol. 43, no. 2, pp. 157–164, 2009.

[11] M. Biebl, W. A. Oldenburg, R. Paz-Fumagalli, J. M. McKinney, and A. G. Hakaim, "Surgical and interventional visceral revascularization for the treatment of chronic mesenteric ischemia—when to prefer which?" *World Journal of Surgery*, vol. 31, no. 3, pp. 562–568, 2007.

[12] M. D. Atkins, C. J. Kwolek, G. M. LaMuraglia, D. C. Brewster, T. K. Chung, and R. P. Cambria, "Surgical revascularization versus endovascular therapy for chronic mesenteric ischemia: a comparative experience," *Journal of Vascular Surgery*, vol. 45, no. 6, pp. 1162–1171, 2007.

[13] G. S. Oderich, T. C. Bower, T. M. Sullivan, H. Bjarnason, S. Cha, and P. Gloviczki, "Open versus endovascular revascularization for chronic mesenteric ischemia: risk-stratified outcomes," *Journal of Vascular Surgery*, vol. 49, no. 6, pp. 1472.e3–1479.e3, 2009.

[14] L. Højgaard and E. Krag, "Chronic ischemic gastritis reversed after revascularization operation," *Gastroenterology*, vol. 92, no. 1, pp. 226–228, 1987.

[15] K. M. Horton and E. K. Fishman, "Multi-detector row CT of mesenteric ischemia: can it be done?" *Radiographics*, vol. 21, no. 6, pp. 1463–1473, 2001.

54

Gastric Schwannoma: A Tumor Must Be Included in Differential Diagnoses of Gastric Submucosal Tumors

Bao-guang Hu,[1] Feng-jie Wu,[1] Jun Zhu,[1] Xiao-mei Li,[2] Yu-ming Li,[1] Yan Feng,[3] and He-sheng Li[1]

[1]*Department of Gastrointestinal Surgery, The Affiliated Hospital of Binzhou Medical University, Binzhou, Shandong, China*
[2]*Centers for Disease Control and Prevention of Binzhou City, Binzhou, Shandong, China*
[3]*Department of Radiology, The Affiliated Hospital of Binzhou Medical University, Binzhou, Shandong, China*

Correspondence should be addressed to Yu-ming Li; PIliym@126.com

Academic Editor: Naohiko Koide

Gastric schwannoma (GS) is a rare neoplasm of the stomach. It accounts for 0.2% of all gastric tumors and is mostly benign, slow-growing, and asymptomatic. Due to its rarity, GS is not widely recognized by clinicians, and the precise differential diagnosis between GS and other gastric submucosal tumors remains difficult preoperatively. The present study reports a case of GS misdiagnosed as gastrointestinal stromal tumor and reviews the clinical, imaging, and pathological features, treatment, and follow-up of 221 patients with GS previously reported in the English literature. Although GS is rare, the case reported in the current study highlights the importance of including GS in differential diagnoses of gastric submucosal tumors. Furthermore, the findings of the review suggest that although many cases are asymptomatic, the most common symptoms are abdominal pain or discomfort, not gastrointestinal bleeding, and malignant GSs present with clinical symptoms more commonly. Although large-sample multicenter studies on the efficacy, safety, and oncological outcomes of minimally invasive techniques are required, the findings presented herein may be helpful for clinicians when diagnosing or treating GS.

1. Introduction

Gastric schwannoma (GS) is a rare submucosal tumor that arises from Schwann cells in the neural plexus of the stomach. It accounts for only 0.2% of all gastric tumors, 6.3% of gastric mesenchymal tumors, and 4% of all benign tumors of the stomach [1]. GS was first described in 1988 in a study by Daimaru et al. [2], in which a series of 24 cases were examined. To date, more than 200 new cases of GS have been reported worldwide, and the findings of imaging findings and analysis of the gross features of GS have been described in some sporadic case reports and the occasional series of GS cases. However, GS is not widely recognized by clinicians, and it remains difficult to accurately distinguish GS from other gastric submucosal tumors preoperatively.

The present study reports the case of a 61-year-old woman with GS and reviews the current knowledge of GS available based on sporadic case reports and the occasional series of case reports in the literature. We hope that the findings will be useful for clinicians during the diagnosis and treatment of GS.

2. Case Report

A 61-year-old woman with a 2-year history of nonspecific epigastric abdominal pain underwent esophagogastroduodenoscopy (EGD) to rule out a digestive ulcer. EGD revealed a submucosal bulge on the anterior wall of the gastric body (Figure 1(a)). The patient then underwent endosonography, which revealed a large submucosal mass measuring 3.7 × 3.2 cm arising from the muscularis propria (the fourth layer). The features of the mass were similar to those of a gastrointestinal stromal tumor (GIST) (Figure 1(b)).

A computed tomography (CT) scan revealed a uniformly enhancing mass located between the left lobe of the liver and the lesser curvature of the gastric body. The mass was partly

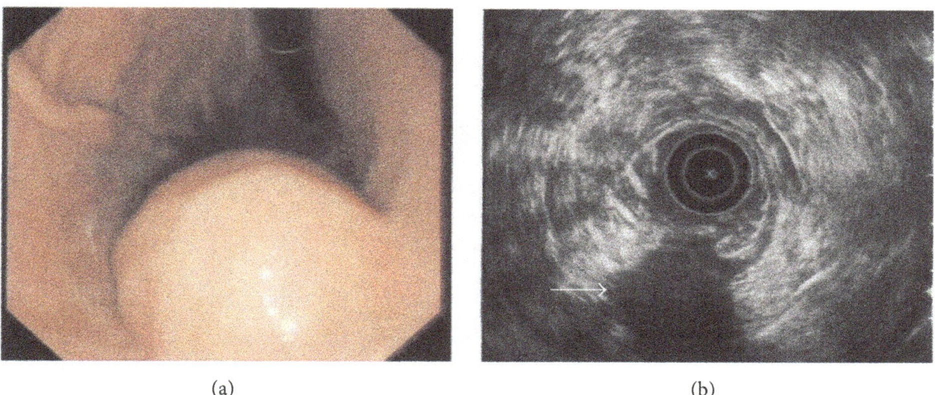

(a) (b)

FIGURE 1: Endoscopic (a) and endosonographic (b) findings in the current case of gastric schwannoma. (a) A round, submucosal mass with an indistinct border was observed at the lesser curvature of the gastric body. (b) On endoscopic ultrasonography, the lesion (white arrow) appeared homogeneous and its echogenicity was lower than that of the normal muscle layer. The mass measured 3.7 × 3.2 cm and originated from the fourth layer.

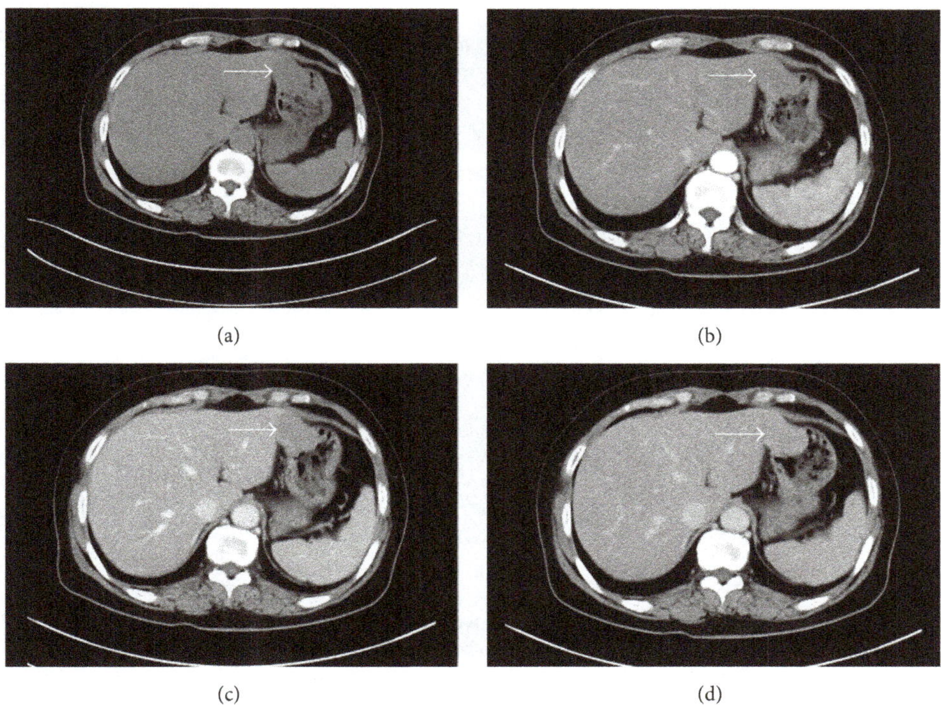

(a) (b) (c) (d)

FIGURE 2: Computed tomography (CT) image of the gastric schwannoma. (a) An oval-shaped mass (white arrow) with a size of 43 × 32 mm was observed in the lesser curvature of the stomach, which exhibited a slightly low density on plain scanning CT imaging. (b) The CT value of the mass was about 38 HU before the injection of contrast medium. The mass showed delayed enhancement with a CT value of 53 HU on arterial-phase enhanced CT scanning. (c) The CT value of the mass was slightly increased (68 HU) on portal venous-phase enhanced CT imaging. (d) The CT value of the mass was increased (78 HU) on delayed enhanced CT scanning after a delay of 3 minutes.

exophytic and partly projected into the gastric lumen, causing smooth indentation, and measured 4.3 × 3.2 cm (Figure 2). The patient's laboratory results were unremarkable. Based on the above data, the patient was given a preoperative diagnosis of GIST arising from the anterior wall of the gastric body.

The patient was then subjected to laparoscopic examination, which showed an exophytic tumor (4 × 3 cm size) arising from the anterior wall of the lesser gastric curvature. The exophytic part of the mass appeared off-white in color and rough, with a concavo-convex surface; however, the margin of the mass on the gastric wall was clear (Figure 3(a)). To achieve an optimal tumor-negative margin, the laparoscopy was converted to a laparotomy, and complete resection of the tumor was performed. Histopathology revealed that

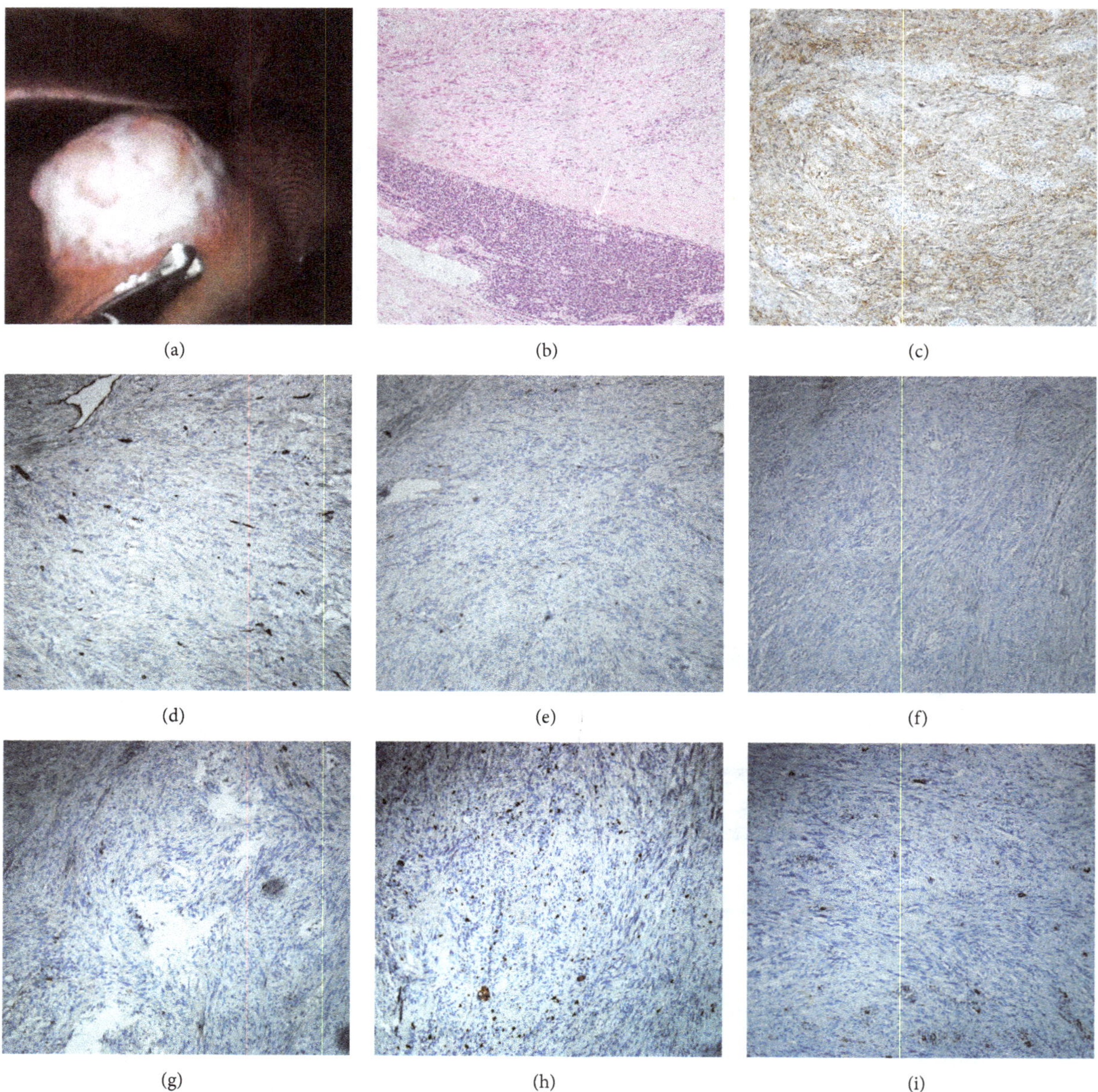

FIGURE 3: Pathological imaging of the mass. (a) An exophytic tumor with size of 4 × 3 cm arising from the anterior wall of the lesser gastric curvature was observed. The exophytic part of the mass appeared off-white in color and rough with a concavo-convex surface; however, the margin of the mass on the gastric wall was clear. (b) Hematoxylin and eosin staining showed that the mass was composed of palisade-arranged spindle cells and peritumoral cuff-like lymphocytic infiltration (white arrow). (c) Immunohistochemical staining of sections showed that the gastric schwannoma was S-100-positive but was negative for (d) CD34, (e) CD117, (f) desmin, (g) DOG1, (h) Ki-67, and (i) SMA. ×100 magnification for all micrographs.

the tumor was composed of spindle cells in a palisading arrangement, and peritumoral cuff-like lymphocytic infiltration was also observed (Figure 3(b)). Immunohistochemical (IHC) staining showed that the spindle cells were positive for S-100 (Figure 3(c)) and negative for CD34, CD117, desmin, DOG1, Ki-67, and smooth muscle actin (SMA) (Figures 3(d)–3(i)), which confirmed a diagnosis of GS. The patient had an uneventful recovery and the 1-year follow-up examination was unremarkable.

3. Discussion

A review of the existing literature identified a total of 221 cases of GS (Table 1). The mean age of the patients was 56.82 ± 13.77 years (range, 10–90 years), and 191 of the 221 patients (86.43%) were aged > 40 years. Thus, it appears that GS predominantly affects adults in the fifth to eighth decades of life. The cases comprised 68 males and 153 females, with an approximate sex ratio of 1 : 2.64. Although the sex ratio in

TABLE 1: Clinical features of GS reported in English literature.

	Benign	Malignant	Overall	P value
Total	211	10	221	
Male/female	63/148	5/5	68/153	0.178
Average age (years)	57.13 ± 13.12	49.78 ± 22.44	56.82 ± 13.77	0.118
Symptoms (cases)				0.695
NA	56	1	57 (34.76%)	
Multiple symptoms	19	3	22 (13.41%)	
Asymptomatic (incidentally found)	69	2	71 (43.29%)	
Abdominal pain or discomfort	32	2	34 (20.73%)	
GI bleeding	19	2	21 (12.80%)	
Palpable mass	5	0	5 (3.05%)	
Poor appetite	5	0	5 (3.05%)	
Dyspepsia	3	0	3 (1.82%)	
Weight loss	2	0	2 (1.22%)	
Nausea or vomiting	1	0	1 (0.6%)	
Location (cases)				0.581
NA	83	3	86 (52.44%)	
Subcardia	2	0	2 (1.22%)	
Fundus	15	0	15 (9.15%)	
Body	82	5	87 (53.05%)	
Antrum	29	2	31 (18.90%)	
Size (diameter, cm)				0.897
Mean size	4.66 ± 2.62	4.66 ± 1.97	4.67 ± 2.60	
Median size	4	4	4	
Follow-up time (months)				0.102
Mean time	78.19 ± 84.85	44.67 ± 38.02	74.67 ± 82.59	
Median time	43	28	38.5	

NA: not available.

certain case series of GS has been reported as ~1 : 4 [1], we hypothesized that the gender predilection may be reduced as more cases are reported. Of the 221 reported cases, detailed clinical information was available for 164 cases. In 71 (43.3%) out of 164 cases, GS was identified incidentally, whereas 22 of the patients (11.6%) initially presented with multiple symptoms [3–21], 34 (20.7%) presented with one symptom, including abdominal pain or discomfort, and 21 cases (12.8%) were reported with gastrointestinal bleeding. These findings indicate that the majority of cases of GS are asymptomatic and that the most common initial symptom is abdominal pain or discomfort, not gastrointestinal bleeding, which differs from the findings of other case series [16]. The other symptoms, which were more rare, included palpable abdominal mass (3.05%), poor appetite (3.05%), dyspepsia (1.82%), weight loss (1.21%), and nausea or vomiting (0.6%). Recently, Yang et al. [21] reported a case of gastroduodenal intussusception due to GS, which, to the best of our knowledge, is the only case reported in English literature. In addition, we found only 1 case in which the patient initially presented with elevated serum carbohydrate antigen 19-9 preoperatively [22].

GS typically grows as a solitary lesion and is commonly located in the body of the stomach. In the current review, we found only 1 case that reported the presence of two GS lesions in the same patient [23]. The most common site of GS among all of the cases was the gastric body (59.3%), followed by the gastric antrum (26.7%) and fundus (12.0%). GS arising from the cardia was rare (2%). Additionally, the tumor size was variable: the greatest diameter size ranged from 0.8 to 15.5 cm, with a mean of 4.69 ± 2.66 cm (median: 4.0 cm).

GSs are usually benign and patients have an excellent prognosis after curative resection. Nevertheless, we identified 10 reported cases of malignant GS in the last several decades [4, 12, 24, 25], which represented 4.5% of all reported GSs. In the cases of malignant GS, 5 patients were male and 5 were females, with a mean age of 49.78 ± 22.44 years (range, 10–73 years). Among these cases, the earliest metastasis and recurrence were detected at 3 months after surgery [12]. These patients commonly presented with clinical symptoms such as abdominal pain and gastrointestinal bleeding. Thus, although this should not be considered definitive criteria by which to classify the tumors as benign or malignant, the presence of such clinical symptoms may provide valuable cues for clinicians.

The features of GS shown by imaging, including CT, magnetic resonance imaging (MRI), and [^{18}F]-fluorodeoxyglucose positron emission tomography (FDG-PET), have been clearly described in several isolated case reports and some case series [26–34]. Briefly, during CT imaging, GS most commonly presented as a well-circumscribed mass with mild enhancement during the arterial phase and strengthened progressive enhancement during the venous and delayed phases. On MRI, GS typically exhibited low signal intensity on T1-weighted images and high signal intensity on T2-weighted images, which could provide further information regarding its relationship with the surrounding structures and the internal features of GS, such as signs of hemorrhage, necrosis, cystic changes, or calcification [29]. FDG-PET was usually used to evaluate the malignant potential of the lesion and to detect the recurrence or metastasis of malignant tumors [32]. Although GS, as a benign lesion, should not be FDG-avid, it was reported in certain studies that GS exhibited a relatively high accumulation of FDG during PET imaging [28, 29, 32, 35, 36] and that FDG accumulation in GS was not significantly different when compared to other submucosal lesions, such as GIST and leiomyoma [37]. Therefore, FDG-PET may be of limited value as preoperative diagnostic technique for the assessment of GS.

Endoscopic ultrasonography (EUS) is considered to be the most reliable procedure for the assessment of patients with gastrointestinal submucosal lesions [38–40], and the EUS features of GS have been systematically summarized in several case series reports [38, 41–44]. In these reports, GS commonly appeared on EUS as a round submucosal lesion arising from the fourth layer, with homogeneous internal echogenicity but without internal echogenic foci. Additionally, the echogenicity of the GS was generally lower than that of the surrounding normal muscle layers [38, 45]. Jung et al. [40] hypothesized that these findings may be helpful for differentiating GS from GIST. However, we were unfortunately unable to do so using EUS in the current described case.

Regarding its gross appearance, GS commonly presents as a yellow-white or off-white, solid, well-circumscribed, and round mural mass. Microscopic examination demonstrates that the typical cytological/morphological features of GS are palisade-arranged spindle cells and peritumoral cuff-like lymphocytic infiltration [46]. On histopathological sections, the spindle cells are predominantly located at the center of the lesion and often appear light red with hematoxylin and eosin staining in the cytoplasm. The nuclei of the spindle cells may exhibit a low degree of atypia and mitotic figures are rarely visible (<15/50 high-power fields); these are considered to be the criteria for classifying the tumor as benign or malignant [16]. On IHC sections, GSs are S-100-positive but are CD34-, CD117-, SMA-, and desmin-negative; detection of these markers is widely considered to be the gold standard for diagnosis of GS [46].

Complete surgical resection is widely considered to be a curative treatment for GS, and laparoscopic or open approaches for wedge resection, subtotal gastrectomy or near-total resection, and total gastrectomy are the treatments of choice [5, 9, 47–51]. As GS rarely metastasizes to the lymph nodes, surgical lymphadenectomy is not routinely performed and is only considered if enlarged lymph nodes are observed. Recently, minimally invasive surgical approaches, including endoscopic submucosal tunneling resection [52, 53], endoscopic enucleation [54], and endoscopic full-thickness resection with [55–57] or without [58–60] laparoscopic assistance, have been actively used as diagnostic tools and therapeutic interventions for GS. Based on short-term follow-up observations, these approaches were not associated with any severe postoperative complications. Nevertheless, to date, no large-sample multicenter studies on the efficacy, safety, and oncological outcomes of these minimally invasive surgical approaches have been published. We therefore suggest that these approaches should not be a first choice and should only be used if the diagnosis of GS is definitively confirmed.

A paper published in 2015 by Hong et al. [17] reviewed 137 cases of GS and did not identify recurrence or metastasis in any patients during a follow-up period ranging from 1 to 336 months. The authors therefore concluded that benign GS does not usually recur and, thus, frequent follow-up with CT imaging is not recommended [17]. For the current review, we retrieved 126 cases that reported detailed follow-up information, ranging from 1 to 420 months, from medical literature published in English. Recurrence and metastasis were only observed in malignant GS and not in benign cases of GS, which was similar to the results reported by Hong et al. [17]. The follow-up times in cases of malignant GS ranged from 5 to 120 months, and only 3 out of 10 patients died due to metastasis or recurrence of GS within 5 years after surgery. The earliest recurrence was detected at 3 months after surgery. In addition, Choi et al. [31] reported that the mean doubling time of GS tumors was nearly 5 years, based on CT images with a series of follow-ups. We therefore suggest that the follow-up should be conducted over a period of at least 5 years for cases of malignant GS. However, further research is necessary in order to better understand the features of malignant GS.

4. Conclusion

Although GS is rare, the case reported in the current study highlights the importance of including GS in differential diagnoses of gastric submucosal tumors. Furthermore, the following points regarding GS should be noted: (i) the magnitude of the gender predilection may be reduced as more cases are reported; (ii) the most common symptom is abdominal pain or discomfort, but not gastrointestinal bleeding; (iii) patients with malignant GS commonly present with some clinical symptoms; (iv) although endoscopic submucosal tunneling resection, endoscopic enucleation, and endoscopic full-thickness resection, with or without laparoscopic assistance, have been actively performed as diagnostic and therapeutic techniques for GS, large-sample multicenter studies on the efficacy, safety, and oncological outcomes are still required.

Abbreviations

GS: Gastric schwannoma
GIST: Gastrointestinal stromal tumor
ESD: Endoscopic submucosal dissection
EGD: Esophagogastroduodenoscopy
CT: Computed tomography
IHC: Immunohistochemistry
MRI: Magnetic resonance imaging

FDG-PET: [^{18}F]-Fluorodeoxyglucose positron emission tomography
EUS: Endoscopic ultrasonography
HPFs: High-power fields
SMA: Smooth muscle actin.

Authors' Contributions

Bao-guang Hu contributed to the concept and manuscript writing. Feng-jie Wu and Jun Zhu contributed to the collection of the clinical data and histological analysis. Yu-ming Li contributed to the critical revision and final approval of the manuscript. Xiao-mei Li, Yan Feng, and He-sheng Li contributed to the collection and analysis of case data and imaging data.

Acknowledgments

The authors thank Professor Nai-guo Liu and his colleagues in clinical laboratory of the Affiliated Hospital of Binzhou Medical University for their kind help in the present study. This work was supported by the Project of Medical and Health Technology Development Program in Shandong Province (Grant no. 2015WS0483) and Scientific Research Starting Foundation of Binzhou Medical University (Grant no. BY2014KYQD37).

References

[1] M. R. Sreevathsa and G. Pipara, "Gastric schwannoma: a case report and review of literature," *Indian Journal of Surgical Oncology*, vol. 6, no. 2, pp. 123–126, 2015.

[2] Y. Daimaru, H. Kido, H. Hashimoto, and M. Enjoji, "Benign schwannoma of the gastrointestinal tract: a clinicopathologic and immunohistochemical study," *Human Pathology*, vol. 19, no. 3, pp. 257–264, 1988.

[3] D. Radulescu, M. Stoian, and M. Sarbu, "Gastric malignant schwannoma," *Revista Medico-Chirurgicala a Societatii de Medici si Naturalisti din Iasi*, vol. 99, pp. 221–225, 1995.

[4] N. R. Bees, C. S. Ng, C. Dicks-Mireaux, and E. M. Kiely, "Gastric malignant schwannoma in a child," *British Journal of Radiology*, vol. 70, pp. 952–955, 1997.

[5] G. Silecchia, A. Materia, A. Fantini et al., "Laparoscopic resection of solitary gastric schwannoma," *Journal of Laparoendoscopic and Advanced Surgical Techniques - Part A*, vol. 7, no. 4, pp. 257–263, 1997.

[6] G. Rymarczyk, M. Hartleb, H. Boldys, M. Kajor, and A. Wodolazski, "Neurogenic tumors of the digestive tract: report of two cases," *Medical Science Monitor*, vol. 6, no. 2, pp. 383–385, 2000.

[7] C. A. Iwamoto, C. F. Garcia, and M. Razzak, "Pathologic quiz case: a 23-year-old woman with a polypoid gastric mass," *Archives of Pathology & Laboratory Medicine*, vol. 127, no. 1, pp. e43–44, 2003.

[8] Y. Fujii, N. Taniguchi, Y. Hosoya et al., "Gastric schwannoma: Sonographic findings," *Journal of Ultrasound in Medicine*, vol. 23, no. 11, pp. 1527–1530, 2004.

[9] A. A. Khan, A. M. P. Schizas, A. B. Cresswell, M. K. Khan, and H. T. Khawaja, "Digestive tract schwannoma," *Digestive Surgery*, vol. 23, no. 4, pp. 265–269, 2006.

[10] Y.-Y. Chen, H.-H. Yen, and M.-S. Soon, "Solitary gastric melanotic schwannoma: sonographic findings," *Journal of Clinical Ultrasound*, vol. 35, no. 1, pp. 52–54, 2007.

[11] A. Agaimy, B. Märkl, J. Kitz et al., "Peripheral nerve sheath tumors of the gastrointestinal tract: a multicenter study of 58 patients including NF1-associated gastric schwannoma and unusual morphologic variants," *Virchows Archiv*, vol. 456, no. 4, pp. 411–422, 2010.

[12] M. Takemura, K. Yoshida, M. Takii, K. Sakurai, and A. Kanazawa, "Gastric malignant schwannoma presenting with upper gastrointestinal bleeding: a case report," *Journal of Medical Case Reports*, vol. 6, article 37, 2012.

[13] L. Voltaggio, R. Murray, J. Lasota, and M. Miettinen, "Gastric schwannoma: a clinicopathologic study of 51 cases and critical review of the literature," *Human Pathology*, vol. 43, no. 5, pp. 650–659, 2012.

[14] W. Yoon, K. Paulson, P. Mazzara, S. Nagori, M. Barawi, and R. Berri, "Gastric schwannoma: a rare but important differential diagnosis of a gastric submucosal mass," *Case Reports in Surgery*, vol. 2012, Article ID 280982, 5 pages, 2012.

[15] J. F. Alvarez and K. Ben-David, "Gastric schwannoma: a rare find," *Journal of Gastrointestinal Surgery*, vol. 17, no. 12, pp. 2179–2181, 2013.

[16] L. Zheng, X. Wu, M. E. Kreis et al., "Clinicopathological and immunohistochemical characterisation of gastric schwannomas in 29 cases," *Gastroenterology Research and Practice*, vol. 2014, Article ID 202960, 7 pages, 2014.

[17] X. Hong, W. Wu, M. Wang, Q. Liao, and Y. Zhao, "Benign gastric schwannoma: how long should we follow up to monitor the recurrence? A case report and comprehensive review of literature of 137 cases," *International Surgery*, vol. 100, no. 4, pp. 744–747, 2015.

[18] M. Manji, A. Ismail, and E. Komba, "Gastric Schwannoma: case report from Tanzania and brief review of literature," *Clinical Case Reports*, vol. 3, no. 7, pp. 562–565, 2015.

[19] D. Özyörük, H. A. Demir, S. Emir, D. Koyuncu, and B. Tunç, "Gastric schwannoma without neurofibromatosis in a 16-year-old adolescent," *Journal of Pediatric Hematology/Oncology*, vol. 37, no. 7, pp. 570–571, 2015.

[20] D. Sousa, M. Allen, A. Pinto et al., "Two synchronous colonic adenocarcinomas, a gastric schwannoma and a mucinous neoplasm of the appendix: a case report," *Journal of Gastrointestinal Cancer*, vol. 46, no. 3, pp. 304–309, 2015.

[21] J.-H. Yang, M. Zhang, Z.-H. Zhao, Y. Shu, J. Hong, and Y.-J. Cao, "Gastroduodenal intussusception due to gastric schwannoma treated by billroth II distal gastrectomy: one case report," *World Journal of Gastroenterology*, vol. 21, no. 7, pp. 2225–2228, 2015.

[22] M. Fukuchi, H. Naitoh, H. Shoji et al., "Schwannoma of the stomach with elevated preoperative serum carbohydrate antigen 19-9: report of a case," *Surgery Today*, vol. 42, no. 8, pp. 788–792, 2012.

[23] G. Tozbikian, Rulong Shen and S. Suster, "Signet ring cell gastric schwannoma: report of a new distinctive morphological variant," *Annals of Diagnostic Pathology*, vol. 12, no. 2, pp. 146–152, 2008.

[24] R. J. L. F. Loffeld, T. G. Balk, J. L. T. Oomen, and A. B. M. M. Van Der Putten, "Upper gastrointestinal bleeding due to a malignant Schwannoma of the stomach," *European Journal of Gastroenterology and Hepatology*, vol. 10, no. 2, pp. 159–162, 1998.

[25] A. Watanabe, H. Ojima, S. Suzuki et al., "An individual with gastric schwannoma with pathologically malignant potential surviving two years after laparoscopy-assisted partial gastrectomy," *Case Reports in Gastroenterology*, vol. 5, no. 2, pp. 502–507, 2011.

[26] H. S. Hong, H. K. Ha, H. J. Won et al., "Gastric schwannomas: radiological features with endoscopic and pathological correlation," *Clinical Radiology*, vol. 63, no. 5, pp. 536–542, 2008.

[27] N. Karabulut, D. R. Martin, and M. Yang, "Gastric schwannoma: MRI findings," *British Journal of Radiology*, vol. 75, no. 895, pp. 624–626, 2002.

[28] I. K. Hong and D. Y. Kim, "F-18 FDG PET/CT of a gastric schwannoma," *Nuclear Medicine and Molecular Imaging*, vol. 45, no. 3, pp. 238–240, 2011.

[29] M. Takeda, Y. Amano, T. Machida, S. Kato, Z. Naito, and S. Kumita, "CT, MRI, and PET findings of gastric schwannoma," *Japanese Journal of Radiology*, vol. 30, no. 7, pp. 602–605, 2012.

[30] S. Fujiwara, K. Nakajima, T. Nishida et al., "Gastric schwannomas revisited: has precise preoperative diagnosis become feasible?" *Gastric Cancer*, vol. 16, no. 3, pp. 318–323, 2013.

[31] J. W. Choi, D. Choi, K.-M. Kim et al., "Small submucosal tumors of the stomach: differentiation of gastric schwannoma from gastrointestinal stromal tumor with CT," *Korean Journal of Radiology*, vol. 13, no. 4, pp. 425–433, 2012.

[32] J. Yap, Y.-T. T. O. Huang, and M. Lin, "Detection of synchronous gastric schwannoma on FDG PET/CT aided by discordant metabolic response," *Clinical nuclear medicine*, vol. 40, no. 5, pp. e287–e289, 2015.

[33] J.-S. Ji, C.-Y. Lu, W.-B. Mao, Z.-F. Wang, and M. Xu, "Gastric schwannoma: CT findings and clinicopathologic correlation," *Abdominal Imaging*, vol. 40, no. 5, pp. 1164–1169, 2015.

[34] Y. R. Choi, S. H. Kim, S.-A. Kim et al., "Differentiation of large (≥5 cm) gastrointestinal stromal tumors from benign subepithelial tumors in the stomach: radiologists' performance using CT," *European Journal of Radiology*, vol. 83, no. 2, pp. 250–260, 2014.

[35] Y. Shimada, S. Sawada, S. Hojo et al., "Glucose transporter 3 and 1 may facilitate high uptake of 18F-FDG in gastric schwannoma," *Clinical Nuclear Medicine*, vol. 38, no. 11, pp. e417–e420, 2013.

[36] D. Komatsu, N. Koide, R. I. Hiraga et al., "Gastric schwannoma exhibiting increased fluorodeoxyglucose uptake," *Gastric Cancer*, vol. 12, no. 4, pp. 225–228, 2009.

[37] Y. Zhang, B. Li, L. Cai, X. Hou, H. Shi, and J. Hou, "Gastric Schwannoma mimicking malignant gastrointestinal stromal tumor and misdiagnosed by 18F-FDG PET/CT," *Hellenic Journal of Nuclear Medicine*, vol. 18, no. 1, pp. 74–76, 2015.

[38] H. Park, D. Son, H. Oh et al., "Endoscopic ultrasonographic characteristics of gastric schwannoma distinguished from gastrointestinal stromal tumor," *Korean Journal of Gastroenterology*, vol. 65, no. 1, p. 21, 2015.

[39] B. Li, T. Liang, L. Wei et al., "Endoscopic interventional treatment for gastric schwannoma: a single-center experience," *International Journal of Clinical and Experimental Pathology*, vol. 7, no. 10, pp. 6616–6625, 2014.

[40] M. K. Jung, S. W. Jeon, C. M. Cho et al., "Gastric schwannomas: endosonographic characteristics," *Abdominal Imaging*, vol. 33, no. 4, pp. 388–390, 2008.

[41] Y. Miyamoto, F. Tsujimoto, and S. Tada, "Ultrasonographic diagnosis of submucosal tumors of the stomach: the 'bridging layers' sign," *Journal of Clinical Ultrasound*, vol. 16, no. 4, pp. 251–258, 1988.

[42] G. H. Kim, K. B. Kim, S. H. Lee et al., "Digital image analysis of endoscopic ultrasonography is helpful in diagnosing gastric mesenchymal tumors," *BMC Gastroenterology*, vol. 14, no. 1, article 7, 2014.

[43] D.-D. Zhong, C.-H. Wang, J.-H. Xu, M.-Y. Chen, and J.-T. Cai, "Endoscopic ultrasound features of gastric schwannomas with radiological correlation: a case series report," *World Journal of Gastroenterology*, vol. 18, no. 48, pp. 7397–7401, 2012.

[44] J. Barbosa, J. Maciel, and M. Amarante Jr., "Endoscopic ultrasonography in the study of extramucosal swellings in the upper digestive tract," *Surgical Endoscopy*, vol. 9, no. 11, pp. 1193–1196, 1995.

[45] T. Okai, T. Minamoto, K. Ohtsubo et al., "Endosonographic evaluation of c-kit-positive gastrointestinal stromal tumor," *Abdominal Imaging*, vol. 28, no. 3, pp. 301–307, 2003.

[46] E. Rodriguez, S. Tellschow, D. M. Steinberg, and E. Montgomery, "Cytologic findings of gastric schwannoma: a case report," *Diagnostic Cytopathology*, vol. 42, no. 2, pp. 177–180, 2014.

[47] Y. Otani, M. Ohgami, N. Igarashi et al., "Laparoscopic wedge resection of gastric submucosal tumors," *Surgical Laparoscopy, Endoscopy & Percutaneous Techniques*, vol. 10, pp. 19–23, 2000.

[48] C. J. Li, M. T. Huang, C. S. Chen, K. W. Tam, C. Y. Chai, and C. H. Wu, "Application of laparoscopic techniques for resection of individual gastric submucosal tumors," *Surgical Laparoscopy, Endoscopy & Percutaneous Techniques*, vol. 17, pp. 425–429, 2007.

[49] H. Y. Yoon, C. B. Kim, Y. H. Lee, and H. G. Kim, "Gastric Schwannoma," *Yonsei Medical Journal*, vol. 49, no. 6, pp. 1052–1054, 2008.

[50] Y. Miyazaki, K. Nakajima, Y. Kurokawa et al., "Clinical significance of surgery for gastric submucosal tumours with size enlargement during watchful waiting period," *European Journal of Cancer*, vol. 49, no. 12, pp. 2681–2688, 2013.

[51] A. Takata, K. Nakajima, Y. Kurokawa et al., "Single-incision laparoscopic partial gastrectomy for gastric submucosal tumors without compromising transumbilical stapling," *Asian Journal of Endoscopic Surgery*, vol. 7, no. 1, pp. 25–30, 2014.

[52] J. Lu, T. Jiao, Y. Li et al., "Heading toward the right direction—Solution package for endoscopic submucosal tunneling resection in the stomach," *PLoS ONE*, vol. 10, no. 3, Article ID e0119870, 2015.

[53] B.-R. Liu, J.-T. Song, L.-J. Kong, F.-H. Pei, X.-H. Wang, and Y.-J. Du, "Tunneling endoscopic muscularis dissection for subepithelial tumors originating from the muscularis propria of the esophagus and gastric cardia," *Surgical Endoscopy and Other Interventional Techniques*, vol. 27, no. 11, pp. 4354–4359, 2013.

[54] C. Sun, Z. He, Z. Zheng et al., "Endoscopic submucosal dissection for gastrointestinal mesenchymal tumors adjacent to the esophagogastric junction: we need to do more," *Journal of Laparoendoscopic and Advanced Surgical Techniques*, vol. 23, no. 7, pp. 570–577, 2013.

[55] N. Abe, H. Takeuchi, O. Yanagida et al., "Endoscopic full-thickness resection with laparoscopic assistance as hybrid NOTES for gastric submucosal tumor," *Surgical Endoscopy*, vol. 23, no. 8, pp. 1908–1913, 2009.

[56] L.-Y. Huang, J. Cui, C.-R. Wu et al., "Endoscopic full-thickness resection and laparoscopic surgery for treatment of gastric

stromal tumors," *World Journal of Gastroenterology*, vol. 20, no. 25, pp. 8253–8259, 2014.

[57] J. S. Barajas-Gamboa, G. Acosta, T. J. Savides et al., "Laparo-endoscopic transgastric resection of gastric submucosal tumors," *Surgical Endoscopy and Other Interventional Techniques*, vol. 29, no. 8, pp. 2149–2157, 2015.

[58] P. H. Zhou, L. Q. Yao, X. Y. Qin et al., "Endoscopic full-thickness resection without laparoscopic assistance for gastric submucosal tumors originated from the muscularis propria," *Surgical Endoscopy and Other Interventional Techniques*, vol. 25, no. 9, pp. 2926–2931, 2011.

[59] C. K. Lee, S.-H. Lee, I.-K. Chung et al., "Endoscopic full-thickness resection of a gastric subepithelial tumor by using the submucosal tunnel technique with the patient under conscious sedation (with video)," *Gastrointestinal Endoscopy*, vol. 75, no. 2, pp. 457–459, 2012.

[60] Y. Feng, L. Yu, S. Yang et al., "Endolumenal endoscopic full-thickness resection of muscularis propria-originating gastric submucosal tumors," *Journal of Laparoendoscopic and Advanced Surgical Techniques*, vol. 24, no. 3, pp. 171–176, 2014.

Asymptomatic Pancreatic Metastasis from Renal Cell Carcinoma Diagnosed 21 Years after Nephrectomy

Megumi Zianne,[1] Naoki Takahashi,[2] Akihiko Tsujibata,[3] Kazuhiro Miwa,[1] Yoshinori Goto,[1] and Yutaka Matano[1]

[1]*Department of Gastroenterology, Komatsu Municipal Hospital, Ishikawa, Japan*
[2]*Department of Gastroenterology, Saitama Cancer Center, Saitama, Japan*
[3]*Department of Pathology, Komatsu Municipal Hospital, Ishikawa, Japan*

Correspondence should be addressed to Naoki Takahashi; naoki19800623@gmail.com

Academic Editor: Hideto Kawaratani

This report presents our experience with a case of pancreatic metastasis of renal cell carcinoma (RCC) at a long-term follow-up after nephrectomy. A 73-year-old man underwent nephrectomy for right RCC 21 years ago; computed tomography (CT) scanning on routine follow-up revealed a solid mass in the tail of the pancreas, and magnetic resonance imaging (MRI) showed some tumors in the head and tail of the pancreas. The patient was asymptomatic and allergic to contrast medium. Therefore we could not perform contrast CT/MRI for further examination to diagnose pancreatic tumors. We undertook endoscopic ultrasonography (EUS) and detected a hypervascular and low echoic mass; tumor tissues were obtained by EUS-guided fine-needle aspiration (EUS-FNA). Pathological diagnosis revealed pancreatic metastasis of clear cell RCC; this was similar to the pathological findings of tumor tissues initially obtained by nephrectomy. EUS-FNA was extremely useful for the definitive diagnosis of a rare type of pancreatic tumor.

1. Introduction

Renal cell carcinoma (RCC) is commonly observed in the field of urology. The incidence of newly developed RCC is estimated at 338,000 per year, and estimated cancer deaths due to RCC are 144,000 per year [1]. In Asia, the incidence of RCC is less frequent compared with that in North Europe and South America. Clear cell RCC is one of the most common histological subtypes of RCC that is characterized by malignant epithelial cells with a clear cytoplasm and a nested or acinar growth pattern [2]. Clear cell RCC initially arises from epithelial cells of proximal convoluted tubules of nephrons and invades the renal sinus before extending into the renal vain. Therefore, vascular invasion is more frequently observed in clear cell RCC compared with other histological types of RCC.

In RCC, pancreatic metastasis is less frequent as compared with metastasis to other organs such as lung, bone, and liver [3]. Enhanced computed tomography (CT) and magnetic resonance imaging (MRI) scan are valuable to discriminate between a metastatic tumor arising from RCC and a primary tumor of the pancreas [4–6]. Endoscopic ultrasound-guided fine-needle aspiration (EUS-FNA) is another significant method to confirm pathological diagnosis of pancreatic tumors before surgical treatment. In this study, we report a case with pancreatic metastasis of RCC at a long-term follow-up after nephrectomy.

2. Case Report

A 73-year-old man had undergone a right nephrectomy with a retroperitoneal approach for RCC in our hospital 21 years earlier, with a pathological diagnosis of clear cell RCC (intermediate type, INF β, G2 > G1, pT3aN0M0, pStage III; UICC 7th edition). Curative resection was confirmed pathologically, and no adjuvant chemotherapy was administered postoperatively. During a routine follow-up assessment by the urology department, a CT scan revealed a slightly low-density mass (27 mm in diameter) in the tail of the pancreas, with no tumor lesions in other organs (Figure 1). Therefore, the patient was referred to the Department of Medical Gastroenterology for intensive evaluation of the

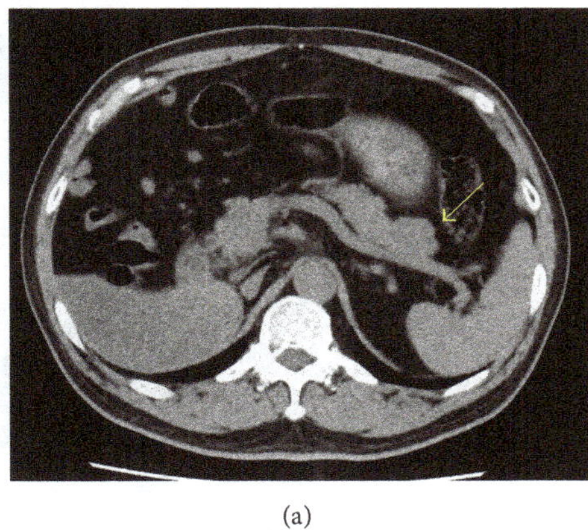

(a)

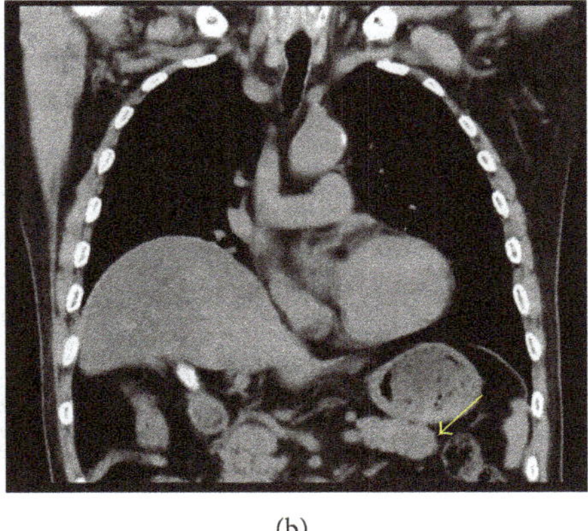

(b)

Figure 1: Abdominal computed tomography imaging demonstrating a 27 mm mass in the tail of the pancreas (yellow arrow).

pancreatic tumor. At the first visit to our department, the patient was asymptomatic, without abdominal pain or weight loss. In addition, there were no abdominal physical findings except for an operative scar in the right lateral region of the abdomen. Laboratory blood test at the first visit showed that blood urea nitrogen (BUN), creatinine, and amylase in serum were mildly elevated, whereas tumor markers such as carcinoembryonic antigen (CEA), carbohydrate antigen 19-9 (CA19-9), and neuron-specific enolase (NSE) in blood were within the normal range. Contrast-enhanced CT/MRI could not be performed because the patient was allergic to the contrast medium. Noncontrast MRI revealed two lesions: central signals were of slightly higher intensity on T1-weighted imaging but showed isointensity on T2-weighted imaging. The marginal capsule of tumors is shown as low-intensity structures on T1- and T2-weighted imaging. The size of the mass in the head and tail of the pancreas was 12 and 24 mm in diameter, respectively. Diffusion-weighted imaging revealed this mass as having high intensity, and magnetic resonance cholangiopancreatography showed no stenosis or irregularity in the pancreatic duct. These MRI imaging scans are summarized in Figure 2. Convex EUS could detect two lesions, which were a hypoechoic and homogenous mass in the head (12 mm diameter) and tail (22 mm diameter) of the pancreas. Color Doppler EUS revealed that these masses had homogeneous hypervascularity. Findings of EUS are shown in Figure 3.

In this case, tumor of pancreas head was not clearly detected by CT scan. EUS is most detected pancreas lesion and EUS-FNA is considered as most safety method as biopsy. We performed EUS-FNA using an EZ shot 22G (Olympus, Tokyo, Japan) to confirm the pathological diagnosis of these masses. Biopsies were performed for each mass, and tumor tissues were gathered from a biopsy specimen of the tail of the pancreas. Tissue smear slides are shown in Figure 4; tumor tissue comprised a cluster of atypical cells with a clear cytoplasm on hematoxylin and eosin (HE) staining, and clear cell RCC was strongly suspected. Immunohistochemical staining was additionally performed to confirm a definitive diagnosis. Immunohistochemistry (IHC) was positive for CD10 and NSE and negative for cytokeratin 7, synaptophysin, and MUC6 (Figure 4). Finally, the pancreatic tumors were pathologically diagnosed as pancreatic metastasis from clear cell RCC.

Curative resection for pancreas lesions was considered as most suitable treatment. On the other hand, surgical resection was very invasive and elderly patients have more risk of any complications after surgery compared with younger patients. In addition, he had taken drugs for the diabetes mellitus and mild nephropathy. After surgery, control of blood sugar level is considered to be worse. We recommended two choices: (1) surgical resection of pancreatic lesions on the basis of previous reports and (2) molecular targeted therapy as a treatment for a metastatic stage of RCC. The patient selected surgical treatment. The findings of the pathological diagnosis of surgical specimens closely resembled those of the diagnosis of clear cell RCC using EUS-FNA. PAX-8 and vimentin were positive in tumor tissues obtained through surgical resection (Figure 4).

3. Discussions

We reported a case of metastatic tumors of the pancreas arising from RCC at a long-term follow-up after curative nephrectomy. Previous case reports of pancreatic metastasis of RCC diagnosed using EUS-FNA after curative nephrectomy exist [7–16]. Owing to the recent development of EUS-FNA, we could obtain a pathological diagnosis by less invasive procedures, without surgical resection, and take an appropriately planned treatment decision. As described in our case report, EUS-FNA may be especially effective for diagnosis of a pancreatic tumor posing difficulties for diagnostic imaging because of a contrast-medium allergy.

Recurrence rates after nephrectomy for RCC are 20%–40% and median time to recurrence is 15–18 months, according to previous reports [17]. Conversely, late recurrences more than 10 years after surgery are more frequently observed in RCCs compared with other malignant tumors. According to a previous meta-analysis that evaluated pancreatic resection for malignant tumors, survival time and recurrence-free interval

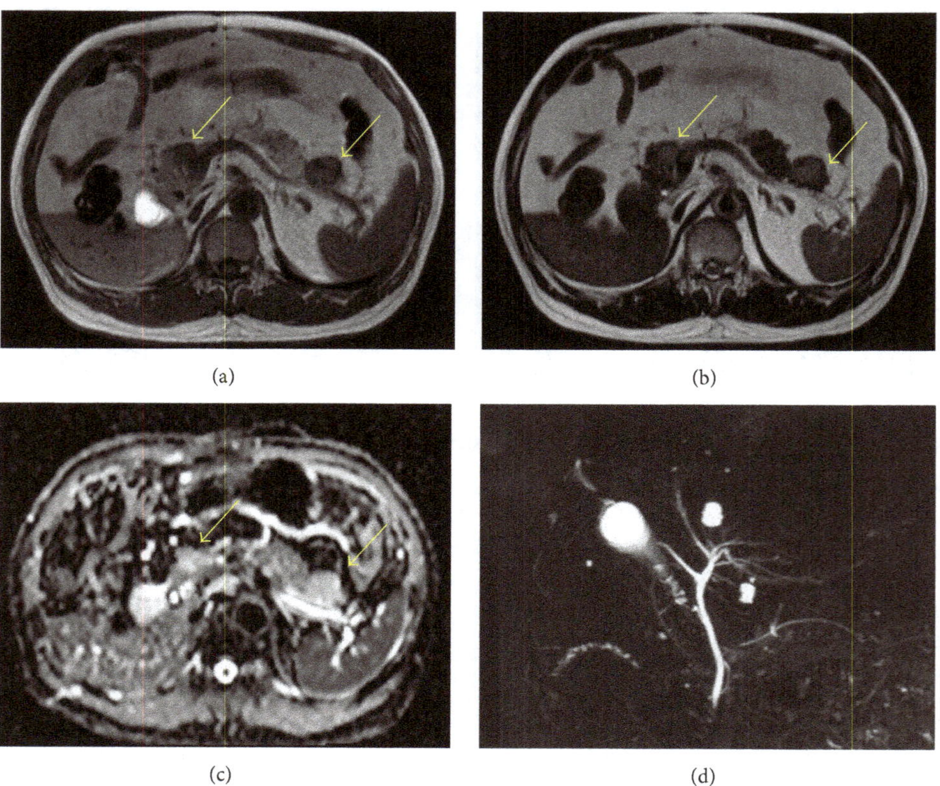

FIGURE 2: *Magnetic resonance imaging sections of pancreas tumors.* Pancreatic tumors were shown as slightly high-intensity regions on T1-weighted imaging and as isointense regions on T2-weighted imaging (yellow arrow: (a), (b)). Diffusion-weighted imaging (DWI) revealed these masses as high-intensity regions (yellow arrow, (c)), and magnetic resonance cholangiopancreatography (MRCP) showed no stenosis and irregularity in the biliary duct and pancreatic duct (d).

after pancreatic resection in RCC were significantly longer than that in other types of tumors [18]. Previous reports indicated that pathological features of most cases with pancreatic metastasis of RCC were a low-grade tumor, and patients with a high-grade tumor were associated with a short survival time [5]. This finding supports the mechanism of late recurrence after nephrectomy for RCC, and the nuclear grade of tumor cells in the present case was also low. Main symptoms at the time of initial recurrence were reported as pain, jaundice, and bleeding in a previous report. Conversely, pancreatic metastasis of RCC is detected without any symptoms in up to 50% of cases [19]. In the present case, there were no symptoms and the pancreatic tumor was incidentally detected by a CT scan 21 years after nephrectomy. Generally, the follow-up period after curative resection for advanced solid tumors is 5 years; however, longer follow-up may be required for patients with high risk of RCC recurrence. Unfortunately, adjuvant treatment after nephrectomy for RCC is controversial, as indicated by a recent phase 3 randomized trial [20, 21]. Therefore, evidences for an appropriate follow-up period after nephrectomy for RCC have not been established by prospective studies.

Metastatic and primary pancreatic tumors need to be differentiated when a pancreatic tumor mass is detected. Pancreatic ductal carcinoma is most frequently observed in solid pancreatic tumors and is usually detected as a hypovascular tumor on a contrast CT scan. On the other hand, the solid pseudopapillary neoplasm, serous cystic neoplasm (solid type), acinar cell carcinoma, endocrine tumor, and metastatic tumor of the pancreas are detected as hypovascular tumors. Frequencies of these hypervascular tumors are rare, and pathological diagnosis is required because treatment strategies differ based on tumor histology. EUS-FNA is effective in providing an accurate diagnosis identifying surgical candidates and avoiding potentially unnecessary surgery.

As treatment for patients with recurrent RCC, surgical resection or molecular targeted therapy is often reported. In an evaluation of the clinical benefit of surgery for pancreatic metastasis from RCC, Tanis et al. gathered individual data of pancreatic metastasis of RCC from a published series and compared survival time between the surgical and nonsurgical groups [22]. The 5-year survival rate was 72.6% in 311 resection patients and 14% in 73 nonresection patients. In addition, extrapancreatic disease is an independent risk factor for recurrence after pancreatic resection. Zerbi et al., moreover, reported that the 5-year survival rate was 88% in 23 resection patients and 47% in 13 nonresection patients in RCC with pancreatic metastasis [23]. All patients who could undergo surgical resection comprised a favorable risk group of MSKCC. Owing to the development of molecular targeted

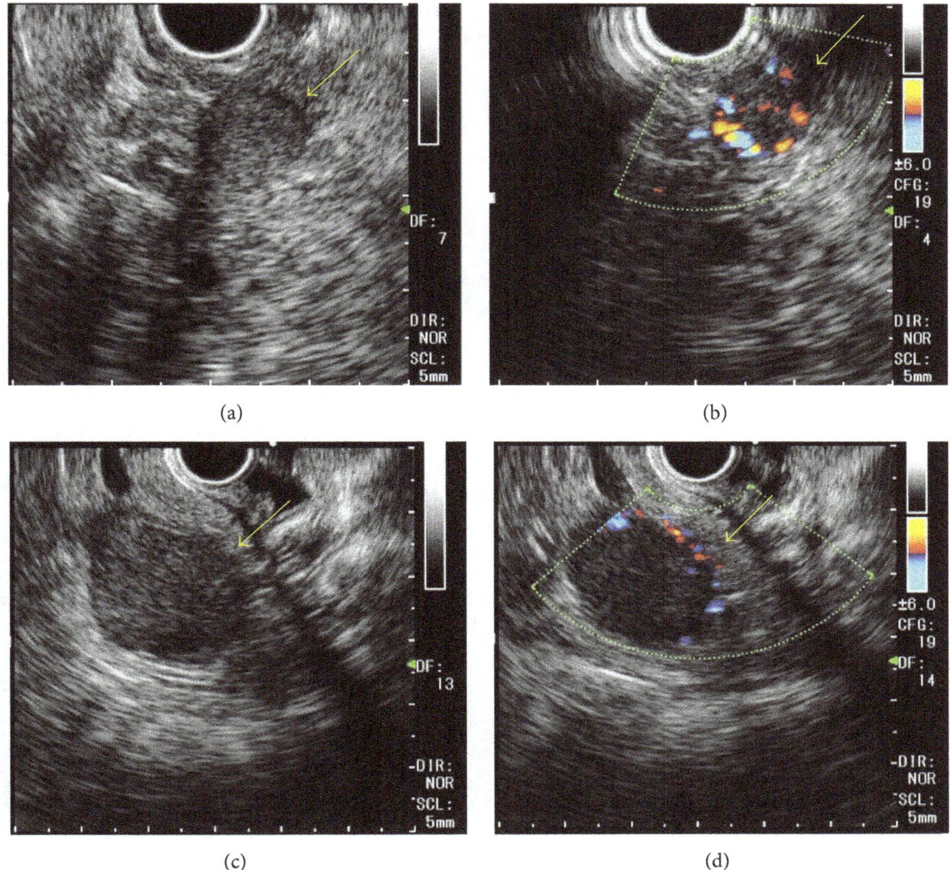

FIGURE 3: *Endoscopic ultrasonography (EUS) imaging sections of pancreas tumors.* Pancreatic tumors are shown by Convex EUS. A tumor in the head of the pancreas is shown as yellow arrows in (a) and (b) and that in the tail of the pancreas is shown as yellow arrows in (c) and (d). Both tumors had similar findings and hypervascularity in tumor was demonstrated by Doppler mode of EUS.

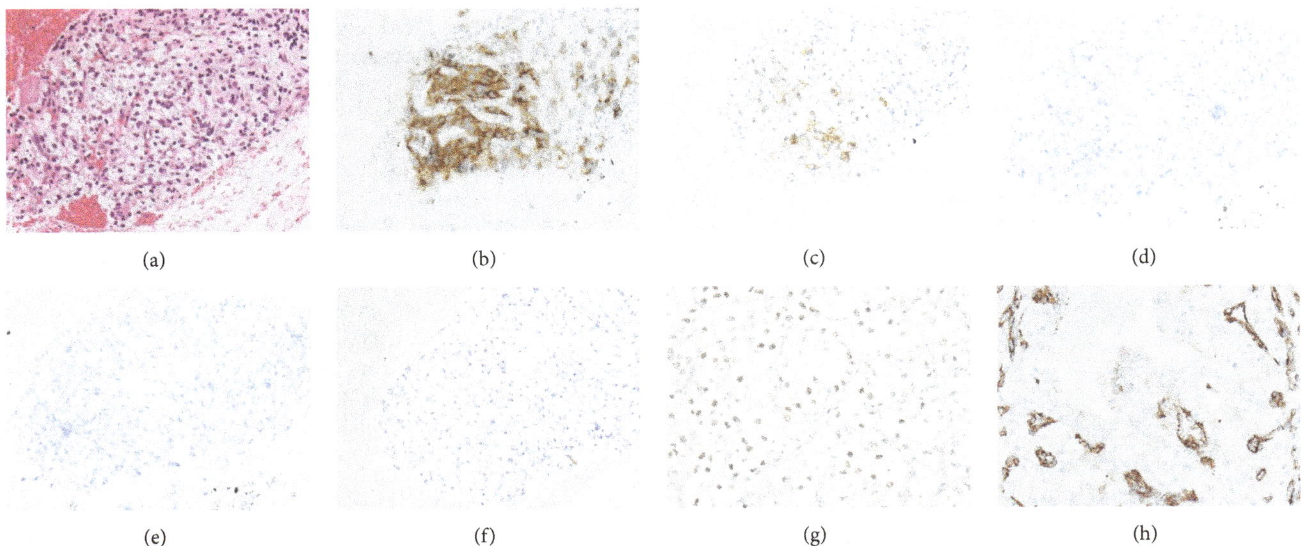

FIGURE 4: *Pathological findings of pancreatic tumor obtained by EUS-FNA and surgical resection.* Tumor tissues were obtained from a tumor of the tail of the pancreas. Tumor tissue comprised a cluster of mild atypical cells with clear cytoplasm on hematoxylin and eosin staining (a). IHC stain of tumor tissue obtained by EUS-FNA showed that CD10 (b) and NSE (c) were positive and synaptophysin (d), MUC6 (e), and cytokeratin 7 (f) were negative. PAX-8 (g) and vintentin (h) were positive in tumor tissue obtained by surgical resection.

therapy, survival time of the nonsurgical group may have recently improved compared with that previously reported.

Molecular targeted drugs markedly improved survival times of RCC patients in the recent decade [24–28]. Furthermore, recent development of immune checkpoint inhibitors provides a new treatment strategy in malignant solid tumors. Among patients previously treated for advanced RCC, nivolumab, a programmed death-1 inhibitor, significantly improved the response rate and overall survival compared with everolimus in a randomized phase 3 trial [29]. If patients with physical complications are considered to be intolerant of surgical treatment, these molecular drugs and immune checkpoint inhibitors may be the first choice of treatment. Because the frequency of severe adverse events of immune checkpoint is well known to be quite lower than that of molecular target inhibitors, even elderly patients can be treated safely by a PD-1 inhibitor.

Immunohistochemical evaluation for the metastatic tumor was effective for the diagnosis of primary tumor. PAX-8 is commonly expressed in epithelial tumors of the thyroid and parathyroid glands, kidney, thymus, and female genital tract [30]. In our study, CT scan showed no tumors in the thyroid gland, parathyroid glands, and thymus. PAX-8 expression strongly indicated the possibility of pancreatic metastasis from RCC. In addition, a previous report indicated that CD10 positivity is useful for pathological diagnosis of clear cell or papillary RCC, and we could eliminate the chromophobe RCC [31]. Pathological finding of clear cell RCC by HE staining is a characteristic feature, and the addition of immunohistochemical evaluation such as PAX-2 or PAX-8, CD10, cytokeratin, vimentin, and epithelial membrane antigen contributes to the definitive diagnosis of a primary lesion in pancreatic metastasis [32].

In conclusion, we report our clinical experience with a case of pancreatic tumor diagnosed by EUS-FNA. Despite a long interval after nephrectomy for RCC, it is necessary to assess the recurrence of RCC. Evidence for an appropriate follow-up period after nephrectomy is not established, and prospective studies evaluating this aspect are required in future. In patients allergic to contrast medium, the vascularity of pancreatic tumors cannot be evaluated by only CT/MRI scan. In such cases, EUS could evaluate the vascularity of tumors and simultaneously obtain tumor tissue samples by EUS-FNA, which is useful for the pathological diagnosis and treatment planning in rare types of pancreatic tumors.

References

[1] R. L. Siegel, K. D. Miller, and A. Jemal, "Cancer statistics, 2015," *CA: Cancer Journal for Clinicians*, vol. 65, no. 1, pp. 5–29, 2015.

[2] D. J. Grignon and M. Che, "Clear cell renal cell carcinoma," *Clinics in Laboratory Medicine*, vol. 25, no. 2, pp. 305–316, 2005.

[3] M. Bianchi, M. Sun, C. Jeldres et al., "Distribution of metastatic sites in renal cell carcinoma: a population-based analysis," *Annals of Oncology*, vol. 23, no. 4, pp. 973–980, 2012.

[4] K. A. Klein, D. H. Stephens, and T. J. Welch, "CT characteristics of metastatic disease of the pancreas," *Radiographics*, vol. 18, no. 2, pp. 369–378, 1998.

[5] R. Ghavamian, K. A. Klein, D. H. Stephens et al., "Renal cell carcinoma metastatic to the pancreas: Clinical and radiological features," *Mayo Clinic Proceedings*, vol. 75, no. 6, pp. 581–585, 2000.

[6] M. Palmowski, N. Hacke, S. Satzl et al., "Metastasis to the pancreas: Characterization by morphology and contrast enhancement features on CT and MRI," *Pancreatology*, vol. 8, no. 2, pp. 199–203, 2008.

[7] M. A. Eloubeidi, D. Jhala, D. C. Chhieng, N. Jhala, I. Eltoum, and C. M. Wilcox, "Multiple late asymptomatic pancreatic metastases from renal cell carcinoma: diagnosis by endoscopic ultrasound-guided fine needle aspiration biopsy with immunocytochemical correlation," *Digestive Diseases and Sciences*, vol. 47, no. 8, pp. 1839–1842, 2002.

[8] D. Béchade, L. Palazzo, M. Fabre, and J.-P. Algayres, "EUS-guided FNA of pancreatic metastasis from renal cell carcinoma," *Gastrointestinal Endoscopy*, vol. 58, no. 5, pp. 784–788, 2003.

[9] H. Kawakami, M. Kuwatani, H. Yamato et al., "Pancreatic metastasis from renal cell carcinoma with intraportal tumor thrombus," *Internal Medicine*, vol. 47, no. 22, pp. 1967–1970, 2008.

[10] I. I. El Hajj, J. K. Leblanc, S. Sherman et al., "Endoscopic ultrasound-guided biopsy of pancreatic metastases: a large single-center experience," *Pancreas*, vol. 42, no. 3, pp. 524–530, 2013.

[11] S. M. Gilani, R. Tashjian, R. Danforth, and L. Fathallah, "Metastatic renal cell carcinoma to the pancreas: diagnostic significance of fine-needle aspiration cytology," *Acta Cytologica*, vol. 57, no. 4, pp. 418–422, 2013.

[12] L. Waters, Q. Si, N. Caraway, D. Mody, G. Staerkel, and N. Sneige, "Secondary tumors of the pancreas diagnosed by endoscopic ultrasound-guided fine-needle aspiration: a 10-year experience," *Diagnostic Cytopathology*, vol. 42, no. 9, pp. 738–743, 2014.

[13] H. H. Okasha, E. H. Al-Gemeie, and R. E. Mahdy, "Solitary pancreatic metastasis from renal cell carcinoma 6 years after nephrectomy," *Endoscopic Ultrasound*, vol. 2, no. 4, pp. 222–224, 2013.

[14] A. L. Smith, S. I. Odronic, B. S. Springer, and J. P. Reynolds, "Solid tumor metastases to the pancreas diagnosed by FNA: a single-institution experience and review of the literature," *Cancer Cytopathology*, vol. 123, no. 6, pp. 347–355, 2015.

[15] A. Alomari, B. Ustun, H. Aslanian, X. Ge, D. Chhieng, and G. Cai, "Endoscopic ultrasound-guided fine-needle aspiration diagnosis of secondary tumors involving the pancreas: An institution's experience," *CytoJournal*, vol. 13, no. 1, article A1, 2016.

[16] R. Pannala, K. M. Hallberg-Wallace, and A. L. Smith, "Endoscopic ultrasound-guided fine needle aspiration cytology of metastatic renal cell carcinoma to the pancreas: a multi-center experience," *CytoJournal*, vol. 13, no. 1, pp. 13–24, 2016.

[17] N. K. Janzen, H. L. Kim, R. A. Figlin, and A. S. Belldegrun, "Surveillance after radical or partial nephrectomy for localized renal cell carcinoma and management of recurrent disease," *The Urologic Clinics of North America*, vol. 30, no. 4, pp. 843–852, 2003.

[18] C. Sperti, G. Pozza, A. R. Brazzale et al., "Metastatic tumors to the pancreas: A systematic review and meta-analysis," *Minerva Chirurgica*, vol. 71, no. 5, pp. 337–344, 2016.

[19] J.-P. Faure, J.-J. Tuech, J.-P. Richer, P. Pessaux, J.-P. Arnaud, and M. Carretier, "Pancreatic metastasis of renal cell carcinoma: Presentation, treatment and survival," *Journal of Urology*, vol. 165, no. 1, pp. 20–22, 2001.

[20] A. Ravaud, R. J. Motzer, H. S. Pandha et al., "Adjuvant sunitinib in high-risk renal-cell carcinoma after nephrectomy," *New England Journal of Medicine*, vol. 375, no. 23, pp. 2246–2254, 2016.

[21] N. B. Haas, J. Manola, R. G. Uzzo et al., "Adjuvant sunitinib or sorafenib for high-risk, non-metastatic renal-cell carcinoma (ECOG-ACRIN E2805): A double-blind, placebo-controlled, randomised, phase 3 trial," *The Lancet*, vol. 387, no. 10032, pp. 2008–2016, 2016.

[22] P. J. Tanis, N. A. van der Gaag, O. R. C. Busch, T. M. van Gulik, and D. J. Gouma, "Systematic review of pancreatic surgery for metastatic renal cell carcinoma," *British Journal of Surgery*, vol. 96, no. 6, pp. 579–592, 2009.

[23] A. Zerbi, E. Ortolano, G. Balzano, A. Borri, A. A. Beneduce, and V. Di Carlo, "Pancreatic metastasis from renal cell carcinoma: Which patients benefit from surgical resection?" *Annals of Surgical Oncology*, vol. 15, no. 4, pp. 1161–1168, 2008.

[24] R. J. Motzer, T. E. Hutson, P. Tomczak et al., "Sunitinib versus interferon alfa in metastatic renal-cell carcinoma," *The New England Journal of Medicine*, vol. 356, no. 2, pp. 115–124, 2007.

[25] B. Escudier, T. Eisen, W. M. Stadler et al., "Sorafenib in advanced clear-cell renal-cell carcinoma," *The New England Journal of Medicine*, vol. 356, no. 2, pp. 125–134, 2007.

[26] R. J. Motzer, B. Escudier, S. Oudard et al., "Efficacy of everolimus in advanced renal cell carcinoma: a double-blind, randomised, placebo-controlled phase III trial," *The Lancet*, vol. 372, no. 9637, pp. 449–456, 2008.

[27] B. I. Rini, B. Escudier, P. Tomczak et al., "Comparative effectiveness of axitinib versus sorafenib in advanced renal cell carcinoma (AXIS): a randomised phase 3 trial," *The Lancet*, vol. 378, no. 9807, pp. 1931–1939, 2011.

[28] R. J. Motzer, T. E. Hutson, D. Cella et al., "Pazopanib versus sunitinib in metastatic renal-cell carcinoma," *The New England Journal of Medicine*, vol. 369, no. 8, pp. 722–731, 2013.

[29] R. J. Motzer, B. Escudier, and D. F. McDermott, "Nivolumab versus everolimus in advanced renal-cell carcinoma," *New England Journal of Medicine*, vol. 373, no. 19, pp. 1803–1813, 2015.

[30] N. G. Ordóñez, "Value of PAX8 immunostaining in tumor diagnosis: a review and update," *Advances in Anatomic Pathology*, vol. 19, no. 3, pp. 140–151, 2012.

[31] A. K. Avery, J. Beckstead, A. A. Renshaw, and C. L. Corless, "Use of antibodies to RCC and CD10 in the differential diagnosis of renal neoplasms," *The American Journal of Surgical Pathology*, vol. 24, no. 2, pp. 203–210, 2000.

[32] P. H. Tan, L. Cheng, and N. Rioux-Leclercq, "Renal tumors: diagnostic and prognostic biomarkers," *The American Journal of Surgical Pathology*, vol. 37, no. 10, pp. 1518–1531, 2013.

Permissions

All chapters in this book were first published in CRGM, by Hindawi Publishing Corporation; hereby published with permission under the Creative Commons Attribution License or equivalent. Every chapter published in this book has been scrutinized by our experts. Their significance has been extensively debated. The topics covered herein carry significant findings which will fuel the growth of the discipline. They may even be implemented as practical applications or may be referred to as a beginning point for another development.

The contributors of this book come from diverse backgrounds, making this book a truly international effort. This book will bring forth new frontiers with its revolutionizing research information and detailed analysis of the nascent developments around the world.

We would like to thank all the contributing authors for lending their expertise to make the book truly unique. They have played a crucial role in the development of this book. Without their invaluable contributions this book wouldn't have been possible. They have made vital efforts to compile up to date information on the varied aspects of this subject to make this book a valuable addition to the collection of many professionals and students.

This book was conceptualized with the vision of imparting up-to-date information and advanced data in this field. To ensure the same, a matchless editorial board was set up. Every individual on the board went through rigorous rounds of assessment to prove their worth. After which they invested a large part of their time researching and compiling the most relevant data for our readers.

The editorial board has been involved in producing this book since its inception. They have spent rigorous hours researching and exploring the diverse topics which have resulted in the successful publishing of this book. They have passed on their knowledge of decades through this book. To expedite this challenging task, the publisher supported the team at every step. A small team of assistant editors was also appointed to further simplify the editing procedure and attain best results for the readers.

Apart from the editorial board, the designing team has also invested a significant amount of their time in understanding the subject and creating the most relevant covers. They scrutinized every image to scout for the most suitable representation of the subject and create an appropriate cover for the book.

The publishing team has been an ardent support to the editorial, designing and production team. Their endless efforts to recruit the best for this project, has resulted in the accomplishment of this book. They are a veteran in the field of academics and their pool of knowledge is as vast as their experience in printing. Their expertise and guidance has proved useful at every step. Their uncompromising quality standards have made this book an exceptional effort. Their encouragement from time to time has been an inspiration for everyone.

The publisher and the editorial board hope that this book will prove to be a valuable piece of knowledge for researchers, students, practitioners and scholars across the globe.

List of Contributors

Yilmaz Bilgic
Department of Gastroenterology, Faculty of Medicine, Inonu University, Malatya, Turkey

Hasan Baki Altinsoy and Ozkan Alatas
Department of Radiology, Elazig Training and Research Hospital, Elazig, Turkey

Nezahat Yildirim
Department of Pathology, Elazig Training and Research Hospital, Elazig, Turkey

Burhan Hakan Kanat
Department of General Surgery, Elazig Training and Research Hospital, Elazig, Turkey

Abdurrahman Sahin
Department of Gastroenterology, Elazig Training and Research Hospital, Elazig, Turkey

Susumu Saigusa, Masaki Ohi, Hiroki Imaoka, Tadanobu Shimura, Ryo Uratani and Yasuhiro Inoue
Department of Surgery, Wakaba Hospital, 28-13 Minami-Chuo, Tsu, Mie 514-0832, Japan
Department of Gastrointestinal and Pediatric Surgery, 2-174 Edobashi, Tsu, Mie 514-8507, Japan

Masato Kusunoki
Department of Gastrointestinal and Pediatric Surgery, 2-174 Edobashi, Tsu, Mie 514-8507, Japan

Keita Saito, Eiki Nomura, Yu Sasaki, Yasuhiko Abe, Nana Kanno, Naoko Mizumoto, Rika Shibuya, Kazuhiro Sakuta, Makoto Yagi, Kazuya Yoshizawa, Daisuke Iwano, Takeshi Sato, Shoichi Nishise and Yoshiyuki Ueno
Department of Gastroenterology, Faculty of Medicine, Yamagata University, 2-2-2 Iida-Nishi, Yamagata 990-9585, Japan

Elhan Tas, Serdar Culcu and Sadik Eryilmaz
General Surgery Clinic, Cizre Dr. Selahattin Cizrelioglu State Hospital, Şırnak, Turkey

Yigit Duzkoylu
General Surgery Clinic, Islahiye State Hospital, Gaziantep, Turkey

Mehmet Mehdi Deniz
General Surgery Clinic, Bayrampasa State Hospital, Istanbul, Turkey

Deniz Yilmaz
Pathology Department, Cizre Dr. Selahattin Cizrelioglu State Hospital, Şırnak, Turkey

Guillermo López-Medina, Alberto Carlos Heredia-Salazar and Daniel Ramón Hernández-Salcedo
Hospital Angeles Clinica Londres, Durango No. 50, Roma Norte, Cuauhtémoc, 06700 Ciudad de México, DF, Mexico

Roxana Castillo Díaz de León
Hospital Angeles Mocel, Gregorio V. Gelati 29, San Miguel Chapultepec, Miguel Hidalgo, 11850 Ciudad de México, DF, Mexico

Matthew P. Soape, Rashmi Verma, J. Drew Payne, Mitchell Wachtel, Fred Hardwicke and Everardo Cobos
Texas Tech University Health Sciences Center, 3601 4th Street, Lubbock, TX 79430, USA

Rintaro Moroi, Katsuya Endo, Masatake Kuhroha, Hisashi Shiga, Yoichi Kakuta, Yoshitaka Kinouchi and Tooru Shimosegawa
Division of Gastroenterology, Department of Internal Medicine, Tohoku University Graduate School of Medicine, 1-1 Seiryo, Aoba-ku, Sendai 980-8574, Japan

Asim Shuja
Department of Medicine, St. Elizabeth's Medical Center, Brighton, MA 02135, USA

Khalid A. Alkimawi
Department Gastroenterology, Tufts Medical Center, 800Washington Street Boston, MA 02111, USA

Ravish Parekh, Ahmed Abdulhamid and Nirmal Kaur
Department of Gastroenterology and Hepatology, Henry Ford Health System, Detroit, MI, USA

Sheri Trudeau
Department of Public Health Sciences, Henry Ford Health System, Detroit, MI, USA

Allon Kahn
Department of Medicine, Mayo Clinic, Scottsdale, AZ, USA

Anitha D. Yadav and M. Edwyn Harrison
Division of Gastroenterology and Hepatology, Mayo Clinic, Scottsdale, AZ, USA

Mitsuo Okada and Hiroshi Sakaeda
Department of Gastroenterology, Chikamori Hospital, Kochi 780-8522, Japan

Keisuke Taniuchi
Department of Gastroenterology, Chikamori Hospital, Kochi 780-8522, Japan
Department of Endoscopic Diagnostics and Therapeutics, Kochi Medical School, Kochi University, Nankoku 783-8505, Japan

Ahmed Dirweesh, Muhammad Khan and Sumera Bukhari
Department of Internal Medicine, Seton Hall University, Hackensack Meridian School of Medicine, Saint Francis Medical Center, Trenton, NJ, USA

Cheryl Rimmer
Department of Pathology, Our Lady of Lourdes Hospital, Willingboro, NJ, USA

Robert Shmuts
Department of Gastroenterology, Our Lady of Lourdes Hospital, Willingboro, NJ, USA

Yaseen Alastal, Tariq A. Hammad, Mohamad Nawras and Basmah W. Khalil
Department of Internal Medicine, University of Toledo Medical Center, Toledo, OH 43614, USA

Osama Alaradi and Ali Nawras
Department of Gastroenterology and Hepatology, University of Toledo Medical Center, Toledo, OH 43614, USA

T. Meira and R. Sousa
GastroenterologyDepartment, Hospital Garcia de Orta E.P.E., Avenida Torrado da Silva, 2801-951 Almada, Portugal

A. Cordeiro
Rheumatology Department, Hospital Garcia de Orta E.P.E., Avenida Torrado da Silva, 2801-951 Almada, Portugal

R. Ilgenfritz and P. Borralho
Anatomical Pathology Department, Hospital Garcia de Orta E.P.E., Avenida Torrado da Silva, 2801-951 Almada, Portugal

Kourosh Alavi, Pradeep R. Atla, Tahmina Haq and Muhammad Y. Sheikh
Division of Gastroenterology and Hepatology, University of California San Francisco, 1st Floor, Endoscopy Suite, 2823 Fresno Street, Fresno, CA 93721, USA

Erin K. Purdy-Payne
University of Central Florida College of Medicine, 6850 Lake Nona Boulevard, Orlando, FL 32827, USA

Jean F. Miner and Brandon Foles
Department of Surgery, Florida Hospital Orlando, 2415 North Orange Avenue, Suite 400, Orlando, FL 32803, USA

Tien-Anh N. Tran
Department of Pathology, Florida Hospital Orlando, 601 E. Rollins Street, Orlando, FL 32803, USA

S. Casiraghi, P. Baggi, A. Vinco and M. Ronconi
Division of General Surgery, Gardone Val Trompia Hospital, Gardone Val Trompia, Italy

P. Lanza and F. Castelli
Department of Infectious and Tropical Diseases, University of Brescia, Brescia, Italy

A. Bozzola and V. Villanacci
Institute of Pathology, Brescia Spedali Civili General Hospital, Brescia, Italy

Samih Nassif
Boston University School of Medicine, 72 East Concord St., Boston, MA 02118, USA

Cecilia Ponchiardi
Department of Pathology and Laboratory Medicine, Boston University School of Medicine, 72 East Concord St., Boston, MA 02118, USA

Teviah Sachs
Boston University School of Medicine, Moakley Building, 3rd Floor, 830 Harrison Avenue, Boston, MA 02118, USA

Soe Lwin, Mardiana binti Kipli and Myat San Yi
Department of Obstetrics and Gynecology, Faculty of Medicine and Health Sciences, UNIMAS, Kota Samarahan, Malaysia

Nina Lau Lee Jing, Haris Suharjono and Lucas Luk Tien Wee
Department of Obstetrics and Gynecology, Sarawak General Hospital, Kuching, Malaysia

Tin Moe Nwe
Department of Basic Health Sciences, Faculty of Medicine and Health Sciences, UNIMAS, Kota Samarahan, Malaysia

Paul J. Belletrutti
Division of Gastroenterology and Hepatology, Department of Medicine, University of Calgary, Calgary, AB, Canada

Takuya Ishikawa
Division of Gastroenterology and Hepatology, Department of Medicine, University of Calgary, Calgary, AB, Canada
Department of Gastroenterology, Nagoya University Graduate School of Medicine, Nagoya, Japan

Hidemi Goto
Department of Gastroenterology, Nagoya University Graduate School of Medicine, Nagoya, Japan

Yoshiki Hirooka
Department of Endoscopy, Nagoya University Hospital, Nagoya, Japan

Carolin J. Teman
Division of Anatomic Pathology and Cytopathology, Department of Pathology and Laboratory Medicine, University of Calgary, Calgary, AB, Canada

Matthew Glover, Zhouwen Tang, Robert Sealock and Shilpa Jain
Baylor College of Medicine, Houston, TX, USA

Seiji Kawano and Hiroyuki Okada
Department of Gastroenterology and Hepatology, Okayama University Graduate School of Medicine, Dentistry and Pharmaceutical Sciences, Okayama 700-8558, Japan

Masaya Iwamuro
Department of Gastroenterology and Hepatology, Okayama University Graduate School of Medicine, Dentistry and Pharmaceutical Sciences, Okayama 700-8558, Japan
Department of General Medicine, Okayama University Graduate School of Medicine, Dentistry and Pharmaceutical Sciences, Okayama 700-8558, Japan

Tadashi Yoshino and Katsuyoshi Takata
Department of Pathology, Okayama University Graduate School of Medicine, Dentistry, and Pharmaceutical Sciences, Okayama 700-8558, Japan

Nobuharu Fujii
Department of Hematology and Oncology, Okayama University Hospital, Okayama 700-8558, Japan

Yoshiro Kawahara
Department of Endoscopy, Okayama University Hospital, Okayama 700-8558, Japan

W. G. P. Kanchana, R. A. A. Shaminda, K. B. Galketiya and R. Heendeniya
Department of Surgery, Teaching Hospital Peradeniya, Peradeniya, Sri Lanka

V. Pinto
Department of Anaesthesiology, Teaching Hospital Peradeniya, Peradeniya, Sri Lanka

D. Walisinghe and S. Wijetunge
Department of Pathology, Teaching Hospital Peradeniya, Peradeniya, Sri Lanka

Antoine Abou Rached, Jowana Saba, Leila El Masri and Mary Nakhoul
Lebanese University, School of Medicine, Lebanon

Carla Razzouk
Saint-Joseph University, School of Medicine, Lebanon

Subhajit Mukherjee and Tanima Jana
Division of Gastroenterology, Hepatology and Nutrition, Department of Internal Medicine, The University of Texas Health Science Center, Houston, TX 77030, USA

Jen-Jung Pan
Division of Gastroenterology and Hepatology, Department of Medicine, University of Arizona College of Medicine, Tucson, AZ 85724, USA

Ashish Lal Shrestha and Pradita Shrestha
Department of General Surgery, United Mission Hospital, Tansen, Palpa, Nepal

Viva Nguyen
Mercer University School of Medicine, Columbus, GA, USA

Henry N. Ngo
Department of Internal Medicine, St. Francis Columbus Clinic, Columbus, GA, USA
Department of Internal Medicine, Mercer University School of Medicine, Columbus, GA, USA

Hamza H. Awad
Department of Community Medicine, Department of Internal Medicine, Mercer University School of Medicine, Macon, GA, USA

Ashish Lal Shrestha and Pradita Shrestha
Department of General Surgery, United Mission Hospital, Tansen, Palpa, Nepal

Fady Daniel and Walid Karaoui
Division of Gastroenterology, Department of Internal Medicine, American University of Beirut Medical Center, Riad El Solh, Beirut 110-72020, Lebanon

Hazem I. Assi and Jean El Cheikh
Division of Hematology and Oncology, Department of Internal Medicine, American University of Beirut Medical Center, Riad El Solh, Beirut 110-72020, Lebanon

Sami Bannoura and Samer Nassif
Pathology and Laboratory Medicine Department, American University of Beirut Medical Center, P.O. Box 11-0236, Riad El Solh, Beirut 110-72020, Lebanon

Masahide Kita, Masaya Iwamuro, Keisuke Hori and Hiroyuki Okada
Department of Gastroenterology and Hepatology, Okayama University Graduate School of Medicine, Dentistry and Pharmaceutical Sciences, Okayama, Japan

Naruto Taira, Tomohiro Nogami, Tadahiko Shien, Hiroyoshi Doihara and Masashi Furukawa
Department of Breast and Endocrine Surgery, Okayama University Hospital, Okayama, Japan

Yoshiro Kawahara
Department of Endoscopy, Okayama University Hospital, Okayama, Japan

Takehiro Tanaka
Department of Pathology, Okayama University Hospital, Okayama, Japan

Pratik Naik and Michael J. Brazeau
Department of Internal Medicine, William Beaumont Army Medical Center (WBAMC), 5005 North Piedras Street, El Paso, TX 79920, USA

James Wang
Division of Gastroenterology, Department of Internal Medicine, William Beaumont Army Medical Center (WBAMC), 5005 North Piedras Street, El Paso, TX 79920, USA

Domingo Rosario
Department of Pathology, William Beaumont Army Medical Center (WBAMC), 5005 North Piedras Street, El Paso, TX 79920, USA

Mouhanna Abu Ghanimeh
Henry Ford Health System, 2799WGrand Blvd, Gastroenterology K-7 Room E-744, Detroit, MI 48202, USA

Omar Abughanimeh and Osama Kaddourah
University of Missouri-Kansas City, School of Medicine, Internal Medicine-Graduate Medical Education, 2411 Holmes Street, M2-302, Kansas City, MO 64108, USA

Sakher Albadarin
Saint Luke's Hospital of Kansas City, Division of Gastroenterology, Mid-America Gastro-Intestinal Consultants, 4401Wornall Rd, Kansas City, MO 64111, USA

John H. Helzberg
University of Missouri of Kansas City/School of Medicine, 2411 Holmes Street, Kansas City, MO 64108, USA Saint Luke's Hospital of Kansas City, 4401 Wornall Rd, Kansas City, MO 64111, USA

Chukwunonso Chime, Charbel Ishak, Kishore Kumar, Venkata Kella and Sridhar Chilimuri
Bronx Care Hospital Health System, Affiliate of Icahn School of Medicine at Mount Sinai, New York, NY, USA

Satoshi Tanida, TsutomuMizoshita, Keiji Ozeki, Takahito Katano, Takaya Shimura, YoshinoriMori, Eiji Kubota, Hiromi Kataoka, Takeshi Kamiya and Takashi Joh
Department of Gastroenterology and Metabolism, Nagoya City University Graduate School of Medical Sciences, Nagoya, Aichi Prefecture 467-8601, Japan

Masaya Takemura
Department of Respiratory Medicine, Allergy and Clinical Immunology, Nagoya City University Graduate School of Medical Sciences, Nagoya, Aichi Prefecture 467-8601, Japan

Satoko Ando, Tatsuhiro Gotoda, Hiromitsu Kanzaki, Seiji Kawano and Hiroyuki Okada
Department of Gastroenterology and Hepatology, Okayama University Graduate School of Medicine, Dentistry and Pharmaceutical Sciences, 2-5-1 Shikata-cho, Kita-ku, Okayama 700-8558, Japan

Masaya Iwamuro
Department of Gastroenterology and Hepatology, Okayama University Graduate School of Medicine, Dentistry and Pharmaceutical Sciences, 2-5-1 Shikata-cho, Kita-ku, Okayama 700-8558, Japan
Department of General Medicine, Okayama University Graduate School of Medicine, Dentistry and Pharmaceutical Sciences, 2-5-1 Shikata-cho, Kita-ku, Okayama 700-8558, Japan

Takehiro Tanaka
Department of Pathology, Okayama University Hospital, Okayama 700-8558, Japan

Yoshiro Kawahara
Department of Endoscopy, Okayama University Hospital, Okayama 700-8558, Japan

Meha Mansi, Nidhi Mahajan and Sonam Mahana
Department of Pathology, Chacha Nehru Bal Chikitsalaya, New Delhi, India

C. R. Gupta and Anup Mohta
Department of Pediatric Surgery, Chacha Nehru Bal Chikitsalaya, NewDelhi, India

Fares Ayoub and Harry Powers
Department of Medicine, University of Florida, Gainesville, FL 32608, USA

Vikas Khullar, Angela Pham and Amitabh Suman
Department of Medicine, Division of Gastroenterology, University of Florida, Gainesville, FL 32608, USA

Shehla Islam
Department of Medicine, Division of Infectious Disease, University of Florida, Gainesville, FL 32608, USA

Mouhanna Abu Ghanimeh
Internal Medicine Department, Division of Gastroenterology, Henry Ford Hospital, Detroit, MI, USA

Ayman Qasrawi and Omar Abughanimeh
Internal Medicine Department, University of Missouri-Kansas City School of Medicine, Kansas City, MO, USA

Sakher Albadarin
Division of Gastroenterology, University of Missouri-Kansas City School of Medicine, Kansas City, MO, USA

John H. Helzberg
Saint Luke's Hospital of Kansas City, University of Missouri-Kansas City School of Medicine, Kansas City, MO, USA

Joseph Bozzay, Diego Vicente, Elliot M. Jessie and Carlos J. Rodriguez
Walter Reed National Military Medical Center, 8901 Rockville Pike, Bethesda, MD 20889, USA

Christienne Shams and Seifeldin Hakim
Division of Gastroenterology and Hepatology, Department of Medicine, William Beaumont Hospital, 3535W.Thirteen Mile Rd, Royal Oak, MI 48073, USA

Mitual Amin
Department of Pathology, William Beaumont Hospital and Oakland University William Beaumont School of Medicine, 3601WThirteen Mile Rd, Royal Oak, MI 48073, USA

Mitchell S. Cappell
Division of Gastroenterology and Hepatology, Department of Medicine, William Beaumont Hospital and Oakland University William Beaumont School of Medicine, 3535W.Thirteen Mile Rd, Royal Oak, MI 48073, USA

Maria Paparoupa and Markus Bruns-Toepler
Department of Pulmonary Diseases, Infectious Diseases, Gastroenterology, Nephrology and Intensive Care Unit, University Hospital of Giessen, Klinikstr. 33, 35392 Giessen, Germany

Syed Hasan, Zubair Khan, Umar Darr, Toseef Javaid, Nauman Siddiqui and Jamal Saleh
Department of Internal Medicine, University of Toledo Medical Center, Toledo, OH, USA

Abdallah Kobeissy and Ali Nawras
Department of Internal Medicine, University of Toledo Medical Center, Toledo, OH, USA
Division of Gastroenterology, University of Toledo, Toledo, OH, USA

Sara Benedicenti, Sarah Molfino, Marie Sophie Alfano, Beatrice Molteni, Paola Porsio, Nazario Portolani and Gian Luca Baiocchi
Department of Clinical and Experimental Sciences, Surgical Clinic, University of Brescia, Brescia, Italy

Muhammad Aziz
Department of Internal Medicine, University of Kansas Medical Center, Kansas City, KS, USA

Asad Pervez and Ajay Bansal
Department of Gastroenterology and Hepatology, University of Kansas Medical Center, Kansas City, KS, USA

Rawish Fatima
Department of Internal Medicine, Dow University of Health Sciences, Karachi, Pakistan

Eric Vecchio, Sehrish Jamot and Jason Ferreira
Rhode Island Hospital and Brown University, USA

Daisuke Takei, Yuusaku Sugihara, Keita Harada, Sakiko Hiraoka and Hiroyuki Okada
Department of Gastroenterology and Hepatology, Okayama University Graduate School of Medicine, Dentistry and Pharmaceutical Sciences, Okayama 700-8558, Japan

Masaya Iwamuro
Department of Gastroenterology and Hepatology, Okayama University Graduate School of Medicine, Dentistry and Pharmaceutical Sciences, Okayama 700-8558, Japan
Department of General Medicine, Okayama University Graduate School of Medicine, Dentistry and Pharmaceutical Sciences, Okayama 700-8558, Japan

Takehiro Tanaka
Department of Pathology, Okayama University Hospital, Okayama 700-8558, Japan

Yoshiro Kawahara
Department of Endoscopy, Okayama University Hospital, Okayama 700-8558, Japan

Masaya Iwamuro, Seiji Kawano and Hiroyuki Okada
Department of Gastroenterology and Hepatology, Okayama University Graduate School of Medicine, Dentistry, and Pharmaceutical Sciences, Okayama 700-8558, Japan

Takehiro Tanaka
Department of Pathology, Okayama University Hospital, Okayama 700-8558, Japan

Kenji Nishida and Tadashi Yoshino
Department of Pathology, Okayama University Graduate School of Medicine, Dentistry, and Pharmaceutical Sciences, Okayama 700-8558, Japan

Yoshiro Kawahara
Department of Endoscopy, Okayama University Hospital, Okayama 700-8558, Japan

Shogen Ohya
Kawaguchi Medical Clinic, Okayama 700-0913, Japan

Chiara Di Renzo, Alessio Pasquale, Alessandra Bertacco and Umberto Cillo
Department of Surgery, Oncology and Gastroenterology, Hepatobiliary Surgery and Liver Transplantation, Padova University, Padova, Italy

Francesco D'Amico and Michele Finotti
Department of Surgery, Oncology and Gastroenterology, Hepatobiliary Surgery and Liver Transplantation, Padova University, Padova, Italy
Department of Surgery, Division of Transplantation and Immunology, Yale University, New Haven, CT, USA

Giorgio Caturegli
Department of Surgery, Division of Transplantation and Immunology, Yale University, New Haven, CT, USA

Gabriel E. Gondolesi
Department of Surgery, Favaloro Foundation, Buenos Aires University, Buenos Aires, Argentina

Heather Katz and Toni O. Pacioles
Department of Hematology/Oncology, Joan C. Edwards School of Medicine, Marshall University, 1600 Medical Center Dr, Huntington, WV 25701, USA

Rahoma E. Saad
Department of Internal Medicine, Joan C. Edwards School of Medicine, Marshall University, 1600 Medical Center Dr, Huntington, WV 25701, USA

Krista Denning
Department of Pathology, Joan C. Edwards School of Medicine, Marshall University, 1600 Medical Center Dr, Huntington, WV 25701, USA

Akshay Sharma, Elisa Akagi and Aji Njie
Resident, Department of Internal Medicine, Sinai-Grace Hospital, Detroit Medical Center/Wayne State University, USA

Sachin Goyal
Fellow, Department of Internal Medicine, Division of Gastroenterology, Detroit Medical Center/Wayne State University, USA

Camelia Arsene
Clinical Research Director, Sinai-Grace Hospital; Associate Program Director, Transitional Medicine Residency Program, Sinai-Grace Hospital, Detroit Medical Center/Wayne State School of Medicine, Detroit, MI, USA

Geetha Krishnamoorthy
Associate Program Director, Department of Internal Medicine, Sinai-Grace Hospital, Detroit Medical Center/Wayne State University, USA

Murray Ehrinpreis
Program Director, Department of Internal Medicine, Division of Gastroenterology, Detroit Medical Center/Wayne State University, USA

Kaci E. Christian, John D. Morris and Guofeng Xie
Division of Gastroenterology and Hepatology, University of Maryland School of Medicine, Veterans Affairs Maryland Health Care System, Baltimore, MD 21201, USA

Haseeb Ahmad Chaudhary, Ibrahim Yusuf Abubeker, Kamran Mushtaq, Khaldun Obeidat and Anand Kartha
Department of Medicine, Hamad Medical Corporation, Doha, Qatar

Saleh Daher and Tawfik Khoury
Division of Gastroenterology and Hepatology, Department of Medicine, Hebrew University-Hadassah Medical Center, Ein Kerem, 91120 Jerusalem, Israel

Ziv Lahav and Ayman Abu Rmeileh
Department of Internal Medicine, Hebrew University-Hadassah Medical Center, 91120 Jerusalem, Israel

Meir Mizrahi
Division of Gastroenterology and Hepatology, Advanced Endoscopy Center, Beth Israel Deaconess Medical Center, Harvard Medical School, 330 Brookline Avenue, Stoneman 458, Boston, MA 02215, USA

Bao-guang Hu, Feng-jie Wu, Jun Zhu, Yu-ming Li and He-sheng Li
Department of Gastrointestinal Surgery, The Affiliated Hospital of Binzhou Medical University, Binzhou, Shandong, China

Xiao-mei Li
Centers for Disease Control and Prevention of Binzhou City, Binzhou, Shandong, China

Yan Feng
Department of Radiology, The Affiliated Hospital of Binzhou Medical University, Binzhou, Shandong, China

Megumi Zianne, Kazuhiro Miwa, Yoshinori Goto and Yutaka Matano
Department of Gastroenterology, Komatsu Municipal Hospital, Ishikawa, Japan

Naoki Takahashi
Department of Gastroenterology, Saitama Cancer Center, Saitama, Japan

Akihiko Tsujibata
Department of Pathology, Komatsu Municipal Hospital, Ishikawa, Japan

Index